a LANGE medical book

Clinical Neurology

TENTH EDITION

Roger P. Simon, MD
Professor of Medicine (Neurology) and Neurobiology
Morehouse School of Medicine
Clinical Professor of Neurology
Emory University
Atlanta, Georgia

Michael J. Aminoff, MD, DSc, FRCP
Distinguished Professor
Department of Neurology
School of Medicine
University of California
San Francisco, California

David A. Greenberg, MD, PhD
Professor Emeritus
Buck Institute for Research on Aging
Novato, California

Mc
Graw
Hill
Education

New York   Chicago   San Francisco   Athens   London   Madrid   Mexico City
Milan   New Delhi   Singapore   Sydney   Toronto

Clinical Neurology, Tenth Edition

2 3 4 5 6 7 8 9   LCR   22 21 20 19 18

ISBN 978-1-259-86172-7
MHID 1-259-86172-4
ISSN 1522-6875

Notice

Medicine is an ever-changing science. As new research and clinical experience broaden our knowledge, changes in treatment and drug therapy are required. The authors and the publisher of this work have checked with sources believed to be reliable in their efforts to provide information that is complete and generally in accord with the standards accepted at the time of publication. However, in view of the possibility of human error changes in medical sciences, neither the editors nor the publisher nor any other party who has been involved in the preparation or publication of this work warrants that the information contained herein is in every respect accurate or complete, and they disclaim all responsibility for any errors or omissions or for the results obtained from use of the information contained in this work. Readers are encouraged to confirm the information contained herein with other sources. For example and in particular, readers are advised to check the product information sheet included in the package of each drug they plan to administer to be certain that the information contained in this work is accurate and that changes have not been made in the recommended dose or in the contraindications for administration. This recommendation is of particular importance in connection with new or infrequently used drugs.

This book was set in Minion pro by Cenveo® Publisher Services.
The editors were Andrew Moyer and Christie Naglieri.
The production supervisor was Rick Ruzycka.
Project management was provided by Neha Bhargava, Cenveo Publisher Services.

McGraw-Hill books are available at special quantity discounts to use as premiums and sales promotions, or for use in corporate training programs. To contact a representative, please visit the Contact Us pages at www.mhprofessional.com.

To our families, as well as to our patients and students over the years.

Contents

v

Preface

Forty years ago, as clinical teachers at the UCSF School of Medicine, we decided that there was a need for a new teaching text that combined the basic and clinical aspects of neurology. Following a lunch meeting, Jack Lange of Lange Medical Publications agreed to the addition of a clinical neurology textbook to the Lange textbook series. He smiled when one of us (RPS) offered to provide the text in two years, noting that no one had produced a textbook in that time. With two coauthors (MJA and DAG) and after some ten years, the text of Clinical Neurology was finally completed and in 1989 the first edition was published. With the publication of the 10th edition and translations in eight languages, our text will have provided nearly 30 consecutive years of neurology teaching material to medical students in the United States and around the world via the print volume (purchased or rented), e-book edition, and AccessMedicine website.

As in each new edition, we have retained and refined the core didactic material relating to the function of the nervous system in health and disease and added new and evolving diagnostic and therapeutic material. Full-color figures illustrate key concepts. Over the years, the book has encompassed the evolution of therapeutics in neurology, particularly for epilepsy and headache and most recently for demyelinating disease. This edition continues to document the expansion of diagnostic and therapeutic approaches to nervous system disease. To those who still believe that there are limited therapeutic options in neurology, we hope that the present volume will help to convince them otherwise. Within just the last year, advances in molecular biology and immunology have led to the approval of new drugs for the treatment of multiple sclerosis (alemtuzumab), spinal muscular atrophy (nusinersen), amyotrophic lateral sclerosis (edaravone), and Huntington's disease (deutetrabenazine). These and other therapeutic advances are included in this new edition.

Over the years, many colleagues have suggested revisions, contributed figures and radiographic material, and read over portions of the book. In this regard, we thank the members of the faculty of UCSF, the University of Pittsburgh, the Oregon Health and Sciences University, and Emory University who helped us, as well as the current and past staff of our publisher, McGraw-Hill, and particularly Andrew Moyer and Christie Naglieri for their assistance with this latest edition. Special thanks are due to Martha Johnson, PhD, for her careful copy-editing of the entire 10th edition and to McGraw-Hill for providing a new index to optimize accessibility.

Roger P. Simon
Michael J. Aminoff
David A. Greenberg

Preface

Neurologic History & Examination

1

HISTORY

Taking a history from a patient with a neurologic complaint is fundamentally the same as taking any history.

Age

Age can be a clue to the cause of a neurologic problem. Epilepsy, multiple sclerosis, and Huntington disease usually have their onset by middle age, whereas Alzheimer disease, Parkinson disease, brain tumors, and stroke predominantly affect older individuals.

Chief Complaint

The chief complaint should be defined as clearly as possible, because it will guide evaluation toward—or away from—the correct diagnosis. The goal is for the patient to describe the nature of the problem in a word or phrase.

Common neurologic complaints include confusion, dizziness, weakness, shaking, numbness, blurred vision, and spells. Each of these terms means different things to different people, so it is critical to clarify what the patient is trying to convey.

A. Confusion

Confusion may be reported by the patient or by family members. Symptoms can include memory impairment, getting lost, difficulty understanding or producing spoken or written language, problems with numbers, faulty judgment, personality change, or combinations thereof. Symptoms of confusion may be difficult to characterize, so specific examples should be sought.

B. Dizziness

Dizziness can mean **vertigo** (the illusion of movement of oneself or the environment), **imbalance** (unsteadiness due to extrapyramidal, vestibular, cerebellar, or sensory deficits), or **presyncope** (light-headedness resulting from cerebral hypoperfusion).

C. Weakness

Weakness is the term neurologists use to mean **loss of power** from disorders affecting motor pathways in the central or peripheral nervous system or skeletal muscle. However, patients sometimes use this term when they mean generalized fatigue, lethargy, or even sensory disturbances.

D. Shaking

Shaking may represent abnormal movements such as tremor, chorea, athetosis, myoclonus, or fasciculation (see Chapter 11, Movement Disorders), but the patient is unlikely to use these terms. Correct classification depends on observing the movements in question or, if they are not present when the history is taken, asking the patient to demonstrate them.

E. Numbness

Numbness can refer to any of a variety of sensory disturbances, including **hypesthesia** (decreased sensitivity), **hyperesthesia** (increased sensitivity), or **paresthesia** ("pins and needles" sensation). Patients occasionally also use this term to signify weakness.

F. Blurred Vision

Blurred vision may represent **diplopia** (double vision), ocular oscillations, reduced visual acuity, or visual field cuts.

G. Spells

Spells imply episodic and often recurrent symptoms such as in **epilepsy** or **syncope** (fainting).

▶ History of Present Illness

The history of present illness should provide a detailed description of the chief complaint, including the following features.

A. Quality and Severity of Symptoms

Some symptoms, such as pain, may have distinctive features. Neuropathic pain—which results from direct injury to nerves—may be described as especially unpleasant (dysesthetic) and may be accompanied by increased sensitivity to pain (hyperalgesia) or touch (hyperesthesia), or by the perception of a normally innocuous stimulus as painful

(allodynia). The severity of symptoms should also be ascertained. Although thresholds for seeking medical attention vary among patients, it is often useful to ask a patient to rank the present complaint in relation to past problems.

B. Location of Symptoms

Patients should be encouraged to localize their symptoms as precisely as possible because location is often critical to neurologic diagnosis. The distribution of weakness, decreased sensation, or pain helps point to a specific site in the nervous system (anatomic diagnosis).

C. Time Course

It is important to determine when the problem began, whether it came on abruptly or insidiously, and if its subsequent course has been characterized by improvement, worsening, or exacerbation and remission (**Figure 1-1**). For episodic disorders, such as headache or seizures, the

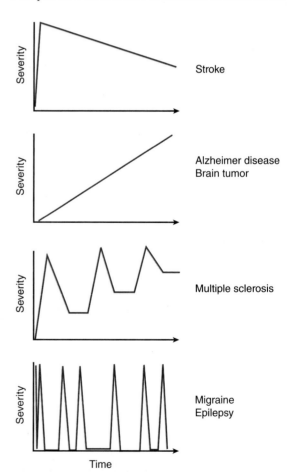

▲ **Figure 1-1.** Temporal patterns of neurologic disease and examples of each.

time course of individual episodes should also be determined.

D. Precipitating, Exacerbating, and Alleviating Factors

Some symptoms may appear to be spontaneous, but in other cases, patients are aware of factors that precipitate or worsen symptoms, and which they can avoid, or factors that prevent symptoms or provide relief.

E. Associated Symptoms

Associated symptoms can assist with anatomic or etiologic diagnosis. For example, neck pain accompanying leg weakness suggests a cervical myelopathy (spinal cord disorder), and fever in the setting of headache suggests meningitis.

▶ Past Medical History

The past medical history may provide clues to the cause of a neurologic complaint.

A. Illnesses

Preexisting illnesses that can predispose to neurologic disease include hypertension, diabetes, heart disease, cancer, and human immunodeficiency virus (HIV) disease.

B. Operations

Open heart surgery may be complicated by stroke or a confusional state. Entrapment neuropathies (disorders of a peripheral nerve due to local pressure) affecting the upper or lower extremity may occur perioperatively.

C. Obstetric History

Pregnancy can worsen epilepsy, partly due to altered metabolism of anticonvulsant drugs, and may increase or decrease the frequency of migraine attacks. Pregnancy is a predisposing condition for idiopathic intracranial hypertension (**pseudotumor cerebri**) and entrapment neuropathies, especially **carpal tunnel syndrome** (median neuropathy) and **meralgia paresthetica** (lateral femoral cutaneous neuropathy). Traumatic neuropathies affecting the obturator, femoral, or peroneal nerve may result from pressure exerted by the fetal head or obstetric forceps during delivery. **Eclampsia** is a life-threatening syndrome in which generalized tonic-clonic seizures complicate the course of pre-eclampsia (hypertension with proteinuria) during pregnancy.

D. Medications

A wide range of medications can cause adverse neurologic effects, including confusional states or coma, headache, ataxia, neuromuscular disorders, neuropathy, and seizures.

E. Immunizations

Vaccination can prevent neurologic diseases such as poliomyelitis, diphtheria, tetanus, rabies, meningococcal or *Haemophilus influenzae* meningitis, and Japanese encephalitis. Rare complications include postvaccination autoimmune encephalitis, myelitis, or neuritis (inflammation of the brain, spinal cord, or peripheral nerves).

F. Diet

Deficiency of vitamin B_1 (thiamin) is responsible for the **Wernicke–Korsakoff syndrome** and polyneuropathy in alcoholics. Vitamin B_3 (niacin) deficiency causes pellagra, which is characterized by dementia. Vitamin B_{12} (cobalamin) deficiency usually results from malabsorption associated with pernicious anemia and produces **combined systems disease** (degeneration of corticospinal tracts and posterior columns in the spinal cord) and dementia (megaloblastic madness). Inadequate intake of vitamin E (tocopherol) can also lead to spinal cord degeneration. Hypervitaminosis A can produce intracranial hypertension (**pseudotumor cerebri**) with headache, visual deficits, and seizures, whereas excessive intake of vitamin B_6 (pyridoxine) is a cause of polyneuropathy. Excessive consumption of fats is a risk factor for stroke. Finally, ingestion of improperly preserved foods containing botulinum toxin causes **botulism**, which presents with descending paralysis.

G. Tobacco, Alcohol, and Other Drug Use

Tobacco use is associated with lung cancer, which may metastasize to the central nervous system or produce paraneoplastic neurologic syndromes. Alcohol abuse can produce withdrawal seizures, polyneuropathy, and nutritional disorders of the nervous system. Intravenous drug use may suggest HIV disease, infection, or vasculitis.

▶ Family History

This should include past or current diseases in the spouse and first- (parents, siblings, children) and second- (grandparents, grandchildren) degree relatives. Several neurologic diseases exhibit Mendelian inheritance, such as Huntington disease (autosomal dominant), Wilson disease (autosomal recessive), and Duchenne muscular dystrophy (X-linked recessive) (**Figure 1-2**).

▶ Social History

Information about the patient's education and occupation helps determine whether cognitive performance is appropriate to the patient's background. The sexual history may indicate risk for sexually transmitted diseases that affect the nervous system, such as syphilis or HIV disease. The travel history can document exposure to infections endemic to particular geographic areas.

Autosomal dominant

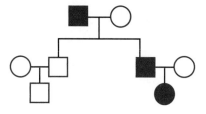

Autosomal recessive

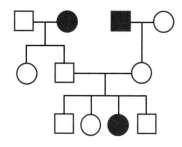

X-linked recessive

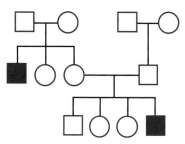

▲ **Figure 1-2.** Simple Mendelian patterns of inheritance. Squares represent males, circles females, and filled symbols affected individuals.

▶ Review of Systems

Non-neurologic complaints elicited in the review of systems may point to a systemic cause of a neurologic problem as described below:

1. **General**—Weight loss may suggest an underlying neoplasm and fever indicate an infection.
2. **Immune**—Acquired immune deficiency syndrome (AIDS) may lead to dementia, myelopathy, neuropathy, myopathy, or infections (eg, toxoplasmosis) or tumors (eg, lymphoma) affecting the nervous system.
3. **Hematologic**—Polycythemia and thrombocytosis may predispose to ischemic stroke, whereas thrombocytopenia and coagulopathy are associated with intracranial hemorrhage.
4. **Endocrine**—Diabetes increases the risk for stroke and polyneuropathy. Hypothyroidism may lead to coma, dementia, or ataxia.

5. **Skin**—Characteristic skin lesions are seen in certain disorders that affect the nervous system, such as neurofibromatosis and postherpetic neuralgia.
6. **Eyes, ears, nose, and throat**—Neck stiffness is a common feature of meningitis and subarachnoid hemorrhage.
7. **Cardiovascular**—Ischemic or valvular heart disease and hypertension are major risk factors for stroke.
8. **Respiratory**—Cough, hemoptysis, or night sweats may be manifestations of tuberculosis or lung neoplasm, which can disseminate to the nervous system.
9. **Gastrointestinal**—Hematemesis, jaundice, and diarrhea may suggest hepatic encephalopathy as the cause of a confusional state.
10. **Genitourinary**—Urinary retention, incontinence, and impotence may be manifestations of peripheral neuropathy or myelopathy.
11. **Musculoskeletal**—Muscle pain and tenderness accompany the myopathy of polymyositis.
12. **Psychiatric**—Psychosis, depression, and mania may be manifestations of several neurologic diseases.

▶ Summary

Upon completion of the history, the examiner should have a clear understanding of the chief complaint, including its location and time course, and familiarity with elements of the past medical history, family and social history, and review of systems that may be related to the complaint. This information should help to guide the general physical and neurologic examinations, which should focus on areas suggested by the history. For example, in an elderly patient who presents with the sudden onset of hemiparesis and hemisensory loss, which is likely to be due to stroke, the general physical examination should stress the cardiovascular system, because a variety of cardiovascular disorders predispose to stroke. On the other hand, if a patient complains of pain and numbness in the hand, much of the examination should be devoted to evaluating sensation, strength, and reflexes in the affected upper extremity.

GENERAL PHYSICAL EXAMINATION

In a patient with a neurologic complaint, the general physical examination should focus on looking for systemic abnormalities often associated with neurologic problems.

▶ Vital Signs

A. Blood Pressure

Elevated blood pressure may indicate chronic **hypertension**, which is a risk factor for stroke and is also seen acutely in the setting of hypertensive encephalopathy,

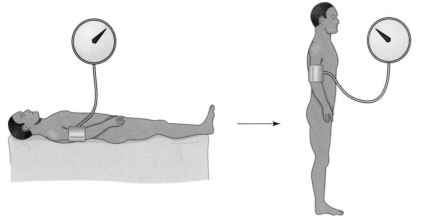

▲ **Figure 1-3.** Test for orthostatic hypotension. Systolic and diastolic blood pressure and heart rate are measured with the patent recumbent (left) and then each minute after standing for 5 min (right). A decrease in systolic blood pressure of ≥20 mm Hg or in diastolic blood pressure of ≥10 mm Hg indicates orthostatic hypotension. When autonomic function is normal, as in hypovolemia, there is a compensatory increase in heart rate, whereas lack of such an increase suggests autonomic failure.

ischemic stroke, or intracerebral or subarachnoid hemorrhage. Blood pressure that drops by ≥20 mm Hg (systolic) or ≥10 mm Hg (diastolic) when a patient switches from recumbent to upright signifies **orthostatic hypotension** (**Figure 1-3**). If the drop in blood pressure is accompanied by a compensatory increase in pulse rate, sympathetic autonomic reflexes are intact, and the likely cause is hypovolemia. However, the absence of a compensatory response is consistent with central (eg, multisystem atrophy) or peripheral (eg, polyneuropathy) disorders of sympathetic function or an effect of sympatholytic (eg, antihypertensive) drugs.

B. Pulse

A rapid or irregular pulse—especially the irregularly irregular pulse of **atrial fibrillation**—may point to a cardiac arrhythmia as the cause of stroke or syncope.

C. Respiratory Rate

The respiratory rate may provide a clue to the cause of a metabolic disturbance associated with coma or a confusional state. Rapid respiration (tachypnea) can be seen in hepatic encephalopathy, pulmonary disorders, sepsis, or salicylate intoxication; depressed respiration is observed with pulmonary disorders and sedative drug intoxication. Tachypnea may also occur in neuromuscular disease affecting the diaphragm. Abnormal respiratory patterns may be observed in coma: Cheyne-Stokes breathing (alternating deep breaths, or hyperpnea, and apnea) can occur in metabolic disorders or with hemispheric lesions, whereas apneustic, cluster, or ataxic breathing (see Chapter 3, Coma) implies a brainstem disorder.

D. Temperature

Fever (hyperthermia) occurs with infection of the meninges (meningitis), brain (encephalitis), or spinal cord (myelitis). Hypothermia can be seen in ethanol or sedative drug intoxication, hypoglycemia, hepatic encephalopathy, Wernicke encephalopathy, and hypothyroidism.

▶ Skin

Jaundice (icterus) suggests liver disease as the cause of a confusional state or movement disorder. Coarse dry skin, dry brittle hair, and subcutaneous edema are characteristic of hypothyroidism. Petechiae are seen in meningococcal meningitis, and petechiae or ecchymoses may suggest a coagulopathy as the cause of subdural, intracerebral, or paraspinal hemorrhage. Bacterial endocarditis, a cause of stroke, can produce a variety of cutaneous lesions, including splinter (subungual) hemorrhages, Osler nodes (painful swellings on the distal fingers), and Janeway lesions (painless hemorrhages on the palms and soles). Hot dry skin accompanies anticholinergic drug intoxication.

▶ Head, Eyes, Ears, & Neck

A. Head

Examination of the head may reveal signs of trauma, such as scalp lacerations or contusions. Basal skull fracture may produce postauricular hematoma (**Battle sign**), periorbital hematoma (**raccoon eyes**), hemotympanum, or cerebrospinal fluid (CSF) otorrhea or rhinorrhea (**Figure 1-4**). Percussion of the skull over a subdural hematoma may cause pain. A bruit heard over the skull is associated with arteriovenous malformations.

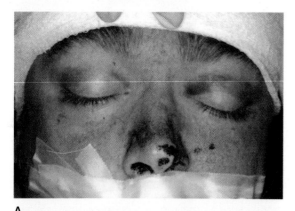

A

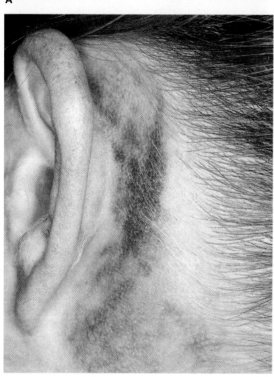

B

▲ **Figure 1-4.** Signs of head trauma include periorbital (raccoon eyes, **A**) or postauricular (Battle sign, **B**) hematoma, each of which suggests basal skull fracture. (Used with permission from Kevin J Knoop (A) and Frank Birinyi (B); from Knoop K, Stack L, Storrow A, Thurman RJ. *Atlas of Emergency Medicine.* 4th ed. New York, NY: McGraw-Hill; 2016).

B. Eyes

Icteric sclerae are seen in liver disease. Pigmented (**Kayser–Fleischer**) corneal rings—best seen by slit-lamp examination—are produced by copper deposits in Wilson disease. Retinal hemorrhages (Roth spots) may occur in

bacterial endocarditis, which may cause stroke. Exophthalmos is observed with hyperthyroidism, orbital or retro-orbital masses, and cavernous sinus thrombosis.

C. Ears

Otoscopic examination shows bulging, opacity, and erythema of the tympanic membrane in otitis media, which may spread to produce bacterial meningitis.

D. Neck

Meningeal signs (**Figure 1-5**), such as neck stiffness on passive flexion or thigh flexion upon flexion of the neck (**Brudzinski sign**), are seen in meningitis and subarachnoid hemorrhage. Restricted lateral movement (flexion or rotation) of the neck may accompany cervical spondylosis. Auscultation of the neck may reveal a carotid bruit, which may be a risk factor for stroke.

▶ Chest & Cardiovascular

Signs of respiratory muscle weakness—such as intercostal muscle retraction and the use of accessory muscles—may

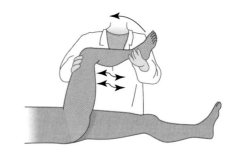

A Kernig sign

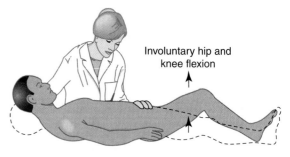

B Brudzinski sign

▲ **Figure 1-5.** Signs of meningeal irritation. Kernig sign (**A**) is resistance to passive extension at the knee with the hip flexed. Brudzinski sign (**B**) is flexion at the hip and knee in response to passive flexion of the neck. (Used with permission from LeBlond RF, DeGowin RL, Brown DD. *DeGowin's Diagnostic Examination.* 9th ed. New York, NY: McGraw-Hill; 2009.)

occur in neuromuscular disorders. Heart murmurs may be associated with valvular heart disease and infective endocarditis, which predispose to stroke.

Abdomen

Abdominal examination may suggest liver disease and is always important in patients with the new onset of back pain, because intra-abdominal processes such as pancreatic carcinoma or aortic aneurysm may present with pain that radiates to the back.

Extremities & Back

Resistance to passive extension of the knee with the hip flexed (**Kernig sign**) (Figure 1-5) is seen in meningitis. Raising the extended leg with the patient supine (straight leg raising, or **Lasègue sign**) stretches the L4-S2 roots and sciatic nerve, whereas raising the extended leg with the patient prone (reverse straight leg raising) stretches the L2-L4 roots and femoral nerve and may reproduce radicular pain with lesions affecting these structures (**Figure 1-6**).

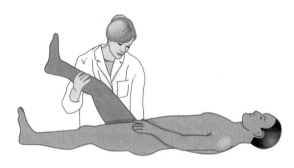

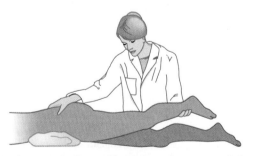

▲ **Figure 1-6.** Signs of lumbosacral nerve root irritation. The straight leg raising or Lasègue sign (top) is pain in an L4-S2 root or sciatic nerve distribution in response to raising the extended leg with the patient supine. The reverse straight leg raising sign (bottom) is pain in an L2-L4 root or femoral nerve distribution in response to raising the extended leg with the patient prone. (Used with permission from LeBlond RF, DeGowin RL, Brown DD. *DeGowin's Diagnostic Examination.* 9th ed. New York, NY: McGraw-Hill, 2009.)

Localized pain with percussion of the spine may be a sign of vertebral or epidural infection. Auscultation of the spine may reveal a bruit due to spinal vascular malformation.

Rectal & Pelvic

Rectal examination can provide evidence of gastrointestinal bleeding, which is a common precipitant of hepatic encephalopathy. Rectal or pelvic examination may disclose a mass lesion responsible for pain referred to the back.

NEUROLOGIC EXAMINATION

The neurologic examination should be tailored to the patient's specific complaint. All parts of the examination—mental status, cranial nerves, motor function, sensory function, coordination, reflexes, and stance and gait—should be covered, but the points of emphasis will differ. The history should have raised questions that the examination can now address. For example, if the complaint is weakness, the examiner seeks to determine its distribution and severity and whether it is accompanied by deficits in other areas, such as sensation and reflexes. The goal is to obtain the information necessary to generate an anatomic diagnosis.

Mental Status

The mental status examination addresses two key questions: (1) Is **level of consciousness** (wakefulness or alertness) normal or abnormal? (2) If the level of consciousness permits more detailed examination, is **cognitive function** normal, and if not, what is the nature and extent of the abnormality?

A. Level of Consciousness

Consciousness is awareness of the internal and external world, and the level of consciousness is described in terms of the patient's apparent state of wakefulness and response to stimuli. A patient with a normal level of consciousness is **awake** (or can be easily awakened), **alert** (responds appropriately to visual or verbal cues), and **oriented** (knows who and where he or she is and the approximate date and time).

Abnormal (depressed) consciousness represents a continuum ranging from mild sleepiness to unarousable unresponsiveness (**coma**, see Chapter 3, Coma). Depressed consciousness short of coma is sometimes referred to as a confusional state, delirium, or stupor, but should be characterized more precisely in terms of the stimulus–response patterns observed. Progressively more severe impairment of consciousness requires stimuli of increasing intensity to elicit increasingly primitive (nonpurposeful or reflexive) responses (**Figure 1-7**).

B. Cognitive Function

Cognitive function involves many spheres of activity, some thought to be localized and others dispersed throughout

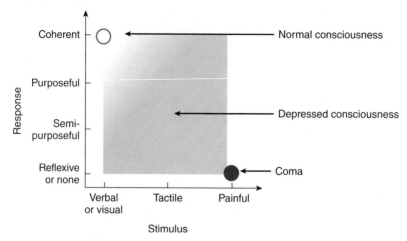

▲ **Figure 1-7.** Assessment of level of consciousness in relation to the patient's response to stimulation. A normally conscious patient responds coherently to visual or verbal stimulation, whereas a patient with impaired consciousness requires increasingly intense stimulation and exhibits increasingly primitive responses.

the cerebral hemispheres. The strategy in examining cognitive function is to assess a range of specific functions and, if abnormalities are found, to evaluate whether these can be attributed to a specific brain region or require more widespread involvement of the brain. For example, discrete disorders of language (**aphasia**) and memory (**amnesia**) can often be assigned to a circumscribed area of the brain, whereas more global deterioration of cognitive function, as seen in **dementia**, implies diffuse or multifocal disease.

1. **Bifrontal or diffuse functions—Attention** is the ability to focus on a particular sensory stimulus to the exclusion of others; **concentration** is sustained attention. Attention can be tested by asking the patient to immediately repeat a series of digits (a normal person can repeat five to seven digits correctly), and concentration can be tested by having the patient count backward from 100 by 7s. Abstract thought processes like **insight** and **judgment** can be assessed by asking the patient to list similarities and differences between objects (eg, an apple and an orange), interpret proverbs (overly concrete interpretations suggest impaired abstraction ability), or describe what he or she would do in a hypothetical situation requiring judgment (eg, finding an addressed envelope on the street). **Fund of knowledge** can be tested by asking for information that a normal person of the patient's age and cultural background would possess (eg, the name of the President, sports stars, or other celebrities, or major events in the news). This is not intended to test intelligence, but to determine whether the patient has been incorporating new information in the recent past. **Affect** is the external expression of internal **mood** and may be manifested by talkativeness or lack thereof, facial expression, and posture. Conversation with the patient may reveal

abnormalities of thought content, such as **delusions** or **hallucinations**, which are usually associated with psychiatric disease, but can also exist in confusional states (eg, alcohol withdrawal).

2. **Memory**—Memory is the ability to register, store, and retrieve information and can be impaired by either diffuse cortical or bilateral temporal lobe disease. Memory is assessed by testing **immediate recall**, **recent memory**, and **remote memory**, which correspond roughly to registration, storage, and retrieval. Tests of **immediate recall** are similar to tests of attention (see earlier discussion) and include having the patient immediately repeat a list of numbers or objects. To test **recent memory**, the patient can be asked to repeat a list of items 3 to 5 minutes later. **Remote memory** is tested by asking the patient about facts he or she can be expected to have learned in past years, such as personal or family data or major historic events. Confusional states typically impair immediate recall, whereas memory disorders (**amnesia**) are characteristically associated with predominant involvement of recent memory, with remote memory preserved until late stages. Personal and emotionally charged memories tend to be preferentially spared, whereas the opposite may be true in **psychogenic amnesia**. Inability of an awake and alert patient to remember his or her own name strongly suggests a psychiatric disorder.

3. **Language**—The key elements of language are comprehension, repetition, fluency, naming, reading, and writing, and all should be tested when a language disorder (**aphasia**) is suspected. There are a variety of aphasia syndromes, each characterized by a particular pattern of language impairment (**Table 1-1**) and often correlating with a specific site of pathology (**Figure 1-8**). **Expressive** (also called **nonfluent**, **motor**, or **Broca**) aphasia

Table 1-1. Aphasia Syndromes.

Type	Fluency	Comprehension	Repetition
Expressive (Broca)	−	+	−
Receptive (Wernicke)	+	−	−
Global	−	−	−
Conduction	+	+	−
Transcortical expressive	−	+	+
Transcortical receptive	+	−	+
Transcortical global	−	−	+
Anomic (naming)	+	+	+

+, preserved; −, impaired
See Figure 1-8 for anatomic correlates.
Modified from Waxman SG. *Clinical Neuroanatomy.* 26th ed. New York, NY: McGraw-Hill; 2010.

is characterized by paucity of spontaneous speech and by the agrammatical and telegraphic nature of the little speech that is produced. Language expression is tested by listening for these abnormalities as the patient speaks spontaneously and answers questions. Patients with this syndrome are also unable to write normally or to repeat (tested with a content-poor phrase such as "no

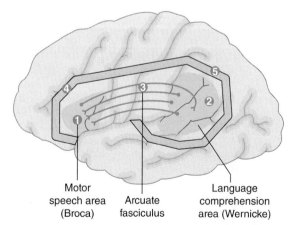

Motor speech area (Broca)   Arcuate fasciculus   Language comprehension area (Wernicke)

▲ **Figure 1-8.** Traditional view of brain areas involved in language function including the language comprehension (Wernicke) area, the motor speech (Broca) area, and the arcuate fasciculus. Lesions at the numbered sites produce aphasias with different features: (1) expressive aphasia, (2) receptive aphasia, (3) conduction aphasia, (4) transcortical expressive aphasia, and (5) transcortical receptive aphasia. See also Table 1-1. (Modified from Waxman SG. *Clinical Neuroanatomy.* 26th ed. New York, NY: McGraw-Hill; 2010.)

ifs, ands, or buts"), but their language comprehension is intact. Thus, if the patient is asked to do something that does not require language expression (eg, "close your eyes"), he or she can do it. The patient is typically aware of the disorder and frustrated by it. In **receptive** (also called **fluent, sensory, or Wernicke) aphasia**, language expression is preserved, but comprehension and repetition are impaired. A large volume of language is produced, but it lacks meaning and may include paraphasic errors (use of words that sound similar to the correct word) and neologisms (made-up words). Comprehension of written language is similarly poor, and repetition is defective. The patient cannot follow oral or written commands, but can imitate the examiner's action when prompted by a gesture to do so. These patients are usually unaware of and therefore not disturbed by their aphasia. **Global aphasia** combines features of expressive and receptive aphasia—patients can neither express, comprehend, nor repeat spoken or written language. Other forms of aphasia include **conduction aphasia**, in which repetition is impaired whereas expression and comprehension are intact; **transcortical aphasia**, in which expressive, receptive, or global aphasia occurs with intact repetition; and **anomic aphasia**, a selective disorder of naming. Language is distinct from **speech**, the final motor step in oral expression of language. A speech disorder (**dysarthria**) may be difficult to distinguish from aphasia, but always spares oral and written language comprehension and written expression.

4. **Sensory integration**—Sensory integration disorders result from parietal lobe lesions and cause misperception of or inattention to sensory stimuli on the side of the body opposite the lesion, even though primary sensory modalities (eg, touch) are intact. Patients with parietal lesions may exhibit various signs. **Astereognosis** is the inability to identify by touch an object placed in the hand, such as a coin, key, or safety pin. **Agraphesthesia** is the inability to identify by touch a number written on the hand. Failure of **two-point discrimination** is the inability to differentiate between a single stimulus and two simultaneously applied, adjacent but separated, stimuli that can be distinguished by a normal person (or on the opposite side). For example, the points of two pens can be applied together on a fingertip and gradually separated until they are perceived as separate objects; the distance at which this occurs is recorded. **Allesthesia** is misplaced (typically more proximal) localization of a tactile stimulus. **Extinction** is the failure to perceive a visual or tactile stimulus when it is applied bilaterally, even though it can be perceived when applied unilaterally. **Neglect** is failure to attend to space or use the limbs on one side of the body. **Anosognosia** is unawareness of a neurologic deficit. **Constructional apraxia** is the inability to draw accurate representations of external space, such as filling in

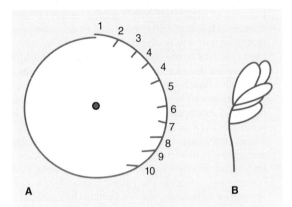

▲ **Figure 1-9.** Unilateral (left-sided) neglect in a patient with a right parietal lesion. The patient was asked to fill in the numbers on the face of a clock (**A**) and to draw a flower (**B**). (Used with permission from Waxman SG. *Clinical Neuroanatomy.* 26th ed. New York, NY: McGraw-Hill; 2010.)

the numbers on a clock face or copying geometric figures (**Figure 1-9**).

5. **Motor integration**—Praxis is the application of motor learning, and **apraxia** is the inability to perform previously learned tasks despite intact motor and sensory function. Tests for apraxia include asking the patient to simulate the use of a key, comb, or fork. Unilateral apraxias are commonly caused by contralateral premotor frontal cortex lesions. Bilateral apraxias, such as gait apraxia, may be seen with bifrontal or diffuse cerebral lesions.

▶ **Cranial Nerves**

A. Olfactory (I) Nerve

The olfactory nerve mediates the sense of smell (olfaction) and is tested by asking the patient to identify common scents, such as coffee, vanilla, peppermint, or cloves. Normal function can be assumed if the patient detects the smell, even if unable to identify it. Each nostril is tested separately. Irritants such as alcohol should not be used because they may be detected as noxious stimuli independent of olfactory receptors.

B. Optic (II) Nerve

The optic nerve transmits visual information from the retina, through the optic chiasm (where fibers from the nasal, or medial, sides of both retinas, conveying information from the temporal, or lateral, halves of both visual fields, cross), and then via the optic tracts to the lateral geniculate nuclei of the thalami. Optic nerve function is assessed separately for each eye and involves inspecting the back of the eye (optic fundus) by direct ophthalmoscopy,

measuring visual acuity, and mapping the visual field as follows:

1. **Ophthalmoscopy** should be conducted in a dark room to dilate the pupils, which makes it easier to see the fundus. Mydriatic (sympathomimetic or anticholinergic) eye drops are sometimes used to enhance dilation, but this should not be done until visual acuity and pupillary reflexes are tested, nor in patients with untreated closed angle glaucoma or an intracranial mass lesion that might lead to transtentorial herniation. In the latter case, the ability to test pupillary reflexes is essential to detect clinical progression. The normal **optic disk (Figure 1-10)** is

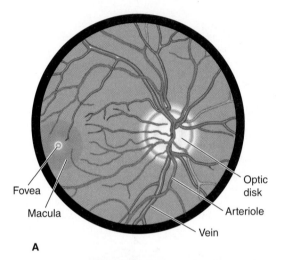

A

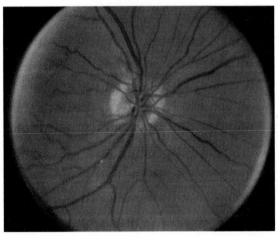

B

▲ **Figure 1-10.** The normal fundus. The diagram (**A**) shows landmarks corresponding to the photograph (**B**). (Photo by Diane Beeston; used with permission from Vaughan D, Asbury T, Riordan-Eva P. *General Ophthalmology.* 15th ed. Stamford, CT: Appleton & Lange; 1999. Copyright © McGraw-Hilll.)

a yellowish, oval structure situated nasally at the posterior pole of the eye. The margins of the disk and the blood vessels that cross it should be sharply demarcated, and the veins should show spontaneous pulsations. The **macula**, an area paler than the rest of the retina, is located about two disk diameters temporal to the temporal margin of the optic disk and can be visualized by having the patient look at the light from the ophthalmoscope. In neurologic patients, the most important abnormality to identify is swelling of the optic disk resulting from increased intracranial pressure (**papilledema**). In early papilledema (**Figure 1-11**), the retinal veins appear engorged, and spontaneous

venous pulsations are absent. The disk may be hyperemic with linear hemorrhages at its borders. The disk margins become blurred, initially at the nasal edge. In fully developed papilledema, the optic disk is elevated above the plane of the retina, and blood vessels crossing the disk border are obscured. Papilledema is almost always bilateral, does not typically impair vision except for enlargement of the blind spot, and is not painful. Another abnormality—**optic disk pallor**—is produced by atrophy of the optic nerve. It can be seen in patients with multiple sclerosis or other disorders of the optic nerve and is associated with defects in visual acuity, visual fields, or pupillary reactivity.

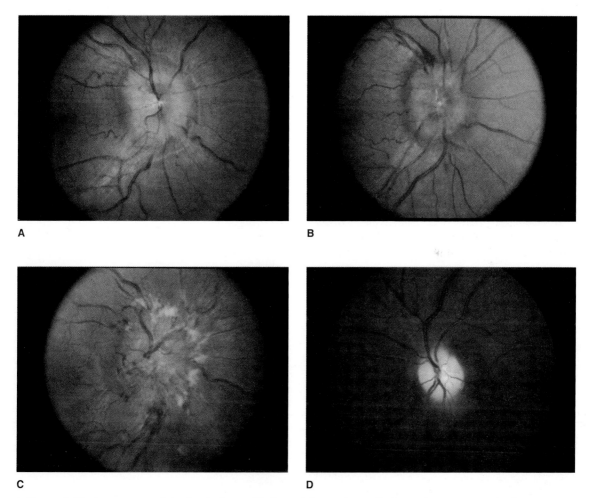

A   B

C   D

▲ **Figure 1-11.** Appearance of the fundus in papilledema. (**A**) In early papilledema, the superior and inferior margins of the optic disk are blurred by the thickened layer of nerve fibers entering the disk. (**B**) Moderate papilledema with disk swelling. (**C**) In fully developed papilledema, the optic disk is swollen, elevated, and congested, and the retinal veins are markedly dilated; swollen nerve fibers (white patches) and hemorrhages can be seen. (**D**) In chronic atrophic papilledema, the optic disk is pale and slightly elevated, and its margins are blurred. (Photos used with permission from Nancy Newman.)

2. **Visual acuity** should be tested with refractive errors corrected, so patients who wear glasses should be examined with them on. Acuity is tested in each eye separately, using a Snellen eye chart approximately 6 m (20 ft) away for distant vision or a Rosenbaum pocket eye chart approximately 36 cm (14 in) away for near vision. The smallest line of print that can be read is noted, and acuity is expressed as a fraction, in which the numerator is the distance at which the line of print can be read by someone with normal vision and the denominator is the distance at which it can be read by the patient. Thus, 20/20 indicates normal acuity, with the denominator increasing as vision worsens. More severe impairment can be graded according to the distance at which the patient can count fingers, discern hand movement, or perceive light. Red–green color vision is often disproportionately impaired with optic nerve lesions and can be tested using colored pens or hatpins or with color vision plates.

3. **Visual fields** are tested for each eye separately, most often using the **confrontation** technique (**Figure 1-12**). The examiner stands at about arm's length from the patient, the patient's eye that is not being tested and the examiner's eye opposite it are closed or covered, and the patient is instructed to fix on the examiner's open eye, superimposing the monocular fields of patient and examiner. Using the index finger of either hand to locate the peripheral limits of the patient's field, the examiner then moves the finger slowly inward in all directions until the patient detects it. The size of the patient's **central scotoma (blind spot)**, located in the temporal half of the visual field, can also be measured in relation to the examiner's. The object of confrontation testing is to determine whether the patient's visual field is coextensive with—or more restricted than—the examiner's. Another approach is to use the head of a hatpin as the visual target. Subtle field defects may be detected by asking the patient to compare the brightness of colored objects presented at different sites in the field or by measuring the fields using a hatpin with a red head as the target. Gross abnormalities can

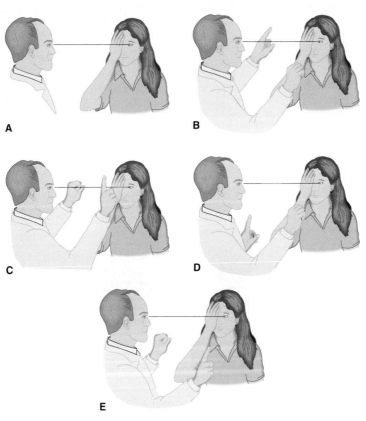

▲ **Figure 1-12.** Confrontation testing of the visual field. (**A**) The left eye of the patient and the right eye of the examiner are aligned. (**B**) Testing the superior nasal quadrant. (**C**) Testing the superior temporal quadrant. (**D**) Testing the inferior nasal quadrant. (**E**) Testing the inferior temporal quadrant. The procedure is then repeated for the patient's other eye.

be detected in less than fully alert patients by determining whether they blink when the examiner's finger is brought toward the patient's eye from various directions. In some situations (eg, following the course of a progressive or resolving defect), the visual fields should be mapped more precisely, using perimetry techniques such as tangent screen or automated perimetry testing. Common visual field abnormalities and their anatomic correlates are shown in **Figure 1-13**.

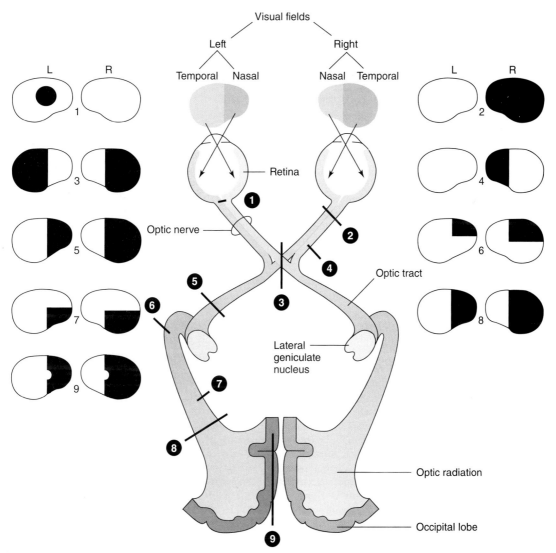

▲ **Figure 1-13.** Common visual field defects and their anatomic bases. 1. **Central scotoma** caused by inflammation of the optic disk (optic neuritis) or optic nerve (retrobulbar neuritis). 2. **Total blindness of the right eye** from a complete lesion of the right optic nerve. 3. **Bitemporal hemianopia** caused by pressure exerted on the optic chiasm by a pituitary tumor. 4. **Right nasal hemianopia** caused by a perichiasmal lesion (eg, calcified internal carotid artery). 5. **Right homonymous hemianopia** from a lesion of the left optic tract. 6. **Right homonymous superior quadrantanopia** caused by partial involvement of the optic radiation by a lesion in the left temporal lobe (Meyer loop). 7. Right homonymous inferior quadrantanopia caused by partial involvement of the optic radiation by a lesion in the left parietal lobe. 8. **Right homonymous hemianopia** from a complete lesion of the left optic radiation. (A similar defect may also result from lesion 9.) 9. **Right homonymous hemianopia (with macular sparing)** resulting from posterior cerebral artery occlusion. Defects are shown in black.

C. Oculomotor (III), Trochlear (IV), and Abducens (VI) Nerves

These three nerves control the action of the intraocular (pupillary sphincter) and extraocular muscles.

1. **Pupils**—The diameter and shape of the pupils in ambient light and their responses to light and accommodation should be ascertained. Normal pupils average ≈3 mm in diameter in a well-lit room, but can vary from ≈6 mm in children to <2 mm in the elderly, and can differ in size from side to side by ≈1 mm (**physiologic anisocoria**). Pupils should be round and regular in shape. Normal pupils constrict briskly in response to direct illumination, and somewhat less so to illumination of the pupil on the opposite side (consensual response), and dilate again rapidly when the source of illumination is removed. When the eyes converge to focus on a nearer object such as the tip of one's nose (**accommodation**), normal pupils constrict. Pupillary constriction (**miosis**) is mediated through parasympathetic fibers that originate in the midbrain and travel with the oculomotor nerve to the eye. Interruption of this pathway, such as by a hemispheric mass lesion producing coma and compressing the oculomotor nerve as it exits the brainstem, produces a dilated (≈7 mm) unreactive pupil. Pupillary dilation is controlled by a three-neuron sympathetic relay, from the hypothalamus, through the brainstem to the T1 level of the spinal cord, to the superior cervical ganglion, and to the eye. Lesions of this pathway result in constricted (≤1 mm) unreactive pupils. Other common pupillary abnormalities are listed in **Table 1-2**.

2. **Eyelids and orbits**—The eyelids (**palpebrae**) should be examined with the patient's eyes open. The distance between the upper and lower lids (interpalpebral fissure) is usually ≈10 mm and approximately equal in the two eyes. The upper lid normally covers 1 to 2 mm of the iris, but this is increased by drooping of the lid (**ptosis**) due to lesions of the levator palpebrae muscle or its oculomotor (III) or sympathetic nerve supply. Ptosis occurs together with miosis (and sometimes defective sweating, or **anhidrosis**, of the forehead) in **Horner syndrome**. Abnormal protrusion of the eye from the orbit (**exophthalmos** or **proptosis**) is best detected by

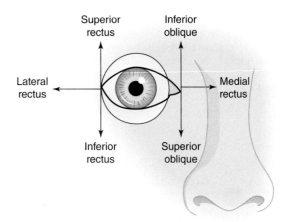

Figure 1-14. The six cardinal positions of gaze for testing eye movement. The eye is adducted by the medial rectus and abducted by the lateral rectus. The adducted eye is elevated by the inferior oblique and depressed by the superior oblique; the abducted eye is elevated by the superior rectus and depressed by the inferior rectus. All extraocular muscles are innervated by the oculomotor (III) nerve except the superior oblique, which is innervated by the trochlear (IV) nerve, and the lateral rectus, which is innervated by the abducens (VI) nerve.

standing behind the seated patient and looking down at his or her eyes.

3. **Eye movements**—Movement of the eyes is accomplished by the action of six muscles attached to each globe, which act to move the eye into the six cardinal positions of gaze (**Figure 1-14**). Equal and opposed actions of these muscles in the resting state place the eye in mid- or primary position (looking directly forward). When the function of an extraocular muscle is disrupted, the eye is unable to move in the direction of action of the affected muscle (**ophthalmoplegia**) and may deviate in the opposite direction because of the unopposed action of other extraocular muscles. When the eyes are thus misaligned, visual images of perceived objects fall at a different place on each retina,

Table 1-2. Common Pupillary Abnormalities.

Name	Appearance	Reactivity (light)	Reactivity (accommodation)	Site of Lesion
Adie (tonic) pupil	Unilateral large pupil	Sluggish	Normal	Ciliary ganglion
Argyll Robertson pupil	Bilateral small, irregular pupils	Absent	Normal	Midbrain
Horner syndrome	Unilateral small pupil and ptosis	Normal	Normal	Sympathetic innervation of eye
Marcus Gunn pupil	Normal	Consensual > direct	Normal	Optic nerve

creating the illusion of double vision or **diplopia**. The extraocular muscles are innervated by the oculomotor (III), trochlear (IV), and abducens (VI) nerves, and defects in eye movement may result from either muscle or nerve lesions. The oculomotor (III) nerve innervates all the extraocular muscles except the superior oblique, which is innervated by the trochlear (IV) nerve, and the lateral rectus, which is innervated by the abducens (VI) nerve. Because of their differential innervation, the pattern of ocular muscle involvement in pathologic conditions can help to distinguish a disorder of the ocular muscles per se from a disorder that affects a cranial nerve.

Eye movement is tested by having the patient look at a flashlight held in each of the cardinal positions of gaze and observing whether the eyes move fully and in a yoked (**conjugate**) fashion in each direction. With normal conjugate gaze, light from the flashlight falls at the same spot on both corneas. Limitations of eye movement and any disconjugacy should be noted. If the patient complains of diplopia, the weak muscle responsible should be identified by having the patient gaze in the direction in which the separation of images is greatest. Each eye is then covered in turn and the patient is asked to report which of the two (near or far) images disappears. The image displaced farther in the direction of gaze is always referable to the weak eye. Alternatively, one eye is covered with translucent red glass, plastic, or cellophane, which allows the eye responsible for each image to be identified. For example, with weakness of the left lateral rectus muscle, diplopia is maximal on leftward gaze, and the leftmost of the two images seen disappears when the left eye is covered.

4. **Ocular oscillations—Nystagmus**, or rhythmic oscillation of the eyes, can occur at the extremes of voluntary gaze in normal subjects. In other settings, however, it may be due to anticonvulsant or sedative drugs, or reflect disease affecting the extraocular muscles or their innervation, or vestibular or cerebellar pathways. The most common form, **jerk nystagmus**, consists of a slow phase of movement followed by a fast phase in the opposite direction (**Figure 1-15**). To detect nystagmus, the eyes are observed in the primary position and in each of the cardinal positions of gaze. If nystagmus is observed, it should be described in terms of the position of gaze in which it occurs, its direction, its amplitude (fine or coarse), precipitating factors such as changes in head position, and associated symptoms, such as vertigo. The direction of jerk nystagmus (eg, leftward-beating nystagmus) is, by convention, the direction of the fast phase. Jerk nystagmus usually increases in amplitude with gaze in the direction of the fast phase (Alexander law). A less common form of nystagmus is **pendular nystagmus**, which usually begins in infancy and is of equal velocity in both directions.

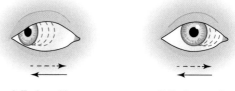

A End-position nystagmus

B Nystagmus in primary position

▲ **Figure 1-15. Nystagmus.** A slow drift of the eyes away from the position of fixation (indicated by the broken arrow) is corrected by a quick movement back (solid arrow). The direction of the nystagmus is named from the quick component. Nystagmus from the primary position is more likely to be pathologic than that from the end position. (Used with permission from LeBlond RF, Brown DD, DeGowin RL. *DeGowin's Diagnostic Examination.* 9th ed. New York, NY: McGraw-Hill; 2009.)

D. Trigeminal (V) Nerve

The trigeminal nerve conveys sensory fibers from the face and motor fibers to the muscles of mastication. Facial touch and temperature sensation are tested, respectively, by touching and by placing the cool surface of a tuning fork on both sides of the face in the distribution of each division of the trigeminal nerve—**ophthalmic** (**V1**, forehead), **maxillary** (**V2**, cheek), and **mandibular** (**V3**, jaw) (**Figure 1-16**). The patient is asked if the sensation is the same on both sides

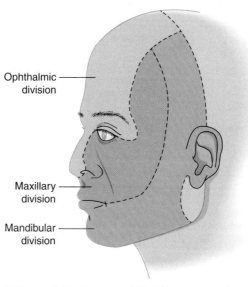

Ophthalmic division

Maxillary division

Mandibular division

▲ **Figure 1-16.** Trigeminal (V) nerve sensory divisions: ophthalmic (V1), maxillary (V2), and mandibular (V3). (Used with permission from Waxman SG. *Clinical Neuroanatomy.* 26th ed. New York, NY: McGraw-Hill; 2010.)

and, if not, on which side the stimulus is felt less well, or as less cool. To test the **corneal reflex**, a wisp of cotton is swept lightly across the cornea overlying the iris (not the surrounding white sclera) on the lateral surface of the eye (out of the subject's view). The normal response, which is mediated by a reflex arc that depends on trigeminal (V1) nerve sensory function and facial (VII) nerve motor function, is bilateral blinking of the eyes. With impaired trigeminal function, neither eye blinks, whereas unilateral blinking implies a facial nerve lesion on the unblinking side. Trigeminal motor function is tested by observing the symmetry of opening and closing of the mouth; on closing, the jaw falls faster and farther on the weak side, causing the face to look askew. More subtle weakness can be detected by asking the patient to clench the teeth and attempting to force the jaw open. Normal jaw strength cannot be overcome by the examiner.

E. Facial (VII) Nerve

The facial nerve supplies the facial muscles and mediates taste sensation from about the anterior two-thirds of the tongue (**Figure 1-17**). To test facial strength, the patient's face should be observed for symmetry or asymmetry of the palpebral fissures and nasolabial folds at rest. The patient is asked to wrinkle the forehead, squeeze the eyes tightly shut (looking for asymmetry in the extent to which the eyelashes protrude), and smile or show the teeth. Again the examiner looks for symmetry or asymmetry. With a peripheral (facial nerve) lesion, an entire side of the face is weak, and the eye cannot be fully closed.

With a central (eg, hemispheric) lesion, the forehead is spared, and some ability to close the eye is retained. This discrepancy is thought to result from dual cortical motor input to the upper face. Bilateral facial weakness cannot be detected by comparison between the two sides. Instead, the patient is asked to squeeze both eyes tightly shut, press the lips tightly together, and puff out the cheeks. If strength is normal, the examiner should not be able to pry open the eyelids, force apart the lips, or force air out of the mouth by compressing the cheeks. Facial weakness may be associated with dysarthria that is most pronounced for *m* sounds. If the patient is normally able to whistle, this ability may be lost with facial weakness. To test taste sensation, cotton-tipped applicators are dipped in sweet, sour, salty, or bitter solutions and placed on the protruded tongue, and the patient is asked to identify the taste.

F. Vestibulocochlear (VIII) Nerve

The vestibulocochlear nerve has two divisions—auditory and vestibular—which are involved in hearing and equilibrium, respectively. Examination should include otoscopic inspection of the auditory canals and tympanic membranes, assessment of auditory acuity in each ear, and Weber and Rinne tests performed with a 512-Hz tuning fork. Auditory acuity can be tested crudely by rubbing thumb and forefinger together approximately 2 in from each ear.

If the patient complains of hearing loss or cannot hear the finger rub, the nature of the hearing deficit should be

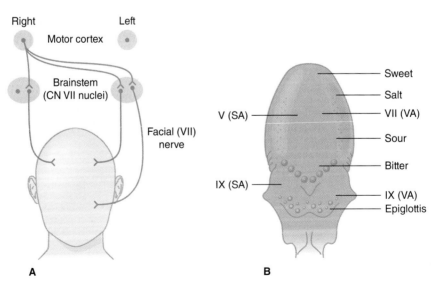

Figure 1-17. Facial (VII) nerve. (**A**) Central and peripheral motor innervation of the face. The motor cortex projects to both sides of the forehead, but only to the contralateral lower face (eyes and below). (**B**) Somatic afferent (SA, touch) and visceral afferent (VA, taste) innervation of the tongue by trigeminal (V), facial (VII) and glossopharyngeal (IX) nerves. (Used with permission from Waxman SG. *Clinical Neuroanatomy*. 26th ed. New York, NY: McGraw-Hill; 2010.)

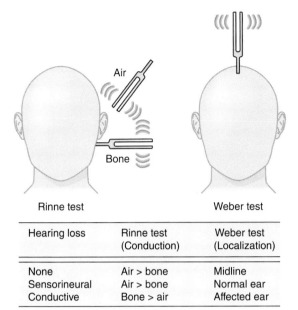

Figure 1-18. Tests for hearing loss.

Hearing loss	Rinne test (Conduction)	Weber test (Localization)
None	Air > bone	Midline
Sensorineural	Air > bone	Normal ear
Conductive	Bone > air	Affected ear

explored. To perform the **Rinne test (Figure 1-18)**, the base of a lightly vibrating tuning fork is placed on the mastoid process of the temporal bone until the sound can no longer be heard; the tuning fork is then moved near the opening of the external auditory canal. In patients with normal hearing or sensorineural hearing loss, air in the auditory canal conducts sound better than bone, and the tone can still be heard. With conductive hearing loss, the patient hears the bone-conducted tone, with the tuning fork on the mastoid process, longer than he or she hears the air-conducted tone. In the **Weber test** (see **Figure 1-18**), the handle of the vibrating tuning fork is placed in the middle of the forehead. With conductive hearing loss, the tone will sound louder in the affected ear; with sensorineural hearing loss, the tone will be louder in the normal ear.

In patients who complain of positional vertigo, the **Nylen–Bárány or Dix–Hallpike maneuver (Figure 1-19)** can be used to try to reproduce the precipitating circumstance. The patient is seated on a table with the head and eyes directed forward and is then quickly lowered to a supine position with the head over the table edge, 45 degrees below horizontal. The test is repeated with the patient's head and eyes turned 45 degrees to the right and again with the head and eyes turned 45 degrees to the left. The eyes are observed for nystagmus, and the patient is asked to note the onset, severity, and cessation of vertigo, if it occurs.

G. Glossopharyngeal (IX) and Vagus (X) Nerves

The glossopharyngeal and vagus nerves innervate muscles of the pharynx and larynx involved in swallowing and phonation. The glossopharyngeal nerve also conveys touch from the posterior one-third of the tongue, tonsils, tympanic membrane, and Eustachian tube, as well as taste from the posterior one-third of the tongue. The vagus nerve contains sensory fibers from the larynx, pharynx, external auditory canal, tympanic membrane, and posterior fossa meninges.

Motor function of these nerves is tested by asking the patient to say "ah" with the mouth open and looking for full and symmetric elevation of the palate. With unilateral weakness, the palate fails to elevate on the affected side; with bilateral weakness, neither side elevates. Patients with palatal weakness may also exhibit dysarthria, which affects especially *k* sounds. Sensory function can be tested by the gag reflex: the back of the tongue is touched on each side in turn using a tongue depressor or cotton-tipped applicator, and differences in the magnitude of gag responses are noted.

H. Spinal Accessory (XI) Nerve

The spinal accessory nerve innervates the sternocleidomastoid and trapezius muscles. The sternocleidomastoid is tested by asking the patient to rotate the head against resistance provided by the examiner's hand, which is placed on the patient's jaw. Sternocleidomastoid weakness results in decreased ability to rotate the head away from the weak side. The trapezius is tested by having the patient shrug the shoulders against resistance and noting any asymmetry.

I. Hypoglossal (XII) Nerve

The hypoglossal nerve innervates the tongue muscles. It can be tested by having the patient push the tongue against the inside of the cheek while the examiner presses on the outside of the cheek. With unilateral tongue weakness, the ability to press against the opposite cheek is reduced. There may be also deviation of the protruded tongue toward the weak side, although facial weakness may result in false-positive tests. Tongue weakness also produces dysarthria with prominent slurring of labial (*l*) sounds. Finally, denervation of the tongue may be associated with wasting (**atrophy**) and twitching (**fasciculation**).

▶ Motor Function

Motor function is governed by both upper and lower motor neurons. **Upper motor neurons** arise in the cerebral cortex and brainstem, and project onto lower motor neurons in the brainstem and anterior horn of the spinal cord. They include projections from cortex to spinal cord (**corticospinal tract**) including the part of the corticospinal tract that crosses (decussates) in the medulla (**pyramidal tract**). The motor examination includes evaluation of muscle bulk, tone, and strength. **Lower motor neurons** project from brainstem and spinal cord, via motor nerves, to innervate skeletal muscle. Lesions of either upper or lower motor neurons produce weakness. As discussed later,

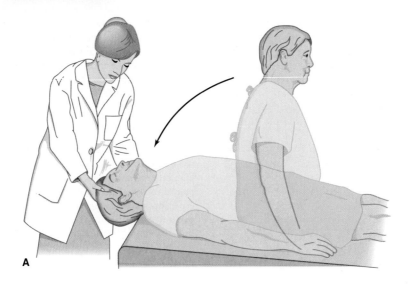

A

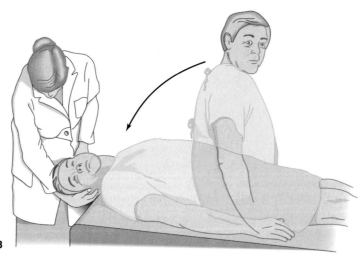

B

▲ **Figure 1-19.** Test for positional vertigo and nystagmus. The patient is seated on a table with the head and eyes directed forward (**A**) and is then quickly lowered to a supine position with the head over the table edge, 45 degrees below horizontal. The patient's eyes are then observed for nystagmus, and the patient is asked to report any vertigo. The test is repeated with the patient's head and eyes turned 45 degrees to the right (**B**), and again with the head and eyes turned 45 degrees to the left.

upper motor neuron lesions also cause increased muscle tone, hyperactive tendon reflexes, and Babinski signs, whereas lower motor neuron lesions produce decreased muscle tone, hypoactive reflexes, muscle atrophy, and fasciculations.

A. Bulk

The muscles should be inspected to determine whether they are normal or decreased in bulk. Reduced muscle bulk (**atrophy**) is usually the result of denervation from lower

motor neuron (spinal cord anterior horn cell or peripheral nerve) lesions. Asymmetric atrophy can be detected by comparing the bulk of individual muscles on the two sides by visual inspection or by using a tape measure. Atrophy may be associated with **fasciculations**—spontaneous muscle twitching visible beneath the skin.

B. Tone

Tone is resistance of a muscle to passive movement at a joint. With normal tone, there is little such resistance.

Abnormally decreased tone (**hypotonia** or **flaccidity**) may accompany muscle, lower motor neuron, or cerebellar disorders. Increased tone takes the form of **rigidity**, in which the increase is constant over the range of motion at a joint, or **spasticity**, in which the increase is velocity-dependent and variable over the range of motion. Rigidity is associated classically with diseases of the basal ganglia and spasticity with diseases affecting the corticospinal tracts. Tone at the elbow is measured by supporting the patient's arm with one hand under the elbow, then flexing, extending, pronating, and supinating the forearm with the examiner's other hand. The arm should move smoothly in all directions. Tone at the wrist is tested by grasping the forearm with one hand and flopping the wrist back and forth with the other. With normal tone, the hand should rest at a 90-degree angle at the wrist; with increased tone the angle is greater than 90 degrees. Tone in the legs is measured with the patient lying supine and relaxed. The examiner places one hand under the knee, and then pulls abruptly upward. With normal or reduced tone, the patient's heel is lifted only momentarily off the bed or remains in contact with the surface of the bed as it slides upward. With increased tone, the leg lifts completely off the bed. Axial tone can be measured by passively rotating the patient's head and observing whether the shoulders also move, which indicates increased tone, or by gently but firmly flexing and extending the neck and noting whether resistance is encountered.

C. Strength

Muscle strength, or power, is graded on a scale according to the force a muscle can overcome: 5, normal strength; 4, decreased strength but still able to move against gravity plus added resistance; 3, able to move against gravity but not added resistance; 2, able to move only with the force of gravity eliminated (ie, horizontally); 1, flicker of movement; 0, no visible muscle contraction. What is normal strength for a young person cannot be expected of a frail, elderly individual, and this must be taken into account in grading muscle strength. Strength is tested by having the patient execute a movement that involves a single muscle or muscle group and then applying a gradually increasing opposing force to determine whether the patient's movement can be overcome (**Figure 1-20**). Where possible, the opposing force should be applied using muscles of similar size (eg, the arm for proximal and the fingers for distal limb muscles). The emphasis should be on identifying differences from side to side, between proximal and distal muscles, or between muscle groups innervated by different nerves or nerve roots. In **pyramidal weakness** (due to lesions affecting the corticospinal tract), there is preferential weakness of extensor and abductor muscles in the upper and flexor muscles in the lower extremity. **Fine finger movements**, such as rapidly tapping the thumb and index finger together, are slowed. With the arms

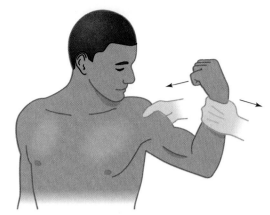

▲ **Figure 1-20.** Technique for testing muscle strength. In the example shown (biceps), the patient flexes the arm and the examiner tries to overcome this movement. (Used with permission from LeBlond RF, Brown DD, DeGowin RL. *DeGowin's Diagnostic Examination.* 9th ed. New York, NY: McGraw-Hill; 2009.)

extended, palms up, and eyes closed, the affected arm falls slowly downward and the hand pronates (**pronator drift**). Bilaterally symmetrical **distal weakness** is characteristic of polyneuropathy, whereas bilaterally symmetrical **proximal weakness** is observed in myopathy. Tests of strength for selected individual muscles are illustrated in the Appendix.

▶ Sensory Function

Somatic sensation is mediated through large sensory fibers that travel from the periphery to the thalamus in the posterior columns of the spinal cord and brainstem medial lemniscus, and small sensory fibers that ascend to the thalamus in the spinothalamic tracts. Light touch sensation is conveyed by both pathways, vibration and position sense by the large-fiber pathway, and pain and temperature sense by the small-fiber pathway. Because most sensory disorders affect distal more than proximal sites, screening should begin distally (ie, at the toes and fingers) and proceed proximally, until the upper border of any deficit is reached. If the patient complains of sensory loss in a specific area, sensory testing should begin in the center of that area and proceed outward until sensation is reported as normal. Comparing the intensity of or threshold for sensation on the two sides of the body is useful for detecting lateralized sensory deficits. When sensory deficits are more limited, such as when they affect a single limb or truncal segment, their distribution should be compared with that of the spinal roots and peripheral nerves (see Chapter 10, Sensory Disorders) to determine whether involvement of a specific root or nerve can explain the deficit observed. Some tests of somatosensory function are illustrated in **Figure 1-21**.

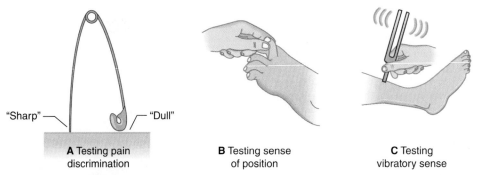

"Sharp"   "Dull"

A Testing pain discrimination   **B** Testing sense of position   **C** Testing vibratory sense

Figure 1-21. Tests of somatosensory function. **(A)** Touch (using finger or dull end of safety pin) and pain (sharp end of safety pin). **(B)** Joint position sense. **(C)** Vibration sense (using 128-Hz tuning fork). (Modified from LeBlond RF, Brown DD, DeGowin RL. *DeGowin's Diagnostic Examination*. 9th ed. New York, NY: McGraw-Hill; 2009.)

A. Light Touch

Touch perception is tested by applying a light stimulus—such as a wisp of cotton, the teased-out tip of a cotton swab, or a brushing motion of the fingertips—to the skin of a patient whose eyes are closed and who is asked to indicate where the stimulus is perceived. If a unilateral deficit is suspected, the patient can be asked to compare how intensely a touch stimulus is felt when applied at the same site on the two sides.

B. Vibration

Vibration sense is tested by striking a low-pitched (128-Hz) tuning fork and placing its base on a bony prominence, such as a joint; the fingers of the examiner holding the tuning fork serve as a normal control. The patient is asked to indicate whether the vibration is felt and, if so, when the feeling goes away. Testing begins distally, at the toes and fingers, and proceeds proximally from joint to joint until sensation is normal.

C. Position

To test joint position sense, the examiner grasps the sides of the distal phalanx of a finger or toe and slightly displaces the joint up or down. The patient, with eyes closed, is asked to report any perceived change in position. Normal joint position sense is exquisitely sensitive, and the patient should detect the slightest movement. If joint position sense is diminished distally, more proximal limb joints are tested until normal position sense is encountered. Another test of position sense is to have the patient close the eyes, extend the arms, and then touch the tips of the index fingers together.

D. Pain

A disposable pin should be used to prick (but not puncture) the skin with enough force for the resulting sensation to be mildly unpleasant. The patient is asked whether the stimulus feels sharp. If a safety pin is used, the rounded end can be used to demonstrate to the patient the intended distinction between a sharp and dull stimulus. Depending on the circumstance, the examiner should compare pain sensation from side to side, distal to proximal, or dermatome to dermatome, and from the area of deficit toward normal regions.

E. Temperature

This can be tested using the flat side of a cold tuning fork or another cold object. The examiner should first establish the patient's ability to detect the cold sensation in a presumably normal area. Cold sensation is then compared on the two sides, moving from distal to proximal, across dermatomes, and from abnormal toward normal areas.

▶ Coordination

Impaired coordination (**ataxia**), which usually results from lesions affecting the cerebellum or its connections, can affect the eye movements, speech, limbs, or trunk. Some tests of coordination are illustrated in **Figure 1-22**.

A. Limb Ataxia

Distal limb ataxia can be detected by asking the patient to perform rapid alternating movements (eg, alternately tapping the palm and dorsum of the hand on the patient's other hand, or tapping the sole of the foot on the examiner's hand) and noting any irregularity in the rate, rhythm, amplitude, or force of successive movements. In the **finger-to-nose test**, the patient moves an index finger back and forth between his or her nose and the examiner's finger; ataxia may be associated with **intention tremor**, which is most prominent at the beginning and end of each movement. Impaired ability to check the force of muscular contraction can also often be demonstrated. When the patient is asked to raise the arms rapidly to a given height—or when the arms, extended and outstretched in

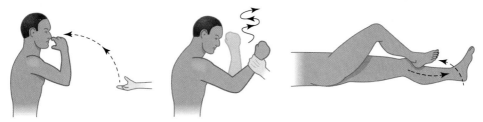

▲ **Figure 1-22.** Tests of cerebellar function: finger-to-nose test (left), test for rebound (center), and heel-knee-shin test (right). (Used with permission from LeBlond RF, Brown DD, DeGowin RL. *DeGowin's Diagnostic Examination.* 9th ed. New York, NY: McGraw-Hill; 2009.)

front of the patient, are displaced by a sudden force—there may be overshooting (**rebound**). This can be demonstrated by having the patient forcefully flex the arm at the elbow against resistance—and then suddenly removing the resistance. If the limb is ataxic, continued contraction without resistance may cause the hand to strike the patient. Ataxia of the lower limbs can be demonstrated by the **heel-knee-shin test**. The supine patient is asked to run the heel of the foot smoothly up and down the opposite shin from ankle to knee. Ataxia produces jerky and inaccurate movement, making it impossible for the patient to keep the heel in contact with the shin.

B. Truncal Ataxia

To detect truncal ataxia, the patient is asked to sit on the side of the bed or in a chair without lateral support, and any tendency to list to one side is noted.

▶ Reflexes

A. Tendon Reflexes

A **tendon reflex** is the reaction of a muscle to being passively stretched by percussion on a tendon and depends on the integrity of both afferent and efferent peripheral nerves and their inhibition by descending central pathways. Tendon reflexes are decreased or absent in disorders that affect any part of the reflex arc, most often by polyneuropathies, and increased by lesions of the corticospinal tract. Tendon reflexes are graded on a scale according to the force of the contraction or the minimum force needed to elicit the response: 4, very brisk, often with rhythmic reflex contractions (**clonus**); 3, brisk but normal; 2, normal; 1, minimal; 0, absent. In some cases, tendon reflexes are difficult to elicit, but may be brought out by having the patient clench the fist on the side not being tested or interlock the fingers and attempt to pull them apart. The main goal of reflex testing is to detect absence or asymmetry. Symmetrically absent reflexes suggest a polyneuropathy; symmetrically increased reflexes may indicate bilateral cerebral or spinal cord disease. The commonly tested tendon reflexes and the nerve roots they involve are: biceps and brachioradialis (C5-6), triceps (C7-8), quadriceps (L3-4), and Achilles (S1-2).

Methods for eliciting these tendon reflexes are shown in **Figure 1-23**.

B. Superficial Reflexes

The **superficial reflexes** are elicited by stimulating the skin, rather than tendons, and are altered or absent in disorders affecting the corticospinal tract. They include the **plantar reflex**, in which stroking the sole of the foot from its lateral border near the heel toward the great toe normally results in plantar flexion of the toes. With corticospinal lesions, the great toe dorsiflexes (**Babinski sign**), which may be accompanied by fanning of the toes, dorsiflexion at the ankle, and flexion at the thigh (**Figure 1-24**). Several superficial reflexes that are normally present in infancy, and subsequently disappear, may reappear with aging or frontal lobe dysfunction. The **palmar grasp** reflex, elicited by stroking the skin of the patient's palm with the examiner's fingers, causes the patient's fingers to close around those of the examiner. The **plantar grasp** reflex consists of flexion and adduction of the toes in response to stimulation of the sole of the foot. The **palmomental reflex** is elicited by scratching the palm of the hand and results in contraction of ipsilateral chin (mentalis) and perioral (orbicularis oris) muscles. The **suck reflex** consists of involuntary sucking movements following stimulation of the lips. The **snout reflex** is elicited by gently tapping the lips and results in their protrusion. In the **rooting reflex**, stimulation adjacent to the lips causes them to deviate toward the stimulus. The **glabellar reflex** is elicited by repetitive tapping on the forehead just above the nose; normal subjects blink only in response to the first several taps, whereas persistent blinking is an abnormal response (**Myerson sign**).

▶ Stance & Gait

The patient should be asked to stand with feet together and eyes open to detect instability from cerebellar ataxia. Next, the patient should close the eyes; instability occurring with eyes closed but not open (**Romberg sign**) is a sign of sensory ataxia. The patient should then be observed walking normally, on the heels, on the toes, and in **tandem** (one foot placed directly in front of the other),

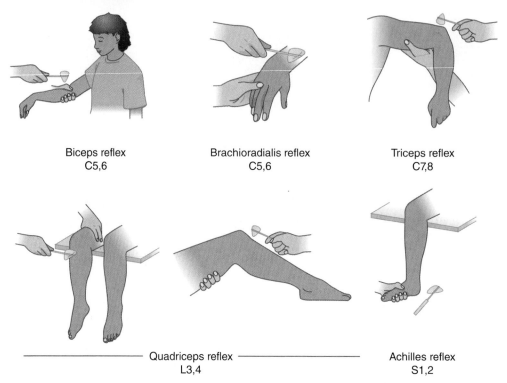

Biceps reflex
C5,6

Brachioradialis reflex
C5,6

Triceps reflex
C7,8

Quadriceps reflex
L3,4

Achilles reflex
S1,2

▲ **Figure 1-23.** Methods to elicit the tendon reflexes. Techniques for eliciting the quadriceps reflex in both seated and supine patients are shown. (Modified with permission from LeBlond RF, Brown DD, DeGowin RL. *DeGowin's Diagnostic Examination.* 9th ed. New York, NY: McGraw-Hill; 2009.)

to identify any of the following classic gait abnormalities (**Figure 1-25**):

1. **Hemiplegic gait**—The affected leg is held extended and internally rotated, the foot is inverted and plantar flexed, and the leg moves in a circular direction at the hip (circumduction).

2. **Paraplegic gait**—The gait is slow and stiff, with the legs crossing in front of each other (scissoring).

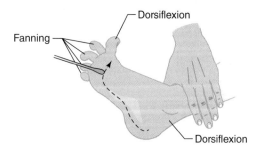

▲ **Figure 1-24.** Extensor plantar reflex (Babinski sign). It is elicited by firmly stroking the lateral border of the sole of the foot. (Modified from LeBlond RF, Brown DD, DeGowin RL. *DeGowin's Diagnostic Examination.* 9th ed. New York, NY: McGraw-Hill; 2009.)

3. **Cerebellar ataxic gait**—The gait is wide-based and may be associated with staggering or reeling, as if one were drunk.

4. **Sensory ataxic gait**—The gait is wide based, the feet are slapped down onto the floor, and the patient may watch the feet.

5. **Steppage gait**—Inability to dorsiflex the foot, often due to a fibular (peroneal) nerve lesion, results in exaggerated elevation of the hip and knee to allow the foot to clear the floor while walking.

6. **Dystrophic gait**—Pelvic muscle weakness produces a lordotic, waddling gait.

7. **Parkinsonian gait**—Posture is flexed, starts are slow, steps are small and shuffling, there is reduced arm swing, and involuntary acceleration (festination) may occur.

8. **Choreic gait**—The gait is jerky and lurching, but falls are surprisingly rare.

9. **Apraxic gait**—Frontal lobe disease may result in loss of the ability to perform a previously learned act (apraxia), in this case the ability to walk. The patient has difficulty initiating walking and may appear to be glued to the floor. Once started, the gait is slow and shuffling. However, there is no difficulty performing the same leg

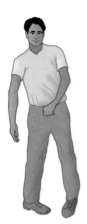 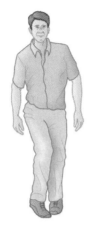 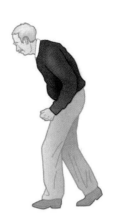 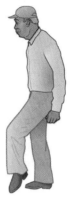 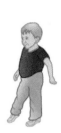

▲ **Figure 1-25.** Gait abnormalities. Left to right: hemiplegic gait (left hemiplegia), paraplegic gait, parkinsonian gait, steppage gait, dystrophic gait. (Modified with permission from *Handbook of Signs & Symptoms*. 4th ed. Ambler, PA: Lippincott Williams & Wilkins; 2009.)

movements when the patient is lying down and the legs are not bearing weight.

10. **Antalgic gait**—One leg is favored over the other in an effort to avoid putting weight on the injured leg and causing pain.

NEUROLOGIC EXAMINATION IN SPECIAL SETTINGS

Although the neurologic examination is always tailored to a patient's specific situation, it is sufficiently distinctive to deserve mention in two special settings: examination of the comatose patient and "screening" examination of a patient without neurologic complaints.

▶ Coma

The comatose patient cannot cooperate for a full neurologic examination. Fortunately, however, a great deal of information can be derived from much more limited examination, focused on three elements: the **pupillary reaction to light**, **eye movements** induced by oculocephalic (head turning) or oculovestibular (cold water caloric) stimulation, and the **motor response to pain**. Examination of the comatose patient is discussed at length in Chapter 3, Coma.

▶ "Screening" Neurologic Examination

1. **Mental status**—Observe whether the patient is awake and alert, confused, or unarousable. Test for orientation to person, place, and time. Screen for aphasia by asking the patient to repeat "no ifs, ands, or buts."

2. **Cranial nerves**—Examine the optic disks for papilledema. Test the visual fields by confrontation. Confirm the patient's ability to move the eyes conjugately in the six cardinal directions of gaze. Have the patient close the eyes tightly and show the teeth to assess facial strength.

3. **Motor function**—Compare the two sides with respect to speed of fine finger movements, strength of extensor muscles in the upper limb, and strength of flexor muscles in the lower limb, to detect corticospinal tract lesions.

4. **Sensory function**—Ask the patient to sketch out any area of perceived sensory deficit. Test light touch and vibration sense in the feet and, if impaired, determine the upper limit of impairment in both the lower and upper limbs.

5. **Reflexes**—Compare the two sides for activity of the biceps, triceps, quadriceps, and Achilles tendon reflexes, as well as the plantar responses.

6. **Coordination, stance, and gait**—Watch the patient stand and walk and note any asymmetry or instability of stance or gait.

DIAGNOSTIC FORMULATION

▶ Principles of Diagnosis

Once the history and examination are completed, evaluation of a neurologic problem proceeds with the formulation of a provisional diagnosis. This is divided into two stages: anatomic diagnosis and etiologic diagnosis. The diagnostic process should always be guided by the **law of parsimony**, or **Occam's razor**: the simplest explanation is most likely to be correct. This means that a single, unifying diagnosis should be sought in preference to multiple diagnoses, each accounting for a different feature of the patient's problem.

▶ Anatomic Diagnosis: Where Is the Lesion?

Anatomic diagnosis takes advantage of neuroanatomic principles to localize a lesion in space. The precision with which localization can be achieved varies, but it should always be possible at least to state the highest and lowest levels of the nervous system at which a lesion could produce the clinical picture under consideration.

A. Central versus Peripheral Nervous System

Making this distinction is typically the first step in anatomic diagnosis. Many symptoms and signs can be produced by both central and peripheral processes, but some symptoms and signs are more definitive. For example, cognitive abnormalities, visual field deficits, hyperreflexia, or extensor plantar responses (Babinski signs) point to the central nervous system, whereas muscle atrophy, fasciculation, or areflexia usually results from peripheral nervous system disorders.

B. Valsalva Doctrine

Unilateral brain lesions typically produce symptoms and signs on the opposite (contralateral) side of the body. This doctrine helps localize most focal cerebral lesions. However, exceptions occur. For example, hemispheric mass lesions that cause transtentorial herniation may compress the contralateral cerebral peduncle in the midbrain, producing hemiparesis on the same side as the mass. Brainstem lesions can produce crossed deficits, with weakness or sensory loss over the ipsilateral face and contralateral limbs. Thus, a unilateral lesion in the pons can cause ipsilateral facial weakness due to involvement of the facial (VII) nerve nucleus, with contralateral weakness of the arm and leg from involvement of descending motor pathways above their crossing (decussation) in the medulla. Wallenberg syndrome, usually due to a stroke in the lateral medulla, is associated with ipsilateral impairment of pain and temperature sensation over the face due to involvement of the descending tract and nucleus of the trigeminal (V) nerve, with contralateral pain and temperature deficits in the limbs from interruption of the lateral spinothalamic tract. Lesions of a cerebellar hemisphere produce ipsilateral symptoms and signs (eg, limb ataxia), due partly to connections with the contralateral cerebral cortex. Finally, the spinal accessory (XI) nerve receives bilateral input from motor cortex, with ipsilateral input predominating, so a cortical lesion can produce ipsilateral sternocleidomastoid muscle weakness.

C. Anatomic Patterns of Involvement

Anatomic diagnosis of neurologic lesions can be facilitated by recognizing patterns of involvement characteristic of disease at different sites (**Figure 1-26**). **Hemispheric lesions** are suggested by contralateral motor and sensory deficits affecting face, arm, and leg, as well as by cognitive or visual field abnormalities. **Brainstem lesions** should be suspected with crossed deficits (motor or sensory involvement of the face on one side of the body and the arm and leg on the other) or cranial nerve (eg, ocular) palsies. **Spinal cord lesions** produce deficits below the level of the lesion and, except for high cervical cord lesions affecting the spinal tract and nucleus of the trigeminal (V) nerve, spare the face. The relative involvement of upper motor neurons, lower motor neurons, and various sensory pathways depends on the site and extent of the spinal lesion in the horizontal plane. **Polyneuropathies** produce distal, symmetric sensory deficits and weakness, which usually affect the lower more than the upper limbs, and are associated with areflexia. **Myopathies** (disorders of muscle) produce proximal weakness, which may affect the face and trunk as well as the limbs, without sensory loss.

▶ Etiologic Diagnosis: What Is the Lesion?

A. Revisit the History

Once an anatomic diagnosis is reached, the next step is to identify the cause. Often the patient's prior history contains

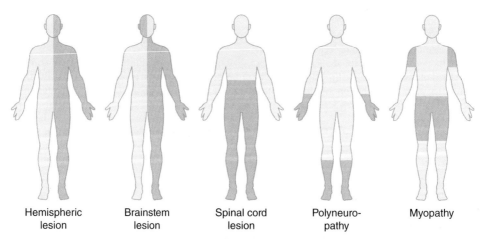

Hemispheric lesion	Brainstem lesion	Spinal cord lesion	Polyneuro-pathy	Myopathy

▲ **Figure 1-26.** Anatomic patterns of involvement (blue) resulting from disorders affecting different sites in the nervous system.

Table 1-3. Etiologic Categories of Neurologic Disease.

Etiologic Category	Examples
Degenerative	Alzheimer disease, Huntington disease, Parkinson disease, amyotrophic lateral sclerosis
Developmental or genetic	Muscular dystrophies, Arnold–Chiari malformation, syringomyelia
Immune	Multiple sclerosis, Guillain–Barré syndrome, myasthenia gravis
Infectious	Bacterial meningitis, brain abscess, viral encephalitis, HIV-associated dementia, neurosyphilis
Metabolic	Hypo/hyperglycemic coma, diabetic neuropathies, hepatic encephalopathy
Neoplastic	Glioma, metastatic carcinoma, lymphoma, paraneoplastic syndromes
Nutritional	Wernicke encephalopathy (vitamin B_1), combined systems disease (vitamin B_{12})
Toxic	Alcohol-related syndromes, intoxication with recreational drugs, side effects of prescription drugs
Traumatic	Sub/epidural hematoma, entrapment neuropathies
Vascular	Ischemic stroke, intracerebral hemorrhage, subarachnoid hemorrhage

clues. Preexisting diseases such as hypertension, diabetes, heart disease, cancer, and AIDS are each associated with a spectrum of neurologic complications. Numerous medications and drugs of abuse (eg, alcohol) have neurologic side effects. The family history may point to a genetic disease.

B. Consider General Categories of Disease

Neurologic disease can be produced by the same kinds of pathologic processes that cause disease in other organ systems (**Table 1-3**). Once a neurologic problem has been

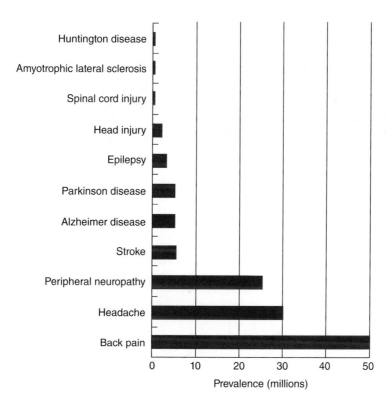

▲ **Figure 1-27.** Prevalence of selected neurologic disorders (US). (Data from Ropper A, Samuels M. *Adams and Victor's Neurology*. 9th ed. New York, NY: McGraw-Hill; 2009.)

localized, these categories can be used to generate a list of possible etiologies.

C. Time Course Is a Clue to Etiology

The time course of a disorder is an important clue to its etiology (see Figure 1-1). For example, only a few processes produce neurologic symptoms that evolve within minutes—typically ischemia, seizure, or syncope. Neoplastic and degenerative processes, by contrast, give rise to progressive, unremitting symptoms and signs, whereas inflammatory and metabolic disorders may wax and wane.

D. Common Diseases Are Common

Sometimes the anatomic syndrome is sufficiently distinctive that the cause is obvious. More often, however, an anatomic syndrome can have multiple etiologies. When this is the case, it is important to remember that common diseases are common and that even unusual presentations of common diseases occur more frequently than classic presentations of rare diseases. **Figure 1-27** illustrates the relative prevalence of several neurologic diseases. It is helpful to appreciate how common different diseases are and whether they affect particular populations (ie, ages, sexes, or ethnic groups) disproportionately. For example, multiple sclerosis usually has its onset between the ages of 20 and 40 years, affects women more often than men, and preferentially affects individuals of north European descent.

LABORATORY INVESTIGATIONS

After the history is taken, the general physical and neurologic examinations are completed, and a preliminary diagnosis is formulated, laboratory investigations are often undertaken to obtain additional diagnostic information. These investigations are addressed in Chapter 2, Investigative Studies.

Investigative Studies

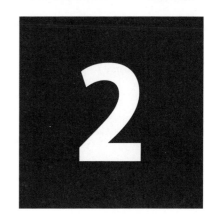

2

(Continued on Next Page)

LUMBAR PUNCTURE

INDICATIONS

1. Diagnosis of meningitis, other infective or inflammatory disorders, subarachnoid hemorrhage, hepatic encephalopathy, meningeal malignancies, paraneoplastic disorders, or suspected intracranial pressure abnormalities.
2. Assessment of therapeutic response in meningitis, infective or inflammatory disorders.
3. Administration of intrathecal medications or radiologic contrast media.
4. Rarely, to reduce cerebrospinal fluid (CSF) pressure.
5. In specialized centers, assessment of biomarkers of certain degenerative diseases, especially Creutzfeldt-Jakob disease and Alzheimer disease, and of narcolepsy.

CONTRAINDICATIONS

1. **Suspected intracranial mass lesion**—Lumbar puncture can hasten incipient transtentorial herniation.
2. **Local infection** over site of puncture. Use cervical or cisternal puncture instead.
3. **Coagulopathy**—Correct clotting-factor deficiencies and thrombocytopenia (platelet count below 50,000/μL or rapidly falling) before lumbar puncture to reduce risk of hemorrhage.
4. **Suspected spinal cord mass lesion**—In this case, remove only a small quantity of CSF to avoid creating a pressure differential above and below the block, which can increase spinal cord compression.

PREPARATION

A. Personnel

With a cooperative patient, one person can perform lumbar puncture. An assistant may be helpful in patient positioning and sample handling especially if the patient is uncooperative or frightened.

B. Equipment and Supplies

The following are usually included in preassembled trays and must be sterile:

1. Gloves
2. Iodine-containing solution for sterilizing the skin
3. Sponges
4. Drapes
5. Lidocaine (1%)
6. Syringe (5 mL)
7. Needles (22- and 25-gauge)
8. Spinal needles (preferably 22-gauge) with stylets
9. Three-way stopcock
10. Manometer
11. Collection tubes
12. Adhesive bandage

C. Positioning

The lateral decubitus position is usually used (**Figure 2-1**) with the patient lying at the edge of the bed facing away from the clinician. Have the patient maximally flex the

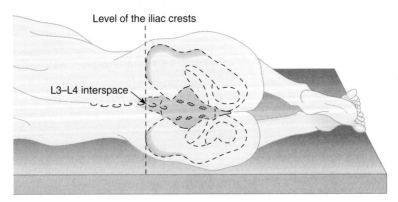

Level of the iliac crests

L3–L4 interspace

▲ **Figure 2-1.** Lateral decubitus position for lumbar puncture.

lumbar spine to open the intervertebral spaces with the spine parallel to the bed surface and hips and shoulders aligned in the vertical plane.

When a seated position is necessary, have the patient sit on the side of the bed, bent over a pillow on a bedside table, and reach over the bed from the opposite side to perform the procedure.

D. Site of Puncture

Most often, puncture is at the L3-L4 (level of posterior iliac crests) or L4-L5 vertebral interspace because the spinal cord (conus medullaris) terminates just above, approximately at L1-L2, in adults. Thus, with puncture below that level, there is no danger of puncturing the cord.

PROCEDURE

1. For blood and CSF glucose level comparison, draw venous blood for glucose determination. Ideally, obtain simultaneous blood and CSF samples after the patient has fasted for at least 4 hours.

2. Place necessary equipment and supplies in easy reach.

3. Wear a mask and sterile gloves.

4. Apply iodine-containing solution to sponges and wipe a wide area surrounding the interspace. Next, wipe the solution off with clean sponges.

5. Drape the area surrounding the sterile field.

6. Anesthetize the skin overlying the puncture site with lidocaine using a 5-mL syringe and a 25-gauge needle. Next, anesthetize the underlying tissues with lidocaine using a 22-gauge needle.

7. With the stylet in place, insert the spinal needle at the midpoint of the interspace. Keep the needle parallel to the bed surface and angled slightly cephalad, or toward the umbilicus. Keep the needle bevel facing upward toward the face of the person performing the procedure.

8. Advance the needle slowly until feeling a pop from penetration of the ligamentum flavum. Withdraw the stylet to check for flow of CSF through the needle, which indicates entry into the CSF space. If no CSF appears, replace the stylet and advance the needle a short distance, continuing until CSF is present. If the needle cannot be advanced, it is likely that bone is in the way. Withdraw the needle partway, keeping it parallel to the surface of the bed, and advance it again at a slightly different angle.

9. After CSF is obtained, reinsert the stylet. Ask the patient to straighten the legs, and attach the stopcock and manometer to the needle. Turn the stopcock to allow CSF to flow into the manometer, and measure opening pressure. Pressure should fluctuate with the phases of respiration.

10. Turn the stopcock to allow CSF collection and note the appearance (clarity and color) of the fluid. Obtain as much fluid in as many tubes as needed for the tests that have been ordered. Typically, collect 1 to 2 mL in each of five tubes for cell count, glucose and protein determination, measurement of the CSF/serum albumin ratio (test of the blood-brain barrier) and IgG index (to exclude neuroinflammatory disorders), the Venereal Disease Research Laboratory (VDRL) test for syphilis, Gram stain, and cultures. Additional specimens may be collected for other tests, such as cryptococcal antigen, other fungal and bacterial antibody studies, polymerase chain reaction for herpes simplex virus and other viruses, oligoclonal bands (when CNS inflammation is a consideration), glutamine (if hepatic encephalopathy is suspected), biomarkers of Creutzfeldt-Jakob disease (increased 14-3-3 protein level) and Alzheimer disease (low $A\beta42$ and high total or phosphorylated tau), hypocretin (very low or absent in narcolepsy with cataplexy), and cytologic study. If the CSF appears bloody, obtain additional fluid so that the cell count can be repeated on the specimen in the last tube collected. Cytologic studies require at least 10 mL of CSF.

11. Replace the stopcock and manometer and record closing pressure.

12. Withdraw the needle and apply an adhesive bandage over the puncture site.

13. Previously, patients were instructed to lie prone or supine for 1 or 2 hours after the procedure to reduce the risk of post-lumbar puncture headache. Current evidence suggests this is unnecessary.

COMPLICATIONS

A. Unsuccessful Tap

Several conditions such as marked obesity, degenerative disease of the spine, previous spinal surgery, recent lumbar puncture, and dehydration can make lumbar puncture difficult to perform. When puncture in the lateral decubitus position is impossible, attempt the procedure with the patient in a sitting position. If the tap is again unsuccessful, have an experienced neurologist or neuroradiologist use an oblique approach, image guidance, or perform lateral cervical or cisternal puncture under image guidance.

B. Arterial or Venous Puncture

If the needle enters a blood vessel rather than the spinal subarachnoid space, withdraw the needle and use a new needle to attempt the tap at a different level. In patients with coagulopathy or taking aspirin or anticoagulants, observe carefully for signs of spinal cord compression (see Chapter 9, Motor Disorders) from spinal subdural or epidural hematoma.

C. Post-Lumbar Puncture Headache

After lumbar puncture, patients may have a mild headache that is worse in the upright position but relieved by recumbency. This will usually resolve spontaneously over hours to days. The frequency of this complication is directly related to the size of the spinal needle, but not to the volume of fluid removed. Vigorous hydration or bed-rest for 1 or 2 hours after the procedure does not reduce the likelihood of headache. The headache usually responds to nonsteroidal anti-inflammatory drugs (NSAIDs) or caf-feine (see Chapter 6, Headache & Facial Pain). Severe and protracted headache can be treated by an autologous blood clot patch, applied by experienced personnel. The use of an atraumatic spinal needle reduces the incidence of post-lumbar puncture headache.

ANALYSIS OF RESULTS

A. Appearance

Note the clarity and color of the CSF as it leaves the spinal needle and any changes in its appearance during the course of the procedure. CSF is normally clear and colorless. It may appear cloudy or turbid with white blood cell counts that exceed approximately 200/μL, but counts as low as about 50/μL may cause light scattering by the suspended cells (Tyndall effect) when the tube is held up to direct sunlight. Color can be imparted to the CSF by hemoglobin (pink), bilirubin (yellow), or rarely, melanin (black).

B. Pressure

With adults in the lateral decubitus position, lumbar CSF pressure is normally between 60 and 180 to 200 mm water. In children, the 90th percentile for opening pressure is 280 mm water. When lumbar puncture is performed with patients seated, they should assume a lateral decubitus posture before CSF pressure is measured. Increased CSF pressure may result from obesity, agitation, or increased intra-abdominal pressure related to position (which may be eliminated by having the patient extend the legs and straighten the back before the opening pressure is recorded). Pathologic conditions associated with the increased CSF pressure include intracranial mass lesions, meningoencephalitis, subarachnoid hemorrhage, and pseudotumor cerebri.

C. Microscopic Examination

This may be undertaken by the person who performed the lumbar puncture or in the clinical laboratory; it always includes a total and differential cell count. Gram stain for bacteria, acid-fast stain for mycobacteria, and cytologic examination for tumor cells may also be indicated. The CSF normally contains up to five mononuclear leukocytes (lymphocytes or monocytes) per microliter, no polymor-phonuclear cells, and no erythrocytes unless the lumbar puncture is traumatic. Normal CSF is sterile, so that in the absence of central nervous system (CNS) infection, no organisms are observed with the above stains.

Table 2-1. Pigmentation of the CSF After Subarach-noid Hemorrhage.

	Appearance	Maximum	Disappearance
Oxyhemoglobin (pink)	0.5-4 hours	24-35 hours	7-10 days
Bilirubin (yellow)	8-12 hours	2-4 days	2-3 weeks

D. Bloody CSF

It is crucial to distinguish between CNS hemorrhage and a traumatic tap. If the blood clears as more fluid is with-drawn, a traumatic tap is likely. This can be confirmed by comparing red cell counts in the first and last tubes of CSF obtained; a marked decrease supports a traumatic tap.

The specimen should also be centrifuged promptly and the supernatant examined. With a traumatic lumbar punc-ture, the supernatant is colorless. In contrast, after CNS hemorrhage, enzymatic degradation of hemoglobin to bili-rubin renders the supernatant yellow (xanthochromic). Xanthochromia may be subtle. Visual inspection requires comparison with a colorless standard (a tube of water) and is best assessed by spectrophotometric quantitation of bilirubin.

Table 2-1 outlines the time course of changes in CSF color after subarachnoid hemorrhage. Blood in the CSF after a traumatic lumbar puncture usually clears within 24 hours and does not clot, whereas after subarachnoid hemorrhage it usually persists for at least 6 days and clot-ting may occur. Crenation (shriveling) of red blood cells is of no diagnostic value. In addition to breakdown of hemo-globin from red blood cells, other causes of CSF xantho-chromia include jaundice with serum bilirubin levels above 4 to 6 mg/dL, CSF protein concentrations exceeding 150 mg/dL, and rarely, the presence of carotene pigments.

White blood cells seen in the CSF early after subarach-noid hemorrhage or with traumatic lumbar puncture result from leakage of circulating whole blood. If the hematocrit and peripheral white blood cell count are within normal limits, there is approximately one white blood cell for every 1,000 red blood cells. If the peripheral white cell count is elevated, this ratio increases proportion-ately. In addition, for every 1,000 red blood cells present in the CSF, the CSF protein concentration increases by approximately 1 mg/dL.

PROCEDURE NOTES

A note describing the lumbar puncture should be recorded in the patient's chart and include:

1. Date and time performed.
2. Name of person or persons performing the procedure.

3. Indication.

4. Position of patient.

5. Anesthetic used.

6. Interspace entered.

7. Opening pressure.

8. Appearance of CSF, including changes in appearance during the procedure.

9. Amount of fluid removed.

10. Closing pressure.

11. Tests ordered; for example: Tube 1 (1 mL), cell count; tube 2 (1 mL), glucose and protein levels; tube 3 (1 mL), microbiologic stains; tube 4 (1 mL), bacterial, fungal, and mycobacterial cultures.

12. Results of any studies, such as microbiologic stains, performed by the operator.

13. Complications, if any.

ELECTROPHYSIOLOGIC STUDIES

ELECTROENCEPHALOGRAPHY

Electrodes placed on the scalp record the electrical activity of the brain. Electroencephalography (EEG) is easy to perform, relatively inexpensive, and helpful in several different clinical contexts (**Figure 2-2**).

EVALUATION OF SUSPECTED EPILEPSY

The EEG is useful in evaluating patients with suspected epilepsy. The presence of electrographic seizure activity (abnormal, rhythmic electrocerebral activity of abrupt onset and termination and showing an evolving pattern) during a behavioral disturbance of uncertain nature establishes the diagnosis beyond doubt. It is often not possible to obtain an EEG during a seizure, because these

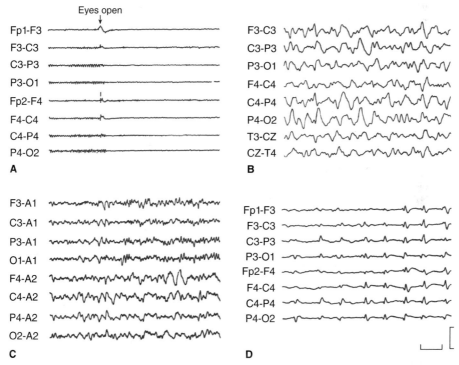

▲ **Figure 2-2.** (**A**) Normal EEG with a posteriorly situated 9-Hz alpha rhythm that attenuates with eye opening. (**B**) Abnormal EEG showing irregular diffuse slow activity in an obtunded patient with encephalitis. (**C**) Irregular slow activity in the right central region, on a diffusely slowed background, in a patient with a right parietal glioma. (**D**) Periodic complexes occurring once every second in a patient with Creutzfeldt-Jakob disease. Horizontal calibration: 1 s; vertical calibration: 200 µV in A, 300 µV in other panels. (Used with permission from Aminoff MJ, ed. *Aminoff's Electrodiagnosis in Clinical Neurology.* 6th ed. Oxford: Elsevier; 2012. Copyright © Elsevier.) Electrode placements are indicated at the left of each panel and are as follows. A, earlobe; C, central; F, frontal; Fp, frontal polar; P, parietal; T, temporal; O, occipital. Right-sided placements are indicated by even numbers, left-sided placements by odd numbers, and midline placements by Z.

occur unpredictably. However, the EEG may be abnormal interictally (at times when the patient is not experiencing clinical attacks) and is therefore still useful diagnostically. The interictal presence of epileptiform activity (abnormal paroxysmal activity containing some spike discharges) is helpful. Such activity occurs occasionally in patients who have never had a seizure, but its prevalence is greater in patients with epilepsy than in normal subjects. Epileptiform activity in the EEG of a patient with episodic behavioral disturbances that could represent seizures on clinical grounds markedly increases the likelihood that attacks are indeed epileptic, thus supporting the clinical diagnosis.

CLASSIFICATION OF SEIZURE DISORDERS

The EEG findings may help in classifying a seizure disorder and thus in selecting appropriate anticonvulsant medication. For example, in patients with the typical absence of petit mal epilepsy (see Chapter 12, Seizures & Syncope), the EEG is characterized both ictally and interictally by episodic generalized spike-wave activity (see Figure 12-3). By contrast, with episodes of impaired external awareness caused by focal seizures, it may be normal or show focal epileptiform discharges interictally. During seizures, abnormal rhythmic activity of variable frequency may occur with a localized or generalized distribution, but sometimes there are no electrographic correlates. A focal or lateralized epileptogenic source is of particular importance if surgical treatment is under consideration.

ASSESSMENT & PROGNOSIS OF SEIZURES

The EEG may guide prognosis and has been used to follow the course of seizure disorders. A normal EEG implies a more favorable prognosis for seizure control, whereas an abnormal background or profuse epileptiform activity implies a poor prognosis. The EEG findings do not, however, provide a reliable guide to the subsequent development of seizures in patients with head injuries, stroke, or brain tumors. EEG findings are sometimes used to determine whether anticonvulsant medication can be discontinued in patients after a seizure-free interval of several years. Although patients with a normal EEG are more likely to be weaned successfully, such findings provide only a general guide, and patients with a normal EEG can have further seizures after withdrawal of antiepileptic medication. Conversely, no further seizures may occur despite a continuing EEG disturbance.

MANAGEMENT OF STATUS EPILEPTICUS

The EEG is of little help in managing tonic–clonic status epilepticus unless patients have received neuromuscular blocking agents and are in a coma induced by medication. The EEG is then useful in indicating the level of anesthesia and determining whether seizures are continuing. Status is characterized by repeated electrographic seizures or continuous epileptiform (spike-wave) activity. Nonconvulsive status may follow control of convulsive status.

In nonconvulsive status epilepticus, the EEG findings provide the only means of making the diagnosis with confidence and in distinguishing the two main types. In absence status epilepticus, continuous spike-wave activity is seen, whereas in focal status, repetitive electrographic seizures are found.

DIAGNOSIS OF OTHER NEUROLOGIC DISORDERS

Certain neurologic disorders produce characteristic but nonspecific EEG abnormalities that help in suggesting, establishing, or supporting the diagnosis. In patients with an acute disturbance of cerebral function, for example, repetitive slow-wave complexes over one or both temporal lobes suggest a diagnosis of herpes simplex encephalitis. Similarly, the presence of periodic complexes in a patient with an acute dementing disorder suggests Creutzfeldt-Jakob disease, subacute sclerosing panencephalitis, or toxicity from lithium, baclofen, or bismuth.

EVALUATION OF ALTERED CONSCIOUSNESS

The EEG slows as consciousness is depressed, depending in part on the underlying etiology. The presence of electrographic seizure activity suggests diagnostic possibilities (eg, nonconvulsive status epilepticus) that might otherwise be overlooked. Serial records permit the prognosis and course to be followed. The EEG response to external stimulation is an important diagnostic and prognostic guide: Electrocerebral responsiveness implies a lighter level of coma. Electrocerebral silence in a technically adequate record implies neocortical death in the absence of hypothermia or drug overdose. In some seemingly comatose patients, consciousness is, in fact, preserved. Although there is quadriplegia and a supranuclear paralysis of the facial and bulbar muscles, the EEG is usually normal and helps in indicating the diagnosis of locked-in syndrome.

MAGNETOENCEPHALOGRAPHY

The magnetic field of electrocerebral activity can be recorded with specialized equipment. The magnetoencephalogram (MEG) is more sensitive than the EEG to activity arising in the cortical sulci, whereas the EEG best detects activity arising at the cortical surface. The MEG has better spatial resolution and can localize activity with more accuracy than the EEG. It is used for localizing abnormal cerebral activity in epilepsy and in localizing the central fissure preoperatively in patients with epilepsy or brain tumors when surgery is planned.

EVOKED POTENTIALS

Noninvasive stimulation of certain afferent pathways elicits spinal or cerebral potentials, which can be used to monitor the functional integrity of these pathways but do not indicate the cause of any lesion involving them. The responses are very small compared with the background EEG activity (noise), which has no relationship to the time of stimulation. The responses to a number of stimuli are therefore recorded and averaged with a computer to eliminate the random noise.

TYPES OF EVOKED POTENTIALS

A. Visual

Monocular visual stimulation with a checkerboard pattern elicits visual evoked potentials, which are recorded from the midoccipital region of the scalp. The most clinically relevant component is the P100 response, a positive peak with a latency of approximately 100 ms. The presence and latency of the response are noted. Although its amplitude can also be measured, alterations in amplitude are far less helpful in recognizing pathology.

B. Auditory

Monaural stimulation with repetitive clicks elicits brainstem auditory evoked potentials, which are recorded at the vertex of the scalp. A series of potentials are evoked in the first 10 ms after the auditory stimulus; these represent the sequential activation of various structures in the subcortical auditory pathway. For clinical purposes, attention is directed at the presence, latency, and interpeak intervals of the first five positive potentials.

C. Somatosensory

Electrical stimulation of a peripheral nerve is used to elicit somatosensory evoked potentials, which are recorded over the scalp and spine. Their configuration and latency depend on the nerve that is stimulated.

INDICATIONS FOR USE

A. Detection of Lesions in Multiple Sclerosis

Evoked potentials can detect and localize lesions in the CNS. This is particularly important in multiple sclerosis, where the diagnosis depends on detecting multifocal CNS lesions. When patients have clinical evidence of only a single lesion, electrophysiologic recognition of abnormalities in other sites helps to establish the diagnosis. When patients with suspected multiple sclerosis present with ill-defined complaints, electrophysiologic abnormalities in the appropriate afferent pathways indicate the organic basis of the symptoms. Although magnetic resonance imaging (MRI) is more useful for detecting lesions, it complements evoked potential studies rather than substituting for them. Evoked potential studies monitor the function rather than anatomic integrity of the afferent pathways and can sometimes reveal abnormalities not detected by MRI (and the reverse also holds true). They also cost less than MRI. In patients with established multiple sclerosis, the evoked

potential findings are sometimes used to follow the course of the disorder or its response to treatment, but their value in this regard is unclear.

B. Detection of Lesions in Other CNS Disorders

Evoked potential abnormalities occur in disorders other than multiple sclerosis; multimodal evoked potential abnormalities may be encountered in certain spinocerebellar degenerations, familial spastic paraplegia, Lyme disease, acquired immunodeficiency syndrome (AIDS), neurosyphilis, and vitamin E or B_{12} deficiency. Their diagnostic value therefore depends on the context in which they are found. Although the findings may permit lesions to be localized within broad areas of the CNS, precise localization may not be possible because the generators of many components are unknown.

C. Assessment and Prognosis After CNS Trauma or Hypoxia

In posttraumatic or postanoxic coma, bilateral absence of cortically generated components of the somatosensory evoked potential implies that cognition will not recover; the prognosis is more optimistic when cortical responses are present on one or both sides. Such studies may be particularly useful in patients with suspected brain death. Somatosensory evoked potentials have also been used to determine the completeness of a traumatic spinal cord lesion; the presence or early return of a response after stimulation of a nerve below the level of the cord injury indicates that the lesion is incomplete and thus suggests a better prognosis than otherwise.

D. Intraoperative Monitoring

The functional integrity of certain neural structures may be monitored by evoked potentials during operative procedures to permit the early recognition of any dysfunction and thereby minimize damage. When the dysfunction relates to a surgical maneuver, it may be possible to prevent or diminish any permanent neurologic deficit by reversing the maneuver.

E. Evaluation of Visual or Auditory Acuity

Visual and auditory acuity may be evaluated by evoked potential studies in patients unable to cooperate with behavioral testing because of age or abnormal mental state.

ELECTROMYOGRAPHY & NERVE CONDUCTION STUDIES

ELECTROMYOGRAPHY

The electrical activity within a discrete region of an accessible muscle can be recorded by inserting a needle electrode into it. The pattern of electrical activity in muscle (**electromyogram** or **EMG**) both at rest and during activity has been characterized, and abnormalities have been correlated with disorders at different levels of the motor unit.

A. Activity at Rest

Spontaneous electrical activity is not present in relaxed normal muscle except in the end-plate region where neuromuscular junctions are located, but various types of abnormal activity occur spontaneously in diseased muscle. **Fibrillation potentials** and **positive sharp waves** (which reflect muscle fiber irritability) are typically—but not always—found in denervated muscle. They are sometimes also found in myopathic disorders, especially inflammatory disorders such as polymyositis. Although **fasciculation potentials**, which reflect the spontaneous activation of individual motor units, are occasionally encountered in normal muscle, they are characteristic of neuropathic disorders, especially those with primary involvement of anterior horn cells (eg, amyotrophic lateral sclerosis). **Myotonic discharges** (high-frequency discharges of potentials from muscle fibers that wax and wane in amplitude and frequency) are found most commonly in disorders such as myotonic dystrophy or myotonia congenita and occasionally in polymyositis or other, rarer disorders. Other types of abnormal spontaneous activity also occur.

B. Activity During Voluntary Muscle Contraction

A slight voluntary contraction of a muscle activates a small number of motor units. The potentials generated by the muscle fibers of individual units within the detection range of the needle electrode can be recorded. Normal motor-unit potentials have clearly defined limits of duration, amplitude, configuration, and firing rates. These limits depend on the muscle under study. In many **myopathic disorders**, there is an increased incidence of small, short-duration, polyphasic motor units in affected muscles, and an excessive number of units may be activated for a specified degree of voluntary activity. In **neuropathic disorders**, motor units are lost; the number of units activated during a maximal contraction is therefore reduced, and units fire faster than normal. In addition, the configuration and dimensions of the potentials may be abnormal, depending on the acuteness of the neuropathic process and on whether reinnervation is occurring (**Figure 2-3**). Variations in the configuration and size of individual motor-unit potentials are characteristic of **disorders of neuromuscular transmission**.

C. Clinical Utility

Lesions can involve the neural or muscle component of the motor unit, or the neuromuscular junction. When the neural component is affected, the pathologic process can be at the level of the anterior horn cells or at some point along the length of the axon as it traverses a nerve root, limb

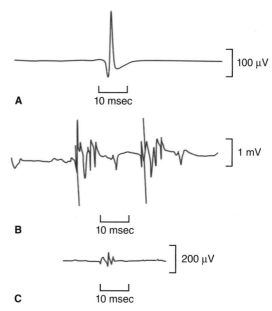

▲ **Figure 2-3.** Motor unit action potentials recorded with a concentric needle electrode. (**A**) Normal potential. (**B**) Long-duration polyphasic potential (shown twice). (**C**) Short-duration, low-amplitude polyphasic potential. (Used with permission from Aminoff MJ. *Electromyography in Clinical Practice.* 4th ed. New York, NY: Churchill Livingstone; 1998. Copyright © Elsevier.)

plexus, and peripheral nerve before branching into its terminal arborizations. Electromyography can detect disorders of the motor units and can indicate the site of the underlying lesion. Neuromuscular disorders can be recognized when clinical examination is unrewarding because the disease is mild or because poor cooperation by the patient or the presence of other symptoms such as pain makes clinical evaluation difficult. The electromyographic findings do not, of themselves, permit an etiologic diagnosis to be reached, and they must be correlated with the clinical findings and the results of other laboratory studies.

The electromyographic findings may provide a guide to prognosis. For example, in an acute disorder of a peripheral or cranial nerve, electromyographic evidence of denervation implies a poorer prognosis for recovery than otherwise.

In contrast to needle electromyography, the clinical utility of surface-recorded electromyography is not established.

NERVE CONDUCTION STUDIES

A. Motor Nerve Conduction Studies

The electrical response of a muscle is recorded to stimulation of its motor nerve at two or more points along its

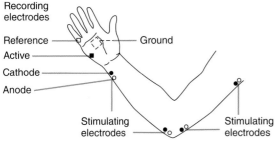

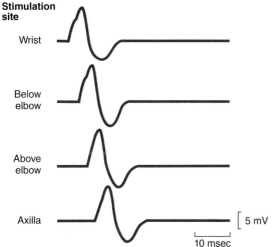

▲ **Figure 2-4.** Arrangement for motor conduction studies of the ulnar nerve. Responses of the abductor digiti minimi to supramaximal stimulation of the nerve at different sites are recorded with a surface electrode. (Used with permission from Aminoff MJ. *Electromyography in Clinical Practice*. 4th ed. New York, NY: Churchill Livingstone; 1998. Copyright © Elsevier.)

course (**Figure 2-4**). This permits conduction velocity to be determined in the fastest-conducting motor fibers between the points of stimulation.

B. Sensory Nerve Conduction Studies

The conduction velocity and amplitude of action potentials in sensory fibers can be determined when these fibers are stimulated at one point and their responses are recorded at another point along the course of the nerve.

C. Indications for Use

Nerve conduction studies can confirm the presence and extent of peripheral nerve damage. They are particularly helpful when clinical examination is difficult (eg, in children). Nerve conduction studies are useful in the following contexts:

1. Determining whether sensory symptoms are caused by a lesion proximal or distal to the dorsal root ganglia (in the latter case, sensory conduction studies of the involved fibers will be abnormal) and whether neuromuscular dysfunction is due to peripheral nerve disease.

2. Detecting subclinical involvement of other peripheral nerves in patients with a mononeuropathy.

3. Determining the site of a focal lesion and providing a guide to prognosis in patients with a mononeuropathy.

4. Distinguishing between a polyneuropathy and a mononeuropathy multiplex. This is important because the causes of these conditions differ.

5. Clarifying the extent to which disabilities in patients with polyneuropathy relate to superimposed compressive focal neuropathies, which are common complications.

6. Following the progression of peripheral nerve disorders and their response to treatment.

7. Indicating the predominant pathologic change in peripheral nerve disorders. In demyelinating neuropathies, conduction velocity is often markedly slowed and conduction block may occur; in axonal neuropathies, conduction velocity is usually normal or slowed only mildly, sensory nerve action potentials are small or absent, and electromyography shows evidence of denervation in affected muscles.

8. Detecting subclinical hereditary disorders of the peripheral nerves in genetic and epidemiologic studies.

F-RESPONSE STUDIES

Stimulation of a motor nerve causes impulses to travel **antidromically** (toward the spinal cord) as well as **orthodromically** (toward the nerve terminals) and leads a few anterior horn cells to discharge. This produces a small motor response (the F wave) considerably later than the direct muscle response elicited by nerve stimulation. The F wave is sometimes abnormal with lesions of the proximal portions of the peripheral nervous system, such as the nerve roots. F-wave studies may be helpful in detecting abnormalities when conventional nerve conduction studies are normal.

REPETITIVE NERVE STIMULATION

DESCRIPTION

The size of the electrical response of a muscle to supramaximal electrical stimulation of its motor nerve correlates with the number of activated muscle fibers. Neuromuscular transmission is tested by recording (with surface electrodes) the response of a muscle to supramaximal stimulation of its motor nerve either repetitively or by single shocks or trains of shocks at selected intervals after a maximal voluntary contraction.

NORMAL RESPONSE

In normal subjects, little or no change occurs in the size of the compound muscle action potential after repetitive stimulation of a motor nerve at 10 Hz or less or with a single stimulus or a train of stimuli delivered at intervals after a 10-second voluntary muscle contraction. Preceding activity in the junctional region influences the amount of acetylcholine released and thus the size of the end-plate potentials elicited by the stimuli. Although the amount of acetylcholine released is increased briefly after maximal voluntary activity and is then reduced, more acetylcholine is normally released than necessary to bring the motor end-plate potentials to the threshold for generating muscle-fiber action potentials.

RESPONSE IN DISORDERS OF NEUROMUSCULAR TRANSMISSION

A. Myasthenia Gravis

In myasthenia gravis, the reduced release of acetylcholine that follows repetitive firing of the motor neuron prevents compensation for the depleted postsynaptic acetylcholine receptors at the neuromuscular junction. Accordingly, repetitive stimulation, particularly between 2 and 5 Hz, may lead to depressed neuromuscular transmission, with a **decrement** in the compound muscle action potential recorded from an affected muscle. Similarly, an electrical stimulus of the motor nerve immediately after a 10-second period of maximal voluntary activity may elicit a muscle response that is slightly larger than before, indicating that more muscle fibers are responding. This postactivation facilitation of neuromuscular transmission is followed by a longer depression that is maximal from 2 to 4 minutes after the conditioning period and lasts up to 10 minutes or so. During this period, the compound muscle action potential is reduced in size.

Decrementing responses to repetitive stimulation at 2 to 5 Hz can also occur in congenital myasthenic syndromes.

B. Myasthenic Syndrome and Botulism

In Lambert–Eaton myasthenic syndrome, defective release of acetylcholine at the neuromuscular junction leads to a very small compound muscle action potential elicited by a single stimulus. With repetitive stimulation at rates of up to 10 Hz, the first few responses may decline in size, but subsequent responses increase, and their amplitude is eventually several times larger than the initial response. Patients with botulism exhibit a similar response to repetitive stimulation but the findings are somewhat more variable, and not all muscles are affected. **Incremental responses** in Lambert–Eaton syndrome and botulism are more conspicuous with high rates of stimulation and may result from the facilitation of acetylcholine release by the progressive accumulation of calcium in the motor nerve terminal.

TESTS OF AUTONOMIC FUNCTION

Autonomic and small-fiber function tests evaluate the control of heart rate, blood pressure, and sweating. Both sympathetic and parasympathetic pathways are assessed. Five simple noninvasive tests of cardiovascular reflexes may be adequate for assessing diabetic (and presumably other) autonomic neuropathies: the heart rate responses to (1) the Valsalva maneuver, (2) standing, and (3) deep breathing; and the blood pressure responses to (4) standing and (5) sustained handgrip. Definite autonomic neuropathy is indicated by an abnormality in two or more tests. Sweating is tested separately. In the thermoregulatory sweat test, the patient is warmed with a radiant heat cradle to increase body temperature by 1°C while the skin is covered with a powder that changes color when moist. This permits the presence and distribution of sweating to be characterized. The sympathetic skin response, that is, the change in voltage at the skin surface following a single electrical stimulus, also can be recorded. This depends on the electrical activity arising from sweat glands and on the reduced electrical resistance of the skin following a noxious stimulus. Quantitative sudomotor axon reflex testing (QSART) assesses postganglionic sympathetic function quantitatively but requires sophisticated and expensive equipment.

POLYSOMNOGRAPHY

DESCRIPTION

The investigation of sleep disorders requires the recording during sleep and wakefulness of multiple physiologic variables, typically the EEG, submental EMG, eye movements, respiratory activity, nasal or oral airflow, oxygen saturation, and the electrocardiogram; a video recording is also made of the patient. Other variables, such as penile tumescence, may be measured depending on the reason for the study.

INDICATIONS FOR USE

1. Diagnosis of sleep-related breathing disorders and their response to various therapeutic maneuvers.
2. Evaluation and diagnosis of patients with suspected narcolepsy. Multiple sleep latency testing is also required, evaluates the time required to fall asleep, and consists of five nap opportunities at 2-hour intervals.
3. Evaluation of periodic limb movements of sleep.

4. Evaluation of insomnia or hypersomnia of uncertain cause.

5. Evaluation of sleep-related symptoms in patients with epilepsy or neuromuscular disorders.

6. Evaluation of organic causes of erectile dysfunction.

CRANIAL IMAGING STUDIES

COMPUTED TOMOGRAPHY

DESCRIPTION

Computed tomographic (**CT**) scanning is a noninvasive, computer-assisted, radiologic means of examining anatomic structures (**Figure 2-5**). It permits the detection of structural intracranial abnormalities with precision, speed, and facility. It is thus of particular use in evaluating patients with progressive neurologic disorders or focal neurologic deficits in whom a structural lesion is suspected, patients with dementia or increased intracranial pressure, and patients with suspected stroke or head injuries. Intravenous administration of an iodinated contrast agent improves the detection and definition of vascular lesions and those associated with a disturbance of the blood–brain barrier. Contrast-enhanced scans may provide more information than unenhanced scans in patients with known or suspected primary or secondary brain tumors, arteriovenous malformations (AVMs), aneurysms, cerebral abscesses, chronic isodense subdural hematomas, or infarctions. Because the contrast agents may affect the kidneys adversely, they should be used with discrimination. Other adverse effects of the contrast agents in common use are pain, nausea, thermal sensations, and anaphylactoid reactions that include bronchospasm and death.

INDICATIONS FOR USE

A. Stroke

CT scan can distinguish infarction from intracranial hemorrhage; it is particularly sensitive in detecting intracerebral hematomas (see Figure 13-20), the location of which may provide a guide to their cause. CT scan occasionally demonstrates a nonvascular cause of the patient's clinical deficit, such as a tumor or abscess.

B. Tumor

CT scans can indicate the site of a brain tumor, the extent of any surrounding edema, whether the lesion is cystic or

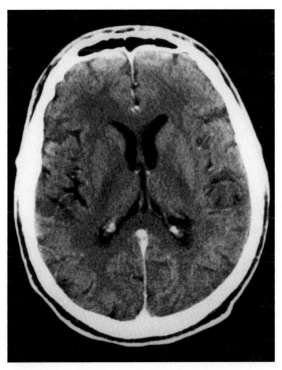
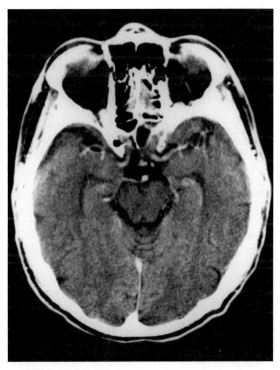

▲ **Figure 2-5.** Contrast-enhanced CT brain scans from a 62-year-old man, showing the normal anatomy. Images are at the level of the lateral ventricles (left) and midbrain (right) (same patient as in Figure 2-6).

solid, and whether it has displaced midline or other normal anatomic structures. It also demonstrates any acute hemorrhagic component.

C. Trauma

CT scans are important for detecting traumatic intracranial (epidural, subdural, subarachnoid, or intracerebral) hemorrhage and bony injuries. They also provide a more precise delineation of associated fractures than do plain x-rays.

D. Dementia

CT scanning may indicate the presence of a tumor or hydrocephalus (enlarged ventricles), with or without accompanying cerebral atrophy. The occurrence of hydrocephalus without cerebral atrophy in demented patients suggests normal pressure or communicating hydrocephalus. Cerebral atrophy can occur in demented or normal elderly subjects.

E. Subarachnoid Hemorrhage

In patients with subarachnoid hemorrhage, the CT scan generally indicates the presence of blood in the subarachnoid space and may even suggest the source of the bleeding (see Figure 6-5). If the CT scan findings are normal despite clinical findings suggestive of subarachnoid hemorrhage, the CSF should be examined to exclude hemorrhage or meningitis. CT angiography (see later) may demonstrate an underlying vascular malformation or aneurysm.

MAGNETIC RESONANCE IMAGING

DESCRIPTION

Magnetic resonance imaging (**MRI**) involves no ionizing radiation. The patient lies within a large magnet that aligns some of the protons in the body along the magnet's axis. The protons resonate when stimulated with radiofrequency energy, producing a tiny echo that is strong enough to be detected. The position and intensity of these radiofrequency emissions are recorded and mapped by a computer. The signal intensity depends on the concentration of mobile hydrogen nuclei (or nuclear-spin density) of the tissues. Spin–lattice (T1) and spin–spin (T2) relaxation times are mainly responsible for the relative differences in signal intensity of the various soft tissues; these parameters are sensitive to the state of water in biologic tissues. Pulse sequences with varying dependence on T1 and T2 selectively alter the contrast between soft tissues (**Figure 2-6**).

The soft-tissue contrast available with MRI makes it more sensitive than CT scanning in detecting certain structural lesions. MRI provides better contrast than CT scans between the gray and white matter of the brain. It is superior for visualizing abnormalities in the posterior fossa

and spinal cord, for subacute and chronic hemorrhage, and for detecting lesions associated with multiple sclerosis or those that cause seizures. In addition to its greater sensitivity, it is also free of bony artifact and permits multiplanar (axial, sagittal, and coronal) imaging with no need to manipulate the position of the patient. Because there are no known hazardous effects, MRI studies can be repeated in a serial manner if necessary. Occasional patients cannot tolerate the procedure without sedation because of claustrophobia.

Gadopentetate dimeglumine (gadolinium-DPTA) is an effective enhancing MRI contrast agent that is stable and well-tolerated intravenously. It is useful in identifying small tumors that, because of their similar relaxation times to normal cerebral tissue, may be missed on unenhanced MRI. It also helps to separate tumor from surrounding edema, identify leptomeningeal disease, and provide information about the blood–brain barrier. Gadolinium has been associated with nephrogenic systemic fibrosis in patients with renal insufficiency, so it should be used judiciously in this setting.

INDICATIONS FOR USE & COMPARISON WITH CT SCAN

A. Stroke

Within a few hours of vascular occlusion, cerebral infarcts may be detected by MRI. Breakdown in the blood–brain barrier (several hours after onset of cerebral ischemia) permits the intravascular content to be extravasated into the extracellular space. This can be detected by T2-weighted imaging and **fluid-attenuated inversion-recovery (FLAIR)** sequences. Diffusion-weighted MRI also has an important role in the early assessment of stroke, as is discussed later, whereas CT scans may be unrevealing for up to 48 hours. Thereafter, the advantage of MRI over CT scanning lessens, except that MRI detects smaller lesions and provides superior imaging of the posterior fossa.

Nevertheless, to determine quickly whether hemorrhage has occurred, CT scanning without contrast is usually the preferred initial study in acute stroke. Hematomas of more than 2 to 3 days' duration, however, are better visualized by MRI. Although MRI can detect and localize vascular malformations, angiography is necessary to define their anatomic features and plan effective treatment. In cases of unexplained hematoma, a follow-up MRI obtained 3 months later may reveal the underlying cause, which is sometimes unmasked as the hematoma resolves.

B. Tumor

Both CT scans and MRI are useful in detecting brain tumors. MRI is the preferred technique because of its greater soft tissue sensitivity, the absence of bone artifacts at the vertex or in the posterior fossa, and the ability to employ advanced imaging techniques such as MR

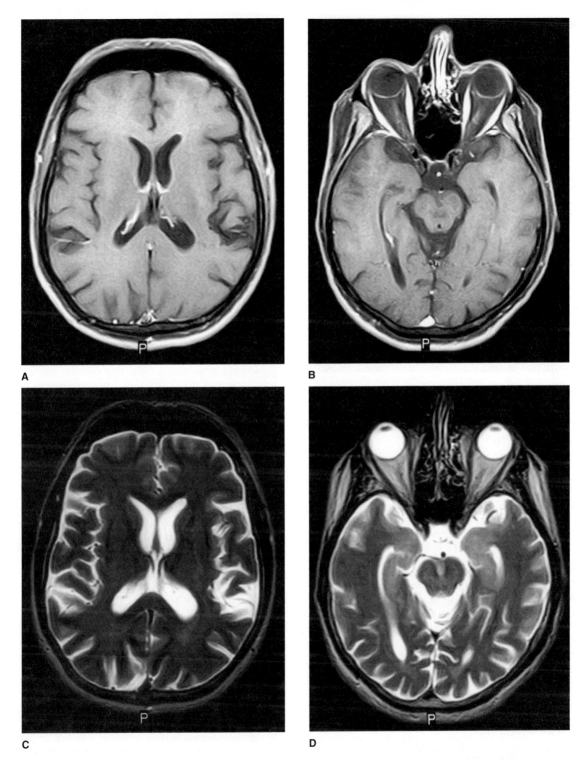

▲ **Figure 2-6.** Brain MR images from a 62-year-old man, showing the normal anatomy. (**A** and **B**) Gadolinium-enhanced T1-weighted (CSF dark) images; (**C** and **D**) T2-weighted (CSF white) images. Images are at the level of the lateral ventricles (**A** and **C**) and midbrain (**B** and **D**).

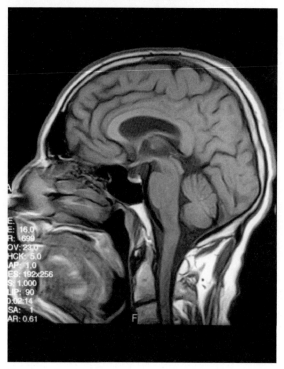

E

▲ **Figure 2-6.** (Continued) A midsagittal T1-weighted image is shown in (**E**). Brain images are from the same patient as in Figure 2-5.

spectroscopy and diffusion and perfusion imaging that better characterize a lesion. MRI or CT scan may detect secondary effects of tumors, such as cerebral herniation, but MRI provides more detailed and sensitive anatomic information. Neither technique, however, permits the type of a tumor to be determined with certainty.

C. Trauma

In the acute phase after head injury, CT scan is preferable to MRI because it requires less time, is superior for detecting intracranial hemorrhage, and may reveal bony injuries. Similarly, spinal MRI should not be used in the initial evaluation of patients with spinal injuries because nondisplaced fractures are often not visualized. For follow-up purposes, however, MRI is helpful for detecting parenchymal pathology of the brain or spinal cord.

D. Dementia

In patients with dementia, either CT scan or MRI can help in demonstrating treatable structural causes, but MRI is more sensitive in demonstrating abnormal white matter signal and associated atrophy.

E. Multiple Sclerosis

Lesions in the cerebral white matter or the cervical cord are best detected by MRI, as lesions may not be visualized on CT scans. The lesions on MRI may have signal characteristics resembling those of ischemic changes, however, and clinical correlation is therefore always necessary. Gadolinium-enhanced MRI permits lesions of different ages to be distinguished. This ability facilitates the diagnosis of multiple sclerosis: The presence of lesions of different ages suggests a multiphasic disease, whereas lesions of similar age suggest a monophasic disorder, such as acute disseminated encephalomyelitis.

F. Infections

MRI is sensitive in detecting white matter edema and probably permits earlier recognition of focal areas of cerebritis and abscess formation than CT scan. Diffusion MR imaging is particularly helpful in detecting areas of reduced diffusion, typical of purulent abscess and encephalitis.

CONTRAINDICATIONS

MRI is contraindicated by the presence of intracranial ferromagnetic aneurysm clips, metallic foreign bodies in the eye, demand-mode pacemakers, and cochlear implants. Many implanted devices are also contraindications for MRI. Patients requiring close monitoring are probably best studied by CT if possible. Furthermore, MRI is difficult in patients with claustrophobia, extreme obesity, uncontrolled movement disorders, or respiratory disorders that require assisted ventilation or carry any risk of apnea. Advances in MRI-compatible mechanical ventilators, pacemakers, and monitoring equipment, however, now allow many critically ill patients to be scanned safely.

DIFFUSION-WEIGHTED MAGNETIC RESONANCE IMAGING

This technique, in which contrast within the image is based on the microscopic motion of water protons in tissue, provides information that is not available on standard MRI or CT. It is particularly important in the assessment of stroke because it can discriminate cytotoxic edema (which occurs in strokes) from vasogenic edema (found with other types of cerebral lesion) and thus reveals cerebral ischemia early and with high specificity. Diffusion-weighted MRI permits reliable identification of acute cerebral ischemia during the first few hours after onset, before it is detectable on standard MRI. This is important because it reveals the true volume of infarcts prior to treatment with thrombolytic agents. However, because diffusion-weighted imaging will be positive in the setting of cytotoxic edema of any cause (eg, brain abscess, highly cellular tumors), clinical correlation is always required. When more than one infarct is found on routine MRI, diffusion-weighted imaging permits the discrimination of acute from older infarcts by the relative increase in signal intensity of the former.

DIFFUSION TENSOR MAGNETIC RESONANCE IMAGING

This technique produces neural tract images by measuring the diffusion of water in tissue. It is important in determining the severity and extent of cerebral involvement after head injury, localizing brain tumors, and planning surgical procedures. White matter changes may be detected that are not seen on conventional MRI.

PERFUSION-WEIGHTED MAGNETIC RESONANCE IMAGING

Blood flow through the brain may be measured using either an injected contrast medium (eg, gadolinium) or an endogenous technique (in which the patient's own blood provides the contrast). Cerebral blood-flow abnormalities can be recognized and the early reperfusion of tissues after treatment can be confirmed. Cerebral ischemia may be detected very soon after clinical onset. Comparison of the findings from diffusion-weighted and perfusion-weighted MRI may have a prognostic role and is currently under study. The distinction of reversible from irreversible ischemic damage is important in this regard. Perfusion-weighted imaging also contributes in distinguishing between various types of brain tumors such as gliomas and metastases.

POSITRON EMISSION TOMOGRAPHY

Positron emission tomography (PET) is an imaging technique that uses positron-emitting radiopharmaceuticals, such as ^{18}F-fluoro-2-deoxy-D-glucose or ^{18}F-L-dopa, to map brain biochemistry and physiology. PET thus complements other imaging methods that provide primarily anatomic information, such as CT scan and MRI, and may demonstrate functional brain abnormalities before structural abnormalities are detectable. PET has proved useful in several clinical settings and is now combined with CT or MR scanners in hybrid machines. When patients with medically refractory epilepsy are being considered for surgical treatment, PET CT scan can identify focal areas of hypometabolism in the temporal lobe as likely sites of the origin of seizures. PET can also be useful in the differential diagnosis of dementia, because common dementing disorders such as Alzheimer disease and frontotemporal dementia exhibit different patterns of abnormal cerebral metabolism. In vivo imaging of amyloid-β (Aβ) with PET facilitates the early diagnosis of Alzheimer disease and provides prognostic information for patients with mild cognitive impairment. PET can help distinguish between clinically similar movement disorders, such as Parkinson

disease and progressive supranuclear palsy, and can provide confirmatory evidence of early Huntington disease. It may also be of value in grading gliomas, selecting tumor biopsy sites, and distinguishing recurrent tumors from radiation-induced brain necrosis. It has been an important tool with which to investigate the functional involvement of different cerebral areas in behavioral and cognitive tasks and is used frequently in patients with suspected metastatic disease. However, PET is more expensive than MR or CT alone, requires administration of radioactive isotopes, and thus exposes subjects to radiation.

SINGLE-PHOTON EMISSION COMPUTED TOMOGRAPHY

In single-photon emission computed tomography (SPECT), chemicals containing isotopes that emit single photons are administered intravenously or by inhalation to image the brain. SPECT has been used, in particular, to measure perfusion, to investigate receptor distribution, and to detect areas of increased metabolism such as occurs with seizures.

A specific contrast agent (^{123}I ioflupane) used with SPECT detects dopamine transporters (DaT) and helps to distinguish parkinsonian syndromes from essential tremor when this is clinically difficult. A DaT scan is also used to confirm a diagnosis of Parkinson disease in patients with ambiguous symptoms.

FUNCTIONAL MAGNETIC RESONANCE IMAGING

Functional MRI (**fMRI**) involves pulse sequences that change in signal intensity in response to alterations in the oxygen concentration of venous blood (blood oxygen level–dependent [BOLD]-fMRI), which correlate with focal cerebral activity. Studies are performed with the subject at rest and then after an activation procedure so that the change in signal intensity reflects the effect of the activation procedure on local cerebral blood flow (**Figure 2-7**). Studies are also performed without a stimulus ("resting state fMRI") to interrogate the brain's functional organization. fMRI studies are indicated for preoperative functional mapping of sensorimotor and language areas in the evaluation of patients with brain tumors, as well as in some cases of epilepsy or vascular malformations.

MAGNETIC RESONANCE SPECTROSCOPY

Magnetic resonance spectroscopy provides information about the chemical composition of tissue. Proton magnetic resonance spectroscopy (^{1}H-MRS) can determine levels of N-acetylaspartate (exclusive to neurons) or choline, creatinine, and lactate (glia and neurons). Measurements of brain concentrations of these metabolites may be useful in detecting specific tissue loss in Alzheimer disease

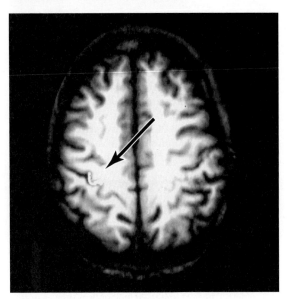

▲ **Figure 2-7.** A functional MR brain image obtained from a patient during rapid finger tapping of the left hand. An increase in relative blood flow in the region of the right motor strip is imaged (arrow) and superimposed on a T1-weighted MR scan. (Used with permission from Waxman SG. *Correlative Neuroanatomy.* 23rd ed. Norwalk, CT: Appleton & Lange; 1996. Copyright © McGraw-Hill.)

or other neurodegenerative disorders; in distinguishing brain tumors from non-neoplastic lesions such as abscesses and in classifying brain tumors; in identifying certain inborn errors of metabolism and leukodystrophies; in prognostication of hypoxic-ischemic brain injury; and in localizing the source of seizures in temporal lobe epilepsy. Phosphorus magnetic resonance spectroscopy (^{31}P-MRS) may be useful in the evaluation of metabolic muscle diseases.

ARTERIOGRAPHY

DESCRIPTION

The intracranial circulation is visualized most satisfactorily by arteriography, in which the major vessels to the head are opacified and radiographed after injection of contrast material through an arterial or venous catheter. Specifically, a catheter is introduced into the femoral or brachial artery and passed into one of the major cervical vessels. A radiopaque contrast material is then injected through the catheter, allowing the vessel (or its origin) to be visualized. Access to the cranial vessels with a catheter also allows for the delivery of certain therapies. The technique, generally performed after noninvasive imaging by CT scan or MRI, has a definite (approximately 1%)

morbidity and mortality associated with it and involves considerable exposure to radiation. It is contraindicated in patients who are allergic to the contrast medium. Stroke may result as a complication of arteriography. Moreover, after the procedure, bleeding may occur at the puncture site, and the catheterized artery (usually the femoral artery) may become occluded, leading to distal ischemic complications. The puncture site and the distal circulation must therefore be monitored.

INDICATIONS FOR USE

The major indications for cerebral arteriography are:

1. Diagnosis of **intracranial aneurysms, arteriovenous malformations (AVMs)**, or **fistulas**. Although these lesions can be visualized by CT scan or MRI, their detailed anatomy and the vessels that feed, drain, or are otherwise implicated in them cannot reliably be defined by these other means. Moreover, arteriography is required for interventional procedures such as embolization, the injection of occlusive polymers, or the placement of detachable balloons or coils to treat certain vascular anomalies.

2. Detection and definition of the underlying lesion in patients with **subarachnoid hemorrhage** who are considered good operative candidates (see Chapter 6, Headache & Facial Pain).

3. Detection and management of vasospasm after subarachnoid hemorrhage.

4. Emergency embolectomy in the setting of ischemic stroke due to large-vessel occlusion. In addition, arteriography can define vascular lesions in patients with **transient cerebral ischemic attacks** or **strokes** if surgical treatment such as carotid endarterectomy is being considered.

5. Evaluation of small vessels, when vasculitis is under consideration.

6. Diagnosis of cerebral **venous sinus thrombosis.**

7. Evaluation of **space-occupying intracranial lesions**, particularly when CT scanning or MRI is unavailable. There may be displacement of the normal vasculature, and in some tumors neovasculature may produce a blush or stain on the angiogram. Meningiomas are supplied from the external carotid circulation. Presurgical embolization of certain tumors reduces their blood supply and decreases the risk of major bleeding during resection.

MAGNETIC RESONANCE ANGIOGRAPHY

Several imaging techniques to visualize blood vessels by MRI depend on the physical properties of flowing blood, thereby allowing visualization of vasculature without the use of intravenous contrast. These properties include the rate at which blood is supplied to the imaged area, its velocity and relaxation time, and the absence of turbulent flow. Magnetic resonance (MR) angiography is a noninvasive technique that is cheaper and less risky than conventional angiography. It has been most useful in visualizing the carotid arteries and proximal portions of the intracranial circulation, where flow is relatively fast. The images are used to screen for stenosis or occlusion of vessels and for large atheromatous lesions. It has particular utility in screening for venous sinus occlusion. Resolution is inferior to that of conventional angiography, and occlusive disease may not be recognized in vessels with slow flow. Moreover, intracranial MR angiograms may be marred by saturation or susceptibility artifacts that result in irregular or discontinuous signal intensity in vessels close to bone. Although current techniques allow visualization of AVMs and aneurysms greater than 3 mm in diameter, conventional angiography remains the "gold standard." Finally, MR angiography may reveal dissection of major vessels: Narrowing is produced by the dissection, and cross-sectional images reveal the false lumen as a crescent of abnormal signal intensity next to the vascular flow void.

CT ANGIOGRAPHY

CT angiography is a minimally invasive procedure that requires a CT scanner capable of acquiring numerous thin, overlapping sections quickly after intravenous injection of a bolus of contrast material. Because the images are acquired within a matter of 5 to 10 seconds, CTA is less likely to be affected by patient movement than MR angiography. A wide range of vessels can be imaged with the technique.

CT angiography of the carotid bifurcation is being used increasingly in patients with suspected disease of the carotid arteries. It can also be used for intracranial imaging and can detect stenotic or aneurysmal lesions. However, sensitivity is reduced for aneurysms less than 3 mm, and the method cannot adequately define aneurysmal morphology in the preoperative evaluation of patients. It is sensitive in visualizing the anatomy in the circle of Willis, the vasculature of the anterior and posterior circulations, and intracranial vasoocclusive lesions, but it may not reveal plaque ulceration or disease of small vessels. It is a reliable alternative to MR angiography, but both techniques are less sensitive than conventional angiography.

In patients with acute stroke, CT angiography provides important information complementary to conventional CT scan studies, revealing the site and length of vascular occlusion and the contrast-enhanced arteries distal to the occlusion as a reflection of collateral blood flow. CT perfusion, in which the relative blood flow to an area of the brain is measured as iodinated contrast passes through over time, can provide additional information regarding the proportion of ischemic to infarcted tissue in this setting.

SPINAL IMAGING STUDIES

PLAIN X-RAYS

Plain x-rays of the spine can reveal congenital, traumatic, degenerative, or neoplastic bony abnormalities or narrowing (stenosis) of the spinal canal. Degenerative changes become increasingly common with advancing age, and their clinical relevance depends on the context in which they are found.

MYELOGRAPHY

Injecting iodinated contrast medium into the subarachnoid space permits visualization of part or all of the spinal subarachnoid system. The cord and nerve roots, which are silhouetted by the contrast material, are visualized indirectly. CSF leaks can be documented and localized. The procedure is relatively safe but carries the risk of headache, vasovagal reactions, persistent CSF leak, nausea, and vomiting. Rarely, confusion and seizures occur. Other rare complications include traumatically induced herniated intervertebral disks due to poor technique and damage to nerve roots.

The contrast agent is absorbed from the CSF and is excreted by the kidneys; approximately 75% is eliminated over the first 24 hours. While current water soluble agents do not cause arachnoiditis, tonic–clonic seizures have sometimes occurred when large amounts of contrast enter the intracranial cavity. Contrast myelography may be followed by a CT scan of the spine while the medium is still in place. This shows the soft tissue structures in or about the spinal cord and provides information complementary to that obtained by the myelogram (see later).

Myelography has largely been replaced by MRI and CT scanning but it is still sometimes performed, particularly in patients with spinal hardware precluding useful MRI studies and in those with suspected CSF fistula.

COMPUTED TOMOGRAPHY

CT scanning after myelography has become a routine procedure and is particularly helpful when the myelogram either fails to reveal any abnormality or provides poor visualization of the area of interest. The myelogram may be normal, for example, when there is a laterally placed disk protrusion; in such circumstances, a contrast-enhanced CT scan may reveal the lesion. It is also useful in visualizing more fully the area above or below an almost complete block in the subarachnoid space and in providing further information in patients with cord tumors.

CT scan is most helpful in defining the bony anatomy of the spine. It is performed routinely after trauma to exclude cervical spine fractures when spinal injury cannot be excluded on clinical grounds. CT scanning may show osteophytic narrowing of neural foramina or the spinal canal in patients with cervical spondylosis and may show spinal stenosis or disk protrusions in patients with neurogenic claudication. In patients with neurologic deficits, however, MRI is generally preferred because it provides more useful information about the spinal canal, neural foramina, and spinal cord.

MAGNETIC RESONANCE IMAGING

Spinal MRI is the best method for visualizing the spinal canal and its contents, and—in most cases—it provides the information obtained previously by myelography. Imaging of the spinal canal by MRI is direct and noninvasive.

Spinal MRI is indicated in the urgent evaluation of patients with suspected spinal cord compression. It permits differentiation of solid from cystic intramedullary lesions. MRI is the preferred imaging method for visualizing cord cavitation and detecting any associated abnormalities at the craniocervical junction. Congenital abnormalities associated with spinal dysraphism are also easily visualized by MRI. In patients with degenerative disk disease, MRI is an important means of detecting cord or root compression (**Figure 2-8**). However, abnormal MRI findings in the

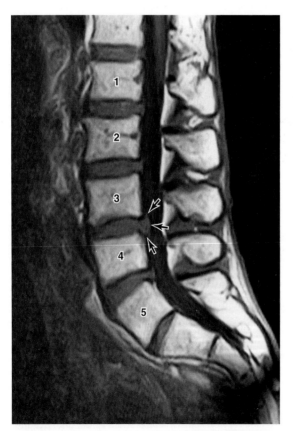

▲ **Figure 2-8.** Spinal MRI showing disk herniation at the L3-L4 level (arrows).

lumbar and cervical spine are common in asymptomatic subjects, especially in middle or later life, and care must therefore be exercised in attributing symptoms such as back pain to anatomic abnormalities that may be coincidental. When a spinal AVM (dural fistula) is suspected but MRI is unrevealing, a myelogram is sometimes helpful, but spinal angiography is often undertaken without proceeding to myelography.

NEUROMUSCULAR IMAGING STUDIES

MRI and ultrasound imaging of peripheral nerves may provide complementary information to clinical examination and electrodiagnostic studies, for example in nerve entrapment syndromes or after nerve injury, but the clinical role of these imaging studies is still being defined. MRI measures of muscle volume and composition and of edema are also being studied, as is their clinical application in patients with muscle disease. Muscle ultrasound is helpful in the identification of specific muscles for chemodenervation procedures, and its role in other clinical contexts is under study.

ULTRASONOGRAPHY

In **2D (B-mode) ultrasonography**, echoes reflected from anatomic structures are plotted on an oscilloscope screen in two dimensions. The resulting brightness at each point reflects the density of the imaged structure. The technique has been used to image the carotid artery and its bifurcation in the neck, permitting evaluation of the extent of extracranial vascular disease. Blood flowing within an artery does not reflect sound, and the lumen of the vessels therefore appears black. The arterial wall can be seen, however, and atherosclerotic lesions can be detected. Note that with severe stenosis or complete occlusion of the internal carotid artery, it may not be possible to visualize the carotid artery bifurcation.

The velocity of blood flow through an artery can be measured by **Doppler ultrasonography**. Sound waves within a certain frequency range are reflected off red blood cells, and the frequency of the echo provides a guide to the velocity of the flow. Any shift in frequency is proportional to the velocity of the red cells and the angle of the beam of sound waves. When the arterial lumen is narrowed, the velocity of flow increases; increased frequencies are therefore recorded by Doppler ultrasonography. Spectral analysis of Doppler frequencies is also used to evaluate the anatomic status of the carotid artery.

Transcranial Doppler studies can be used to detect intracranial arterial lesions or vasospasm (eg, after subarachnoid hemorrhage) and to assess the hemodynamic consequences of extracranial disease of the carotid arteries.

Duplex instruments perform a combination of both B-mode imaging and Doppler ultrasonography, thereby simultaneously providing information about the structure and the hemodynamics of the circulation in a color-coded format. The technique is commonly used to screen asymptomatic patients at high risk of carotid artery disease. Depending on the quality of the study, a CT angiogram may be necessary to confirm the extent and severity of disease. Symptomatic patients with suspected atheromatous lesions of the cervical carotid artery are best studied by magnetic resonance or computed tomographic angiography to determine whether carotid endarterectomy is indicated. Duplex ultrasound is also useful for follow-up after carotid endarterectomy or stenting to detect recurrent stenosis. The role of ultrasonography in neuromuscular disease, referred to earlier, is currently under study.

BIOPSIES

BRAIN BIOPSY

Biopsy of brain tissue is sometimes useful when less invasive methods, such as imaging studies, fail to provide a diagnosis. Brain lesions most amenable to biopsy are those that can be localized by imaging studies; are situated in superficial, surgically accessible sites; and do not involve critical brain regions, such as the brainstem or the areas of cerebral cortex involved in language or motor function. Cerebral disorders that can be diagnosed by biopsy include primary and metastatic brain tumors, inflammatory conditions such as vasculitis or sarcoidosis, infectious disorders such as brain abscess, and certain degenerative diseases such as Creutzfeldt-Jakob disease, although MRI has largely supplanted biopsy in the diagnosis of this disorder.

MUSCLE BIOPSY

Histopathologic examination of a biopsy specimen of a weak muscle can indicate whether the weakness is neurogenic or myopathic. In neurogenic disorders, atrophied fibers occur in groups, adjacent to groups of larger uninvolved fibers. In myopathies, atrophy occurs in a random pattern; the nuclei of muscle cells may be centrally situated, rather than in their normal peripheral location; and fibrosis or fatty infiltration may also be found. Examination of a muscle biopsy specimen may also permit certain inflammatory diseases of muscle, such as polymyositis, to be recognized and treated.

In some patients with a suspected myopathy, although the electromyographic findings are normal, examination of a muscle biopsy specimen reveals the nature of the underlying disorder. Conversely, electromyographic abnormalities suggestive of a myopathy are sometimes found in patients in whom the histologic or histochemical studies fail to establish a diagnosis of myopathy. The two approaches are therefore complementary.

NERVE BIOPSY

Nerve biopsy is not required to establish a diagnosis of peripheral neuropathy. The nature of any neuropathologic abnormalities, however, can sometimes suggest the underlying cause, such as a metabolic storage disease (eg, Fabry disease, Tangier disease), infection (eg, leprosy), inflammatory change, vasculitis, or neoplastic involvement. The findings are not always of diagnostic relevance, and nerve biopsy itself can be performed only on accessible nerves. It is rarely undertaken on more than a single occasion.

ARTERY BIOPSY

In patients with suspected giant cell arteritis, temporal artery biopsy may help to confirm the diagnosis, but the pathologic abnormalities are usually patchy in distribution. Therefore, a normal study should not exclude the diagnosis or lead to withdrawal of treatment.

SKIN BIOPSY

In patients with suspected small-fiber neuropathy, punch skin biopsy may be performed to determine the number, density, and length of small nerve fibers in the epidermis. The most common biopsy site is the lateral calf, for which normative values have been established.

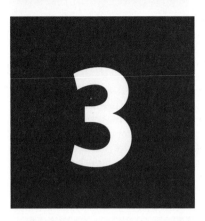

Coma

Coma is a sleep-like state with no purposeful response to the environment and from which the patient cannot be aroused. The eyes are closed and do not open spontaneously. The patient does not speak, and there is no purposeful movement of the face or limbs. Verbal stimulation produces no response. Painful stimulation may produce no response or nonpurposeful reflex movements mediated through spinal cord or brainstem pathways. Coma results from a disturbance in the function of the **brainstem**

reticular activating system above the mid pons or of **both cerebral hemispheres (Figure 3-1)**.

 APPROACH TO DIAGNOSIS

The approach to diagnosis of the comatose patient consists first of emergency measures to stabilize the patient and treat presumptively certain life-threatening disorders, followed by efforts to establish an etiologic diagnosis.

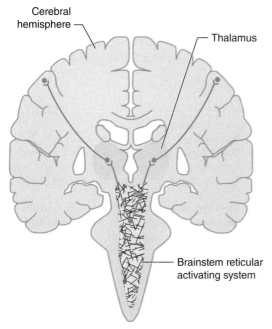

Cerebral hemisphere

Thalamus

Brainstem reticular activating system

▲ **Figure 3-1.** Anatomic basis of coma. Consciousness is maintained by the normal functioning of the brainstem reticular activating system above the mid pons and its bilateral projections to the thalamus and cerebral hemispheres. Coma results from lesions that affect either the reticular activating system or both hemispheres.

EMERGENCY MANAGEMENT

1. Ensure patency of the airway and adequacy of ventilation and circulation (**Table 3-1**). Adequacy of **ventilation** can be established by the absence of cyanosis, a respiratory rate greater than 8/min, the presence of breath sounds on auscultation of the chest, and the results of arterial blood gas studies. If any of these suggest inadequate ventilation, the patient should be ventilated mechanically. Measurement of the pulse and blood pressure provides a rapid assessment of the status of the **circulation**. Circulatory embarrassment should be treated with intravenous fluid replacement, pressors, and anti-arrhythmic drugs, as indicated.

2. Insert an intravenous catheter and withdraw blood for determination of serum glucose and electrolytes, hepatic and renal function tests, prothrombin time, partial thromboplastin time, complete blood count, and drug screen.

3. Begin an intravenous infusion and administer dextrose, thiamine, and naloxone. Every comatose patient should be given 25 g of **dextrose** intravenously, typically as 50 mL of a 50% dextrose solution, to treat possible hypoglycemic coma. Because administration of dextrose alone may precipitate or worsen Wernicke encephalopathy (see Chapter 4, Confusional States) in thiamine-deficient patients, all comatose patients should also receive 100 mg of **thiamine** by the intravenous route. To treat possible opiate overdose, the opiate antagonist **naloxone**, 0.4 to 1.2 mg intravenously, should also be administered routinely to comatose patients. The benzodiazepine antagonist **flumazenil**, 1 to 10 mg intravenously, may be useful when benzodiazepine overdose contributes to coma. However, it should not be used in patients with a history of seizures, chronic benzodiazepine abuse, or suspected co-ingestion of tri- or tetracyclic antidepressants. The latter should be suspected if the electrocardiogram (ECG) shows sinus tachycardia at a rate of 130/min or more, QTc interval greater than 0.5 seconds, and QRS duration greater than 0.1 seconds.

4. Withdraw arterial blood for blood gas and pH determinations. In addition to assisting in the assessment

Table 3-1. Emergency Management of the Comatose Patient.

Immediately	Next	Later
Ensure adequacy of airway, ventilation, and circulation	If signs of meningeal irritation are present (see Figure 1-5), perform LP to rule out meningitis. Obtain a history if possible	ECG
Draw blood for serum glucose, electrolytes, liver and renal function tests, PT, PTT, and CBC	Perform detailed general physical and neurologic examination	Correct hyper- or hypothermia
Start IV and administer 25 g of dextrose, 100 mg of thiamine, and 0.4-1.2 mg of naloxone IV	Order CT scan of head if history or findings suggest structural lesion or subarachnoid hemorrhage	Correct severe acid–base and electrolyte abnormalities
Draw blood for arterial blood gas determinations		Chest X-ray
Treat seizures (see Chapter 12, Seizures & Syncope)		Blood and urine toxicology studies; EEG

CBC, complete blood count; IV, intravenous; LP, lumbar puncture; PT, prothrombin time; PTT, partial thromboplastin time.

Table 3-2. Metabolic Coma: Differential Diagnosis by Acid–Base Abnormalities.

Respiratory acidosis
Sedative drug intoxication
Pulmonary encephalopathy
Respiratory alkalosis
Hepatic encephalopathy
Salicylate intoxication
Sepsis
Metabolic acidosis
Diabetic ketoacidosis
Uremic encephalopathy
Lactic acidosis
Methanol intoxication
Ethylene glycol intoxication
Isoniazid intoxication
Salicylate intoxication
Sepsis (terminal)
Metabolic alkalosis
Coma unusual

Data from Plum F, Posner JB. *The Diagnosis of Stupor and Coma.* 3rd ed. Vol 19: *Contemporary Neurology Series.* Philadelphia, PA: FA Davis; 1980.

of ventilatory status, these studies can provide clues to metabolic causes of coma **(Table 3-2)**.

5. Institute treatment for seizures, if present. Persistent or recurrent seizures in a comatose patient should be considered to represent status epilepticus and treated accordingly, as described in Chapter 12, Seizures & Syncope (see particularly Table 12-6).

HISTORY & EXAMINATION

HISTORY

The most crucial aspect of the history is the time over which coma develops.

1. A **sudden onset** of coma suggests a vascular origin, especially a brainstem stroke or subarachnoid hemorrhage.
2. **Rapid progression** from hemispheric signs, such as hemiparesis, hemisensory deficit, or aphasia, to coma within minutes to hours is characteristic of intracerebral hemorrhage.
3. A more **protracted course** leading to coma (days to a week or more) is seen with tumor, abscess, or chronic subdural hematoma.
4. Coma preceded by a **confusional state or agitated delirium**, without lateralizing signs or symptoms, is

probably due to a metabolic derangement or infection (meningitis or encephalitis).

GENERAL PHYSICAL EXAMINATION

▶ Signs of Trauma

1. Inspection of the head may reveal signs of **basilar skull fracture**, including the following:
   A. **Raccoon eyes**—Periorbital ecchymoses (see Figure 1-4).
   B. **Battle sign**—Swelling and discoloration overlying the mastoid bone behind the ear (see Figure 1-4).
   C. **Hemotympanum**—Blood behind the tympanic membrane.
   D. **Cerebrospinal fluid (CSF) rhinorrhea or otorrhea**—Leakage of CSF from the nose or ear. CSF rhinorrhea must be distinguished from other causes of rhinorrhea, such as allergic rhinitis. Glucose concentration does not reliably distinguish CSF from nasal mucus, but beta-2 transferrin is a reliable marker of CSF. High-resolution scanning is then used for localization.
2. Palpation of the head may demonstrate a **depressed skull fracture** or **swelling of soft tissues** at the site of trauma.

▶ Blood Pressure

Elevated blood pressure in a comatose patient may reflect long-standing hypertension, which predisposes to intracerebral hemorrhage or stroke. In the rare condition of hypertensive encephalopathy, the blood pressure exceeds 250/150 mm Hg in chronically hypertensive patients; it may be lower in children or after acute elevation of blood pressure in previously normotensive patients (eg, in acute renal failure). Elevated blood pressure may also be a consequence of the process causing the coma, as in intracerebral or subarachnoid hemorrhage or, rarely, brainstem stroke.

▶ Temperature

Hypothermia occurs in coma caused by ethanol or sedative drug intoxication, hypoglycemia, Wernicke encephalopathy, hepatic encephalopathy, myxedema and exposure. Coma with hyperthermia is seen in heat stroke, status epilepticus, malignant hyperthermia related to inhalational anesthetics, anticholinergic drug intoxication, pontine hemorrhage, and certain hypothalamic lesions.

▶ Signs of Meningeal Irritation

Signs of meningeal irritation (eg, nuchal rigidity or the Brudzinski sign [see Figure 1-5]) can be invaluable in the prompt diagnosis of meningitis or subarachnoid hemorrhage, but these signs are lost in deep coma, so their absence does not exclude these conditions.

Optic Fundi

Examination of the optic fundi may reveal papilledema or retinal hemorrhages compatible with chronic or acute hypertension, or an elevation in intracranial pressure (see Figure 1-11). Subhyaloid (superficial retinal) hemorrhages in an adult strongly suggest subarachnoid hemorrhage (see Figure 6-3).

NEUROLOGIC EXAMINATION

The neurologic examination is central to etiologic diagnosis in the comatose patient. Pupillary size and reactivity, reflex eye movements (oculocephalic and oculovestibular reflexes), and the motor response to pain should be evaluated in detail (**Figure 3-2**).

Pupils

1. **Normal pupils**—Normal pupils are typically 3 to 4 mm in diameter (but larger in children and smaller in the elderly) and equal in size bilaterally; they constrict briskly and symmetrically in response to light. Normally reactive pupils in a comatose patient are characteristic of a metabolic cause.

2. **Thalamic pupils**—Slightly smaller (~2 mm) reactive pupils are present in the early stages of thalamic (diencephalic) compression from mass lesions, perhaps because of interruption of the descending sympathetic pathways.

3. **Fixed, dilated pupils**—Pupils greater than 7 mm in diameter and fixed (unreactive to light) usually result from compression of the oculomotor (III) cranial nerve (and associated sympathetic, pupillodilator nerve fibers) anywhere along its course, from the midbrain to the orbit, but may also be seen in anticholinergic or sympathomimetic drug intoxication. The most common cause of a fixed, dilated pupil in a comatose patient is transtentorial herniation of the medial temporal lobe from a supratentorial mass.

4. **Fixed, midsized pupils**—Pupils fixed at approximately 5 mm in diameter are the result of brainstem damage at

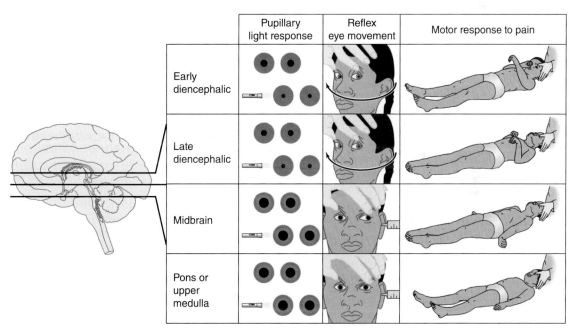

▲ **Figure 3-2.** Neurologic signs in coma with downward transtentorial herniation. In the **early diencephalic** phase, the pupils are small (approximately 2 mm in diameter) and reactive, reflex eye movements are intact, and the motor response to pain is purposeful or semipurposeful (localizing) and often asymmetric. The **late diencephalic** phase is associated with similar findings, except that painful stimulation results in decorticate (flexor) posturing, which may also be asymmetric. With **midbrain** involvement, the pupils are fixed and midsized (approximately 5 mm in diameter), reflex adduction of the eyes is impaired, and pain elicits decerebrate (extensor) posturing. Progression to involve the **pons or medulla** also produces fixed, midsized pupils, but these are accompanied by loss of reflex abduction as well as adduction of the eyes and by no motor response or only leg flexion upon painful stimulation. Note that although a lesion restricted to the pons produces pinpoint pupils as a result of the destruction of descending sympathetic (pupillodilator) pathways, downward herniation to the pontine level is associated with midsized pupils. This happens because herniation also interrupts parasympathetic (pupilloconstrictor) fibers in the oculomotor (III) nerve.

the midbrain level, which interrupts both sympathetic, pupillodilator and parasympathetic, pupilloconstrictor nerve fibers.

5. **Pinpoint pupils**—Pinpoint pupils (1-1.5 mm in diameter) in a comatose patient usually indicate opioid overdose or, less commonly, a focal structural lesion in the pons with the associated defects in horizontal eye movements that usually accompany pontine lesions. Pinpoint pupils may appear unreactive to light except when viewed with a magnifying glass. Structural versus opioid causes can be distinguished by the administration of naloxone (see earlier). Pinpoint pupils can also be caused by organophosphate poisoning, miotic eye drops, or neurosyphilis (Argyll Robertson pupils).

6. **Asymmetric pupils**—Asymmetry of pupillary size (anisocoria) of a difference of 1 mm or less in diameter is a normal finding that occurs in 20% of the population. In such physiologic anisocoria, each pupil constricts to a similar extent in response to light, and extraocular movements are unimpaired. In contrast, a pupil that constricts less rapidly or to a lesser extent than its contralateral fellow usually implies a structural lesion affecting the midbrain, oculomotor nerve, or eye.

▶ Eye Movements

1. **Pathways tested**—The neuronal pathways examined by testing eye movements begin at the pontomedullary junction (vestibular [VIII] nerve and nucleus), synapse in the caudal pons (horizontal gaze center and abducens [VI] nerve nucleus), ascend through the central core of the brainstem reticular activating system (medial longitudinal fasciculus), and arrive at the contralateral midbrain (oculomotor [III] nucleus and nerve; **Figure 3-3**).

2. **Methods of testing**—In the comatose patient, eye movements are tested by stimulating the vestibular system (semicircular canals of the middle ear) by passive head rotation (the **oculocephalic reflex**, or **doll's-head maneuver**) or using the stronger stimulus of ice-water irrigation against the tympanic membrane (**oculovestibular reflex**, or **cold-water caloric** testing) (see Figure 3-3).

   The doll's-head (oculocephalic) maneuver is performed by rotating the head horizontally to elicit horizontal eye movements and vertically to elicit vertical movements. The eyes should move in the direction opposite to that of head rotation. This may be an inadequate stimulus for inducing eye movements, however, and the reflex may be overridden in conscious patients.

   Cold-water caloric (oculovestibular) stimulation is a more potent stimulus and is performed by irrigating

one tympanic membrane with ice water. Otoscopic examination should always be undertaken before this maneuver is attempted, because it is contraindicated if the tympanic membrane is perforated. In conscious patients, unilateral cold water irrigation produces nystagmus with the fast phase directed away from the irrigated side. In comatose patients with intact brainstem function, unilateral ice water irrigation results in tonic deviation of the eyes toward the irrigated side. An absent or impaired response to caloric stimulation with 50 mL of ice water is indicative of peripheral vestibular disease, a structural lesion involving the posterior fossa (cerebellum or brainstem), or intoxication with sedative drugs.

3. **Normal movements**—A comatose patient with intact brainstem function has full conjugate horizontal eye movements, which occur either spontaneously (as "roving eye movements") or during the doll's-head maneuver, or as tonic conjugate deviation of both eyes toward the side of the ice-water irrigation during cold-water caloric testing. Full horizontal eye movements in a comatose patient exclude a structural lesion in the brainstem as the cause of coma and suggest either a nonstructural (eg, metabolic) cause or, less commonly, bilateral hemispheric lesions.

4. **Abnormal movements**
   a. With lesions affecting the oculomotor (III) nerve or nucleus, such as hemispheric mass lesions causing downward transtentorial herniation at the midbrain level (see Figure 3-2), cold-water caloric testing fails to produce adduction of the contralateral eye, whereas the ipsilateral eye abducts normally.
   b. Complete unresponsiveness to cold-water caloric testing in a comatose patient implies either a structural lesion of the brainstem affecting the pons or a metabolic disorder that affects the brainstem preferentially, such as sedative drug intoxication.
   c. Downward deviation of one or both eyes in response to unilateral cold-water caloric testing also suggests sedative drug intoxication.

▶ Motor Response to Pain

The motor response to pain is assessed by applying strong pressure on the supraorbital ridge, sternum, or nail beds. The response to such stimuli can indicate whether the condition causing coma affects the brain symmetrically (as is typical of metabolic and other diffuse disorders) or asymmetrically (as in unilateral structural lesions). The motor response to pain may also help to localize the anatomic level of cerebral dysfunction (Figure 3-2) or provide a guide to the depth of coma as described below:

1. With cerebral dysfunction of only moderate severity, patients may localize an offending stimulus by reaching toward the site of stimulation. Although such

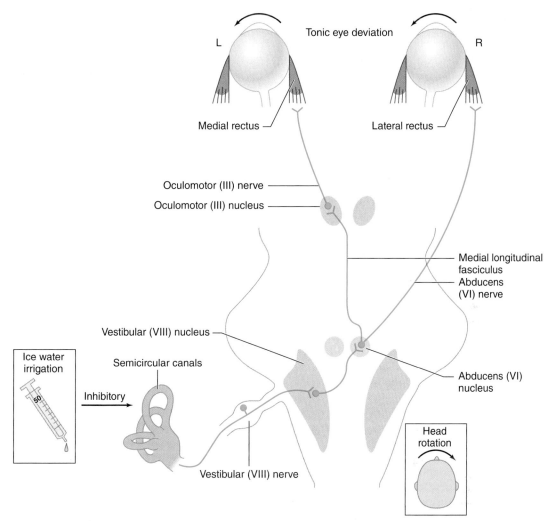

▲ **Figure 3-3.** Brainstem pathways mediating reflex conjugate horizontal eye movements. In a comatose patient with intact brainstem function, irrigation of the tympanic membrane with ice water inhibits the vestibuloocular pathways shown, resulting in tonic deviation of both eyes toward the irrigated side; head rotation causes eye deviation away from the direction of rotation.

"semipurposeful" localizing responses can be difficult to distinguish from the flexion/decorticate reflex response described below, movements that involve limb abduction almost never represent reflex movements.

2. A **decorticate** response to pain (flexion of the arm at the elbow, adduction at the shoulder, and extension and internal rotation of the leg and ankle) is classically associated with lesions that involve the thalamus directly or large hemispheric masses that compress the thalamus from above.

3. A **decerebrate** response (extension at the elbow, internal rotation at the shoulder and forearm, and leg extension)

tends to occur when brain dysfunction has descended to the level of the midbrain. Thus, decerebrate posturing generally implies more severe brain dysfunction than decorticate posturing, although neither response localizes the site of dysfunction precisely.

4. Bilateral symmetric posturing may be seen in both structural and metabolic disorders.

5. Unilateral or asymmetric posturing suggests structural disease in the contralateral cerebral hemisphere or brainstem.

6. In patients with pontine and medullary lesions, there is usually no response to pain, but occasionally some flexion at the knee (a spinal reflex) is noted.

Table 3-3. Glasgow Coma Scale.

Score	Eye Opening	Verbal Response	Motor Response
1	None	None	None
2	To pain	Vocal but not verbal	Extension
3	To voice	Verbal but not conversational	Flexion
4	Spontaneous	Conversational but disoriented	Withdraws from pain
5	—	Oriented	Localizes pain
6	—	—	Obeys commands

Adapted from Teasdale G, Jennett B. Assessment of coma and impaired consciousness. A practical scale. *Lancet*. 1974;2:81-84.

▶ Glasgow Coma Scale

The pupillary, eye movement, and motor responses described earlier are sometimes translated to a numerical scale so that changes in the examination (and thus the numerical score) may be more easily noticed over time and compared between different examiners (**Table 3-3**).

PATHOPHYSIOLOGIC ASSESSMENT

The most important step in evaluating a comatose patient is to decide whether the cause is a structural brain lesion (for which emergency neurosurgical intervention may be required) or a diffuse disorder caused by a metabolic disturbance, meningitis, or seizures (for which immediate medical treatment may be needed).

▶ Supratentorial Structural Lesions

When coma results from a supratentorial mass lesion, the history and physical findings early in the course usually point to dysfunction of one cerebral hemisphere. Symptoms and signs include contralateral hemiparesis, contralateral hemisensory loss, aphasia (with dominant, usually left, hemisphere lesions), and agnosia (indifference to or denial of the deficit, with injury to the nondominant hemisphere).

As the mass expands (commonly from associated edema), the patient becomes increasingly lethargic due to compression of the contralateral hemisphere or thalamus. Stupor progresses to coma, but findings on examination often remain asymmetric. With rostral–caudal (downward) progression of brain injury, the thalamus, midbrain, pons, and medulla become sequentially involved, and the neurologic examination reveals dysfunction at successively lower anatomic levels (see Figure 3-2). This segmental pattern of rostral-caudal involvement strongly

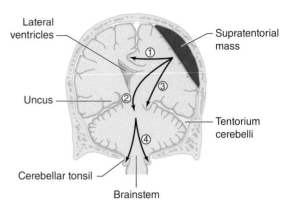

▲ **Figure 3-4.** Anatomic basis of herniation syndromes. An expanding supratentorial mass lesion may cause brain tissue to be displaced into an adjacent intracranial compartment, resulting in (1) cingulate herniation under the falx, (2) downward transtentorial (central) herniation, (3) uncal herniation over the edge of the tentorium, or (4) cerebellar tonsillar herniation into the foramen magnum. Coma and ultimately death result when (2), (3), or (4) produces brainstem compression.

supports the diagnosis of a supratentorial mass with downward transtentorial herniation (**Figure 3-4**) and dictates the need for neurosurgical intervention. At the fully developed midbrain level (midsized, unreactive pupils), chances of survival without severe neurologic impairment decrease rapidly, especially in adults. Once the pontine level of dysfunction is reached (unreactive pupils, and absent horizontal eye movements), a fatal outcome is inevitable.

Supratentorial mass lesions may cause herniation of the medial portion of the temporal lobe (the uncus) over the edge of the cerebellar tentorium (see Figure 3-4). This exerts direct pressure on the upper brainstem and produces signs of oculomotor (III) nerve and midbrain compression, such as ipsilateral pupillary dilatation and impaired adduction of the eye (**uncal syndrome**), which may precede loss of consciousness. Neurosurgical decompression must occur early in the course of oculomotor (III) nerve involvement if functional recovery is to occur.

▶ Subtentorial Structural Lesions

Coma of sudden onset with focal signs of brainstem dysfunction strongly suggests a subtentorial structural lesion. Abnormal pupillary function and impaired eye movement are the findings most suggestive of a subtentorial structural lesion, especially if these abnormalities are asymmetric. Midbrain lesions cause loss of pupillary function: the pupils are midsized (approximately 5 mm in diameter) and unreactive to light. Pontine hemorrhage, pontine infarction, or compression of the pons by adjacent cerebellar

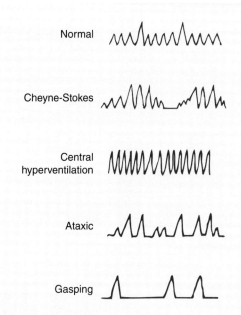

Normal

Cheyne-Stokes

Central
hyperventilation

Ataxic

Gasping

Figure 3-5. Ventilatory patterns in coma. Cheyne–Stokes respiration and central hyperventilation are seen with metabolic disturbances and with structural lesions at a variety of sites in the brain. They are therefore not useful for anatomic localization of disorders producing coma. Ataxic and gasping ventilatory patterns are most commonly seen with pontomedullary lesions.

focal signs, such as hemiparesis, hemisensory loss, or aphasia, and—except in some cases of subarachnoid hemorrhage—consciousness is lost only gradually, typically after a period of progressive somnolence or agitated delirium.

A symmetric neurologic examination is the rule, although hypoglycemia, hyperosmolar nonketotic hyperglycemia, and hepatic encephalopathy may sometimes be accompanied by focal signs, such as hemiparesis, which may alternate from side to side. Asterixis, myoclonus, and tremor preceding coma are important clues that suggest metabolic disease. Symmetric decorticate or decerebrate posturing can be seen with hepatic, uremic, anoxic, hypoglycemic, or sedative drug-induced coma.

Reactive pupils in the presence of otherwise impaired brainstem function are the hallmark of metabolic encephalopathy. Although coma with intact pupillary reaction can also be seen early in transtentorial herniation (see Figure 3-2), the latter is associated with asymmetric neurologic findings, such as hemiparesis. A few metabolic causes of coma can also impair pupillary light reflexes, including massive barbiturate overdose with apnea and hypotension, acute anoxia, marked hypothermia, anticholinergic poisoning (large pupils), and opioid overdose (pinpoint pupils), but even in these settings, completely unreactive pupils are uncommon.

Ventilatory patterns in metabolic coma vary widely (see Figure 3-5), but measuring arterial blood gases and pH may help to establish an etiologic diagnosis. Arterial blood gas abnormalities in coma are outlined in Table 3-2.

Summary

The relationship between neurologic signs and the pathophysiology of coma is summarized in **Table 3-4.** Examining pupil size and reactivity and testing reflex eye movements and the motor response to pain help determine whether brain function is disrupted at a discrete anatomic level (**structural lesion**) or in a diffuse manner (**metabolic coma**).

Supratentorial structural lesions compromise the brain in an orderly way, producing dysfunction at progressively lower anatomic levels. In patients with metabolic coma, such localization is not possible, and scattered, anatomically inconsistent findings may be seen. An impressive example of the anatomically discordant findings characteristic of metabolic coma is the retention of pupillary reactivity in the face of otherwise depressed brainstem functions—including paralysis of eye movements, respiratory depression, flaccid muscle tone, and unresponsiveness to painful stimuli—after sedative drug overdose. The same degree of low brainstem dysfunction produced by a supratentorial mass lesion would first compromise the more rostrally situated midbrain structures that mediate pupillary reactivity before affecting the lower brainstem centers controlling eye movement and ventilation.

hemorrhage or infarction produces pinpoint pupils. Brainstem lesions may also be associated with conjugate gaze deviation away from the side of the lesion (and toward a hemiparesis) (see Figure 7-17), or disconjugate eye movements such as internuclear ophthalmoplegia (Figure 7-15) (selective impairment of eye adduction). Motor responses are generally not helpful in separating subtentorial from supratentorial lesions. Ventilatory patterns associated with subtentorial lesions are abnormal but variable and may be ataxic or gasping (**Figure 3-5**). Because the fully developed syndrome of transtentorial herniation from a supratentorial mass is characterized by extensive brainstem dysfunction, its differentiation from a primary subtentorial process may be impossible except by history.

Diffuse Encephalopathies

Diffuse encephalopathies that result in coma (often termed **metabolic coma**) include not only metabolic disorders such as hypoglycemia and drug intoxication, but other processes that affect the brain diffusely, such as meningitis, subarachnoid hemorrhage, and seizures.

The clinical presentation of diffuse encephalopathy is distinct from that of a mass lesion. There are usually no

Table 3-4. Pathophysiologic Assessment of the Comatose Patient.

	Supratentorial Structural Lesion	Subtentorial Structural Lesion	Diffuse Encephalopathy/Meningitis
Pupil size and light reaction	Usually normal size (3-4 mm) and reactive; large (>7 mm) and unreactive with transtentorial herniation	Midsized (about 5 mm) and unreactive with midbrain lesion; pinpoint (1-1.5 mm) and unreactive with pontine lesion	Usually normal size (3-4 mm) and reactive; pinpoint (1-1.5 mm) and sometimes unreactive with opiates; large (>7 mm) and unreactive with anticholinergics
Reflex eye movements	Normal (gaze preference toward side of lesion may occur)	Impaired adduction with midbrain lesion; impaired adduction and abduction with pontine lesion	Usually normal; impaired by sedative drugs or Wernicke encephalopathy
Motor responses	Usually asymmetric; may be symmetric after transtentorial herniation	Asymmetric (unilateral lesion) or symmetric (bilateral lesion)	Usually symmetric; may rarely be asymmetric with hypoglycemia, hyperosmolar nonketotic hyperglycemia, or hepatic encephalopathy

CAUSES OF COMA

SUPRATENTORIAL STRUCTURAL LESIONS

SUBDURAL HEMATOMA

Subdural hematoma is a collection of blood in the subdural space between the dura mater and the arachnoid. Because subdural hematoma is resectable, it must always be considered early in any comatose patient with a suspected supratentorial mass lesion. Subdural hematoma is more common in older patients, because cerebral atrophy stretches cortical veins bridging the subdural space, rendering them more susceptible to laceration from shearing injury or spontaneous rupture.

Trauma is the most common cause, and in the acute stage after head injury, focal neurologic deficits are often conspicuous. The severity of injury needed to produce a subdural hematoma becomes less with advancing age; in perhaps 25% of cases no history of trauma is present.

The most common clinical features are headache and altered consciousness, but symptoms and signs may be absent, nonspecific, or nonlocalizing, especially with chronic subdural hematomas that appear months or years after injury (**Table 3-5**). The classic history of waxing and waning signs and symptoms occurs too infrequently to be relied on for diagnosis. Hemiparesis, when present, is contralateral to the lesion in approximately 70% of cases. Pupillary dilation, when present, is ipsilateral in approximately 90% of cases. The frequency of bilateral hematomas may make clinical localization difficult, as may coexisting cerebral contusion.

Diagnosis is by computed tomography (CT) scan or magnetic resonance imaging (MRI) (**Figure 3-6**).

Treatment of subdural hematoma causing coma is by surgical evacuation.

Table 3-5. Clinical Features of Subdural Hematoma.

	Acute[1] (82 Cases) (%)	Subacute[2] (91 Cases) (%)	Chronic[3] (216 Cases) (%)
Symptoms			
Depressed consciousness	100	88	47
Vomiting	24	31	30
Weakness	20	19	22
Confusion	12	41	37
Headache	11	44	81
Speech disturbance	6	8	6
Seizures	6	3	9
Vertigo	0	4	5
Visual disturbance	0	0	12
Signs			
Depressed consciousness	100	88	59
Pupillary inequality	57	27	20
Motor asymmetry	44	37	41
Confusion and memory loss	17	21	27
Aphasia	6	12	11
Papilledema	1	15	22
Hemianopia	0	4	3
Facial weakness	0	3	3

[1]Within 3 days of trauma.
[2]4-20 days after trauma.
[3]More than 20 days after trauma.
Data from McKissock W, Richardson A, Bloom WH. Subdural hematoma, a review of 389 cases. *Lancet.* 1960;1:1365-1370.

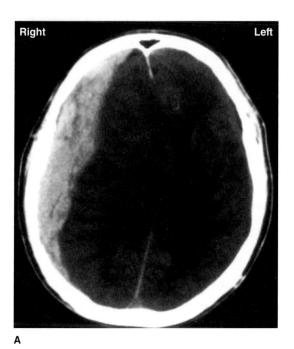 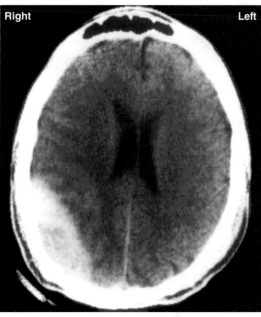

A   B

▲ **Figure 3-6.** (**A**) Subdural hematoma. Unenhanced CT scan showing a large, high-density crescentic mass over the right cerebral hemisphere, with shift of the lateral ventricles across the midline. (**B**) Epidural hematoma. Unenhanced CT scan showing a large, high-density lens-shaped mass in the right parietooccipital region. Fracture of the occipital bone was seen on bone windows.

EPIDURAL HEMATOMA

Epidural hematoma typically results from head trauma associated with a lateral skull fracture and tearing of the middle meningeal artery and vein. Patients may or may not lose consciousness initially. There is often a lucid interval of several hours before the onset of coma, during which time headache, vomiting, obtundation, seizures, and focal neurologic signs may occur. The diagnosis is made by CT scan or MRI (see Figure 3-6), which classically shows a hyper intense, biconvex, lens-shaped mass compressing the cerebral hemisphere. Prompt surgical evacuation of the hematoma is essential to prevent a fatal outcome.

CEREBRAL CONTUSION

Cerebral contusion is bruising of the brain caused by head trauma. It may be associated with initial unconsciousness from which the patient recovers. Edema surrounding the contusion may cause the level of consciousness to fluctuate, and seizures and focal neurologic signs may develop. Patients must be carefully monitored for neurologic deterioration related to progressive edema and herniation.

Lumbar puncture is unnecessary and potentially dangerous. CT scan or MRI are the diagnostic procedures of choice. In contrast to subdural and epidural hematomas, cerebral contusions rarely require surgery.

INTRACEREBRAL HEMORRHAGE

▶ Etiology

The most common cause of nontraumatic intracerebral hemorrhage is chronic hypertension. This and other causes are discussed in more detail in Chapter 13, Stroke.

▶ Clinical Findings

Intracerebral hemorrhage usually occurs while the patient is awake. Hemorrhage is not preceded by transient prodromal symptoms, such as the transient ischemic attacks (TIAs) often associated with cerebral infarction (see Chapter 13, Stroke).

Headache occurs in many cases and can be moderate to severe. If present, headache may be localized to the site of hemorrhage or generalized. Nausea and vomiting are common. Altered consciousness may progress steadily to stupor or coma over minutes to hours.

On examination, patients are nearly always hypertensive (blood pressure 170/90 mm Hg or higher), even in the late stages of transtentorial herniation. The funduscopic examination usually shows vascular changes associated with chronic hypertension. Nuchal rigidity is common. Gaze deviation—toward the side of a putaminal or lobar hemorrhage or downward and medially in thalamic hemorrhage—may occur. Hemiparesis is frequent because of the proximity of common hemorrhage sites, such as the basal ganglia and thalamus, to the internal capsule, which conveys descending motor fibers from the cerebral cortex.

Seizures occur in approximately 10% of cases and are often focal. Neurologic deficits do not fluctuate spontaneously.

▶ Investigative Studies

CT brain scan without contrast or MRI shows intraparenchymal blood and confirms the diagnosis (see Figure 13-20).

▶ Treatment

1. **Blood pressure**—Systolic blood pressure should be reduced to 140 mm Hg or less to limit hematoma expansion, but excessive blood pressure reduction should be avoided, as it may compromise blood flow in brain tissue adjacent to the hemorrhage.

2. **Cerebral edema**—The mass effect of intracerebral hemorrhage is typically compounded by progressive cerebral edema, which becomes evident at approximately 24 hours and maximal within 5 to 6 days. Cerebral edema may be treated with mannitol or intravenous hypertonic saline (**Table 3-6**), but this is usually only useful as a temporizing measure prior to surgery, when indicated, and alone rarely alters the eventual outcome.

3. **Surgical treatment**—Evacuation of the clot may be appropriate in cases (approximately 10%) in which

hemorrhage is located superficially in the cerebral hemisphere and produces a mass effect. However, most hemorrhages are deep within the brain and less accessible to surgery.

▶ Prognosis

Early mortality from intracerebral hemorrhage is high, with approximately 25% of patients dying within 72 hours. However, those who survive may be left with surprisingly mild deficits as the clot resolves over a period of weeks to months.

BRAIN ABSCESS

Brain abscess is an uncommon disorder, accounting for only 2% of intracranial masses but occurring more frequently in immunosuppressed patients.

▶ Etiology

The common conditions predisposing to brain abscess, in approximate order of frequency, are blood-borne metastasis from distant systemic (especially pulmonary) infection, direct extension from parameningeal sites (otitis, cranial osteomyelitis, mastoiditis, sinusitis), an unknown source, infection associated with recent or remote head trauma or craniotomy, and infection associated with cyanotic congenital heart disease.

The most frequently cultured organisms are *Streptococcus* species (30%), *Staphylococcus* species (20%) (local rates

Table 3-6. Drug Therapy for Cerebral Edema.

Drug	Dose	Route	Indications and Comments
Glucocorticoids			
Dexamethasone	10-100 mg, then 4 mg 4 times daily	Intravenous or orally	
Prednisone	60 mg, then 25 mg 4 times daily	Orally	Dexamethasone preferred for lowest mineralocorticoid effect. Antacid treatment indicated. Effective for edema associated with brain tumor or abscess; not indicated for intracerebral hemorrhage or infarction.
Methylprednisolone	60 mg, then 25 mg 4 times daily	Intravenous or orally	
Hydrocortisone	300 mg, then 130 mg 4 times daily	Intravenous or orally	
Osmotic diuretic agents			
Mannitol	1.5-2 g/kg over 30 min–1 h	20% intravenous solution	Effective acutely. Major dehydrating effect on normal tissue; osmotic effect short-lived, and more than two intravenous doses rarely effective. Hypertonic saline has both osmotic and vasoregulatory effects.
Hypertonic saline	3% continuous infusion or 23.4% or 29.2% by 20 mL bolus	Intravenously	Continuous infusion of 3% hypertonic saline to target a serum sodium of 145-155 mEq/L; boluses of hypertonic saline may be more effective than other osmotic agents.

of methicillin-resistant staph vary widely), and gram-negative enteric bacteria (15%). Abscess formation in neurosurgical or head trauma patients is more likely to be staphylococcal, and abscess from infections promoting contiguous spread (otitis, sinusitis) is more commonly streptococcal. Multiple organisms are present in the majority of abscesses. Patients immunocompromised by HIV coinfection are subject to *Toxoplasma gondii* and tuberculosis abscess; solid organ or stem cell transplant patients are at risk for fungal brain abscess, mainly *Aspergillus* and *Candida* species.

Clinical Findings

The course is that of an expanding mass lesion, usually presenting with headache and focal neurologic deficits in a conscious patient with a mean symptom duration of approximately one week. Presentation with seizure occurs in 25% of patients. Coma may develop over days and rarely over hours. Common presenting signs and symptoms are shown in **Table 3-7**. It is important to note that common correlates of infection may be absent: Temperature is normal in 40% of patients, and the peripheral white blood cell count is below 10,000/μL in 20%.

Investigative Studies

The diagnosis is strongly supported by finding a mass lesion with a contrast-enhanced rim on CT scan or MRI or an avascular mass on angiography. Diffusion-weighted MRI differentiates abscess from tumor. A single abscess, most commonly in the frontal or temporal lobe, occurs in 80% of patients. CSF reveals an increased opening pressure in 75% of patients, pleocytosis of 25 to 500 or more white cells/μL (depending on the proximity of the abscess to the

Table 3-7. Brain Abscesses: Presenting Features in 123 Cases.

Fever	58%
Headache	55%
Disturbed consciousness	48%
Hemiparesis	48%
Nausea, vomiting	32%
Nuchal rigidity	29%
Dysarthria	20%
Seizures	19%
Sepsis	17%
Visual disturbances	15%

Data from Lu CH, Chang WN, Lin YC, et al. Bacterial brain abscess: microbiological features, epidemiological trends and outcomes. *Q J Med.* 2002;95:501-509.

ventricular surface and its degree of encapsulation), and elevated protein level (45-500 mg/dL) in approximately 60% of patients. CSF and blood cultures are each positive in a quarter of cases. Marked clinical deterioration may follow lumbar puncture in patients with brain abscess; therefore, lumbar puncture should not be performed if brain abscess is suspected based on other studies.

Treatment

Treatment of pyogenic brain abscess can be with antibiotics alone or combined with surgical drainage. Surgical therapy should be strongly considered when there is a significant mass effect or the abscess is near the ventricular surface, because catastrophic rupture into the ventricular system may occur.

Medical treatment alone is indicated for surgically inaccessible, multiple, or early abscesses. If the causal organism is unknown, broad-spectrum antibiotic coverage is indicated. The first-line recommendation in North America is a third-generation cephalosporin plus metronidazole. If staphylococcal infection is suspected, vancomycin should be added. Glucocorticoids (see Table 3-6) are commonly used to reduce edema surrounding the abscess. The response to medical treatment should be assessed by clinical examination and serial CT or MRI scans. When medically treated patients do not improve, needle aspiration of the abscess is indicated to identify the organisms present.

STROKE (CEREBRAL INFARCTION)

Embolic or thrombotic occlusion of one carotid artery does not cause coma directly, because bilateral hemispheric lesions are required for consciousness to be lost. However, cerebral edema after massive hemispheric infarction can compress the contralateral hemisphere or cause transtentorial herniation, either of which can produce coma. Edema becomes maximal within 48 to 72 hours after infarction, and may cause progression of the original neurologic deficit and ultimately stupor and coma. Cerebral hemorrhage is excluded by CT scan or MRI.

The use of corticosteroids and dehydrating agents to treat cerebral edema associated with stroke has produced no clear benefit. Stroke is discussed in more detail in Chapter 13, Stroke.

BRAIN TUMOR

Clinical Findings

Primary or metastatic brain tumors (see Chapter 6, Headache & Facial Pain) rarely present with coma, although they can do so when hemorrhage into the tumor or tumor-induced seizures occur. More often, coma occurs late in the clinical course of brain tumor, and there is a history of headache, focal neurologic deficits, and altered consciousness. Papilledema is a presenting sign in 25% of cases.

Investigative Studies

If brain tumor is suspected, a head CT scan or MRI should be obtained. It may or may not be possible to determine the nature of the tumor by its imaging appearance alone; biopsy may be required. Chest X-ray or CT scan is useful, because lung carcinoma is the most common source of intracranial metastasis and because other tumors that metastasize to the brain commonly involve the lungs first.

Treatment

In contrast to their lack of therapeutic effect on cytotoxic edema resulting from cerebral ischemia, corticosteroids (see Table 3-6) are often remarkably effective in reducing tumor-associated vasogenic brain edema from leaking capillaries with resultant improvement in related neurologic deficits. Specific approaches to the treatment of tumors include excision, radiotherapy, and chemotherapy, depending on the site and nature of the lesion.

SUBTENTORIAL STRUCTURAL LESIONS

BASILAR ARTERY THROMBOSIS OR EMBOLIC OCCLUSION

Clinical Findings

These relatively common vascular syndromes (discussed in more detail in Chapter 13, Stroke) produce coma by impairing blood flow to the brainstem reticular activating system. Patients are typically middle-aged to elderly and often have a history of hypertension, atherosclerotic vascular disease, or TIAs. Thrombosis usually affects the middle portion, and embolic occlusion the top, of the basilar artery. Virtually all patients present with some alteration of consciousness, and 50% are comatose at presentation. Focal neurologic signs are present from the outset.

Pupillary abnormalities vary with the site of the lesion and include midsized fixed pupils with midbrain involvement and pinpoint pupils with pontine lesions. Vertically skewed deviation of the eyes is common, and horizontal eye movements may be absent or asymmetric during doll's-head or cold-water caloric testing. Conjugate eye deviation, if present, is directed away from the side of the lesion and toward the hemiparesis (see Figure 7-17). Vertical eye movements may be impaired or intact. Symmetric or asymmetric signs, such as hemiparesis, hyperreflexia, and Babinski responses, may be present. There is no blood in the CSF.

Treatment & Prognosis

Conventional treatment involves antiplatelet agents or anticoagulation for progressive subtotal basilar artery thrombosis, despite the absence of clear evidence of efficacy for either strategy. The prognosis depends directly on the degree of brainstem injury as represented by depth of decreased consciousness or coma. Eligible patients should be treated with intravenous t-PA. For complete occlusion, endovascular thrombectomy should be considered, and some patients with prolonged symptoms (even beyond 6 hours from onset) may benefit, especially if symptoms have been progressive or fluctuating.

Additional discussion is found in Chapter 13, Stroke.

PONTINE HEMORRHAGE

Pontine hemorrhage occurs almost exclusively in hypertensive patients, but only approximately 6% of hypertensive intracerebral hemorrhages are at this site. The sudden, "apoplectic" onset of coma is the hallmark of this syndrome. Physical examination reveals many of the findings noted in basilar artery infarction, but preceding transient ischemic episodes do not occur. Features especially suggestive of pontine involvement include pinpoint pupils, loss of horizontal eye movements, and ocular bobbing (spontaneous, brisk, periodic, mainly conjugate, downward movements of the eyes, with slower return to the primary position). Hyperthermia, with temperature elevations to 39.5°C (103°F) or more, occurs in most patients who survive for more than a few hours. The diagnosis is made by CT scan or MRI. CSF is grossly bloody and under increased pressure, but lumbar puncture is not indicated. There is no effective treatment. Pontine hemorrhage is considered in greater detail in Chapter 13, Stroke.

CEREBELLAR HEMORRHAGE OR INFARCTION

The clinical presentation of cerebellar hemorrhage or infarction ranges from sudden onset of coma with rapid evolution to death to a syndrome in which headache, dizziness, vomiting, and inability to stand progress to coma over hours or even several days. Acute deterioration may occur without warning; this emphasizes the need for careful observation and early treatment of all patients. CT scan or MRI confirms the diagnosis.

Surgical decompression may produce dramatic reduction of symptoms, and with proper surgical treatment, lethargic or even stuporous patients may survive with minimal or no residual deficits and intact intellect. Current treatment guidelines emphasize surgical hematoma evacuation in potentially salvageable patients, and this includes those in deep coma. Salvageability likely decreases with longer duration of coma.

Additional discussion of these disorders can be found in Chapter 13, Stroke.

POSTERIOR FOSSA SUBDURAL & EPIDURAL HEMATOMAS

These very uncommon lesions have similar clinical pictures and are important to recognize because they are treatable. Occipital trauma typically precedes the onset of brainstem involvement by hours to many weeks. Physical findings result from extra-axial (extrinsic) compression of the brainstem and include ataxia, nystagmus, vertigo, vomiting, and progressive obtundation. Nuchal rigidity may be present, as may papilledema in more chronic cases. CT scans of the skull often reveal a fracture line crossing the transverse or sigmoid sinus. The source of the hematoma is the traumatic tearing of these vessels. Examination of the CSF is not helpful. Treatment is by surgical decompression.

DIFFUSE ENCEPHALOPATHIES

MENINGITIS & ENCEPHALITIS

Meningitis and encephalitis may be manifested by an acute confusional state (Chapter 4) or coma and are characteristically associated with fever and headache. In meningitis, signs of meningeal irritation are also typically present and should be sought meticulously so that lumbar puncture, diagnosis, and treatment can be undertaken promptly. These signs include resistance of the neck to full forward flexion, knee flexion during passive neck flexion, and flexion of the neck or contralateral knee during passive elevation of the extended straight leg (see Figure 1-5). Meningeal signs may be absent in encephalitis without meningeal involvement and in meningitis occurring at the extremes of age, in patients who are deeply comatose, or in those who are immunosuppressed. Findings on neurologic examination are usually symmetric, but focal features may be seen in certain infections, such as herpes simplex encephalitis or bacterial meningitis complicated by vasculitis. CSF findings and treatment are considered in Chapter 4, Confusional States. If signs of meningeal irritation are present, CSF examination should not be delayed in order to obtain a CT scan.

SUBARACHNOID HEMORRHAGE

In subarachnoid hemorrhage, discussed in detail in Chapter 6, Headache & Facial Pain, symptoms begin suddenly and almost always include headache, which is typically, but not invariably, severe. Consciousness is frequently lost, either transiently or permanently, at onset. Decerebrate posturing or, rarely, seizures may occur at this time. Other than oculomotor (III) or abducens (VI) nerve palsies, prominent focal neurologic signs are uncommon, although bilateral extensor plantar responses occur frequently. Subarachnoid blood causes meningeal irritation and meningeal signs. Examination of the optic fundi may show acute hemorrhages from suddenly increased intracranial pressure or the more classic superficial subhyaloid hemorrhages (see Figure 6-3). The CSF is bloody and the CT brain scan shows blood in the subarachnoid space (see Figure 6-5).

HYPOGLYCEMIA

▶ Etiology

Hypoglycemic encephalopathy and coma usually result from insulin overdose. Other causes include alcoholism, severe liver disease, oral hypoglycemic agents, insulin-secreting neoplasms (insulinoma), and large retroperitoneal tumors.

▶ Clinical Findings

As the blood glucose level declines, signs of sympathetic nervous system hyperactivity (tachycardia, sweating, and anxiety) appear and may warn patients of hypoglycemia. These prodromal symptoms may be absent, however, in patients with diabetic autonomic neuropathy. Neurologic findings in hypoglycemia include seizures, focal neurologic signs that may alternate sides, delirium, stupor, and coma. Progressive hypothermia is common.

▶ Investigative Studies

There is no precise correlation between blood glucose levels and symptoms; thus, a level of 30 mg/dL can be associated with coma in one patient, delirium in a second, and hemiparesis with preserved consciousness in a third. Coma, stupor, and confusion have been reported with blood glucose concentrations of 2 to 28, 8 to 59, and 9 to 60 mg/dL, respectively.

▶ Treatment

Permanent brain damage from hypoglycemia can be avoided if glucose is rapidly administered intravenously, orally, or by nasogastric tube. Because hypoglycemia is so easily treated and because a delay in treatment can have tragic consequences, every patient presenting with altered consciousness (acute confusional state, coma, or psychosis) should have blood drawn for subsequent glucose determination and immediately receive 50 mL of 50% dextrose intravenously. This allows blood to be analyzed without delaying therapy.

▶ Prognosis

The duration of hypoglycemia that will result in permanent damage to the brain is variable. Hypoglycemic coma may be tolerated for 60 to 90 minutes, but once the stage of flaccidity with hyporeflexia has been reached, glucose must be administered within 15 minutes if recovery is to be expected. If the brain has not been irreparably damaged, full recovery should occur within seconds after intravenous administration of glucose and within 10 to 30 minutes after nasogastric administration. Rapid and complete recovery is the rule, but improvement to full normality may sometimes take hours to several days. Any lingering signs or symptoms suggest irreversible brain damage from hypoglycemia or an additional neuropathologic process.

GLOBAL CEREBRAL ISCHEMIA

Global cerebral ischemia produces encephalopathy and coma, which occur most often after cardiac arrest. The pupils dilate rapidly, and there may be tonic, often opisthotonic, posturing with a few seizure-like tonic–clonic movements. Fecal incontinence is common.

If cerebral perfusion is promptly reestablished, recovery can occur and begins at the brainstem level with the return of reflex eye movements and pupillary function. Reflex motor activity (extensor or flexor posturing) then gives way to purposive movements, and consciousness is regained.

Prognosis is related to the rapidity with which brain function returns (**Table 3-8**). Patients without pupillary reactivity within 1 day—or those who fail to regain consciousness within 4 days—have a poor prognosis.

Persistent impairment of brainstem function (unreactive pupils) in adults after the return of cardiac function essentially precludes meaningful recovery. Incomplete recovery may occur, leading to the return of brainstem function and wakefulness (ie, eye opening with sleep–wake cycles) without higher-level intellectual functions. The condition of such patients—awake but not aware—has been termed **persistent vegetative state** (see later). Although such an outcome is possible after other major brain insults such as trauma, bihemispheric stroke, or subarachnoid hemorrhage, global ischemia is the most common cause.

Table 3-8. Prognostic Signs in Normothermic Coma From Global Cerebral Ischemia.

	Probability of Recovering Independent Function (%)			
	Time Since Onset of Coma (days)			
Sign	0	1	3	7
No verbal response	13	8	5	6
No eye opening	11	6	4	0
Unreactive pupils	0	0	0	0
No spontaneous eye movements	6	5	2	0
No caloric responses	5	6	6	0
Extensor posturing	18	0	0	0
Flexor posturing	14	3	0	0
Absent motor responses	4	3	0	0

Data from Levy DE, Caronna JJ, Singer BH, Lapinski RH, Frydman H, Plum F. JAMA. 1985 Mar 8;253(10):1420-6.

The advent of therapeutic hypothermia (now termed Targeted Temperature Management [TTM]) to treat patients in coma after resuscitation from cardiac arrest has improved prognosis but has also required a reassessment of the prognostic indicators summarized in Table 3-8 for normothermic patients. Debate exists about whether prognostic assessment at 72 hours after rewarming (therefore 96 hours post-arrest) allows sufficient time for accurate assessment, and many advocate a longer observation period. Loss of pupillary light reflex remains a grave prognostic sign, while motor responsiveness, prognostic in normothermic anoxia 3 days out, is of uncertain significance in hypothermia-treated patients. A combination of brainstem signs, EEG findings, and the results of somatosensory-evoked potential studies is increasingly used for prognostication in many centers.

DRUG INTOXICATION

▶ Sedative Drugs

Sedative drug overdose is the most common cause of coma in many series; barbiturates and benzodiazepines are the prototypical drugs.

Coma is preceded by a period of intoxication marked by prominent nystagmus in all directions of gaze, dysarthria, and ataxia. Shortly after consciousness is lost, the neurologic examination may briefly suggest a structural lesion affecting motor pathways, with hyperreflexia, ankle clonus, extensor plantar responses, and (rarely) decorticate or decerebrate posturing. However, the characteristic feature of sedative-hypnotic overdose is the absence of eye movements on doll's-head or cold-water caloric testing, with preserved pupillary reactivity. Rarely, concentrations of barbiturates or other sedative drugs sufficient to produce severe hypotension and respiratory depression requiring pressors and ventilatory support can also compromise pupillary reactivity, resulting in pupils 2 to 3 mm in diameter that are nonreactive to light. Bullous skin eruptions and hypothermia are also characteristic of barbiturate-induced coma.

The electroencephalogram (EEG) may be flat—and in overdose with long-acting barbiturates may remain isoelectric for 24 hours or more—yet full recovery will occur with support of cardiopulmonary function.

Treatment should be supportive, centered on maintaining adequate ventilation and circulation. Barbiturates are dialyzable, but with shorter-acting barbiturates, morbidity and mortality rates are lower in more conservatively managed patients. The benzodiazepine-receptor antagonist **flumazenil** (0.2-0.3 mg intravenously, repeated once, then 0.1-mg intravenous dosing to maximum of 1 mg) can be used to reverse sedative drug intoxication in some cases, but can precipitate status epilepticus by unmasking tricyclic antidepressant–induced seizures in patients with mixed overdose.

Ethanol

Ethanol overdose produces a syndrome similar to that seen with sedative drug overdose, although nystagmus during wakefulness, early impairment of lateral eye movements, and progression to coma are not as common. Peripheral vasodilation is prominent, as are tachycardia, hypotension, and hypothermia. Stupor is typically associated with blood ethanol levels of 250 to 300 mg/dL and coma with levels of 300 to 400 mg/dL, but alcoholic patients who have developed tolerance to the drug may remain awake and even apparently sober with considerably higher levels.

Opioids

Opioid overdose is characterized by pupillary constriction (which can also be produced by miotic eye drops, pontine hemorrhage, Argyll Robertson pupils, and organophosphate poisoning). The diagnosis of opioid intoxication is confirmed by rapid pupillary dilation and awakening after intravenous administration of 0.4 to 1.2 mg of the opioid antagonist naloxone. The duration of action of naloxone is typically 1 to 4 hours. Repeated doses may therefore be necessary after intoxication with long-acting opioids such as methadone.

HEPATIC ENCEPHALOPATHY

Clinical Findings

Hepatic encephalopathy leading to coma can occur in patients with severe liver disease, especially those with portacaval shunting. Jaundice need not be present. Coma may be precipitated by an acute insult, especially gastrointestinal hemorrhage. The production of ammonia by colonic bacteria may contribute to coma pathogenesis. Neuronal depression may result from multiple pathophysiologic mechanisms: an increase in inhibitory γ-aminobutyric acid–mediated neurotransmission from elevated levels of endogenous benzodiazepine-receptor agonists in the brain, perhaps via neuroinflammation and by way of brain edema in fulminant (acute) hepatic failure. As in other metabolic encephalopathies, the patient presents with either somnolence or delirium. Asterixis may be especially prominent. Muscle tone is often increased, hyperreflexia is common, and alternating hemiparesis and decorticate or decerebrate posturing have been described. Generalized and focal seizures occur but are infrequent. More details are provided in Chapter 4, Confusional States.

Investigative Studies

A helpful diagnostic clue is the nearly invariable presence of hyperventilation with resultant respiratory alkalosis; however, serum bicarbonate levels are rarely depressed below 16 mEq/L. The CSF is usually normal but may appear yellow (xanthochromic) in patients with serum bilirubin levels greater than 4 to 6 mg/dL. The diagnosis is confirmed by an elevated CSF glutamine concentration. Coma is usually associated with concentrations above 50 mg/dL but may occur with values as low as 35 mg/dL. Hepatic encephalopathy is treated by controlling gastrointestinal bleeding or systemic infection, decreasing protein intake to less than 20 g/d, and decreasing intracolonic pH with lactulose (30 mg orally 2-3 times per day or titrated to produce 2-4 bowel movements daily). Abdominal cramping may occur during the first 48 hours of lactulose treatment. Production of ammonia by colonic bacteria may be reduced with neomycin 6 g/d orally in three or four divided doses. Rifaximin, a nonabsorbable antibiotic, can be used as a lactulose adjunct to attenuate ammonia from colonic bacteria.

HYPEROSMOLAR STATES

Coma with focal seizures is a common presentation of the hyperosmolar state, which is most often associated with nonketotic hyperglycemia. Hyperosmolar nonketotic hyperglycemia is discussed in Chapter 4, Confusional States.

HYPONATREMIA

Hyponatremia can cause neurologic symptoms if serum sodium levels fall below 120 mEq/L, especially when the serum sodium level falls rapidly. Delirium and seizures are common presenting features. Hyponatremia is considered in detail in Chapter 4, Confusional States.

HYPOTHERMIA

All patients with temperatures below 26°C (79°F) are comatose, whereas mild hypothermia (>32.2°C [90°F]) does not cause coma. Causes of coma with hypothermia include hypoglycemia, drug intoxication (sedatives, tricyclics, phenothiazines), Wernicke encephalopathy, hypothyroidism (myxedema), and in the elderly, hypothermia associated with sepsis. Exposure can also produce hypothermia, such as may occur when a structural brain lesion causes acute coma out of doors or in another unheated area; therefore, structural lesions should not be excluded from consideration in the differential diagnosis of coma with hypothermia.

On physical examination, the patient is obviously cold to the touch but may not be shivering (which ceases at temperatures <32.5°C [90.5°F]). Neurologic examination shows the patient to be unresponsive to pain, with diffusely increased muscle tone. Pupillary reactions may be sluggish or even absent.

The ECG may show prolonged PR, QRS, and QT intervals; bradycardia; and characteristic J-point elevation (Osborn waves). Serum creatine kinase may be elevated in the absence of myocardial infarction. Arterial blood gas values and pH must be corrected for temperature, otherwise, falsely high PO_2 and PCO_2 and falsely low pH values will be reported. EEG shows burst suppression at 22°C (71°F) and is isoelectric at 18-20°C (64-68°F).

Treatment is aimed at the underlying disease responsible for hypothermia and at restoration of normal body temperature. The optimal method and speed of rewarming are controversial, but passive rewarming with blankets in a warm room is an effective and simple treatment. Ventricular fibrillation may occur during rewarming. Because warming produces vasodilation and can lead to hypotension, intravenous fluids may be required.

Most patients who recover from hypothermia do so without neurologic sequelae. Except in myxedema, there is no direct correlation between recorded temperature and survival. Death, when it occurs, is caused by the underlying disease process responsible for hypothermia or by ventricular fibrillation, to which the human myocardium becomes especially susceptible at temperatures less than 30°C (86°F); myocardial sensitivity is maximal below 21 to 24°C (70-75°F).

HYPERTHERMIA

At body temperatures exceeding 42 to 43°C (107.6-109.4°F), the brain's metabolic activity cannot meet the increased energy demands, and coma ensues. There is associated multi-organ system immunological and inflammatory involvement. The most common cause of hyperthermia is exposure to elevated environmental temperatures with or without associated exertion (**heat stroke**). Additional causes include status epilepticus, idiosyncratic reactions to halogenated inhalational anesthetics (**malignant hyperthermia**) or antipsychotic drugs (**neuroleptic malignant syndrome**), anticholinergic drugs, hypothalamic damage, and delirium tremens. Patients surviving pontine hemorrhage for more than a few hours have centrally mediated temperature elevations ranging from 38.5 to 42.8°C (101.3-109°F).

The neurologic examination in hyperthermia reveals reactive pupils and a diffuse increase in muscle tone, as well as coma. Tonic/clonic seizures can occur.

Treatment is immediate reduction of body temperature to 39°C (102.2°F) by sponging the patient with ice water and alcohol and using an electric fan or cooling blanket. Care must be taken to prevent overhydration, because cooling results in vasoconstriction that may produce pulmonary edema in volume-expanded patients.

SEIZURE OR PROLONGED POSTICTAL STATE

Status epilepticus should always be considered in the differential diagnosis of coma. Motor activity may be restricted to repetitive movements of part of a single limb or one side of the face. Although these signs of seizure activity can be subtle, they must not escape notice: Status epilepticus requires urgent treatment (see Chapter 12, Seizures & Syncope).

Coma may also be due to a prolonged postictal state, which is also discussed in Chapter 12.

OTHER DIFFUSE ENCEPHALOPATHIES

Rare causes of coma include multifocal disorders that present as metabolic coma because of their diffuse effect upon the brain: disseminated intravascular coagulopathy, sepsis, pancreatitis, vasculitis, thrombotic thrombocytopenic purpura, fat emboli, hypertensive encephalopathy, and diffuse micrometastases.

▼ DIFFERENTIAL DIAGNOSIS

Coma can be confused with a variety of psychiatric and neurologic disorders.

PSYCHOGENIC UNRESPONSIVENESS

Psychogenic unresponsiveness is a diagnosis of exclusion that should be made only on the basis of compelling evidence. It may be a manifestation of schizophrenia (catatonic type), somatoform disorders (conversion disorder or somatization disorder), or malingering.

The general physical examination reveals no abnormalities; neurologic examination generally reveals symmetrically decreased muscle tone, normal reflexes, and a normal (flexor) response to plantar stimulation. The pupils are 2 to 3 mm in diameter or occasionally larger and respond briskly to light. Lateral eye movements on doll's-head testing may or may not be present because visual fixation can suppress this reflex. The slow conjugate roving eye movements of metabolic coma cannot be imitated, however, and, if present, are incompatible with a diagnosis of psychogenic unresponsiveness. Likewise, the slow, often asymmetric and incomplete eye closure commonly seen after the eyes of a comatose patient are passively opened cannot be voluntarily reproduced. The patient with psychogenic unresponsiveness usually exhibits some voluntary muscle tone in the eyelids during passive eye opening. A helpful confirmatory test is irrigation of the tympanic membrane with cold water. Brisk nystagmus is the characteristic response in conscious patients, whereas no nystagmus occurs in coma. The EEG in psychogenic unresponsiveness is that of a normal awake person.

PERSISTENT VEGETATIVE STATE

Some patients who are comatose because of cerebral hypoxia, global cerebral ischemia, head trauma, or bilateral hemispheric strokes (**Figure 3-7**) regain wakefulness but not awareness. If this persists for at least 1 month, it is termed a **persistent vegetative state**. Such patients exhibit spontaneous eye opening and sleep–wake cycles, which distinguish them from patients in coma, and have intact brainstem and autonomic function. However, they neither comprehend nor produce language, and they make no purposeful motor responses. This condition may persist

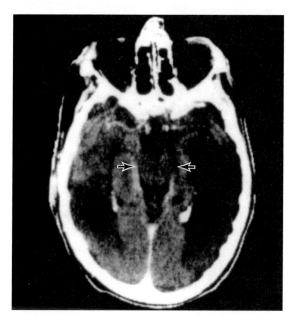

▲ **Figure 3-7.** CT brain scan (contrast-enhanced) of a patient with bilateral middle cerebral artery infarcts who is in a persistent vegetative state. The reticular activating system in the intact midbrain (**arrows**) allows wakefulness, but the bihemispheric lesions preclude awareness.

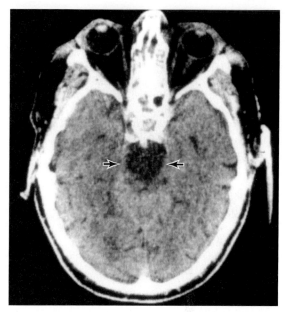

▲ **Figure 3-8.** CT brain scan (contrast-enhanced) of a man with basilar artery occlusion who exhibits the "locked-in" syndrome. The pontine infarction (**arrows**) is below the level of the reticular activating system, allowing wakefulness, but the bilateral descending motor tracts have been transected.

for years. Recovery of consciousness from nontraumatic causes is rare after 3 months, and recovery from traumatic causes is rare after 12 months. A subset of these patients may have minimal but definite evidence of environmental awareness, which has been referred to as a **minimally conscious state**. Late recovery of responsiveness with severe residual disability has been reported.

LOCKED-IN SYNDROME

Because the portion of the reticular formation responsible for consciousness lies above the level of the mid pons, functional transection of the brainstem below this level—by pontine infarction (**Figure 3-8**), hemorrhage, central pontine myelinolysis, tumor, or encephalitis—can interrupt descending neural pathways to produce an akinetic and mute state, with preserved consciousness. Such patients appear comatose but are awake and alert although mute and quadriplegic. Decerebrate posturing or flexor spasms may be seen. The diagnosis is made by noting that voluntary eye opening, vertical eye movements, ocular convergence, or some combination of these volitional midbrain-mediated movements is preserved. During the examination of any apparently comatose patient, the patient should be told to "open your eyes," "look up," "look down," and "look at the tip of your nose" to elicit such

movements. The EEG is normal. Outcome is variable and related to the underlying cause and the extent of the brainstem lesion. Mortality, usually from pneumonia, is approximately 70% when the cause is a vascular disturbance and approximately 40% in nonvascular cases. Survivors may recover partially or completely over a period of weeks to months.

BRAIN DEATH

Current standards for the determination of brain death, developed by the President's Commission for the Study of Ethical Problems in Medicine and Biomedical and Behavioral Research (1981), are summarized here. Irreversible cessation of all brain function is required for a diagnosis of brain death. The diagnosis of brain death in children younger than 5 years must be made with caution.

CESSATION OF BRAIN FUNCTION

▶ **Unresponsiveness**

The patient must be unresponsive to sensory input, including speech and pain.

The presence of seizures or decorticate/decerebrate posturing is incompatible with brain death.

▶ Absent Brainstem Reflexes

Pupillary, corneal, and oropharyngeal responses are absent, and attempts to elicit eye movements with doll's-head and cold-water caloric testing are unsuccessful. Respiratory responses are also absent, with no ventilatory effort after the patient's PCO_2 is permitted to rise to 60 mm Hg for maximal ventilatory stimulation, while oxygenation is maintained by giving 100% oxygen by a cannula inserted into the endotracheal tube (apnea test).

IRREVERSIBILITY OF BRAIN DYSFUNCTION

The cause of coma must be known, it must be adequate to explain the clinical picture, and it must be irreversible. Sedative drug intoxication, hypothermia (<32.2°C [90°F]), neuromuscular blockade, and shock must be ruled out because these conditions can produce a clinical picture that resembles brain death, but in which neurologic recovery may still be possible.

PERSISTENCE OF BRAIN DYSFUNCTION

The criteria for brain death described in the preceding section must persist for an appropriate length of time, as follows:

1. Six hours with a confirmatory isoelectric (flat) EEG, performed according to the technical standards of the American Electroencephalographic Society.
2. Twelve hours without a confirmatory isoelectric EEG.
3. Twenty-four hours for anoxic brain injury without a confirmatory isoelectric EEG.

ADDITIONAL CONFIRMATORY TESTS

Demonstrating the absence of cerebral blood flow confirms brain death without a waiting period. Cerebral angiography provides the most unequivocal assessment, although Doppler techniques and technetium imaging are used in some centers.

Confusional States

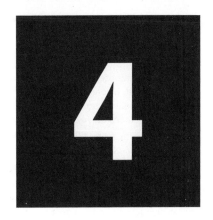

4

A confusional state, sometimes referred to as **encephalopathy** or **delirium,** is a state in which the level of consciousness is depressed, but to a lesser extent than in coma (unarousable unresponsiveness; see Chapter 3, Coma). In confusional states, responses to stimulation are at least semi-purposeful, whereas in coma, patients fail to respond to even painful stimulation or do so only in reflex fashion. Thus, the difference between a confusional state and coma is largely one of degree, and the causes overlap extensively.

▼ APPROACH TO DIAGNOSIS

Evaluation of a patient with altered consciousness is aimed first at characterizing the **nature** of the disorder (confusional state, coma, or a more chronic condition, such as dementia) and second at determining the **cause.**

A confusional state is most readily distinguished from dementia by the time course of impairment: confusional states are acute or subacute in onset, typically developing over hours to days, whereas dementia is a chronic disorder that evolves over months or years.

Certain causes of confusional state must be identified urgently because they may lead rapidly to severe structural brain damage or death, which prompt treatment can prevent: examples include hypoglycemia, bacterial meningitis, subarachnoid hemorrhage, traumatic intracranial hemorrhage, and Wernicke encephalopathy (**Table 4-1**).

HISTORY

▶ History of Present Illness

The history should establish the time course of the disorder and provide clues to its nature and cause.

Confusional states are acute to subacute in onset, whereas dementias are chronic disorders. In either case, a relative or friend may be the best source of information about the patient's previous level of functioning, the time when dysfunction became evident, and the nature of observed changes.

▶ Past History

Preexisting conditions that predispose to confusional states should be noted, such as alcoholism (intoxication or withdrawal, or Wernicke encephalopathy), other drug abuse (intoxication or infection), diabetes (hypo- or hyperglycemia), heart disease (stroke), epilepsy (seizures or postictal state), and head trauma (concussion, intracranial hemorrhage). A thorough medication history is also important, because many therapeutic drugs can impair consciousness as a side effect.

GENERAL PHYSICAL EXAMINATION

Findings on general physical examination of a confused patient that suggest specific causes are listed in **Table 4-2.**

NEUROLOGIC EXAMINATION

▶ Mental Status Examination

The mental status examination of a patient with a possible confusional state should focus on confirming that the level of consciousness is depressed by evaluating the following functions.

A. **Wakefulness**—In confusional states, the patient often appears sleepy; this may alternate with apparent hyperalertness.

Table 4-1. Most Urgent Causes of Confusional States.

Cause	Clinical Evidence	Laboratory Confirmation	Treatment
Hypoglycemia	Tachycardia, sweating, and dilated pupils, sometimes progressing to mimic herniation, with or without lateralized signs	Low blood glucose	IV dextrose
Acute bacterial meningitis	Headache, fever, Brudzinski or Kernig sign (stiff neck)	CSF pleocytosis, positive Gram stain, low glucose, and increased protein	IV antibiotics
Subarachnoid hemorrhage	Headache, hypertension, retinal hemorrhages, Brudzinski or Kernig sign (stiff neck)	Non-clearing red blood cells in CSF; subarachnoid blood and aneurysm or other vascular malformation on CT scan or MRI	Surgical ablation of aneurysm or other vascular malformation
Traumatic intracranial hemorrhage	Headache, hypertension, lateralized neurologic signs	Epidural, subdural, or intracerebral hemorrhage on CT scan or MRI	Surgical evacuation of epidural or subdural (or in some cases intracerebral) hematoma
Wernicke encephalopathy	Ophthalmoplegia, ataxia	Macrocytic anemia may be present	IV thiamine and dextrose

Table 4-2. General Physical Examination in Confusional States.

Finding	Most Suggestive of
Vital signs	
Fever	Infectious meningitis, anticholinergic or sympathomimetic intoxication, ethanol or sedative drug withdrawal, sepsis
Hypothermia	Ethanol or sedative drug intoxication, hepatic encephalopathy, hypoglycemia, hypothyroidism, sepsis
Hypertension	Anticholinergic or sympathomimetic intoxication, ethanol or sedative drug withdrawal, hypertensive encephalopathy, subarachnoid hemorrhage
Tachycardia	Anticholinergic or sympathomimetic intoxication, ethanol or sedative drug withdrawal, hyperthyroidism, sepsis
Bradycardia	Hypothyroidism
Hyperventilation	Hepatic encephalopathy, hyperglycemia, sepsis
Head and neck	
Neck stiffness	Meningitis, subarachnoid hemorrhage
Battle sign or raccoon eyes	Head trauma
Hemotympanum	Head trauma
CSF oto- or rhinorrhea	Head trauma
Skin and mucous membranes	
Jaundice	Hepatic encephalopathy, malaria
Petechial rash	Meningococcal meningitis, disseminated intravascular coagulation, thrombotic thrombocytopenic purpura
Chest, abdomen, and rectal	
Heart murmur	Stroke
Ascites	Hepatic encephalopathy
Rectal bleeding	Hepatic encephalopathy

B. **Arousability**—In mild confusional states, the patient may be arousable when spoken to or lightly shaken. As consciousness is further impaired, the intensity of stimulation required for arousal increases, the duration of arousal declines, and the responses elicited become less purposeful.

C. **Orientation**—With a confusional state, the patient loses orientation to time and later to place.

D. **Attention**—Confused patients are inattentive, as demonstrated by the inability to immediately repeat a list of numbers or words.

E. **Memory**—Confusion impairs short-term memory so that the patient cannot remember a brief list of items when asked to repeat them after a delay of several minutes.

An important pitfall to avoid is mistaking **receptive or fluent (Wernicke) aphasia** for confusion. Although patients with receptive aphasia cannot comprehend written or spoken language and may speak incomprehensibly, they appear normally awake and alert, can respond appropriately to nonverbal commands (such as gestures), and usually have associated right-sided neurologic abnormalities such as hemiparesis, hemisensory deficit, and visual field deficits.

▶ Signs of Diffuse Versus Focal Disorders Causing Confusional States

Certain neurologic findings help distinguish diffuse (including metabolic) from focal (including mass) lesions as the likely cause of a confusional state.

A. **Diffuse disorders**—Suggestive findings include fever or hypothermia, nystagmus, tremor, asterixis, and myoclonus.

B. **Focal disorders**—Suggestive findings include signs of head trauma, papilledema, hemiparesis, focal seizures, asymmetric hyperreflexia, and unilateral Babinski signs.

▶ Signs of Specific Disorders Causing Confusional States

Neurologic findings that suggest specific causes of a confusional state are listed in **Table 4-3**.

LABORATORY INVESTIGATIONS

Laboratory tests that suggest specific causes of a confusional state are listed in **Table 4-4**. Cerebrospinal fluid (CSF) profiles in disorders associated with confusional states are given in **Table 4-5**.

▼ CAUSES OF CONFUSIONAL STATES

DRUGS

Many drugs can cause confusional states, especially when taken in greater than customary doses, in combination with other drugs, by patients with altered drug metabolism from hepatic or renal failure, by the elderly, or in those with preexisting cognitive impairment. Evaluation of any patient with a confusional state should always include a

Table 4-3. Neurologic Examination in Confusional States.

Finding	Most Suggestive of
Cranial nerves	
Papilledema	Hypertensive encephalopathy, intracranial mass
Dilated pupils	Ethanol or sedative drug withdrawal, anticholinergic or sympathomimetic intoxication
Constricted pupils	Opioid intoxication
Nystagmus or ophthalmoplegia	Ethanol, sedative drug, dissociative anesthetic or entactogen intoxication; Wernicke encephalopathy; vertebrobasilar ischemia
Motor function	
Tremor	Ethanol or sedative drug withdrawal, sympathomimetic intoxication, hyperthyroidism
Asterixis	Metabolic encephalopathy
Hemiparesis	Hypoglycemia, hyperglycemia, vascular disorders, head trauma
Coordination	
Ataxia	Ethanol or sedative drug intoxication, Wernicke encephalopathy, vertebrobasilar ischemia
Other	
Seizures	Ethanol or sedative drug withdrawal, hypoglycemia, hyperglycemia, head trauma

thorough review of prescribed and over-the-counter medications. Recreational and psychotherapeutic drugs are the most likely to produce altered consciousness (**Table 4-6**).

ALCOHOL INTOXICATION

Ethyl alcohol (ethanol) intoxication produces a confusional state with nystagmus, dysarthria, and limb and gait ataxia. In nonalcoholics, signs correlate roughly with blood alcohol levels, but chronic alcoholics, who have developed tolerance, may have very high levels without appearing intoxicated. Laboratory studies useful in confirming the diagnosis include blood alcohol levels and serum osmolality, which exceeds the calculated osmolality (2 × serum sodium + 1/20 serum glucose + 1/3 serum urea nitrogen) by 22 mOsm/L for every 100 mg/dL of alcohol. Intoxicated patients are at high risk for head trauma and hypoglycemia, and chronic alcoholism increases the risk of bacterial meningitis. Alcohol intoxication requires no treatment unless a withdrawal syndrome ensues, but thiamine

(200-500 mg three times daily by the intravenous route, for 3 days or until a normal diet is restored) should be given to prevent malnutrition-related Wernicke encephalopathy (discussed later in this chapter).

ALCOHOL WITHDRAWAL

Three common withdrawal syndromes are recognized (**Figure 4-1**). Patients with these syndromes are also at risk for Wernicke encephalopathy and should be given thiamine.

▶ Tremulousness & Hallucinations

This self-limited condition occurs within 2 days after cessation of drinking and is characterized by tremulousness, agitation, anorexia, nausea, insomnia, tachycardia, and hypertension. Confusion, if present, is mild. Illusions and hallucinations, usually visual, occur in approximately 25% of patients. Lorazepam (1-4 mg) or diazepam (5-20 mg), given intravenously every 5-15 minutes until calm and hourly thereafter to maintain light sedation, will terminate the syndrome and prevent more serious consequences of withdrawal.

▶ Seizures

Alcohol withdrawal seizures occur within 48 hours of abstinence and within 7-24 hours in approximately two-thirds of cases. Roughly 40% of patients who experience seizures have a single seizure; more than 90% have between one and six seizures. In approximately 85% of cases, the interval between the first and last seizures is 6 hours or less. Treatment is not usually required, as seizures cease spontaneously in most cases, but lorazepam 2 mg intravenously

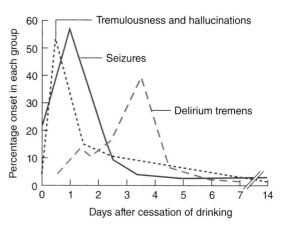

▲ **Figure 4-1.** Alcohol withdrawal syndromes in relation to the time since cessation of drinking. (Data from Victor M, Adams RD. The effect of alcohol on the nervous system. *Res Publ Assoc Res Nerv Ment Dis.* 1952;32: 526-573.)

Table 4-4. Laboratory Studies in Confusional States.

Test	Finding	Most Suggestive of
Blood		
WBC	Increased	Meningitis, encephalitis, sepsis
Hematocrit	Decreased	Wernicke encephalopathy, vitamin B12 deficiency, malaria, systemic lupus erythematosus, thrombotic thrombocytopenic purpura
Platelets	Decreased	Alcohol intoxication or withdrawal, vitamin B12 deficiency, disseminated intravascular coagulation, thrombotic thrombocytopenic purpura
PT and PTT	Increased	Hepatic encephalopathy, disseminated intravascular coagulation
Arterial blood gases	Metabolic acidosis	Diabetic ketoacidosis, lactic acidosis (postictal, shock, sepsis), toxins (methanol, ethylene glycol, salicylates, paraldehyde), uremia
	Respiratory acidosis	Pulmonary insufficiency, sedative drug overdose
	Respiratory alkalosis	Hepatic encephalopathy, pulmonary insufficiency, salicylates, sepsis
Sodium	Decreased	Hyponatremia
Urea nitrogen and creatinine	Increased	Uremia
Glucose	Increased or decreased	Hyperglycemia, hypoglycemia
Osmolality	Increased	Alcohol intoxication, hyperglycemia
Liver enzymes, ammonia	Increased	Hepatic encephalopathy
Thyroid hormones	Increased or decreased	Hyperthyroidism, hypothyroidism
Calcium	Increased or decreased	Hypercalcemia, hypocalcemia
Drug screen	Positive	Drug intoxication
Cultures	Positive	Acute bacterial meningitis, sepsis
FTA or MHA-TP	Positive	Syphilitic meningitis
HIV antibody titer	Positive	HIV infection
Urine, gastric aspirate		
Drug screen	Positive	Drug intoxication
Stool		
Occult blood	Positive	Hepatic encephalopathy
ECG		
	Tachyarrhythmia	Anticholinergic or sympathomimetic intoxication
Cerebrospinal fluid (see Table 4-5)		
CT brain scan or MRI		
	Various	Cerebral infarction, intracranial hemorrhage, head trauma, toxoplasmosis, herpes simplex encephalitis, subarachnoid hemorrhage
EEG		
	Epileptiform activity	Complex partial seizures, postictal state
	Triphasic waves	Hepatic encephalopathy
	Periodic complexes	Herpes simplex encephalitis

CT, computed tomography; EEG, electroencephalogram; FTA, fluorescent treponemal antibody; MHA-TP, microhemagglutination-*Treponema pallidum;* MRI, magnetic resonance imaging; PT, prothrombin time; PTT, partial thromboplastin time; WBC, white blood cells.

Table 4-5. Cerebrospinal Fluid (CSF) Profiles in Confusional States.

	Appearance	OP	RBC	WBC	Glucose	Protein[1]	Other	Cultures
Normal	Clear, colorless	70-200 mm H₂O	0/µL	≤5 mononuclear/µL	≥45 mg/dL	≤45 mg/dL	–	–
Acute bacterial meningitis	Cloudy	↑	Normal	↑↑ (PMN)	↓↓	↑↑	Gram stain, PCR, culture +	+
Tuberculous meningitis	Normal or cloudy	↑	Normal	↑ (MN)	→	↑	AFB stain, PCR +	±
Syphilitic meningitis	Normal or cloudy	Normal or ↑	Normal	↑ (MN)	→	↑	VDRL +	–
Fungal meningitis	Normal or cloudy	Normal or ↑	Normal	↑ (MN)	→	↑	India ink prep, cryptococcal antigen + (*Cryptococcus*)	±
Viral meningitis/encephalitis	Normal	Normal or ↑	Normal[2]	↑ (MN)[3]	Normal[4]	Normal or ↑	PCR +	±
Parasitic meningitis/encephalitis	Normal or cloudy	Normal or ↑	Normal	↑ (MN, E)	Normal	Normal or ↑	Organisms on wet mount	±
Leptomeningeal metastases	Normal or cloudy	Normal or ↑	Normal	Normal or ↑ (MN)	↓↓	Normal or ↑	Cytology +	–
Subarachnoid hemorrhage	Pink or red (supernatant yellow)	↑	↑	Normal or ↑ (PMN)[5]	Normal or ↓[5]	↑	–	–
Hepatic encephalopathy	Normal	Normal	Normal	Normal	Normal	Normal	Glutamine ↑	–

E, eosinophils often present; MN, mononuclear (lymphocytic or monocytic) predominance; OP, opening pressure; PCR, polymerase chain reaction; PMN, polymorphonuclear predominance; RBC, red blood cells; WBC, white blood cells; +, positive; –, negative; ±, can be positive or negative.
[1] Lumbar cerebrospinal fluid.
[2] Red blood cell count may be elevated in herpes simplex encephalitis.
[3] PMN predominance may be seen early in course.
[4] Glucose may be decreased in herpes or mumps infections.
[5] Pleocytosis and low glucose, sometimes seen several days after hemorrhage, reflect chemical meningitis caused by subarachnoid blood.

Table 4-6. Drug-Induced Confusional States.

Drug Class	Examples	Mechanism of Action	Intoxication Syndrome[1]				Antidote
			Level of Consciousness	Respiratory Depression	Pupils	Eye Movements	
Alcohols	Ethanol	GABA$_A$ receptor potentiator	Depressed	±	Normal	Nystagmus	None
Sedatives	Barbiturates Benzodiazepines	GABA$_A$ receptor agonists	Depressed or comatose	+	Normal	Impaired	Flumazenil (benzodiazepines)
Opiates	Heroin Oxycodone Hydrocodone	μ-Opiate receptor agonists	Depressed or comatose	+	Constricted	Normal	Naloxone
Anticholinergics	Tricyclic antidepressants	Muscarinic acetylcholine receptor antagonists	Agitated	−	Dilated	Normal	Physostigmine
Sympathomimetics	Dextroamphetamine Methamphetamine Cocaine	Catecholamine reuptake inhibitors and releasers	Agitated	−	Dilated	Normal	Haloperidol Phentolamine
Hallucinogens	LSD	Serotonin receptor agonists	Agitated	−	Normal or dilated	Normal	None
Dissociative anesthetics	Phencyclidine (PCP) Ketamine	NMDA receptor antagonists	Euphoric, agitated, depressed, or comatose	−	Normal	Nystagmus	None
Entactogens	MDMA (Ecstasy)	Serotonin and dopamine reuptake inhibitors and releasers	Euphoric	−	Dilated	Nystagmus	None
Synthetic cathinones (bath salts)	Mephedrone Methylone MDPV	Catecholamine reuptake inhibitors and releasers	Agitated	−	Dilated	Normal	None
γ-Hydroxybutyrate and prodrugs	γ-Hydroxybutyrate (GHB) γ-Butyrolactone 1,4-Butanediol	γ-Hydroxybutyrate and GABA$_B$ receptor agonists	Euphoric, agitated, depressed or comatose	−	Normal	Normal	None
Inhalants	Toluene Xylene	Unknown	Euphoric, depressed, or comatose	−	Normal	Normal	None
Synthetic cannabinoids (Spice, K2)	JWH-018 AMB-FUBINACA	CB1 cannabinoid receptor agonists	Agitated or depressed	−	Normal	Normal	None

[1]The most distinctive findings are (1) normal pupils with impaired eye movements in sedative-hypnotic overdose and (2) constricted pupils with intact eye movements in opiate overdose.

may reduce the number of seizures that occur. Unusual features such as focal seizures, prolonged duration of seizures (>6-12 hours), more than six seizures, status epilepticus, or a prolonged postictal state should prompt a search for other causes or complicating factors, such as head trauma or infection. The patient should be observed for 6-12 hours after the onset of seizures to make certain that atypical features suggesting another cause do not develop.

▶ Delirium Tremens

This most serious ethanol withdrawal syndrome typically begins 3-5 days after cessation of drinking and lasts for up to 72 hours. It is characterized by confusion, agitation, fever, sweating, tachycardia, hypertension, and hallucinations. Death may result from concomitant infection, pancreatitis, cardiovascular collapse, or trauma. Treatment consists of lorazepam or diazepam as described previously for tremulousness and hallucinations and correction of fluid and electrolyte abnormalities and hypoglycemia, if present. β-adrenergic receptor blockade with atenolol (50-100 mg/d) may be useful for patients with persistent hypertension or tachycardia.

SEDATIVE DRUG INTOXICATION

Sedative drugs include barbiturates, benzodiazepines, propofol, methaqualone, glutethimide, and chloral hydrate. The distinctive clinical features of sedative drug intoxication are a confusional state or coma with respiratory depression, reactive pupils, and **impaired eye movements**. Other common findings include hypotension, hypothermia, nystagmus, ataxia, dysarthria, and hyporeflexia; decerebrate or decorticate posturing can also occur. The differential diagnosis of altered consciousness with impaired eye movements includes structural brainstem lesions, but these usually affect the pupils as well. Sedative drug ingestion can be confirmed by toxicologic analysis of blood, urine, or gastric aspirate, but blood levels of short-acting sedatives do not correlate with clinical severity.

Management is directed at supporting respiratory and circulatory function while the drug is being cleared, primarily by hepatic metabolism. Patients with benzodiazepine intoxication can also be treated with flumazenil, 1 to 5 mg intravenously over 2 to 10 minutes, repeated every 20 to 30 minutes as needed.

Complications of sedative drug intoxication include aspiration pneumonia, hypotension, and renal failure. However, barring such complications, patients who arrive at the hospital with adequate cardiopulmonary function should survive without sequelae.

SEDATIVE DRUG WITHDRAWAL

Sedative drug withdrawal can produce confusional states, seizures, or a syndrome resembling delirium tremens. The likelihood and severity of these complications depend on the duration of drug intake and the dose and half-life of the drug, and are greatest in patients taking large doses of intermediate- or short-acting drugs for at least several weeks. Withdrawal syndromes typically develop 1 to 3 days after cessation of short-acting sedatives but may not appear until 1 week or more with longer-acting drugs. Sedative drug withdrawal can be confirmed by the failure of a normally sedating or hypnotic dose to produce signs of sedative drug intoxication (sedation, nystagmus, dysarthria, or ataxia). Symptoms and signs of withdrawal are usually self-limited, but myoclonus and seizures—most common in patients taking several times a drug's sedative dose daily—may require treatment.

OPIATES

Opiates (narcotics) include morphine, heroin, codeine, hydromorphone, oxycodone, hydrocodone, meperidine, fentanyl, and methadone. These drugs can produce analgesia, mood changes, confusional states, coma, respiratory depression, pulmonary edema, nausea and vomiting, pupillary constriction, hypotension, urinary retention, and reduced gastrointestinal motility. Chronic use is associated with tolerance and physical dependence.

The cardinal features of opiate overdose are **pinpoint pupils**, which usually constrict in bright light, and respiratory depression. Pinpoint pupils can also occur in pontine hemorrhage, but opiate overdose can be distinguished by the patient's response to the opiate antagonist **naloxone** and the preservation of horizontal eye movements. After administration of naloxone, pupillary dilation and full recovery of consciousness usually occur promptly. When large doses of opiates or multiple drug ingestions are involved, however, slight dilation of the pupils may be the only observable effect.

Treatment consists of intravenous administration of naloxone, 0.4-2.0 mg every 2-3 minutes, to a maximum of 10 mg. Ventilatory support is sometimes also required. An intranasal naloxone preparation is available but its effect is slower in onset. Because the action of naloxone may be as short as 1 hour—and many opiates are longer-acting—naloxone should be readministered as the patient's condition dictates. With appropriate treatment, patients should recover uneventfully.

ANTICHOLINERGICS

Muscarinic anticholinergic drugs are used to treat parkinsonism (eg, trihexyphenidyl), motion sickness (eg, dimenhydrinate), allergies (eg, diphenhydramine), gastrointestinal disturbances (eg, dicyclomine), and psychiatric disease (eg, antipsychotics, tricyclic antidepressants). Overdose with any of these agents can produce a confusional state with agitation, hallucinations, fixed and dilated pupils, blurred vision, dry skin and mucous membranes, flushing, fever, urinary retention, and tachycardia

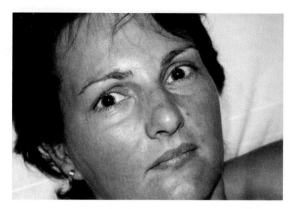

▲ **Figure 4-2.** Pupillary dilation and facial flushing in anticholinergic drug overdose. (Used with permission from Dodt C: Iatrogenic anticholinergic overdose. Dtsch Arztebl Int 2017; 114: 167.)

(**Figure 4-2**). In some cases, the diagnosis can be confirmed by toxicologic analysis of blood or urine. Symptoms usually resolve spontaneously, but treatment with the cholinesterase inhibitor physostigmine may be required if life-threatening cardiac arrhythmias occur. However, because physostigmine may produce bradycardia and seizures, it is rarely used.

SYMPATHOMIMETICS

Sympathomimetics include cocaine, amphetamine, methamphetamine, dextroamphetamine, methylphenidate, phentermine, fenfluramine, ephedrine, and antidepressants. Sympathomimetic intoxication can produce a confusional state with hallucinations, motor hyperactivity, stereotypic behavior, and paranoid psychosis. Examination shows tachycardia, hypertension, and dilated pupils. Hyperthermia, tremor, seizures, and cardiac arrhythmias may also occur, and cocaine or amphetamine use can be associated with stroke. Agitation is treated with benzodiazepines, psychosis with haloperidol, and hypertension with sodium nitroprusside or phentolamine.

HALLUCINOGENS

Hallucinogens include lysergic acid diethylamide (LSD), psilocybin, mescaline, ibogaine, and bufotenin. They do not usually produce confusional states that come to medical attention, but may cause anxiety, panic, hypertension, hyperthermia, and seizures. Benzodiazepines can be used to treat anxiety.

DISSOCIATIVE ANESTHETICS

Dissociative anesthetics include phencyclidine (PCP) and ketamine. Intoxication can produce drowsiness, agitation, disorientation, amnesia, hallucinations, paranoia, and violent behavior. Neurologic examination may show large or small pupils, horizontal and vertical nystagmus, ataxia, increased muscle tone, analgesia, hyperreflexia, and myoclonus. In severe cases, complications include hypertension, malignant hyperthermia, status epilepticus, coma, and death. Benzodiazepines may be useful for sedation and for treating muscle spasms, and antihypertensives, anticonvulsants, and dantrolene (for malignant hyperthermia) may be required. Symptoms and signs usually resolve within 24 hours.

ENTACTOGENS

Entactogens (also termed empathogens) are recreational drugs that evoke sensations of connectedness or empathy. Most, including MDMA (ecstasy), are amphetamine derivatives. Altered consciousness requiring medical attention is unusual, but jaw clenching, bruxism, and nystagmus are common, and adverse effects similar to those of hallucinogens (discussed previously) can occur. In addition, hyponatremia may result from a combination of drug-induced antidiuretic hormone release and polydipsia. Rhabdomyolysis and acute kidney injury are reported, and imaging studies are consistent with MDMA-induced damage to serotonergic nerve terminals in the brain.

SYNTHETIC CATHINONES

Synthetic cathinones are analogs of a stimulant alkaloid found in the khat plant. They are related to amphetamines and found in preparations sold as "bath salts". Clinical manifestations of cathinone intoxication include agitation, tachycardia, hypertension, and seizures. Psychosis and bizarre or violent behavior can occur.

γ-HYDROXYBUTYRATE

γ-Hydroxybutyrate and its prodrugs (eg, γ-butyrolactone and 1,4-butanediol) are so-called date-rape drugs, sometimes used to induce rapid somnolence or unconsciousness in prospective victims. Bradycardia and myoclonus may occur. In addition to assault, adverse effects include vomiting with aspiration and depressed respiration.

INHALANTS

These include volatile solvents (eg, glue), volatile nitrites (eg, amyl nitrite), anesthetics (eg, ether, chloroform, nitrous oxide), and propellants. Their pharmacologic actions are diverse, but most can produce euphoria followed by depression, and sometimes respiratory compromise. Withdrawal may be associated with irritability, anxiety, tremor, and seizures. There is no specific treatment.

SYNTHETIC CANNABINOIDS

Synthetic cannabinoids (eg, Spice, K2) are analogs of Δ^9-tetrahydrocannabinol (THC), the principal psychoactive constituent of marijuana, with more potent and purer agonist effects on CB1 cannabinoid receptors. As a consequence, they are much more likely than marijuana to produce adverse effects, including tachycardia, agitation, drowsiness, nausea, vomiting, and hallucinations.

ENDOCRINE & METABOLIC DISORDERS

HYPOGLYCEMIA

Hypoglycemia is an especially important cause of a confusional state, because its prompt recognition and treatment can prevent rapid progression from a reversible to an irreversible stage.

The most common cause of hypoglycemia is **insulin overdose** in diabetic patients (**Table 4-7**), but oral hypoglycemic drugs, alcoholism, malnutrition, hepatic failure, insulinoma, and non–insulin-secreting fibromas, sarcomas, or fibrosarcomas may also be responsible. Neurologic symptoms develop over minutes to hours. Although no strict correlation between blood glucose levels and the severity of neurologic dysfunction can be demonstrated, prolonged hypoglycemia at levels of 30 mg/dL or lower invariably leads to irreversible brain damage.

▶ Clinical Findings

Early signs of hypoglycemia include tachycardia, sweating, and pupillary dilation, which may be followed by a confusional state with somnolence or agitation at blood glucose levels less than ~50 mg/dL and by coma at under ~30 mg/dL. Neurologic dysfunction progresses in a rostral-caudal fashion (see Chapter 3, Coma) and may mimic a mass lesion causing transtentorial herniation. Coma ensues with spasticity, extensor plantar responses, and decorticate or decerebrate posturing. Signs of brainstem dysfunction then appear, including abnormal eye movements and loss of pupillary reflexes. Respiratory depression, bradycardia, hypotonia, and hyporeflexia signal that irreversible brain damage is imminent. Hypoglycemic coma may be associated with focal neurologic signs and focal or generalized seizures.

▶ Treatment

The diagnosis is confirmed by measuring blood glucose levels, but intravenous glucose (50 mL of 50% dextrose) should be given *immediately*, without waiting for the blood glucose level to be measured. Improvement in the level of consciousness occurs within minutes after glucose administration in patients with reversible hypoglycemic encephalopathy. In hypoglycemia caused by sulfonylurea antidiabetic drugs (eg, tolbutamide, glipizide, or glyburide), administration of glucose may stimulate insulin secretion, antagonizing the therapeutic effect. In such cases, octreotide (50-75 μg subcutaneously or intravenously) should be given to inhibit insulin release. Doubt as to whether encephalopathy in a diabetic is due to hypoglycemia or hyperglycemia should never delay dextrose administration, since the consequences of worsening hyperglycemia are less dire than those of failing to treat hypoglycemia.

HYPERGLYCEMIA

Two hyperglycemic syndromes, **diabetic ketoacidosis** (hyperglycemia, ketosis, and metabolic acidosis) and **hyperosmolar nonketotic hyperglycemia** (hyperglycemia and hyperosmolarity) (Table 4-7), can produce encephalopathy or coma, and may be the presenting manifestation of diabetes. Impaired cerebral metabolism, intravascular coagulation, and brain edema contribute to pathogenesis. Whereas the severity of hyperosmolarity correlates well with depression of consciousness, the degree of systemic acidosis does not.

Table 4-7. Features of Hypo- and Hyperglycemic Encephalopathies.

	Hypoglycemia	Diabetic Ketoacidosis	Hyperosmolar Nonketotic State
Precipitating factors	Antidiabetic overtreatment Concurrent illness Nutritional inadequacy	Antidiabetic noncompliance Infection New diagnosis	Infection Antidiabetic noncompliance New diagnosis
Blood glucose (mg/dL)	<60	>250	>600
Serum osmolality (mOsm/L)	<300	<320	>320
Ketosis	–	+	–
Metabolic acidosis	–	+	–
Confusion	Common	Uncommon	Common
Focal neurologic signs	+	–	+
Seizures	+	–	+

+, present; –, absent

Clinical Findings

Symptoms include blurred vision, dry skin, anorexia, polyuria, and polydipsia. Physical examination may show hypotension and other signs of dehydration, especially in hyperosmolar nonketotic hyperglycemia. Deep, rapid (Kussmaul) respiration characterizes diabetic ketoacidosis. Impairment of consciousness varies from mild confusion to coma. Focal neurologic signs and generalized or focal seizures are common in hyperosmolar nonketotic hyperglycemia. Laboratory findings are summarized in Table 4-7.

Treatment

Treatment is with intravenous fluids, regular insulin, potassium (if <5 mmol/L in blood), and bicarbonate (if arterial blood pH < 6.9); antibiotics are added for concurrent infection. Fluids should be given as 0.9% saline (1-2 L over 1-2 hours), followed by 0.9% or 0.45% saline (250-500 mL/hour) until blood glucose reaches ~200 mg/dL, and then 5% dextrose in 0.9% saline. Regular insulin is administered as a bolus of 0.1 U/kg, followed by continuous infusion at 0.1 U/kg/h; this is reduced to 0.05 U/kg/h when blood glucose reaches ~250 mg/dL and adjusted thereafter to maintain blood glucose at ~200 mg/dL. Blood glucose, electrolytes, urea nitrogen, and pH should be followed closely. Mortality is <1% in diabetic ketoacidosis but 5-16% in hyperosmolar nonketotic hyperglycemia; causes include delayed treatment due to misdiagnosis, sepsis, cardiovascular complications, and renal failure.

HYPOTHYROIDISM

The most common cause of hypothyroidism is Hashimoto thyroiditis. Symptoms and signs include fatigue, depression, weight gain, constipation, bradycardia, dry skin, and hair loss (**Figure 4-3**). Cognitive disturbances include flat affect, psychomotor retardation, agitation, and psychosis (**myxedema madness**); profound hypothyroidism can produce a confusional state, coma, or dementia. Findings on examination include hypothermia, dysarthria, deafness, and ataxia, but the most characteristic neurologic abnormality is delayed relaxation of the tendon reflexes. Untreated, hypothyroidism can progress to seizures, coma, and death.

Blood-test abnormalities include elevated thyroid-stimulating hormone (TSH) levels, low serum free tetraiodothyronine (T_4) levels, and antithyroglobulin and antithyroperoxidase antibodies. Hypoglycemia, hyponatremia, and respiratory acidosis may be present. CSF protein is typically elevated, and CSF pressure is occasionally increased. Treatment is of the underlying thyroid disorder. With severe myxedema madness or coma (myxedema crisis), this involves administration of levothyroxine (T_4; 500 μg, then 50-100 μg intravenously daily) and sometimes liothyronine (T_3; 10-20 μg, then 10 μg intravenously every 4-6 hours for 48 hours), with hydrocortisone (100 mg, then 25-50 mg intravenously every 8 hours) for adrenal insufficiency, which often coexists.

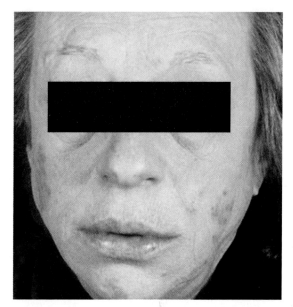

▲ **Figure 4-3.** Clinical features of hypothyroidism. The patient shows a lack of facial expression, together with pallor, dry skin, loss of hair in the lateral eyebrows, facial puffiness, and broadening of the nose. (Used with permission from Wolff K, Goldsmith LA, Katz SI, et al. *Fitzpatrick's Dermatology in General Medicine.* 7th ed. New York, NY: McGraw-Hill; 2007.)

HYPERTHYROIDISM

Hyperthyroidism (**thyrotoxicosis**) is most often due to Graves disease and produces anxiety, palpitations, sweating, and weight loss. Physical examination may show goiter, warm moist skin, and pretibial myxedema. Acute exacerbation of hyperthyroidism (**Figure 4-4**) may cause a confusional state, coma, or death. In younger patients, agitation, hallucinations, and psychosis are common (**activated thyrotoxic crisis**), whereas those older than age 50 tend to be apathetic and depressed (**apathetic thyrotoxic crisis**). Seizures may occur. Neurologic examination shows exophthalmos, restricted eye movements, exaggerated physiologic action tremor, and hyperreflexia; ankle clonus and extensor plantar responses are rare. The diagnosis is confirmed by low serum TSH, elevated free T_3, antithyroglobulin and antithyroperoxidase antibodies, and increased ^{123}I uptake on thyroid scan. Treatments include propranolol 60 mg orally once or twice daily, increasing gradually to 320 mg daily; methimazole 30-60 mg orally daily or propylthiouracil 75-150 mg orally four times daily; iodinated contrast agents; radioactive iodine (unless ophthalmopathy is present); and thyroidectomy. Adjustments to treatment must be made for pregnant or lactating patients. Factors precipitating thyrotoxic crisis (eg, medications or tumors) should also be investigated and corrected.

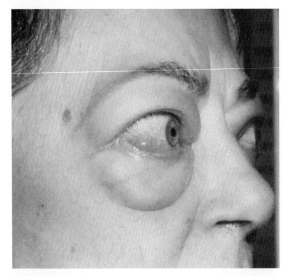

A

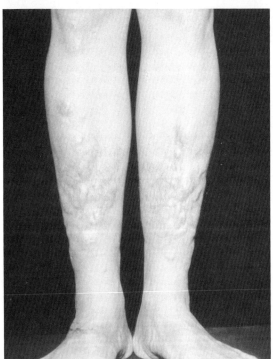

B

▲ **Figure 4-4.** Clinical features of hyperthyroidism. The patient shows (**A**) ophthalmopathy with exophthalmos (proptosis), and (**B**) pretibial myxedema. (Used with permission from Brunicardi CF, Andersen DK, Billiar TR, et al. *Schwartz's Principles of Surgery.* 9th ed. New York: McGraw Hill, 2009.)

HYPOADRENALISM

Causes of adrenocortical insufficiency include autoimmunity (**Addison disease**), tuberculosis, adrenal hemorrhage (Waterhouse–Friderichsen syndrome), and withdrawal from corticosteroids. Hypoadrenalism produces fatigue, weakness, weight loss, anorexia, hyperpigmentation of the skin, hypotension, nausea and vomiting, abdominal pain, and diarrhea or constipation. Neurologic manifestations include confusional states, seizures, or coma. Blood tests show decreased cortisol, sodium, glucose, and bicarbonate; increased potassium; and eosinophilia. Treatment of acute adrenocortical insufficiency is with hydrocortisone (100–300 mg intravenously in 0.9% saline, followed by 50–100 mg every 6 hours until oral replacement is possible), and correction of hypovolemia, hypoglycemia, electrolyte disturbances, and any precipitating illness.

HYPERADRENALISM

Hyperadrenalism (**Cushing syndrome**) usually results from administration of exogenous glucocorticoids, but may also be due to ACTH-secreting pituitary adenomas (**Cushing disease**) or adrenal tumors. Clinical features include moon facies with facial flushing (**Figure 4-5**), truncal obesity, hirsutism, menstrual irregularities, hypertension, weakness, cutaneous striae, acne, and ecchymoses.

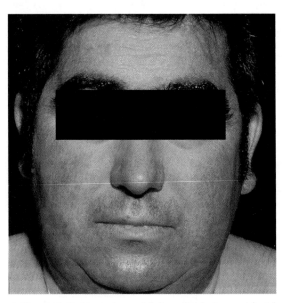

▲ **Figure 4-5.** Moon (round, full, puffy) facies and facial flushing in Cushing syndrome. (Used with permission from Wolff K, Johnson RA, Saavedra A, Roh E. *Fitzpatrick's Color Atlas and Synopsis of Clinical Dermatology.* 8th ed. New York, NY: McGraw-Hill; 2017.)

Neuropsychiatric disturbances are common and include depression or euphoria, anxiety, irritability, memory impairment, psychosis, delusions, and hallucinations. The diagnosis can be confirmed by a dexamethasone suppression test, 24-hour urinary free cortisol, late night salivary cortisol assay, or midnight serum cortisol level. Measurement of serum adrenocorticotropic hormone (ACTH) distinguishes adrenal from pituitary causes of hyperadrenalism, and magnetic resonance imaging (MRI) is used to localize pituitary or other ACTH-secreting tumors. Treatment depends on the cause and includes tapering of exogenous corticosteroids, transphenoidal resection or stereotactic radiotherapy of pituitary adenomas, and laparoscopic resection of cortisol-secreting adrenal neoplasms or ectopic ACTH-secreting tumors.

ELECTROLYTE DISORDERS

HYPONATREMIA

▶ Clinical Findings

Hyponatremia (serum sodium <135 mEq/L), particularly when acute, produces brain swelling from hypoosmolality of the extracellular fluid and resulting water influx into cells. If uncorrected this can lead to brain herniation and death. Causes of acute (evolving over 24-48 hours) hyponatremia include psychogenic polydipsia, exercise-associated hyponatremia, and entactogen drugs (eg, ecstasy). Hyponatremia produces headache, lethargy, confusion, weakness, muscle cramps, nausea, and vomiting. Neurologic signs include confusional state or coma, papilledema, tremor, asterixis, rigidity, extensor plantar responses, focal or generalized seizures, and occasionally focal neurologic deficits. Neurologic complications are usually associated with serum sodium levels less than 120 mEq/L (**Figure 4-6**),

but may be seen after a rapid fall to 130 mEq/L; conversely, chronic hyponatremia with levels as low as 110 mEq/L may be asymptomatic.

▶ Treatment

Treatment includes correction of the underlying cause of hyponatremia and administration of hypertonic (3%) saline to raise the serum sodium concentration to 125-130 mmol/L, at a rate not exceeding 4-6 mmol/L/d. Serum sodium should be monitored at ~2-h intervals. Furosemide (20 mg intravenously) may be added, but vasopressin receptor antagonists (eg, tolvaptan, conivaptan) have no established role in the treatment of acute or severe symptomatic hyponatremia. Excessively rapid correction of hyponatremia may lead to **osmotic demyelination syndrome** (formerly **central pontine myelinolysis**), a disorder of white matter characterized by a confusional state, paraparesis or quadriparesis, dysarthria, dysphagia, hyper- or hyporeflexia, and extensor plantar responses. Severe cases can result in the locked-in syndrome (see Chapter 3, Coma), coma, or death. MRI may show pontine and extrapontine white matter lesions. There is no treatment for osmotic demyelination syndrome, so prevention is essential and may best be achieved by adhering to the guidelines given above for gradual correction of hyponatremia.

HYPERCALCEMIA

Hypercalcemia may result from primary hyperparathyroidism (serum calcium ≥10.5 mg/dL or 2.6 mmol/L) or from neoplasms associated with bone metastases, especially lung cancer, breast cancer, or multiple myeloma (serum calcium ≥14 mg/dL or 3.5 mmol/L). Symptoms include thirst, polyuria, constipation, nausea and vomiting, abdominal pain, anorexia, and flank pain from nephrolithiasis. Neurologic symptoms are always present with

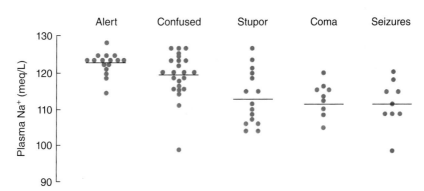

▲ **Figure 4-6.** Relationship between serum sodium concentration and neurologic manifestations of hyponatremia. (Adapted with permission from Arieff AI, Llach F, Massry SG. Neurologic manifestations and morbidity of hyponatremia: correlation with brain water and electrolytes. *Medicine.* 1976;55:121-129.)

serum calcium levels higher than ~17 mg/dL (8.5 mEq/L) and include headache, weakness, and lethargy.

Physical examination may show dehydration, abdominal distention, focal neurologic signs, myopathic weakness, and a confusional state that can progress to coma. Seizures are rare. The myopathy spares bulbar muscles, and tendon reflexes are usually normal. The diagnosis is confirmed by an elevated serum calcium level and sometimes by increased parathyroid hormone levels and a shortened QT interval on the electrocardiogram (ECG). Severe hypercalcemia in patients with normal cardiac and renal function is treated by vigorous intravenous hydration with 0.45% or 0.9% saline and usually requires central venous pressure monitoring. Bisphosphonates (eg, zoledronic acid) are added to treat hypercalcemia associated with malignancy.

HYPOCALCEMIA

Hypocalcemia (total serum calcium <8.5 mg/dL or 2.1 mmol/L; ionized calcium <4.6 mg/dL or 1.15 mmol/L) can be due to chronic kidney disease, hypoparathyroidism, hypomagnesemia, pancreatitis, or vitamin D deficiency. Symptoms include irritability, delirium, psychosis with hallucinations, depression, nausea and vomiting, abdominal pain, and paresthesias of the circumoral region and distal extremities. The most characteristic physical signs are those of overt or latent **tetany**. These include contraction of facial muscles in response to percussion of the facial (VII) nerve anterior to the ear (**Chvostek sign**) and **carpopedal spasm (Figure 4-7)**, which may occur spontaneously or after tourniquet-induced limb ischemia (**Trousseau sign**). Cataracts and papilledema are sometimes present, and chorea is reported. Seizures or laryngospasm can be life threatening. The ECG may show a prolonged QT interval.

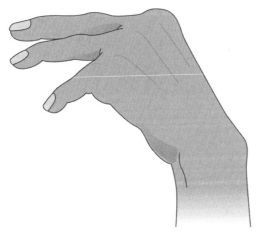

▲ **Figure 4-7.** Carpal spasm, a sign of tetany (neuronal hyperexcitability) in hypocalcemia. (Used with permission from Gardner DG, Shoback D. *Greenspan's Basic & Clinical Endocrinology*, 8th ed. New York, NY: McGraw-Hill, 2007.)

Treatment of severe symptomatic hypocalcemia is with intravenous calcium gluconate, 10-15 mg/kg of elemental calcium over 4-6 hours followed by infusion to maintain serum calcium at 7-8.5 mg/dL. Concomitant magnesium deficiency should also be corrected. Seizures are sometimes treated acutely with phenytoin or phenobarbital, but long-term anticonvulsant therapy is not indicated.

NUTRITIONAL DISORDERS

WERNICKE ENCEPHALOPATHY

Wernicke encephalopathy is usually a complication of chronic alcoholism, but can also result from gastrointestinal tract disease, hyperemesis gravidarum, malnutrition, bariatric surgery, cancer, or intravenous feeding. It is caused by deficiency of **thiamine** (vitamin B_1). Pathologic features include neuronal loss, demyelination, and gliosis in periventricular gray matter. Proliferation of small blood vessels and petechial hemorrhages may be seen. The areas most commonly involved are the medial thalamus, mammillary bodies, periaqueductal gray matter, cerebellar vermis, and oculomotor, abducens, and vestibular nuclei.

▶ Clinical Findings

The classic syndrome comprises the triad of **ophthalmoplegia**, **ataxia**, and **confusional state**. The most common ocular abnormalities are nystagmus, abducens (VI) nerve palsy, and horizontal or combined horizontal–vertical gaze palsy. Ataxia affects gait primarily, with ataxia of the arms and dysarthria uncommon. The mental status examination reveals global confusion with a prominent disorder of immediate recall and recent memory. The confusional state progresses to coma in a small percentage of patients. Most patients have associated neuropathy with absent ankle jerks. Hypothermia and hypotension may occur. Pupillary abnormalities, including mild anisocoria, or a sluggish reaction to light, are occasionally seen. The peripheral blood smear may show macrocytic anemia, and MRI may show atrophy of the mammillary bodies (**Figure 4-8**).

▶ Treatment

Treatment is prompt administration of thiamine, 500 mg intravenously, before or with dextrose (which, if given alone, can exacerbate the disorder). Parenteral thiamine is continued for several days. The maintenance requirement for thiamine, approximately 1 mg/d, is usually available in the diet, although enteric absorption of thiamine is impaired in alcoholics.

After treatment, ocular abnormalities usually begin to improve within 1 day and ataxia and confusion within 1 week. Ophthalmoplegia, vertical nystagmus, and acute confusion are entirely reversible, usually within 1 month. Horizontal nystagmus and ataxia, however, resolve

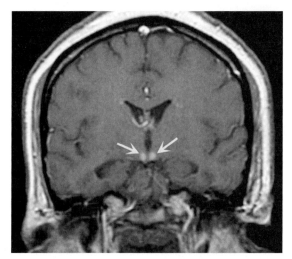

▲ **Figure 4-8.** Coronal T1-weighted MRI with contrast showing abnormal enhancement of the mammillary bodies (**arrows**) in a patient with Wernicke encephalopathy. (Used with permission from Fauci A, Braunwald E, Kasper D, et al. *Harrison's Principles of Internal Medicine.* 17th ed. New York, NY: McGraw-Hill, 2008.)

completely in only approximately 40% of cases. The major long-term complication of Wernicke encephalopathy is Korsakoff syndrome (see Chapter 5, Dementia & Amnestic Disorders).

VITAMIN B₁₂ DEFICIENCY

Vitamin B_{12} deficiency usually results from autoimmune destruction of gastric parietal cells leading to defective secretion of intrinsic factor (**pernicious anemia**); malabsorption due to achlorhydria, gastritis, gastrectomy, proton pump inhibitors, or H_2 antihistamines; or dietary inadequacy in vegans or vegetarians. Neurologic abnormalities include polyneuropathy, subacute combined degeneration of the corticospinal tracts and dorsal columns of the spinal cord (**combined systems disease**), optic neuropathy, and cognitive dysfunction ranging from mild confusion to dementia or psychosis (**megaloblastic madness**).

▶ Clinical Findings

The presentation is usually with **macrocytic anemia** or orthostatic lightheadedness but may also be neurologic. Distal paresthesias, gait ataxia, a bandlike sensation of tightness around the trunk or limbs, and **Lhermitte sign** (an electric shock-like sensation along the spine precipitated by neck flexion) may be present. Physical examination may show low-grade fever, glossitis, lemon-yellow discoloration of the skin, and cutaneous hyperpigmentation. Cerebral involvement produces confusion, depression, agitation, or psychosis with hallucinations. Spinal cord

involvement causes impaired vibratory and joint position sense, sensory gait ataxia, and spastic paraparesis with extensor plantar responses. Associated peripheral nerve involvement may lead to loss of tendon reflexes in the legs and urinary retention.

▶ Laboratory Findings

Hematologic abnormalities in vitamin B_{12} deficiency (**Figure 4-9**) include macrocytic anemia, leukopenia with hypersegmented neutrophils, and thrombocytopenia with giant platelets. The diagnosis is based on detecting a serum cobalamin level <148 pmol/L or 200 ng/L, but folate levels

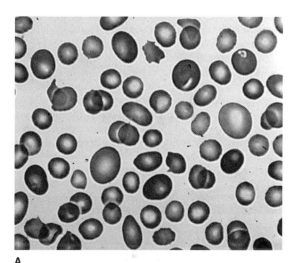

A

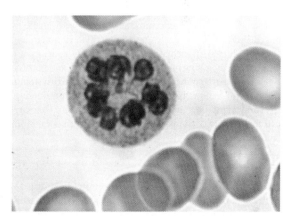

B

▲ **Figure 4-9.** Peripheral blood smear from a patient with vitamin B_{12} deficiency showing oval macrocytes (**A**) and hypersegmented neutrophil (**B**). (Used with permission from Kaushansky K, Lichtman M, Beutler E, Kipps T. *Williams Hematology.* 8th ed. New York, NY: McGraw-Hill, 2010.)

must also be determined, because folate deficiency can confound vitamin B_{12} measurement and mimic hematologic features of vitamin B_{12} deficiency. Pernicious anemia can be distinguished from other causes of vitamin B_{12} deficiency by testing blood for anti-intrinsic factor antibodies, which are highly specific but insensitive; anti-parietal cell antibodies are too nonspecific to be diagnostically useful. T1-weighted MRI may show gadolinium enhancement of the posterior spinal cord in B_{12} myelopathy (discussed in Chapter 10, Sensory Disorders) and deep T2-signal abnormalities in B_{12} encephalopathy, which resolve with treatment.

▶ Treatment

Treatment should begin as soon as blood is drawn to determine the vitamin B_{12} level. **Cyanocobalamin** is given by either the intramuscular route (1,000 μg immediately, then 8-10 times over the following 1-2 weeks, and then monthly for life) or orally (1,000-2,000 μg immediately, then daily for life), unless a correctable underlying cause is found. The reversibility of neurologic complications depends on their duration, and abnormalities present for more than 1 year are less likely to resolve with treatment. Encephalopathy may begin to clear within 24 hours after the first vitamin B_{12} dose, but full neurologic recovery, when it occurs, may take several months.

ORGAN SYSTEM FAILURE

HEPATIC ENCEPHALOPATHY

Hepatic encephalopathy occurs as a complication of alcoholic cirrhosis, portosystemic shunting, chronic active hepatitis, or fulminant hepatic necrosis after viral hepatitis. The syndrome may be chronic and progressive or acute in onset; in the latter case, gastrointestinal hemorrhage, systemic infection, dehydration, and sedative drugs are frequent precipitating factors. Liver disease impairs hepatocellular detoxifying mechanisms and causes portosystemic shunting of venous blood, leading to hyperammonemia. Cerebral symptoms may result from ammonia toxicity, cytotoxic edema, altered GABAergic neurotransmission, and inflammation.

▶ Clinical Findings

Physical examination shows systemic signs of liver disease, such as jaundice, ascites, fetor hepaticus, gynecomastia, palmar erythema, spider angiomas, and caput medusae. Cognitive disturbances include somnolence, agitation, and coma. Ocular reflexes are usually brisk. Nystagmus, tonic downward ocular deviation, or disconjugate eye movements may be seen. A helpful indicator of metabolic disturbance (including, but not limited to, liver disease) is **asterixis (Figure 4-10)**—a flapping tremor of the outstretched, dorsiflexed hands or feet that results from

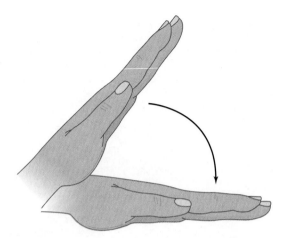

▲ **Figure 4-10.** Asterixis, a flapping tremor of the outstretched hands or feet, is often associated with hepatic encephalopathy, but can be seen in a variety of metabolic disorders.

impaired postural control. Other motor abnormalities in hepatic encephalopathy include tremor, myoclonus, paratonic rigidity, spasticity, decorticate or decerebrate posturing, and extensor plantar responses. Focal neurologic signs and focal or generalized seizures may occur.

▶ Laboratory Findings

Laboratory studies may show elevated serum bilirubin, transaminases, ammonia, prothrombin time (PT) and partial thromboplastin time (PTT); respiratory alkalosis; and elevated CSF glutamine. The electroencephalogram (EEG) may be diffusely slow with triphasic waves.

▶ Treatment

Underlying factors that may have precipitated acute decompensation should be corrected, and, when indicated, coagulopathy should be reversed with fresh-frozen plasma or vitamin K. Encephalopathy is treated with **lactulose**, a nonabsorbable disaccharide that decreases colonic pH and ammonia absorption (20-30 g orally 2-4 times daily, or 200 g in 1 L of saline rectally for 30-60 min every 4-6 hours), and **rifaximin**, a poorly absorbed antibiotic that reduces ammonia-forming bacteria in the colon (550 mg orally, twice daily). Dietary protein should not be severely restricted. Liver transplantation is required in some cases. Prognosis in hepatic encephalopathy correlates best with the severity of hepatocellular rather than neurologic dysfunction.

UREMIA

Renal failure, particularly when acute or rapidly progressive, may produce encephalopathy or coma with hyperventilation and prominent motor manifestations, including tremor, asterixis, myoclonus, and tetany. Focal or generalized seizures, focal neurologic signs, and decorticate or decerebrate posturing may occur. Laboratory abnormalities include elevated serum urea nitrogen, creatinine, and potassium and metabolic acidosis, but their severity correlates poorly with symptoms. The EEG is diffusely slow and may show triphasic waves or paroxysmal spikes or sharp waves.

Acute management includes relief of urinary tract obstruction if present, hydration, protein and salt restriction, and treatment of complications such as seizures. Long-term management includes dialysis or kidney transplantation. Although dialysis reverses the encephalopathy, clinical improvement often lags behind normalization of serum urea nitrogen and creatinine. Dialysis itself can produce an encephalopathy (**dialysis disequilibrium syndrome**) that is thought to result from hypo-osmolality leading to brain edema. This can be avoided by more gradual correction of uremia.

PULMONARY ENCEPHALOPATHY

Patients with lung disease or brainstem or neurologic disorders that affect respiratory function may develop encephalopathy related to hypoventilation. Symptoms include headache, confusion, and somnolence. Examination shows papilledema, asterixis or myoclonus, and a confusional state or coma. Tendon reflexes are often decreased, but pyramidal signs may be present, and seizures occur occasionally. Arterial blood gases show respiratory acidosis. Treatment involves ventilatory support to decrease hypercapnia and maintain adequate oxygenation.

ORGAN TRANSPLANTATION

Bone-marrow or solid-organ transplantation may be associated with an acute confusional state related to surgical complications, immunosuppressive drug treatment, stroke, opportunistic infection, reconstitution of the immune system, lymphoproliferative disorders, or transplant rejection. The problems encountered depend on the time in relation to transplantation and on the organ transplanted.

Surgical complications that may produce encephalopathy include hypotension, hypoxia, thromboembolism, and air embolism, which are most common with heart and liver transplants.

Drugs used for pretransplantation conditioning or preventing transplant rejection can cause acute confusional states by direct effects on the nervous system or as a consequence of immunologic impairment. Calcineurin inhibitors (eg, cyclosporine, tacrolimus) produce encephalopathy that may be associated with seizures, tremor, visual disturbances, weakness, sensory symptoms, or ataxia. MRI may show abnormalities in the occipital and posterior parietal white matter (**posterior reversible encephalopathy syndrome**). Symptoms are often associated with excessively high drug levels in the blood and may improve with dosage reduction or substitution of mycophenolate mofetil or an mTOR inhibitor (eg, sirolimus, everolimus). Corticosteroids can produce psychosis, and corticosteroid withdrawal is sometimes associated with lethargy, headache, myalgia, and arthralgia. The monoclonal antibody muromonab-CD3 may cause encephalopathy, aseptic meningitis, and seizures. Busulfan can produce encephalopathy and seizures. Gabapentin, valproate, and leviracetam are recommended to treat seizures in transplant recipients because of their relative lack of pharmacokinetic interaction with other drugs typically given to these patients.

Infections causing confusional states are most prominent after bone marrow transplantation but are also common after transplantation of other organs. They are comparatively rare in the first month after transplantation and, when they occur, usually reflect preexisting infection in the recipient or in the donor organ, or a perioperative complication. Within this period, the most frequent organisms are gram-negative bacteria, herpes simplex virus, and fungi. Opportunistic infections are more common between 1 and 6 months after transplant and include acute *Listeria* meningitis or encephalitis, human herpes virus 6 limbic encephalitis, chronic meningitis from *Cryptococcus* or *Mycobacterium tuberculosis*, and brain abscesses related to infection with *Aspergillus, Nocardia*, or *Toxoplasma*. Past 6 months, varicella-zoster virus, progressive multifocal leukoencephalopathy, *Toxoplasma, Cryptococcus, Listeria*, or *Nocardia* infection may be seen.

Immune reconstitution inflammatory syndrome (IRIS) related to transplantation is typically seen following reduction of immunosuppressive therapy and institution of antibiotics for an opportunistic infection. Neurologic involvement may produce headache, increased intracranial pressure, and CSF pleocytosis. Treatment is with corticosteroids. A similar syndrome occurs in patients with human immunodeficiency virus infection receiving combination antiretroviral therapy.

Posttransplant lymphoproliferative disorder is related to immunosuppression and may be associated with primary central nervous system (CNS) lymphoma.

Transplant rejection may also produce encephalopathy, especially in recipients of kidney transplants.

MENINGITIS, ENCEPHALITIS, & SEPSIS

ACUTE BACTERIAL MENINGITIS

Acute bacterial meningitis is a leading cause of confusional states and one in which early diagnosis is crucial to a good outcome. Predisposing conditions include systemic (especially respiratory) or parameningeal infection, head trauma, anatomic meningeal defects, prior neurosurgery, cancer, alcoholism, and immunodeficiency states. The great majority of cases in adults are due to *Streptococcus pneumoniae* or *Neisseria meningitidis* infection, but the etiologic organism varies with age and with the presence of predisposing conditions (**Table 4-8**).

Table 4-8. Causes and Empirical Antibiotic Treatment of Acute Bacterial Meningitis.

Age or Condition	Etiologic Agents	Antibiotics of Choice
Neonate	S. agalactiae E. coli L. monocytogenes	Ampicillin[1] + Ceftriaxone[2] or cefotaxime[3]
Child	S. pneumoniae N. meningitidis H. influenzae	Ceftriaxone[2] or cefotaxime[3] + Vancomycin[4]
Adult <50 y	S. pneumoniae N. meningitidis	Ceftriaxone[5] or cefotaxime[6] + Vancomycin[4]
Adult >50 y	S. pneumoniae N. meningitidis L. monocytogenes	Ceftriaxone[5] or cefotaxime[6] + Vancomycin[5] + Ampicillin[7]
Immunosuppression	S. pneumoniae L. monocytogenes Gram-negative bacilli	Ceftriaxone[5] or cefotaxime[6] + Vancomycin[4] + Ampicillin[7]
Head trauma, neurosurgery, or CSF shunt	Staphylococci Gram-negative bacilli S. pneumoniae	Vancomycin[4] + Ceftazidime[8]

[1]Ampicillin dose for neonates is 50 mg/kg IV every 6-8 hours.
[2]Ceftriaxone dose for neonates and children is 50-100 mg/kg IV every 12 hours.
[3]Cefotaxime dose for neonates and children is 50 mg/kg IV every 6-12 hours.
[4]Vancomycin dose is 15 mg/kg IV every 6 hours to maximum of 4 g per day.
[5]Ceftriaxone dose for adults is 2 g IV every 12 hours.
[6]Cefotaxime dose for adults is 2 g IV every 4-6 hours.
[7]Ampicillin dose for adults is 2 g IV every 4 hours.
[8]Ceftazidime dose is 50-100 mg/kg (to maximum of 2 g) IV every 8 hours.

▶ Pathogenesis & Pathology

Bacteria typically gain access to the CNS by colonizing the mucous membranes of the nasopharynx, leading to local tissue invasion, bacteremia, and hematogenous seeding of the subarachnoid space. *Listeria* is an exception in that it is ingested. Bacteria can also spread to the meninges directly, through anatomic defects in the skull or from parameningeal sites such as the paranasal sinuses or middle ear.

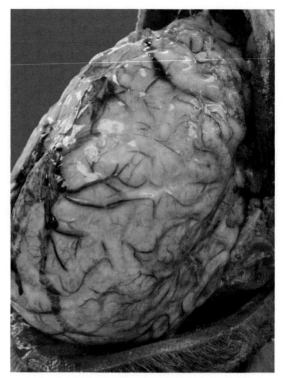

▲ **Figure 4-11.** Acute bacterial meningitis showing purulent exudate over the cerebral convexities. (Used with permission from Kemp WL, Burns DK, Brown TG. *Pathology: The Big Picture.* New York, NY: McGraw-Hill; 2008. Fig. 11-23A.)

The low levels of antibody and complement present in the cerebrospinal fluid are inadequate to contain the infection. The resulting inflammatory response is associated with release of inflammatory cytokines that promote blood–brain barrier permeability, vasogenic cerebral edema, changes in cerebral blood flow, and perhaps direct neurocellular toxicity.

Acute bacterial meningitis is characterized by leptomeningeal and perivascular infiltration with polymorphonuclear leukocytes and an inflammatory exudate (**Figure 4-11**). These tend to be most prominent over the cerebral convexities in *Streptococcus pneumoniae* and *Haemophilus* infection and over the base of the brain with *Neisseria meningitidis*. Brain edema, hydrocephalus, and cerebral infarction may occur, although bacterial invasion of the brain parenchyma is rare.

▶ Clinical Findings

At presentation, most patients have had symptoms for 1 to 7 days. These include fever, confusion, vomiting, headache, and neck stiffness, but the full syndrome is not usually present (**Table 4-9**).

Table 4-9. Findings in Acute Bacterial Meningitis.

Feature	Percentage of Patients
Clinical findings	
Headache[1]	87
Neck stiffness[1]	83
Fever (≥38°C)[1]	77
Altered mental status[1]	69
Focal neurologic deficit	33
Skin rash	26
Papilledema	3
At least 2 of classic tetrad ([1]above)	95
Neck stiffness + fever + altered mental status	44
Laboratory findings	
CSF pressure >200 mm water	82
CSF WBC ≥100/μL	92
CSF WBC ≥1,000/μL	78
Positive blood culture	66
Abnormal head CT scan[2]	34

[1]Classic tetrad.
[2]Most commonly brain edema, sinusitis or otitis, recent infarct, or hydrocephalus.
Data from van de Beek D, de Gans J, Spanjaard L, Weisfelt M, Reitsma JB, Vermeulen M. Clinical features and prognostic factors in adults with bacterial meningitis. *N Engl J Med.* 2004;351:1849-1859.

Physical examination may show fever and signs of systemic or parameningeal infection, such as skin abscess or otitis. A petechial rash is seen in 50% to 60% of patients with *N. meningitidis* meningitis (**Figure 4-12**). Signs of meningeal irritation (**meningismus**) are seen in approximately 80% of cases, but are often absent in the very young and very old, or with immunosuppression or profoundly impaired consciousness. These signs include neck stiffness on passive flexion, thigh flexion on flexion of the neck (**Brudzinski sign**), and resistance to passive extension of the knee with the hip flexed (**Kernig sign**) (see Figure 1-5). The level of consciousness, when altered, ranges from mild confusion to coma. Focal neurologic signs, seizures, and cranial nerve palsies may occur. Papilledema is rare.

Laboratory Findings

Peripheral blood may show polymorphonuclear leukocytosis from systemic infection or leukopenia caused by immunosuppression. The causative organism can be cultured from the blood in approximately two-thirds of cases. Images of the chest, sinuses, or mastoid bones may indicate a primary site of infection. A brain CT or MRI scan may show contrast enhancement of the cerebral convexities, the base of the brain, or the ventricular ependyma. The EEG is usually diffusely slow.

Prompt **lumbar puncture** and CSF examination are critical in all cases of suspected meningitis. CSF pressure is elevated in approximately 90% of cases, and the appearance of the fluid ranges from slightly turbid to grossly purulent. CSF white cell counts of 1,000 to 10,000/μL are usual, consisting chiefly of polymorphonuclear leukocytes, although mononuclear cells may predominate in *Listeria monocytogenes* meningitis. Protein concentrations of 100 to 500 mg/dL are most common. The CSF glucose level is lower than 40 mg/dL in approximately 80% of cases and may be too low to measure. Gram-stained smears of CSF identify the causative organism in 70% to 80% of cases. CSF culture, which is positive in approximately 80% of cases, provides a definitive diagnosis and allows determination of antibiotic sensitivity. The polymerase chain reaction is also useful, including for culture-negative or partially treated bacterial meningitis.

Differential Diagnosis

Signs of meningeal irritation may also be seen with nonbacterial meningitis and subarachnoid hemorrhage. However, the combination of an acute to subacute course (days rather than weeks), polymorphonuclear pleocytosis, and low CSF glucose point to a bacterial cause. Early viral meningitis can produce polymorphonuclear pleocytosis and symptoms identical to those of bacterial meningitis, but a repeat lumbar puncture after 6 to 12 hours should demonstrate a shift to lymphocytic predominance in viral meningitis, and the CSF glucose level is normal. Subarachnoid hemorrhage is distinctive in that lumbar puncture yields bloody CSF, which does not clear as increasing amounts of CSF are removed.

Prevention

Vaccines are available for three bacteria that can cause meningitis: *H. influenzae* type b, *N. meningitidis*, and

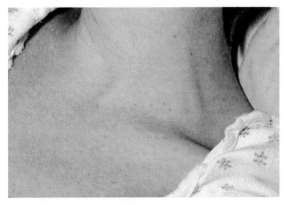

▲ **Figure 4-12.** Petechial skin rash in meningococcemia with meningococcal meningitis.

Table 4-10. Vaccines Against Acute Bacterial Meningitis.

Agent	Recommended Vaccination Schedule
H. influenzae type b	Ages 2, 4, 6, and 12-15 months
N. meningitidis (serogroups A,C,W135,Y)	Age 11-12 years
N. meningitidis (serogroup B)	Age 16-18 years
S. pneumoniae	Ages 2, 4, 6, and 12-15 months Age ≥ 65 years

Data from US Centers for Disease Control and Prevention (www.cdc.gov/vaccines).

S. pneumoniae. Current recommendations for vaccination are listed in **Table 4-10**. The risk of contracting *H. influenzae* or *N. meningitidis* meningitis can be reduced in household and other close contacts of affected patients by prophylactic administration of rifampin 20 mg/kg/d orally given as a single daily dose for 4 days (*H. influenzae*) or as two divided doses for 2 days (*N. meningitidis*).

Treatment

Unless the physical examination shows focal neurologic abnormalities or papilledema, suggesting a mass lesion, lumbar puncture should be performed immediately; if the CSF is not clear and colorless, antibiotic treatment (see next paragraph) is started without delay. When focal signs or papilledema are present, blood and urine should be taken for culture, antibiotics begun, and a brain CT scan obtained. If the scan shows no focal lesion that would contraindicate lumbar puncture, the puncture is then performed.

The initial choice of antibiotics is empirical, based on the patient's age and predisposing factors (see Table 4-8). Therapy is adjusted as indicated when the Gram stain, PCR, or culture and sensitivity results become available (**Table 4-11**). Lumbar puncture can be repeated to assess the response to therapy. CSF should be sterile after 24 hours, and a decrease in pleocytosis and in the proportion of polymorphonuclear leukocytes should occur within 3 days.

Dexamethasone, given immediately before the onset of antibiotic treatment and continued for 4 days, may improve outcome and decrease mortality in immunocompetent patients with confirmed bacterial meningitis.

Prognosis

Complications of acute bacterial meningitis include headache, seizures, hydrocephalus, syndrome of inappropriate secretion of antidiuretic hormone (SIADH), residual neurologic deficits (including cognitive disturbances and cranial—especially VIII—nerve abnormalities), and death. A CT or MRI scan will confirm suspected hydrocephalus, and fluid and electrolyte status should be carefully monitored to detect SIADH. *N. meningitidis* infections may be complicated by adrenal hemorrhage related to meningococcemia (Waterhouse–Friderichsen syndrome), resulting in hypotension and often death.

Morbidity and mortality from acute bacterial meningitis are high. Fatalities occur in approximately 20% of affected adults, and more often in low-income countries and with some pathogens (eg, *S. pneumoniae*, gramnegative bacilli) compared to others (eg, *H. influenzae*, *N. meningitidis*). Factors that worsen prognosis include extremes of age, delay in diagnosis and treatment, complicating illness, stupor or coma, seizures, and focal neurologic signs.

TUBERCULOUS MENINGITIS

Tuberculous meningitis should be considered in patients who present with a confusional state, especially if there is a history of pulmonary tuberculosis, alcoholism, corticosteroid treatment, HIV infection, or other conditions associated with impaired immune responses. It should also be considered in patients from regions (eg, Asia, Africa) or groups (eg, the homeless and inner-city drug users) with a high incidence of tuberculosis.

Pathogenesis & Pathology

Tuberculous meningitis usually results from reactivation of latent infection with *Mycobacterium tuberculosis*. Primary infection, typically acquired by inhaling bacillus-containing droplets, may be associated with metastatic dissemination of blood-borne bacilli from the lungs to the meninges and the surface of the brain. Here the organisms remain in a dormant state in tubercles that can rupture into the subarachnoid space at a later time, resulting in tuberculous meningitis.

The main pathologic finding is a basal meningeal exudate containing primarily mononuclear cells (**Figure 4-13**). Tubercles may be seen on the meninges and surface of the brain. The ventricles may be enlarged as a result of hydrocephalus, and their surfaces may show ependymal exudate or granular ependymitis. Arteritis can result in cerebral infarction, and basal inflammation and fibrosis can compress cranial nerves.

Clinical Findings

Symptoms usually have been present for less than 4 weeks at the time of presentation and include headache, fever, neck stiffness, vomiting, and lethargy or confusion. Weight loss, visual impairment, diplopia, focal weakness, and seizures may also occur. A history of contact with known cases of tuberculosis is usually absent.

Table 4-11. Treatment of Acute Bacterial Meningitis of Known Cause.

Etiologic Agents	Antibiotics of Choice	Treatment Duration
CSF Gram stain		
Gram-positive cocci	Vancomycin[1] + Ceftriaxone[2] or cefotaxime[3]	[4]
Gram-negative cocci	Penicillin G[5]	[4]
Gram-positive bacilli	Ampicillin[f] or penicillin G[5] + Gentamicin[7]	[4]
Gram-negative bacilli	Ceftriaxone,[2] cefotaxime,[3] or ceftazidime,[8] + Gentamicin[7]	[4]
CSF culture or PCR		
S. pneumoniae	Vancomycin[1] + Ceftriaxone[2] or cefotaxime[3]	10-14 days
H. influenzae	Ceftriaxone[2]	7 days
N. meningitidis	Penicillin G[5]	7 days
L. monocytogenes	Ampicillin[6] + Gentamicin[7]	21 days
S. agalactiae	Penicillin G[5]	14-21 days
Gram-negative enteric bacilli	Ceftriaxone[2] or cefotaxime[3] + Gentamicin[7]	21-28 days
Pseudomonas aeruginosa, Acinetobacter	Ceftazidime[8] + Gentamicin[7]	21-28 days
Actinomyces israelii	Penicillin G[9]	6-12 months
Nocardia species	Trimethoprim/sulfamethoxazole[10] + Ceftriaxone[11] + Amikacin[12]	12 months

[1]Vancomycin dose is 15 mg/kg IV every 6 hours to maximum of 4 g per day; rifampin 600 mg PO or IV per day should be substituted for vancomycin in patients receiving dexamethasone.
[2]Ceftriaxone dose for children is 50-100 mg/kg IV every 12 hours; dose for adults is 2 g IV every 12 hours.
[3]Cefotaxime dose for neonates is 50 mg/kg IV every 6 hours; dose for adults is 2 g IV every 12 hours.
[4]When CSF culture results are known, modify treatment based on organism and antibiotic sensitivity.
[5]Penicillin G dose is 300,000 units/kg/d IV to maximum 24 million units/d.
[6]Ampicillin dose for children is 100 mg/kg IV every 8 hours; dose for adults is 2 g IV every 4 hours.
[7]Gentamicin dose is 1.5 mg/kg IV loading followed by 1-2 mg/kg IV every 8 hours.
[8]Ceftazidime dose is 50-100 mg/kg (to maximum of 2 g) IV every 8 hours.
[9]Penicillin G dose is 18-24 million units intravenously daily for 4-6 weeks, then 500 mg orally 4 times daily.
[10]Trimethoprim/sulfamethoxazole dose is 5-10/25-50 mg/kg IV twice daily for several weeks, then PO.
[11]Ceftriaxone dose is 2 g IV daily for several weeks, then PO.
[12]Amikacin dose is 15 mg/kg IV daily for several weeks, then PO.

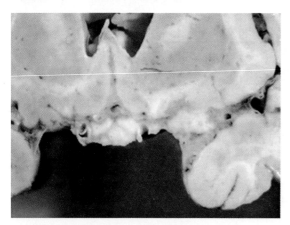

▲ **Figure 4-13.** Basilar meningitis showing inflammatory exudate surrounding cranial nerves and blood vessels at the base of the brain, as seen in tuberculous or fungal meningitis. (Used with permission from Kemp WL, Burns DK, Brown TG. *Pathology: The Big Picture.* New York, NY: McGraw-Hill; 2008. Fig 11-25.)

Fever, signs of meningeal irritation, and a confusional state are the most common findings on physical examination, but all may be absent. Papilledema, ocular palsies, and hemiparesis or paraparesis are sometimes seen. Complications include hyponatremia, hydrocephalus, brain edema, visual loss, cranial nerve (especially III, IV, and VI) palsies, spinal subarachnoid block, and stroke, which usually affects the internal capsule, basal ganglia, or thalamus.

Only one-half to two-thirds of patients show a positive skin test for tuberculosis or evidence of active or healed tubercular infection on chest X-ray; chest CT is more sensitive. The diagnosis is established by CSF analysis. CSF pressure is usually increased, and the fluid is typically clear and colorless. Lymphocytic and mononuclear cell pleocytosis of 50 to 500 cells/mL is most often seen, but polymorphonuclear pleocytosis can occur early and may give an erroneous impression of bacterial meningitis. CSF protein is usually more than 100 mg/dL and may exceed 500 mg/dL, particularly in patients with spinal subarachnoid block. The glucose level is usually decreased and may be less than 20 mg/dL. Acid-fast bacillus (AFB) smears of CSF (**Figure 4-14**) should be performed in all cases of suspected tuberculous meningitis, but they are positive in only a minority of cases. PCR of CSF is diagnostically helpful. Culturing *M. tuberculosis* from the CSF usually takes several weeks and requires large quantities of spinal fluid for maximum yield, so it is useful in confirming a presumptive diagnosis of tuberculous meningitis, but not in deciding to begin treatment. A CT or MRI scan may show enhancement of the basal cisterns and cortical meninges or hydrocephalus.

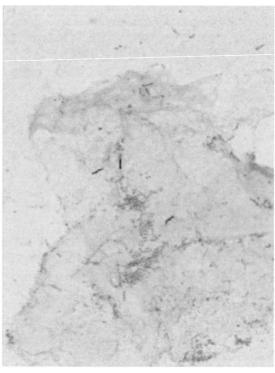

▲ **Figure 4-14.** Acid-fast bacillus (AFB) stain showing *Mycobacterium tuberculosis* bacilli (red rods).

▶ Differential Diagnosis

Many other conditions can cause a subacute to chronic confusional state with mononuclear cell pleocytosis (**Table 4-12**). These can usually be distinguished based on the history, associated physical findings, and appropriate laboratory studies.

▶ Treatment

Treatment should be started as early as possible; it should not be withheld while awaiting culture results. The decision to treat is based on the CSF findings described previously; lymphocytic pleocytosis and decreased glucose are particularly suggestive, even if AFB smears are negative.

Four antituberculous drugs are used for the 2-month initiation phase of therapy: isoniazid 300 mg, rifampin 600 mg, pyrazinamide 1,500 mg, and ethambutol 1,200 mg, each given orally once daily. During the subsequent, 7- to 12-month continuation phase, only isoniazid and rifampin are used, at the same doses. Adverse drug effects, drug resistance, concurrent HIV infection, and pregnancy may necessitate modifying the treatment regimen. Pyridoxine 50 mg/d can decrease the likelihood of isoniazid-induced polyneuropathy or seizures.

Table 4-12. Causes of Chronic Meningitis.

Cause	Features
Infectious	
Bacteria	
Partially treated acute bacterial meningitis	History of antibiotic treatment
Tuberculosis	Positive CSF acid-fast stain and AFB culture
Syphilis	Positive CSF VDRL
Lyme disease	History of tick bite, erythema migrans, facial (VII) nerve palsy, painful polyradiculopathy, positive serology
Leptospirosis	Myalgia, conjunctival reddening, positive serology
Brucellosis	Exposure to livestock, enzootic areas
Mycoplasma	Cough, abnormal chest X-ray
Viruses (HIV, EBV, HSV2)	Positive HIV or EBV serology, Mollaret cells in CSF (HSV2)
Fungi	Positive CSF India ink stain, cryptococcal antigen, or CSF culture
Parasites	Blood smear (malaria), peripheral or CSF eosinophilia, CT or MRI scan (toxoplasmosis, cysticercosis), positive serology
Parameningeal infection	Sinusitis, otitis, dental infection, CSF leak
Noninfectious	
Neoplastic meningitis	Low CSF glucose, positive cytology
Chemical meningitis	
Subarachnoid hemorrhage	CSF xanthochromia
Drugs (NSAIDs, antimicrobials, IVIG, immunosuppressants, allopurinol, lamotrigine, intrathecal agents, vaccination)	History of treatment
Uveomeningitis[1]	
Sarcoidosis	Erythema nodosum, dyspnea, facial (VII) nerve palsy, hilar adenopathy, positive biopsy
Behçet syndrome	Painful orogenital ulcers, erythema nodosum-like skin lesions, abducens (VI) nerve palsy, ataxia, corticospinal signs
Wegener granulomatosis	Upper and lower respiratory tract disease, glomerulonephritis, cranial neuropathy, mononeuritis multiplex
Vogt–Koyanagi–Harada syndrome	Deafness, tinnitus, alopecia, poliosis, vitiligo
Sjögren syndrome	Xerostomia, xerophthalmia, trigeminal (V) neuropathy, positive Schirmer test, positive ANA (SSB/La), lip biopsy
Fabry disease	Exercise-induced neuropathic pain, periumbilical angiokeratomas, stroke
Hypertrophic pachymeningitis	Cranial neuropathies

AFB, acid-fast bacilli; ANA, antinuclear antibody; CSF, cerebrospinal fluid; CT, computed tomography; EBV, Epstein–Barr virus; HIV, human immunodeficiency virus; IVIG, intravenous immunoglobulin; MRI, magnetic resonance imaging; NSAIDs, nonsteroidal anti-inflammatory drugs; VDRL, Venereal Disease Research Laboratory.
[1]Includes inflammatory disorders of the iris (iritis), ciliary body (cyclitis), or choroid (choroiditis).

Corticosteroids (eg, prednisone, 60 mg/d orally, tapered gradually over 3-4 weeks) reduce mortality from tuberculous meningitis. Aspirin 75-150 mg/d may confer an additional anti-inflammatory effect. Antifungal therapy (see later) should be added unless fungal meningitis has been excluded.

Ventriculoperitoneal shunting or endoscopic third ventriculostomy can be useful to relieve hydrocephalus. Treatment of tuberculous meningitis in patients with HIV infection is similar except that the benefit of corticosteroids is less clearly established. Delaying the onset of retroviral therapy for

2 months after beginning treatment of tuberculous meningitis in patients with HIV infection yields a similar rate of survival with fewer adverse effects.

Prognosis

Even with appropriate treatment, approximately one-third of patients with tuberculous meningitis succumb. Adverse prognostic factors include age less than 5 or more than 50 years, coma, seizures, and concomitant HIV infection. Neurologic sequelae include cognitive disturbances, visual loss, motor deficits, and cranial nerve palsies.

SYPHILITIC MENINGITIS

Syphilitic meningitis usually occurs within 2 years after primary syphilitic infection. It is most common in young adults, and patients with HIV infection are at particular risk for developing this and other forms of neurosyphilis.

In approximately one-fourth of patients with *Treponema pallidum* infection, treponemes gain access to the CNS, where they produce meningitis that is usually asymptomatic. Asymptomatic neurosyphilis is associated with CSF pleocytosis, elevated protein, and positive serologic tests for syphilis.

Clinical Findings

In a few patients, syphilitic meningitis is a clinically apparent acute or subacute disorder. At presentation, symptoms such as headache, nausea and vomiting, stiff neck, mental disturbances, focal weakness, seizures, deafness, and visual impairment usually have been present for up to 2 months.

Physical examination may show signs of meningeal irritation, confusion or delirium, papilledema, hemiparesis, and aphasia. The cranial nerves most frequently affected are (in order) the facial (VII), acoustic (VIII), oculomotor (III), trigeminal (V), abducens (VI), and optic (II) nerves, but other nerves may be involved as well. Fever is typically absent.

The diagnosis is established by CSF findings. Opening pressure is normal or slightly elevated. Pleocytosis is lymphocytic or mononuclear in character, with white blood cell counts usually in the range of 100 to 1,000/mL. Protein level may be mildly or moderately elevated (<200 mg/dL) and glucose mildly decreased. CSF Venereal Disease Research Laboratory (VDRL) and serum fluorescent treponemal antibody (FTA) or microhemagglutination-*Treponema pallidum* (MHA-TP) tests are usually positive. Protein electrophoretograms of CSF may show discrete γ-globulin bands (oligoclonal bands) not visible in normal CSF.

Treatment

Syphilitic meningitis is usually a self-limited disorder, but treatment is required to avoid more advanced vascular and parenchymatous neurosyphilis (tabes dorsalis, general paresis, optic neuritis, myelitis). Treatment is with aqueous penicillin G 2 to 4×10^6 units intravenously every 4 hours for 10 to 14 days. For penicillin-allergic patients, ceftriaxone 2 g intravenously daily for 14 days or doxycycline 200 mg orally twice daily for 21 to 28 days can be substituted. The CSF should be examined every 6 months until all findings are normal. Another course of therapy must be given if the CSF cell count or protein remains elevated.

LYME DISEASE

Clinical Findings

Lyme disease is a tick-borne disorder due to infection with the spirochete *Borrelia burgdorferi* (or, outside the United States, other *Borrelia* species). Most cases occur during the summer. Primary infection may be manifested by an expanding erythematous annular skin lesion (**erythema migrans**) (**Figure 4-15**), which usually appears 1-2 weeks after detachment of the tick (*Ixodes scapularis* or *Ixodes pacificus*). Less distinctive symptoms include fatigue, headache, fever, neck stiffness, joint or muscle pain, anorexia, sore throat, and nausea. Neurologic involvement (neuroborreliosis), which occurs in 10-15% of cases, may be delayed for up to 10 weeks. It is characterized by meningitis or meningoencephalitis and disorders of the cranial or peripheral nerves or nerve roots; bilateral facial weakness from involvement of cranial nerve VII is particularly common. Cardiac abnormalities (conduction defects, myocarditis, pericarditis, cardiomegaly, or heart failure) can also occur at this stage. Lyme meningitis produces prominent headache accompanied by signs of meningeal irritation,

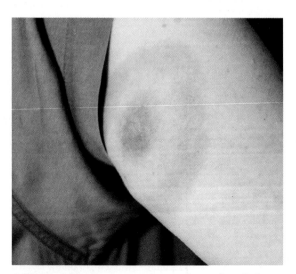

▲ **Figure 4-15.** Erythema migrans due to *Borrelia burgdorferi* (Lyme disease). (Used with permission from James Gathany, Public Health Image Library, US Centers for Disease Control and Prevention.)

photophobia, pain when moving the eyes, nausea, and vomiting. When encephalitis is present, it is usually mild and characterized by insomnia, emotional lability, or impaired concentration and memory. European Lyme disease differs clinically from that seen in the United States in that the infective organism is *Borrelia garinii or Borrelia afzelii,* erythema migrans is not a feature, and painful radiculopathy (Bannwarth syndrome) is common.

Laboratory Findings

The CSF usually shows a lymphocytic pleocytosis with 100 to 200 cells/mL, slightly elevated protein, and normal glucose. Oligoclonal immunoglobulin G (IgG) bands may be detected. Definitive diagnosis is usually made by serologic testing for *B. burgdorferi,* using enzyme-linked immunosorbent assay (ELISA) for screening followed by western blot to confirm positive ELISA results.

Treatment

Preventive measures include avoiding tick-infested areas and using insect repellents and protective clothing when avoidance is impossible. Treatment of Lyme disease with neurologic involvement is with ceftriaxone (2 g/d intravenously) or doxycycline (100 mg/d orally) for 2 to 3 weeks.

Symptoms of acute Lyme disease typically resolve within 10 days in treated cases. Untreated or inadequately treated infections may lead to recurrent oligoarthritis; memory, language, and other cognitive disturbances; focal weakness; and ataxia. In such cases, a CT scan or MRI may show hydrocephalus, lesions in white matter resembling those seen in multiple sclerosis, or abnormalities suggestive of cerebral infarction. Subtle chronic cognitive or behavioral symptoms should not be attributed to Lyme encephalitis in the absence of serologic evidence of *B. burgdorferi* exposure, CSF abnormalities, or focal neurologic signs. The peripheral neurologic manifestations of Lyme disease are discussed in Chapter 10, Sensory Disorders.

VIRAL MENINGITIS & ENCEPHALITIS

Viral infections of the meninges (**meningitis**), brain parenchyma (**encephalitis**), or both (**meningoencephalitis**) often present as acute confusional states. The most common causative agents are listed in **Table 4-13**. Clues in the history that suggest a specific virus or virus family include the time of year, recent travel, contact with insects or other animals, sexual contacts, and immunosuppression. Some viruses (eg, herpesviruses) can cause either meningitis or encephalitis, but others preferentially affect the meninges (eg, enteroviruses) or brain parenchyma (eg, many arthropod-borne—or arbo—viruses). Herpes simplex and human immunodeficiency virus infections have special features that merit distinct consideration, and are therefore discussed separately.

Pathology

Viral infections can affect the CNS in three ways—hematogenous dissemination of a systemic viral infection (eg, arthropod-borne viruses), neuronal spread of the virus by axonal transport (eg, herpes simplex, rabies), and autoimmune postinfectious demyelination (eg, varicella, influenza). Pathologic changes in viral meningitis consist of an inflammatory meningeal reaction mediated by lymphocytes. Encephalitis is characterized by perivascular cuffing, lymphocytic infiltration, and microglial proliferation mainly involving subcortical gray matter regions. Intranuclear or intracytoplasmic inclusions are often seen.

Clinical Findings

Clinical manifestations of viral meningitis include fever, headache, neck stiffness, photophobia, pain with eye movement, and mild impairment of consciousness. Patients usually do not appear as ill as those with bacterial meningitis. Systemic manifestations of viral infection, including skin rash, pharyngitis, lymphadenopathy, pleuritis, carditis, jaundice, organomegaly, diarrhea, or orchitis, may suggest a particular etiologic agent. Viral encephalitis, which involves the brain directly, causes more marked alteration of consciousness than viral meningitis, and may also produce seizures and focal neurologic signs.

Laboratory Findings

CSF analysis is the most important laboratory test. CSF pressure is normal or increased, and a lymphocytic or monocytic pleocytosis is present, with cell counts usually less than 1,000/mL. Higher counts can be seen in lymphocytic choriomeningitis or herpes simplex encephalitis. A polymorphonuclear pleocytosis can occur early in viral meningitis, whereas red blood cells may be seen with herpes simplex encephalitis. Protein level is normal or slightly increased (usually 80-200 mg/dL). Glucose is usually normal, but may be decreased in mumps, herpes zoster, or herpes simplex encephalitis. Gram stains and other tests for bacterial, tuberculous, syphilitic and fungal infection are negative. Oligoclonal bands and CSF protein electrophoresis abnormalities may be present. An etiologic diagnosis often can be made from CSF by virus isolation, polymerase chain reaction, or detection of antiviral antibodies.

Blood counts may show a normal white cell count, leukopenia, or mild leukocytosis. Atypical lymphocytes in blood smears and a positive heterophile test suggest infectious mononucleosis. Serum amylase is frequently elevated in mumps; abnormal liver function tests are associated with both hepatitis viruses and infectious mononucleosis. The EEG is diffusely slow, especially if there is direct cerebral involvement.

Table 4-13. Causes of Viral Meningitis and Encephalitis.

	Virus	Season or Geography	Vector	Features
Meningitis				
Enterovirus	Echo, coxsackie, enterovirus 71	Summer, fall	Human	Rash, gastroenteritis, carditis
Herpesvirus	Herpes simplex type 2 (HSV2)	—	Human	Neonates
	Varicella-zoster virus (VZV)	—	Human	Immunosuppression; rash
	Epstein–Barr virus (EBV)	—	Human	Teenagers; infectious mononucleosis syndrome
Arbovirus	West Nile	Summer	Mosquito	May also cause encephalitis, flaccid paralysis
	Toscana	Southern Europe	Sandfly	May also cause encephalitis
	Tick-borne	Eurasia	Tick	May also cause encephalitis
Other	Human immunodeficiency virus (HIV)	—	Human	Immunosuppression
	Mumps	Winter, spring	Human	Especially boys; parotitis, orchitis, oophoritis, pancreatitis
	Lymphocytic choriomeningitis	Fall, winter	Mouse	Pharyngitis, pneumonia; marked CSF pleocytosis, low CSF glucose; transmissible by organ transplantation
Encephalitis				
Herpesvirus	Herpes simplex type 1 (HSV1)	—	Human	Focal (especially temporal lobe); treatable with acyclovir
	Varicella-zoster virus (VZV)	—	Human	Immunosuppression; rash
	Epstein–Barr virus (EBV)	—	Human	Teenagers; infectious mononucleosis syndrome
Arbovirus	Japanese	Asia	Mosquito	Common; vaccine available; high mortality
	St. Louis	Western hemisphere	Mosquito	Common in US
	California	North America	Mosquito	Common in US; includes La Crosse encephalitis
	Western equine	Western hemisphere	Mosquito	Children
	Eastern equine	Western hemisphere	Mosquito	Children
	Venezuelan equine	Western hemisphere	Mosquito	Children
	Powassan	Northeast US	Tick	Seizures (in children), focal neurologic signs
	Dengue	Southeast Asia, Western Pacific	Mosquito	May cause hemorrhagic fever
	Chikungunya	Africa	Mosquito	Arthralgia
	Zika	Pacific Islands, Americas	Mosquito	May also cause microcephaly & Guillain–Barré syndrome; can be sexually transmitted
Other	Rabies	—	Dog, bat, raccoon, skunk, fox	Postexposure prophylaxis available; fatal once symptoms (hyperexcitability, autonomic dysfunction, hydrophobia) appear
	Ebola	West Africa	Human, bat	Vomiting, diarrhea, hemorrhage, persistent neurologic deficits

Differential Diagnosis

The differential diagnosis of meningitis with mononuclear cell pleocytosis includes partially treated bacterial meningitis; syphilitic, tuberculous, fungal, parasitic, and neoplastic meningitis; and acute disseminated encephalomyelitis after infections (see later). Evidence of systemic viral infection and CSF wet mounts, stained smears, cultures, and cytology can distinguish among these possibilities. When suspected early viral meningitis is associated with a polymorphonuclear pleocytosis of less than 1,000 white blood cells/mL and normal CSF glucose, one of two strategies can be used. The patient can be treated for bacterial meningitis until the results of CSF cultures are known, or treatment can be withheld and lumbar puncture repeated in 6 to 12 hours. If the meningitis is viral in origin, the second sample should show a mononuclear cell pleocytosis.

Prevention & Treatment

Vaccines are available against varicella-zoster virus and Japanese encephalitis, and postexposure prophylaxis against rabies can be achieved through active immunization by vaccine combined with passive immunization using human rabies-immune globulin. No specific treatment is available for most causes of viral meningitis or encephalitis. Exceptions include herpes simplex and human immunodeficiency viruses (discussed in the following sections); varicella-zoster, which responds to acyclovir (10-15 mg/kg intravenously every 8 hours for 14 days); and cytomegalovirus, which is treated with a 21-day course of ganciclovir (5 mg/kg intravenously twice daily) and foscarnet (60 mg/kg intravenously every 8 hours), followed by maintenance therapy for 3 to 6 weeks with either drug. Corticosteroids are of no proven benefit except in immune-mediated postinfectious syndromes. Headache and fever can be treated with acetaminophen or nonsteroidal anti-inflammatory drugs. Seizures usually respond to phenytoin or phenobarbital. Supportive measures in comatose patients include mechanical ventilation and intravenous or nasogastric feeding.

Prognosis

Symptoms of viral meningitis usually resolve spontaneously within 2 weeks regardless of the causative agent, although residual deficits may be seen. The outcome of viral encephalitis varies with the specific virus—for example, eastern equine and HSV infections are associated with severe morbidity and high mortality rates. Mortality rates as high as 20% have also been reported in immune-mediated encephalomyelitis after measles infections.

HERPES SIMPLEX VIRUS ENCEPHALITIS

Herpes simplex virus (HSV) type 1 (oral herpes) is the most common cause of sporadic fatal encephalitis in the United States. Most cases involve patients <3 or >50 years of age. The virus migrates along nerve axons to sensory ganglia, where it persists in a latent form and may be subsequently reactivated. HSV type 1 encephalitis can result from either primary infection or reactivation of latent infection. Neonatal HSV encephalitis usually results from acquisition of HSV type 2 (genital herpes) during passage through the birth canal of a mother with active genital lesions. CNS involvement by HSV type 2 in adults usually causes meningitis, rather than encephalitis.

Pathology

HSV type 1 encephalitis is an acute, necrotizing, asymmetric hemorrhagic process with lymphocytic and plasma cell reaction and usually involves the medial temporal and inferior frontal lobes. Intranuclear inclusions may be seen in neurons and glia. Patients who recover may show cystic necrosis of the involved regions.

Clinical Findings

The clinical syndrome may include headache, stiff neck, vomiting, behavioral disorders, memory loss, anosmia, aphasia, hemiparesis, and focal or generalized seizures. Active herpes labialis is seen occasionally, but does not reliably implicate HSV as the cause of encephalitis. HSV encephalitis is usually rapidly progressive over several days and may result in coma or death. The most common sequelae in patients who survive are memory and behavior disturbances, reflecting the predilection of HSV for limbic structures.

Laboratory Findings

The CSF in HSV type 1 encephalitis most often shows increased pressure, lymphocytic or mixed lymphocytic and polymorphonuclear pleocytosis (50-100 white blood cells/mL), mild protein elevation, and normal glucose; red blood cells, xanthochromia, and decreased glucose are seen in some cases. However, CSF pleocytosis may not be found in immunocompromised patients. The virus generally cannot be isolated from the CSF, but can be detected by the polymerase chain reaction and serologic testing. The EEG may show periodic slow-wave complexes arising from one or both temporal lobes. MRI is more sensitive than CT for early detection of edema and mass effect in one or both temporal lobes and cingulate gyrus (**Figure 4-16**). However, imaging studies may also be normal, especially early in the course.

Differential Diagnosis

The symptoms and signs are not specific for herpes virus infection, and may also be observed with brain abscess, tuberculosis, varicella-zoster virus encephalitis, and autoimmune limbic encephalitis. Detection of viral DNA in CSF using PCR is highly sensitive and specific, so brain biopsy is no longer required for definitive diagnosis of HSV encephalitis.

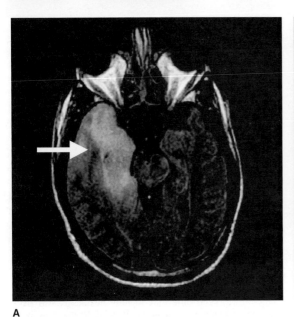
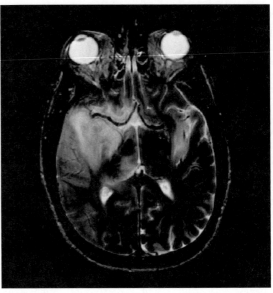

A   **B**

▲ **Figure 4-16.** MRI in herpes simplex encephalitis. FLAIR I (**A**) and T2 (**B**) sequences show mild mass effect, loss of gray-white differentiation caused by edema, and characteristic involvement of the temporal lobe (**arrow**). T2 image shows involvement on the other side as well. (Used with permission from Jason Handwerker.)

▶ Treatment

Treatment is with **acyclovir**, 10 mg/kg intravenously every 8 hours for 14 to 21 days. Complications include erythema at the infusion site, gastrointestinal disturbances, headache, skin rash, tremor, seizures, and encephalopathy or coma. Treatment is started as early as possible, without waiting for laboratory confirmation of the diagnosis, because outcome is greatly influenced by the severity of dysfunction at the time treatment is initiated.

▶ Prognosis

Patients younger than age 30 and those who are only lethargic at the onset of treatment are more likely to survive than are older or comatose patients. With acyclovir treatment, mortality is <10% in immunocompetent but >30% in immunocompromised patients.

HUMAN IMMUNODEFICIENCY VIRUS INFECTION

Acquired immune deficiency syndrome (AIDS) is caused by human immunodeficiency virus type 1 (HIV-1) and is characterized by opportunistic infections, malignant neoplasms (eg, non-Hodgkin lymphoma, Kaposi sarcoma), and a variety of neurologic disturbances. Transmission occurs through sexual activity or transfer of virus-contaminated blood or blood products, such as by intravenous drug users who share needles. HIV enters the brain

and spinal cord directly or in circulating HIV-infected lymphocytes or monocytes, yielding detectable levels of HIV RNA in CSF within ~1 week of viral exposure. Within the CNS, the virus infects microglia, perivascular macrophages, astrocytes and endothelial cells, and increases blood-brain barrier permeability. Neurotoxicity is an indirect result of these alterations.

Neurologic complications of HIV infection per se include meningitis, dementia (see Chapter 5, Dementia & Amnestic Disorders), myelopathy (see Chapter 10, Sensory Disorders), neuropathy (see Chapter 10), myopathy (see Chapter 9, Motor Disorders), and stroke (see Chapter 13, Stroke). Patients with systemic HIV infection are also at increased risk of neurologic involvement from opportunistic infections and tumors. Moreover, antiretroviral treatment of HIV may cause paradoxical clinical worsening of (or unmask) opportunistic infections, especially cryptococcal meningitis, tuberculous meningitis, and progressive multifocal leukoencephalopathy (**immune reconstitution inflammatory syndrome**; see *Organ Transplantation* earlier in this chapter).

A. HIV-1 Meningitis

Around the time of HIV-1 seroconversion, patients can develop a syndrome characterized by headache, fever, signs of meningeal irritation, cranial nerve (especially VII) palsies, other focal neurologic abnormalities, or seizures. An acute confusional state with impaired concentration and memory disturbance may also be present. HIV-1 meningitis is associated with mononuclear CSF pleocytosis of up to approximately 200 cells/μL with normal or slightly elevated protein and normal glucose levels. HIV may be detectable in CSF by polymerase chain reaction. Symptoms usually resolve spontaneously within about 1 month. Other causes of pleocytosis associated with HIV infection, including cryptococcal meningitis and cerebral toxoplasmosis, must be excluded. Treatment of newly diagnosed HIV disease, including meningitis, should include a combination of two nucleoside reverse transcriptase inhibitors plus a third drug from one of the following categories: integrase strand transfer inhibitor, non-nucleoside reverse transcriptase inhibitor, or protease inhibitor with pharmacokinetic enhancer. Recommended regimens for specific clinical situations can be found at https://aidsinfo.nih.gov/guidelines.

B. Cryptococcal Meningitis or Meningoencephalitis

Cryptococcus neoformans causes subacute meningitis or meningoencephalitis in patients with HIV infection. Clinical features include headache, confusion, stiff neck, fever, nausea and vomiting, seizures, and cranial nerve palsies. CSF cell counts, protein, and glucose may be normal, so CSF India ink staining and cryptococcal antigen titers should always be obtained. CT or MRI scans may show meningeal enhancement, intraventricular or intraparenchymal cryptococcomas, gelatinous pseudocysts, abscesses, hydrocephalus, or small vessel ischemic infarcts. Treatment consists of induction for at least 2 weeks with liposomal amphotericin B (0.7-1 mg/kg intravenously 4 times daily) and flucytosine (25 mg/kg orally 4 times daily), followed upon clinical improvement and negative CSF culture by consolidation with fluconazole (400 mg orally daily for 8 weeks), and then maintenance with fluconazole (200 mg orally daily) until the patient is asymptomatic with CD4 cell counts >100/μL. Increased intracranial pressure should be managed by daily lumbar puncture or ventriculoperitoneal shunting. Corticosteroids are not recommended. Survival is improved by delaying antiretroviral therapy until 5 weeks after the start of treatment for cryptococcal meningitis.

C. Cerebral Toxoplasmosis

In patients with HIV infection, cerebral toxoplasmosis produces cerebral abscesses and, less commonly, diffuse encephalitis or chorioretinitis. Presenting symptoms include fever, headache, altered mental status, focal neurologic abnormalities, and seizures. Movement disorders may also occur due to the predilection of *Toxoplasma* abscesses for the basal ganglia. Blood and CSF serology and PCR can be diagnostically helpful, but lumbar puncture may be inadvisable in the presence of mass lesions. Thus, imaging studies are typically relied upon for presumptive diagnosis of cerebral toxoplasmosis. MRI is more sensitive than CT scanning and typically reveals one or more ring-enhancing supratentorial lesions at cortical

gray-white matter junctions or in the basal ganglia. Because intracerebral mass lesions in HIV-infected patients are typically due to toxoplasmosis or primary central nervous system lymphoma (see later), and since toxoplasmosis is more readily treatable, patients with HIV infection and intracerebral mass lesions should be treated for toxoplasmosis. Treatment is with pyrimethamine (200 mg then 75-100 mg orally daily), sulfadiazine (1-1.5 g orally four times daily), and folinic acid (10-50 mg orally daily), continued until 1-2 weeks after clinical resolution. In patients with CD4$^+$ cell counts <100/μL, maintenance therapy should then be instituted with pyrimethamine (25-50 mg orally daily), sulfadiazine (0.5-1 g orally four times daily), and folinic acid (10-50 mg orally daily). Absence of a response to treatment for toxoplasmosis should prompt brain biopsy for diagnosis of possible lymphoma.

D. Cytomegalovirus Encephalitis

Cytomegalovirus infection can result in encephalitis, myelitis, polyradiculitis, or retinitis in patients with HIV infection. Clinical features of encephalitis include fever, headache, confusion, seizures, cranial nerve palsies, and ataxia. CSF cell count, protein, and glucose are variable; diagnosis is by PCR testing of CSF. Treatment is with ganciclovir (5 mg/kg) and foscarnet (90 mg/kg), both given intravenously twice daily until improvement occurs (~3-6 weeks).

E. Progressive Multifocal Leukoencephalopathy

This demyelinating disorder is caused by infection with JC virus. Altered mental status may be accompanied by focal neurologic signs, including hemianopsia, ataxia, or hemiparesis, and seizures. Headache and fever are usually absent. CT or MRI scan shows one or more white matter lesions, which may be bilateral. The CSF typically shows mild lymphocytic pleocytosis, elevated protein, and normal glucose, and polymerase chain reaction may provide evidence for JC virus infection. There is no proven effective treatment.

F. Primary CNS Lymphoma

Primary CNS lymphoma is the most common brain tumor associated with HIV infection. Clinical features include confusion, hemiparesis, aphasia, seizures, cranial nerve palsies, and headache; signs of meningeal irritation are uncommon. CSF commonly shows elevated protein and mild mononuclear pleocytosis, and glucose may be low; cytology is rarely positive. MRI is more sensitive than CT scanning and shows single or multiple contrast-enhancing lesions, which may not be distinguishable from those seen in toxoplasmosis. Patients with HIV infection and one or more intracerebral mass lesions that fail to respond to treatment for toxoplasmosis within 3 weeks should undergo brain biopsy for diagnosis of lymphoma. Recommended first-line treatment includes high-dose methotrexate, which may be combined with rituximab or autologous stem-cell transplantation, reserving whole-brain radiotherapy for relapses.

FUNGAL MENINGITIS

In a small fraction of patients with systemic fungal infections (mycoses), fungi invade the CNS to produce meningitis or focal intraparenchymal lesions (**Table 4-14**). Several fungi are opportunistic organisms that cause infection in patients with cancer or HIV infection, those receiving immunosuppressive drugs, and other debilitated hosts. Intravenous drug abuse is a potential route for infection with *Candida* and *Aspergillus*. Diabetic acidosis is strongly correlated with rhinocerebral mucormycosis. In contrast, meningeal infections with *Coccidioides*, *Blastomyces*, and *Actinomyces* usually occur in previously healthy individuals. *Cryptococcus* (the most common cause of fungal meningitis in the United States) and *Histoplasma* infection can occur in either healthy or immunosuppressed patients. Cryptococcal meningitis is the most common fungal infection of the nervous system in patients with HIV infection. Geographic factors are also important in the epidemiology of certain mycoses: *Blastomyces* is seen especially in the Mississippi River Valley, *Coccidioides* in the southwestern United States, and *Histoplasma* in the eastern and midwestern United States.

▶ Pathogenesis & Pathology

Fungi reach the CNS by hematogenous spread from the lungs, heart, gastrointestinal or genitourinary tract, or

Table 4-14. Causes of Fungal Meningitis.

Name	Opportunistic	Systemic Involvement	Distinctive CSF Findings	Treatment
Aspergillus species	+	Lungs, nasal sinuses	Polymorphonuclear pleocytosis	Voriconazole 6 mg/kg intravenously every 12 hours for 2 doses, then 4 mg/kg intravenously or 200 mg orally twice daily
Blastomyces dermatitidis	–	Lungs, skin, bones, joints, viscera	Polymorphonuclear pleocytosis	Amphotericin B (liposomal) 5 mg/kg intravenously daily for 4-6 weeks, then Itraconazole 200 mg orally 2-3 times daily for 3 days, then 200 mg orally twice daily for 12 months
Candida species	+	Mucous membranes, skin, esophagus, genitourinary tract, heart	Polymorphonuclear or mononuclear pleocytosis; may be Gram-positive	Amphotericin B (liposomal) 3-5 mg/kg intravenously daily ± Flucytosine 25 mg/kg orally four times daily, then 400 mg orally daily for 8 weeks, then maintenance with Fluconazole 400-800 mg orally daily
Coccidioides immitis	–	Lungs, skin, bones	Eosinophilic pleocytosis; positive complement fixation	Fluconazole 400-800 mg intravenously or orally daily for 1 year
Cryptococcus neoformans	± (HIV)	Lungs, skin, bones, joints	Lymphocytic pleocytosis, viscous fluid, positive India ink prep and cryptococcal antigen	Amphotericin B (liposomal) 3-5 mg/kg intravenously daily + Flucytosine 25 mg/kg orally four times daily, then 400 mg orally daily for 8 weeks, then maintenance with Fluconazole 200 mg orally daily
Histoplasma capsulatum	±	Lungs, skin, mucous membranes, heart, viscera	Lymphocytic pleocytosis	Amphotericin B (liposomal) 5 mg/kg/d intravenously for 4-6 weeks, then Itraconazole 200 mg orally 2-3 times daily for 12 months
Mucor species	+ (diabetes)	Orbits, paranasal sinuses	–	Amphotericin B (liposomal) 3-10 mg/kg intravenously daily for 10-12 weeks, correction of hyperglycemia and acidosis, and wound debridement

skin, or by direct extension from parameningeal sites such as the orbits or paranasal sinuses. Invasion of the meninges from a contiguous focus of infection is particularly common in mucormycosis but may also occur in aspergillosis and actinomycosis.

Pathologic findings in fungal infections of the nervous system include a primarily mononuclear basal meningeal exudative reaction (see Figure 4-13), focal abscesses or granulomas in the brain or spinal epidural space, cerebral infarction related to vasculitis, and ventricular enlargement caused by communicating hydrocephalus.

▶ Clinical Findings

Fungal meningitis is usually a subacute illness resembling tuberculous meningitis. Common symptoms include headache and lethargy or confusion. Nausea and vomiting, visual loss, seizures, or focal weakness may also occur, and fever may be absent. Facial or eye pain, nasal discharge, proptosis, or visual loss should prompt urgent consideration of *Mucor* infection in diabetic patients with acidosis.

Careful examination of the skin, orbits, sinuses, and chest may reveal evidence of systemic fungal infection. Neurologic examination may show signs of meningeal irritation, a confusional state, papilledema, visual loss, ptosis, exophthalmos, ocular or other cranial nerve palsies, and focal neurologic abnormalities such as hemiparesis. Because some fungi (eg, *Cryptococcus*) can cause spinal cord compression, there may be evidence of spine tenderness, paraparesis, pyramidal signs in the legs, or loss of sensation over the legs and trunk.

▶ Laboratory Findings

Blood cultures should be obtained. Serum glucose and arterial blood gas levels should be determined in diabetic patients. The urine should be examined for *Candida*. Chest X-ray may show hilar lymphadenopathy, patchy or miliary infiltrates, cavitation, or pleural effusion in several fungal infections. The CT scan or MRI may demonstrate intracerebral mass lesions associated with *Cryptococcus* (**Figure 4-17**) or other organisms, a contiguous infectious source in the orbit or paranasal sinuses, or hydrocephalus.

CSF pressure may be normal or elevated. The fluid is usually clear, but may be viscous in cryptococcal infection. Lymphocytic pleocytosis of up to 1,000 cells/mL is common, but a normal cell count or polymorphonuclear pleocytosis can be seen in early fungal meningitis, immunosuppressed patients, or *Aspergillus* infection. CSF protein may be normal initially, but subsequently rises, usually not exceeding 200 mg/dL; higher levels (up to 1 g/dL) suggest subarachnoid block. Glucose is normal or decreased, but rarely below 10 mg/dL. Microscopic examination of Gram-stained and acid-fast smears and India ink preparations may reveal the infecting organism. Fungal cultures of CSF and other body fluids and tissues should be obtained, but are often negative. In suspected mucormycosis, biopsy of the affected tissue (usually

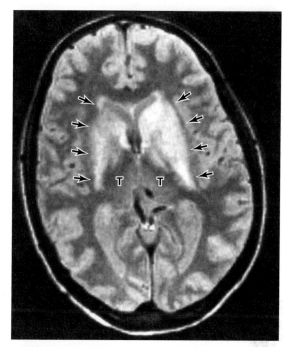

▲ Figure 4-17. T2-weighted MRI in cryptococcal meningitis. Note the bilateral increase in signal in the basal ganglia (**arrows**) with relative sparing of the thalami (**T**). This is caused by gelatinous fungal pseudocysts in the territory of the lenticulostriate arteries. (Used with permission from A. Gean.)

nasal mucosa) is essential. Useful CSF serologic studies include cryptococcal antigen and *Coccidioides* complement-fixing antibody. Cryptococcal antigen is more sensitive than India ink for detecting *Cryptococcus* and should always be looked for in both CSF and serum when that organism is suspected, as in patients with HIV infection.

▶ Differential Diagnosis

Fungal meningitis may mimic brain abscess and other subacute or chronic meningitides, such as those caused by tuberculosis or syphilis. CSF findings and CT or MRI scans are useful in differential diagnosis.

▶ Treatment & Prognosis

Treatment of fungal meningitis is summarized in Table 4-14. In addition to antibiotics, CSF drainage is used to control intracranial pressure in cryptococcal meningitis. Mortality is high, complications of treatment are common, and neurologic sequelae are frequent.

PARASITIC INFECTIONS

Protozoal, helminthic, and rickettsial infections may cause CNS disease, particularly in immunosuppressed patients (including those with HIV infection), and in certain regions of the world. The relationship of these infections to host immunity and recommended treatments are summarized in **Table 4-15**.

A. Malaria

Malaria, the most common human parasitic infection, is caused by the protozoan *Plasmodium falciparum* or other

Table 4-15. Parasitic Infections of the Central Nervous System.

Parasite	Opportunistic	Treatment
Protozoa		
Plasmodium falciparum (malaria)	–	Quinidine/artesunate/quinine[1] then Doxycycline[2] or Tetracycline[3] or Clindamycin[4]
Toxoplasma gondii	±	Pyrimethamine[5] and Sulfadiazine[6]
Naegleria fowleri (primary amebic meningoencephalitis)	–	Amphotericin B[7] + Rifampin[7] + Fluconazole[7] + Azithromycin[7] + Miltefosine[8]
Acanthamoeba or *Hartmannella* species (granulomatous amebic encephalitis)	+	Pentamidine[9] ± Sulfadiazine[9] ± Flucytosine[9] ± Fluconazole[9] ± Miltefosine[8]
Helminths		
Taenia solium (cysticercosis)	–	Albendazole[10] + Praziquantel[10] ± Dexamethasone[11] ± Surgery[12]
Angiostrongylus cantonensis (eosinophilic meningitis)	–	Dexamethasone[11] ± CSF removal
Rickettsia		
Rickettsia rickettsii (Rocky Mountain spotted fever)	–	Chloramphenicol[13] **or** Doxycycline[2]

[1]Quinidine dose is 10 mg/kg IV, then 0.02 mg /kg/min IV. Quinine dose is 20 mg/kg IV in 5% dextrose over 4 hours, then 10 mg/kg over 2-4 hours every 8 hours. Where available, artesunate (2.4 mg/kg IV at 0, 12, 24, 48, and 72 hours) may be preferred. When oral treatment becomes tolerated, can switch to quinine sulfate (650 mg PO three times daily) for the remainder of a 7-day course.
[2]Doxycycline dose is 100 mg PO twice daily for 7 days.
[3]Tetracycline dose is 250 mg PO four times daily for 7 days.
[4]Clindamycin dose is 20 mg/kg/d in 3 divided doses for 7 days.
[5]Pyrimethamine dose is 200 mg PO once, then 50-75 mg/d PO for 3-6 weeks.
[6]Sulfadiazine dose is 1-1.5 g PO four times daily for 3-6 weeks.
[7]Amphotericin B dose is 0.25 mg/kg IV over 4-6 hours, then 0.5-1.5 mg/kg/d IV. An alternative is 1 mg/kg once daily IV plus up to 0.5 mg/d by the intraventricular route. Rifampin dose is 10 mg/kg IV once daily. Fluconazole dose is 12 mg/kg IV once daily. Azithromycin dose is 500 mg IV once daily. However, treatment is rarely effective.
[8]Miltefosine dose is 50 mg PO 2-3 times daily.
[9]Pentamidine dose is 4 mg/kg IV once daily. Sulfadiazine dose is 1.5 g PO every 6 hours. Flucytosine dose is 37.5 mg/kg PO every 6 hours. Fluconazole dose is 12 mg/kg IV once daily. Miltefosine dose is 50 mg PO 2-3 times daily. Used in various combinations but rarely effective.
[10]Albendazole dose is 15 mg/kg PO daily for 10-15 days. Praziquantel dose is 50 mg/kg PO daily for 10 days.
[11]Dexamethasone dose is 6 mg PO daily for 10-15 days.
[12]Shunting for or excision of intraventricular, subarachnoid, spinal, or ocular cysts.
[13]Chloramphenicol dose is 12.5 mg/kg PO four times daily for 1 week.

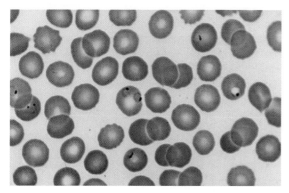

▲ **Figure 4-18.** Peripheral blood smear from a patient with *Plasmodium falciparum* malaria, showing parasites (dark spots) within red blood cells. (Used with permission from Kaushansky K, Lichtman M, Beutler E, Kipps T. *Williams Hematology.* 8th ed. New York, NY: McGraw-Hill, 2010.)

Plasmodium species and is transferred to humans by the female *Anopheles* mosquito. Clinical features include fever, chills, myalgia, nausea and vomiting, anemia, renal failure, hypoglycemia, and pulmonary edema. Cerebral involvement occurs when plasmodia reach the CNS in infected red blood cells and occlude cerebral capillaries. Neurologic involvement becomes apparent weeks after infection. In addition to acute confusional states, cerebral malaria can produce coma, focal neurologic abnormalities, and seizures. The most common findings on neurologic examination of affected adults are bilateral pyramidal signs (especially extensor plantar responses), sustained upgaze, signs of meningeal irritation, and decorticate or decerebrate posturing. The diagnosis is made by finding plasmodia in red blood cells on thick and thin peripheral blood smears (**Figure 4-18**). The CSF may show increased pressure, xanthochromia, mononuclear pleocytosis, or mildly elevated protein. Antibiotic treatment is given in Table 4-15. In addition, the ECG should be monitored for QTc segment prolongation during intravenous quinidine administration, and hypoglycemia may require IV administration of dextrose. Mannitol and corticosteroids are not helpful and may be deleterious. The mortality rate in cerebral malaria is about 20%.

B. Toxoplasmosis

Toxoplasmosis results from ingestion of *Toxoplasma gondii* cysts in raw meat or cat excrement and is usually asymptomatic. Symptomatic disease is associated with reactivation of latent infection in the setting of HIV infection, underlying malignancy, or immunosuppressive therapy. Systemic manifestations include skin rash, lymphadenopathy, myalgias, arthralgias, carditis, pneumonitis, and splenomegaly. CNS involvement can cause abscesses or encephalitis, and symptoms and signs include headache, altered mental status, seizures, and focal deficits. The CSF

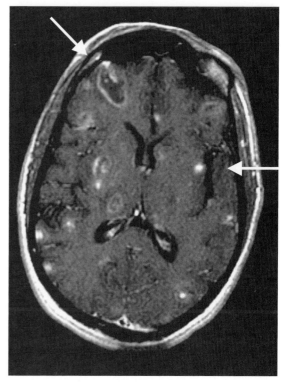

▲ **Figure 4-19.** T1-weighted, gadolinium-enhanced MRI in cerebral toxoplasmosis complicating HIV infection. Note the multiple calcifications (**arrow, right**) and ring-enhanced lesions (**arrow, left**) in the basal ganglia and cerebral cortex.

may show mild mononuclear cell pleocytosis or slight protein elevation, and the organism may be seen on wet mounts of centrifuged CSF. MRI is superior to CT scanning for demonstrating the characteristic ring-enhancing lesions (**Figure 4-19**). Diagnosis can be made by detection of anti-*Toxoplasma* IgG antibodies. Folinic acid 10 mg orally daily should accompany antibiotic treatment (Table 4-15) to prevent pyrimethamine-induced leukopenia and thrombocytopenia.

C. Primary Amebic Meningoencephalitis

The free-living ameba *Naegleria fowleri* causes primary amebic meningoencephalitis in previously healthy young persons exposed to warm, polluted fresh water. Amebas gain entry to the CNS through the cribriform plate, producing a diffuse meningoencephalitis that affects the base of the frontal lobes and posterior fossa. It is characterized by headache, fever, nausea and vomiting, signs of meningeal irritation, and disordered mental status. The CSF shows a polymorphonuclear pleocytosis with elevated protein and low glucose; highly motile, refractile trophozoites can sometimes be seen on CSF wet mounts. The disease is usually fatal but occasional recovery has been reported with antibiotic treatment (Table 4-15).

D. Granulomatous Amebic Encephalitis

Granulomatous amebic encephalitis results from infection with *Acanthamoeba/Hartmanella* species and commonly occurs with chronic illness or immunosuppression. The disorder typically lasts 1 week to 3 months and is characterized by subacute or chronic meningitis and granulomatous encephalitis. The cerebellum, brainstem, basal ganglia, and cerebral hemispheres are affected. An acute confusional state is the most common clinical finding. Fever, headache, meningeal signs, seizures, hemiparesis cranial nerve palsies, cerebellar ataxia, and aphasia may be seen. CSF pleocytosis is lymphocytic or polymorphonuclear, protein is elevated, and glucose is low or normal. Sluggishly motile trophozoites may be seen on CSF wet mounts. Despite treatment (Table 4-15), the disease is usually fatal.

E. Cysticercosis

Cysticercosis is the most common helminthic infection of the CNS and is observed most often in Mexico, Central and South America, Africa, and Asia. Infection follows ingestion of larvae of the pork tapeworm *Taenia solium*. Larvae form single or multiple cysts in the brain, ventricles, and subarachnoid space, and neurologic manifestations result from mass effect, obstruction of CSF flow, or inflammation. Seizures are the most common manifestation of parenchymal brain disease; obstructive hydrocephalus is associated with intraventricular lesions; communicating hydrocephalus, meningitis, and stroke result from subarachnoid involvement; myelopathy or radiculopathy may complicate spinal cysticercosis; and visual impairment is observed with ocular infection. Ophthalmoscopic examination may show ocular cysts, and there may be peripheral blood eosinophilia, soft tissue calcifications, or parasites in the stool. The CSF shows a lymphocytic pleocytosis with eosinophils sometimes present (**Table 4-16**). Opening pressure is often increased, but if it is decreased, imaging studies should be performed to detect possible spinal subarachnoid block. CSF protein is 50 to 100 mg/dL and glucose is 20 to 50 mg/dL in most cases. CT scan or MRI is the most useful diagnostic test and may show contrast-enhanced mass lesions (sometimes containing live parasites) with surrounding edema, intracerebral calcifications, or ventricular enlargement (**Figure 4-20**).

Treatment depends on symptoms and the site of involvement. Patients with seizures and calcified cysts should be treated with anticonvulsants. Cysts containing viable parasites or persistent or multiple enhancing lesions are usually treated with anticonvulsants, antihelminthic drugs (Table 4-15), and corticosteroids. Intraventricular,

Table 4-16. Causes of CSF Eosinophilia.

Parasitic CNS infections
Angiostrongylus cantonensis (eosinophilic meningitis)
Gnathostoma spinigerum (gnathostomiasis)
Baylisascaris procyonis
Taenia solium (cysticercosis)
Other helminthic infections
Other CNS infections
Coccidioides immitis meningitis
Neurosyphilis
Tuberculous meningitis
Noninfectious causes
Hematologic malignancies (Hodgkin disease, non-Hodgkin lymphoma, eosinophilic leukemia)
Medications (ciprofloxacin, ibuprofen)
Foreign matter in subarachnoid space (antibiotics, myelography dye, ventriculoperitoneal shunts)
Idiopathic hypereosinophilic syndrome

Data from Lo Re V III, Gluckman SJ. Eosinophilic meningitis. *Am J Med.* 2003;114:217-223.

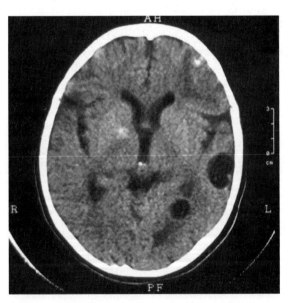

▲ **Figure 4-20.** Neurocysticercosis. Noncontrast head CT showing new (cystic, black) and old (calcified, white) lesions. (Used with permission from Seth W. Wright, MD, and Universidad Peruana Cayetano Heredia, Lima, Peru.)

ocular, and spinal cysts may be amenable to surgical removal, and hydrocephalus is treated by ventriculoperitoneal shunting. Patients with ocular cysts should not be given antihelminthics.

F. *Angiostrongylus cantonensis* Meningitis

Angiostrongylus cantonensis (rat lungworm) is endemic to Southeast Asia, Hawaii, and other Pacific islands. Infection is transmitted by ingestion of raw or undercooked snails, shellfish, or frogs and produces meningitis with peripheral blood and CSF eosinophilia (Table 4-16). Symptoms include headache, neck stiffness, paresthesia, vomiting, and nausea. Lymphocytic CSF pleocytosis, CSF eosinophilia, brain CT or MRI, and ELISA can aid in diagnosis. Rarely, worms can be found in the eye or CSF. The acute illness usually resolves spontaneously in 1 to 2 weeks, although corticosteroids, analgesics, and reduction of CSF pressure by repeated lumbar puncture may be helpful.

G. Rickettsiae

Rickettsiae are intracellular parasitic gram-negative bacteria transmitted to humans by tick, flea, or louse bites. They cause a variety of diseases that can affect the nervous system and produce meningitis or encephalitis, including Rocky Mountain spotted fever, typhus, tsutsugamushi fever, and Q fever. Neurologic manifestations include headache, encephalopathy, coma, and death. Most rickettsial infections respond to antibiotics (Table 4-15).

ACUTE DISSEMINATED ENCEPHALOMYELITIS

Acute disseminated encephalomyelitis is an immune-mediated monophasic demyelinating disorder that typically occurs within 1 month after a bacterial or viral (usually upper respiratory) infection. Children are affected most often. Deficits evolve over 2-5 days. Clinical features include fever, seizures, confusion or coma, and focal neurologic deficits (eg, optic or other cranial neuropathies, hemiparesis, ataxia). MRI shows multifocal demyelinating lesions affecting primarily the supratentorial white matter, although gray matter and spinal cord can also be involved. The CSF may show lymphocytic or, less commonly, polymorphonuclear pleocytosis, but oligoclonal bands are absent. In a more fulminant variant, **acute hemorrhagic leukoencephalitis**, MRI shows bihemispheric demyelinating lesions associated with hemorrhage and edema, and the CSF may contain red blood cells. Treatment of both acute disseminated encephalomyelitis and acute hemorrhagic leukoencephalitis is with methylprednisolone 30 mg/kg/d (up to 1 g/d) intravenously for 5 days, followed by prednisone 1-2 mg/kg/d orally tapered over 4 to 6 weeks. Outcome in acute disseminated encephalomyelitis is usually good, but acute hemorrhagic leukoencephalitis has a high mortality.

SARCOIDOSIS

Sarcoidosis is an idiopathic inflammatory disorder that produces noncaseating granulomas and prominently affects the lungs. Neurologic involvement occurs in 5-15% of cases and causes basal meningitis or intraparenchymal mass lesions. Clinical findings include cranial (especially facial) neuropathy, confusion, seizures, hydrocephalus, myelopathy, stroke, and endocrine disorders from hypothalamic or pituitary involvement. Laboratory abnormalities include elevated serum levels of angiotensin-converting enzyme, increased CSF protein and mononuclear pleocytosis, and positive Kveim test. High-resolution chest CT is more sensitive than chest X-ray for detecting hilar adenopathy or interstitial lung disease. Brain MRI may show meningeal enhancement, intraparenchymal lesions, or hydrocephalus. Treatment is with prednisone 20 to 60 mg orally daily, tapered over 1 to 6 months. In severe cases, this may be preceded by methylprednisolone 1 g intravenously daily for 3 to 5 days. Addition of azathioprine, methotrexate, hydroxychloroquine, cyclosporine A, mycophenolate mofetil, infliximab, or adalimumab may improve the response to treatment and reduce the likelihood of relapse.

LEPTOMENINGEAL METASTASES

Diffuse metastatic seeding of the leptomeninges may complicate systemic cancer (especially carcinoma of the breast, carcinoma of the lung, lymphoma, leukemia, carcinoma of the gastrointestinal tract, and melanoma) or primary brain tumors (especially glioma, medulloblastomas, and pineal tumors), producing disorders of the brain or spinal cord, including cognitive dysfunction. Two varieties of leptomeningeal metastasis are observed and may coexist: **diffuse or nonadherent** metastasis, consisting of free-floating cells in the subarachnoid space, and **nodular** metastasis, characterized by contrast-enhancing adherent tumor nodules. Neoplastic meningitis usually occurs 3 months to 5 years after the diagnosis of cancer, but may precede it. Abnormal neurologic signs are often more striking than the symptoms and usually suggest involvement at multiple levels of the neuraxis. Diffuse or nonadherent metastasis is diagnosed by CSF cytology (**Table 4-17**), whereas diagnosis of nodular metastasis depends on cranial and spinal MRI with contrast (**Figure 4-21**). Treatment depends on the type of leptomeningeal metastasis and the presence or absence of parenchymal brain metastasis and systemic disease. Treatment options include intrathecal and systemic chemotherapy (eg, methotrexate, cytosine arabinoside) and local or whole-brain radiotherapy. In treated cases, the average duration of survival is 3-6 months, but this is influenced by tumor type. Prognosis in leptomeningeal metastasis is best for leukemia and lymphoma, intermediate for breast cancer, and worst for non-small cell lung cancer and melanoma.

Table 4-17. Presenting Features of Leptomeningeal Metastases.

Feature	Percentage of Patients
Symptoms	
Gait disturbance	46
Headache	38
Altered mentation	25
Weakness	22
Back pain	18
Nausea or vomiting	12
Radicular pain	12
Paresthesia	10
Signs	
Lower motor neuron weakness	78
Absent tendon reflex	60
Cognitive disturbance	50
Extensor plantar response	50
Dermatomal sensory deficit	50
Ophthalmoplegia	30
Facial weakness	25
Hearing loss	20
Neck meningeal signs	16
Seizures	14
Papilledema	12
Facial sensory deficit	12
Leg meningeal signs	12
Laboratory findings	
MRI positive	77
CSF pleocytosis	64
CSF protein >50 mg/dL	59
CSF opening pressure >160 mm CSF	50
CSF cytology positive	47
CSF glucose <40 mg/dL	31
Both MRI and CSF cytology positive	24
CSF normal	3

CSF, cerebrospinal fluid; MRI, magnetic resonance imaging.
Data from DeAngelis LM, Posner JB. *Neurologic Complications of Cancer.* 2nd ed. Oxford, UK: Oxford; 2008, and Clarke JL, Perez HR, Jacks LM, Panageas KS, Deangelis LM. Leptomeningeal metastases in the MRI era. *Neurology.* 2010;74:1449-1454.

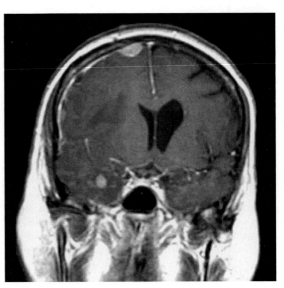

▲ **Figure 4-21.** Gadolinium-enhanced T1 coronal MRI showing meningeal spread of breast cancer. There are contrast-enhancing (white) focal lesions in the meninges on the left, diffuse meningeal enhancement, and mass effect from a hemispheric lesion on the left.

SEPSIS-ASSOCIATED ENCEPHALOPATHY

Systemic sepsis can produce an encephalopathy that may be related to impaired cerebral blood flow, disruption of the blood–brain barrier, or cerebral edema. Gram-negative infections are the most common cause. Bacteremia, liver failure, or kidney failure may be present. Neurologic manifestations include confusional states or coma, seizures, focal neurologic deficits, rigidity, myoclonus, and asterixis. CSF examination is essential to exclude meningitis. The EEG is often abnormal. Therapy involves supportive measures, such as assisted ventilation, and treatment of the underlying infection. Mortality is high, but can be reduced by prompt diagnosis and treatment.

ANTIBIOTIC-ASSOCIATED ENCEPHALOPATHY

Antibiotics can cause confusional states characterized by encephalopathy with seizures or myoclonus (cephalosporins, penicillin), psychosis (quinolones, macrolides, procaine penicillin), or vertigo and cerebellar ataxia (metronidazole). Renal failure may be a predisposing factor, especially with cephalosporins. Symptoms typically resolve within about 1 week after the drug is discontinued, or about 2 weeks with metronidazole.

VASCULAR DISORDERS

Vascular causes of acute confusional states include disorders of the blood vessels, heart, or blood.

HYPERTENSIVE ENCEPHALOPATHY

A sudden increase in blood pressure, with or without pre-existing chronic hypertension, may result in encephalopathy and headache, which develop over a period of hours to days. Patients at risk include those with acute glomerulonephritis or eclampsia. Impaired autoregulation of cerebral blood flow (**Figure 4-22**), vasospasm, and intravascular coagulation have all been proposed as contributing factors. Vomiting, visual disturbances, focal neurologic deficits, and focal or generalized seizures can occur. Blood pressure in excess of 250/150 mm Hg is usually required to precipitate the syndrome in patients with chronic hypertension, but previously normotensive patients may be affected at lower pressures. Retinal arteriolar spasm is almost invariable, and papilledema, retinal hemorrhages, and exudates are usually present. Lumbar puncture may show normal or elevated CSF pressure and protein. Areas of edema, located especially in parieto-occipital white matter, are seen on CT scan and MRI (**Figure 4-23**) and are reversible with treatment.

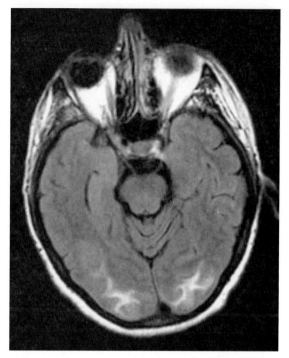

▲ **Figure 4-23.** Axial FLAIR MRI in hypertensive encephalopathy showing increased signal (white) in the subcortical occipital white matter and occipital cortex bilaterally. These findings may represent reversible vasogenic edema.

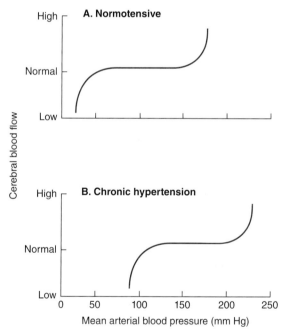

▲ **Figure 4-22.** Cerebrovascular autoregulation. (**A**) Cerebral blood flow is normally held constant over a wide range of blood pressures. At very low pressures, cerebral hypoperfusion occurs, producing syncope. Pressures above the autoregulatory range can cause hypertensive encephalopathy. (**B**) Chronic hypertension shifts the autoregulatory range to higher blood pressures. Hypoperfusion and syncope can occur at normal pressures, and pressures associated with hypertensive encephalopathy are higher.

The diagnosis of hypertensive encephalopathy is established when lowering the blood pressure results in rapid resolution of symptoms. This is accomplished with sodium nitroprusside, given by continuous intravenous infusion at an initial rate of 0.25 μg/kg/min and increased to as much as 10 μg/kg/min as required. The patient must be carefully monitored and the infusion rate adjusted to maintain a therapeutic effect without producing hypotension. Mean arterial blood pressure should be reduced by no more than 25% in the first 2 hours of treatment, and a target of 160/100 mm Hg should be aimed for in the following 4 hours. Treatment should be terminated immediately if neurologic function worsens. Untreated hypertensive encephalopathy can result in renal failure, stroke, coma, or death, but prompt treatment usually produces full clinical recovery.

Stroke and subarachnoid hemorrhage can also produce encephalopathy with acutely elevated blood pressure; when focal neurologic abnormalities are also present, stroke is most likely.

The clinical syndrome of hypertensive encephalopathy overlaps with **posterior reversible encephalopathy syndrome (PRES)**, which is defined by subcortical, most often parieto-occipital white matter changes, consistent with edema, seen on CT or MRI. Patients often have a history of immunosuppressive drug treatment; most but not all have increased blood pressure at presentation. Presenting features include headache, altered mental status, seizures, and visual deficits. Treatment includes discontinuing drugs that may have precipitated the disorder and treating elevated blood pressure if present.

PRES, in turn, overlaps with **reversible cerebral vasoconstriction syndrome (RCVS)**, which is often associated with the use of vasoconstrictive, serotonergic antidepressant, or illicit recreational drugs. Blood pressure is sometimes elevated. The most distinctive clinical feature of RCVS is onset with thunderclap headache, but it may also produce seizures or focal neurologic deficits. CT or MRI may be normal, or may show border zone infarcts, intracerebral hemorrhage, or vasogenic edema. The characteristic imaging abnormality is multifocal vasoconstriction on angiography. Treatment is with nimodipine. The disorder is typically self-limited with resolution within ~1 month. RCVS is discussed in Chapter 13 in the differential diagnosis of stroke.

SUBARACHNOID HEMORRHAGE

Subarachnoid hemorrhage, usually due to rupture of a cerebral aneurysm, must receive early consideration in the differential diagnosis of an acute confusional state. Subarachnoid hemorrhage may produce encephalopathy, coma, meningeal signs, and focal neurologic deficits, but the most prominent symptom is usually headache. For this reason, the disorder is discussed in Chapter 6, Headache & Facial Pain.

VERTEBROBASILAR ISCHEMIA

An embolus to the top of the basilar artery that subsequently breaks up and sends fragments distally can produce ischemia affecting the territory of both posterior cerebral arteries. This condition (**top of the basilar syndrome**) may cause an acute confusional state accompanied by pupillary (sluggish responses to light and accommodation), visual (homonymous hemianopia, cortical blindness), visuomotor (impaired convergence, paralysis of upward or downward gaze, diplopia), and behavioral (hypersomnolence, peduncular hallucinosis) abnormalities. Vertebrobasilar ischemia is discussed in more detail in Chapter 13, Stroke.

NONDOMINANT HEMISPHERIC INFARCTION

Agitated confusion of sudden onset can result from infarction (usually embolic) in the territory of the inferior division of the nondominant (usually right) middle cerebral artery. If the superior division is spared, there is no associated hemiparesis. Agitation may be so pronounced as to suggest drug intoxication or withdrawal, but autonomic hyperactivity is absent. The diagnosis is confirmed by brain CT scan or MRI. Rarely, isolated anterior cerebral artery infarcts or posterior cerebral artery infarcts cause acute confusion.

SYSTEMIC LUPUS ERYTHEMATOSUS

Systemic lupus erythematosus (SLE) is an autoimmune disorder that causes skin rash, arthritis, serositis, nephritis, anemia, leukopenia, and thrombocytopenia. In addition, SLE produces neurologic involvement in about one-half of patients and is the most common autoimmune cause of encephalopathy. Clinically active systemic disease need not be present for neurologic symptoms to occur. The pathophysiology of nervous system involvement is unclear, but may involve vasculopathy resulting in blood-brain barrier defects and neurotoxic effects of autoantibodies and cytokines. Neuropathologic findings include fibrinoid degeneration of arterioles and capillaries, microinfarcts, and intracerebral hemorrhages, but true vasculitis of cerebral blood vessels is rare. Clinical features include headache, cognitive impairment, mood disorders, seizures, stroke, acute confusional states, chorea, transverse myelitis, and aseptic meningitis. Seizures are usually generalized but may be focal. Laboratory abnormalities include anti-phospholipid, anti-ribosomal P protein, anti-glutamate receptor, and anti-endothelial cell antibodies and a false-positive serologic test for syphilis. CSF shows mild elevation of protein or a modest, usually mononuclear, pleocytosis in some cases. MRI may show white or gray matter lesions, brain atrophy, and ischemic or hemorrhagic strokes.

In patients with SLE, encephalopathy can be caused by a variety of factors, including coagulopathy, infection, uremia, emboli from endocarditis, and corticosteroid therapy. Cerebral lupus is treated with corticosteroids, beginning at 60 mg/d of prednisone or the equivalent. In patients already receiving steroids, the dose should be increased by the equivalent of 5 to 10 mg/d of prednisone. After symptoms resolve, steroids should be tapered to a maintenance dose of 5 to 10 mg/d. Treatments used in refractory cases or to reduce exposure to steroids include cyclophosphamide, azathioprine, mycophenolate mofetil, rituximab, plasma exchange, and intravenous immunoglobulin. Seizures are treated with anticonvulsants. Neurologic symptoms of SLE improve in >80% of patients treated with corticosteroids, but may also resolve without treatment. Cerebral involvement in SLE has not been shown to adversely affect the overall prognosis.

VASCULITIS

Acute confusional states can occur in primary central nervous system vasculitis, primary systemic vasculitis, and vasculitis secondary to systemic infection or neoplasm.

Primary central nervous system vasculitis, sometimes referred to as granulomatous angiitis, is usually manifested by headache and encephalopathy; it may also cause seizures or stroke (discussed in Chapter 13, Stroke). There is no involvement of other organs, and laboratory studies reveal no evidence of systemic vasculitis. The CSF usually shows mild lymphocytic pleocytosis and elevated protein. MRI may demonstrate bilateral, multifocal infarcts or diffuse changes consistent with ischemic demyelination. Angiography shows beading of small to medium-sized arteries due to multifocal narrowing. This finding also occurs in reversible cerebral vasoconstriction syndrome (see *Hypertensive Encephalopathy* earlier in this chapter). Definitive diagnosis of primary central nervous system vasculitis is by angiography or brain biopsy. Treatment is with methylprednisolone, 1 g/d intravenously for 3-5 days, followed by prednisone, 1/mg/kg/d orally for 1 month and then tapered over 1 year. Addition of cyclophosphamide, 2 mg/kg/d orally for 3 to 6 months, followed by azathioprine, 2 mg/kg/d orally for 2 to 3 years, may be associated with a lower relapse rate.

Large vessel systemic vasculitis (eg, giant cell or Takayasu arteritis) produces ischemic optic neuropathy and stroke, rather than confusional states. Medium-size vessel systemic vasculitis due to **polyarteritis nodosa** can cause encephalopathy, focal neurologic deficits, and seizures, but these occur late in the course, when the diagnosis is likely already known. Small vessel systemic vasculitis due to **cryoglobulinemia**, **Henoch-Schönlein purpura**, or **granulomatosis with polyangiitis** (formerly known as **Wegener granulomatosis**) can also produce encephalopathy. These diseases are diagnosed based on the pattern of systemic involvement and by laboratory tests. Treatment of systemic vasculitis affecting the central nervous system is similar to that described above for primary central nervous system vasculitis.

COMPLICATIONS OF CARDIAC SURGERY

Cardiac surgery, including coronary artery bypass grafting and valve repair or replacement, is associated with neurologic complications, especially stroke and encephalopathy. Several factors—embolization, hypoperfusion, arrhythmia, metabolic disturbances, and pharmacologic agents—may contribute. Evaluation should include a review of medications, search for metabolic derangements, and CT scan or MRI to detect perioperative stroke. Sedatives and other psychoactive medications should be avoided. Postoperative encephalopathy is typically transient, but some patients show more persistent cognitive dysfunction, which affects memory disproportionately and lasts for weeks to months. Cognitive decline that continues for years after cardiac surgery is likely due to another cause.

DISSEMINATED INTRAVASCULAR COAGULATION

Disseminated intravascular coagulation (DIC) results from pathologic activation of the coagulation and fibrinolytic systems in the setting of an underlying disorder such as sepsis, malignancy, or trauma. The principal manifestation is hemorrhage. Common findings in the brain include small multifocal infarctions and petechial hemorrhages involving gray and white matter. Subdural hematoma, subarachnoid hemorrhage, and hemorrhagic infarction in the distribution of large vessels may also occur.

Neurologic manifestations are common and include confusional states, coma, focal signs, and seizures. They may precede hematologic abnormalities, which include hypofibrinogenemia, thrombocytopenia, fibrin degradation products, and prolonged prothrombin time. Microangiopathic hemolytic anemia may also occur. The differential diagnosis includes thrombotic thrombocytopenic purpura (see later), which is distinguished by its tendency to occur in previously healthy individuals and its association with normal plasma fibrinogen and normal or only slightly elevated fibrin degradation products. Treatment is directed at the underlying disease and correction of anemia, thrombocytopenia, and coagulopathy. Prognosis is related to the severity of the underlying disease.

THROMBOTIC THROMBOCYTOPENIC PURPURA

TTP (Moschcowitz disease) is a rare multisystem disorder defined by the pentad of thrombocytopenic purpura, microangiopathic hemolytic anemia, neurologic dysfunction, fever, and renal disease. It is caused by autoantibodies against or mutations in the gene for the metalloprotease ADAMTS13. This allows multimers of von Willebrand factor to accumulate in the plasma, where they stimulate platelet aggregation. The result is platelet-fibrin thrombus formation with occlusion of small blood vessels, especially at arteriolar-capillary junctions. Pathologic findings in the brain include disseminated microinfarcts and, less frequently, petechial hemorrhages that are present mainly in gray matter.

Patients usually present with altered consciousness, headache, focal neurologic signs, or seizures, or with cutaneous purpura, ecchymoses, or petechiae. Neurologic symptoms may be fleeting and recurrent. Hematologic studies show Coombs-negative hemolytic anemia, thrombocytopenia, and normal or only slightly abnormal PT, PTT, fibrinogen, and fibrin degradation products. Compared with DIC (see preceding section), TTP is suggested by a platelet count of <20,000/μL and PT within 5 seconds of the upper limit of the normal range. There may be hematuria, proteinuria, or azotemia. CSF is usually normal. The diagnosis can be made by gingival biopsy or splenectomy.

Treatment includes daily plasma exchange to provide ADAMTS13 and remove autoantibodies, rituximab (375 mg/m^2 intravenously weekly for 4 weeks), or both. With treatment, mortality is 10% to 20%.

HEAD TRAUMA

Blunt head trauma can produce a confusional state or coma. Acceleration or deceleration forces and physical deformation of the skull can cause shearing of white matter with axonal injury, contusion from contact between the inner surface of the skull and the polar regions of the cerebral hemispheres, torn blood vessels, vasomotor changes, brain edema, and increased intracranial pressure.

CONCUSSION

Concussion is a syndrome that follows head trauma and is characterized by transient confusion, memory impairment, or incoordination. Other symptoms, which include headache, fatigue, irritability, dizziness, nausea, vomiting, blurred vision, and imbalance, tend to resolve after 1 to 2 days but persist for weeks to months (postconcussion syndrome) in ~15% of patients. Because a concussion may increase the risk of subsequent concussion, athletes who sustain a concussion while playing sports should delay their return to play until postconcussive symptoms have resolved and they have gradually resumed normal activity over about 1 week.

INTRACRANIAL HEMORRHAGE

Traumatic intracranial hemorrhage can be epidural, subdural, or intracerebral. **Epidural hematoma (Figure 4-24)** most often results from a lateral skull fracture that lacerates the middle meningeal artery or vein. Patients may or may not lose consciousness initially, but in either event a lucid interval lasting several hours to 1 to 2 days is followed by the rapid evolution, over hours, of headache, progressive obtundation, hemiparesis, and finally ipsilateral pupillary dilatation from uncal herniation. Death may follow if treatment is delayed.

Subdural hematoma after head injury can be acute, subacute, or chronic. In each case, headache and altered consciousness are the principal manifestations. Delay in diagnosis and treatment may lead to a fatal outcome. In contrast to epidural hematoma, the time between trauma and the onset of symptoms is typically longer, the hemorrhage tends to be located over the cerebral convexities, and associated skull fractures are uncommon.

Intracerebral contusion (bruising) or **intracerebral hemorrhage** related to head injury is usually located at the frontal or temporal poles. Blood typically enters the CSF, resulting in signs of meningeal irritation and sometimes hydrocephalus. Focal neurologic signs are usually absent or subtle.

The diagnosis of posttraumatic intracranial hemorrhage is made by CT scan or MRI. Epidural hematoma tends to appear as a biconvex, lens-shaped, extra-axial mass that may cross the midline or the tentorium but not the cranial sutures. Subdural hematoma is typically crescent-shaped and may cross the cranial sutures but not the midline or tentorium. Midline structures may be displaced contralaterally.

Epidural and subdural hematomas are treated by surgical evacuation. The decision to operate for intracerebral hematoma depends on the clinical course and location. Evacuation, decompression, or shunting for hydrocephalus may be indicated.

SEIZURES

POSTICTAL STATE

Generalized tonic-clonic (grand mal) seizures are typically followed by a transient confusional state (postictal state) that resolves within 1 to 2 hours. Sleepiness and confusion are usually prominent, but coma, agitation, amnesia, aphasia, or psychosis may occur. When postictal confusion does not clear rapidly, an explanation for the prolonged postictal state must be sought. This occurs in three settings: status epilepticus, an underlying structural brain abnormality (eg, stroke, intracranial hemorrhage), or an underlying diffuse cerebral disorder (eg, dementia, meningitis or encephalitis, metabolic encephalopathy). Patients with an unexplained prolonged postictal state should be evaluated with blood chemistry studies, lumbar puncture, EEG, and CT scan or MRI.

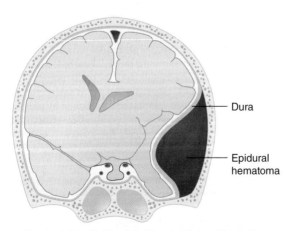
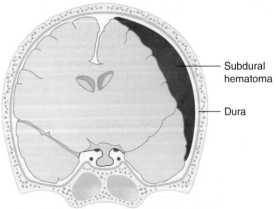

▲ **Figure 4-24.** Epidural (left) and subdural (right) hematomas. (Used with permission from Waxman SG. *Clinical Neuroanatomy.* 26th ed. New York, NY: McGraw-Hill, 2009.)

COMPLEX PARTIAL SEIZURES

Complex partial seizures—also termed temporal lobe seizures, psychomotor seizures, or focal seizures with impairment of consciousness or awareness—produce alterations in consciousness characterized by confusion or other cognitive, affective, psychomotor, or psychosensory symptoms. Such symptoms include withdrawal, agitation, and automatisms such as staring, repetitive chewing, swallowing, lip-smacking, or picking at clothing. Spells are typically brief and stereotypical, and psychomotor manifestations may be obvious to the observer (see Chapter 12, Seizures & Syncope). The diagnosis is made or confirmed by EEG.

NONCONVULSIVE STATUS EPILEPTICUS

Nonconvulsive (focal or absence) status epilepticus can produce confusion or coma, personality change, aphasia, subtle motor activity, or nystagmus. The diagnosis is established by a favorable clinical or EEG response to the administration of anticonvulsants (eg, lorazepam 4 mg or diazepam 10 mg given intravenously).

PSYCHIATRIC DISORDERS

Symptoms similar to those associated with acute confusional states—including incoherence, agitation, distractibility, hypervigilance, delusions, and hallucinations—can also be seen in a variety of psychiatric disorders. These include psychotic disorders, bipolar disorders, depressive disorders, anxiety disorders, and somatic disorders. Such diagnoses may be mistakenly assigned to patients with acute confusional states; conversely, patients with psychiatric disturbances may be thought, incorrectly, to have neurologic disease.

Unlike acute confusional states, psychiatric disorders are rarely acute in onset but typically develop over a period of at least several weeks. The history may reveal previous psychiatric disease or hospitalization or a precipitating psychologic stress. Physical examination may show abnormalities related to autonomic overactivity, including tachycardia, tachypnea, and hyperreflexia, but no definitive signs of neurologic dysfunction. Routine laboratory studies are normal in the psychiatric disorders listed previously, but are useful for excluding organic disorders.

Although the mental status examination in acute confusional states is often characterized by disorientation and fluctuating consciousness, patients with psychiatric disorders tend to maintain a consistent degree of cognitive impairment, appear awake and alert, have intact memory, and are oriented to person, place, and time. Disturbances in the content and form of thought (eg, delusions), perceptual abnormalities (eg, hallucinations), and flat or inappropriate affect are common, however. Psychiatric consultation should be sought regarding diagnosis and management.

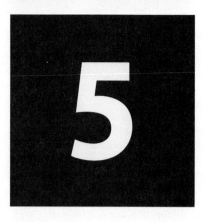

Dementia & Amnestic Disorders

5

Dementia is an acquired, generalized, and usually progressive impairment of the content of consciousness. Dementia differs from other disorders of cognitive function, such as coma (see Chapter 3, Coma) or confusional states (see Chapter 4, Confusional States), in that in dementia, the level of consciousness (wakefulness or arousal) is preserved.

Although the prevalence of dementia increases with advancing age (**Figure 5-1**), dementia is not an invariable consequence of aging, and results instead from diseases involving the cerebral cortex, its subcortical connections, or both. Normal aging may be associated with minor alterations in neurologic function (**Table 5-1**) and with neuroanatomic changes, such as enlargement of cerebral

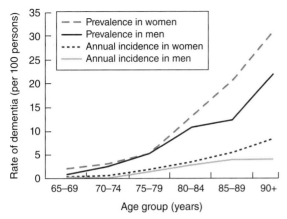

▲ **Figure 5-1.** Relationship between advancing age and incidence and prevalence of dementia. (Data from Lobo A et al. Prevalence of dementia and major subtypes in Europe. *Neurology.* 2000;54[suppl 5]:S4; Fratiglioni L et al. Incidence of dementia and major subtypes in Europe. *Neurology.* 2000;54[suppl 5]:S10.)

Table 5-1. Neurologic Changes in Normal Aging.

Cognitive
Slowed information processing
Impaired learning and recall of new information
Reduced spontaneous word finding and verbal fluency
Increased reaction time
Neuro-ophthalmologic
Small, sluggishly reactive pupils
Impaired upgaze
Impaired convergence
Motor
Atrophy of intrinsic hand and foot muscles
Increased muscle tone
Flexion (stooped) posture
Small-stepped or broad-based gait
Sensory
Reduced visual acuity
Reduced auditory acuity
Reduced gustatory acuity
Reduced olfactory acuity
Reduced vibration sense
Reflexes
Primitive reflexes
Absent abdominal reflexes
Absent ankle reflexes

ventricles and cortical sulci seen on computed tomography (CT) or magnetic resonance imaging (MRI) scans. However, these alone do not imply cognitive deficits. The term **mild cognitive impairment (MCI)** is sometimes used to describe deficits that are more severe than are customarily seen with normal aging but are insufficient to warrant a diagnosis of dementia. Nevertheless, patients with MCI have an increased risk (approximately 10% per year) of developing dementia.

Whereas dementia affects multiple spheres of cognitive function, more limited cognitive disorders may also occur. These include deficits in language function (aphasia) or motor (apraxia) or sensory integration, which are considered in Chapter 1, Neurologic History & Examination. **Memory disturbance (amnestic disorder or amnesia)**, another example of a circumscribed cognitive defect, is discussed later in this chapter. Memory may also be impaired in normal aging and in dementia, but in the former impairment is mild, and in the latter it is accompanied by defects in other spheres, such as reasoning, judgment, behavior, or language. Some causes of dementia, notably Alzheimer disease, produce early and disproportionate impairment of memory and, at least in the early stages of disease, may be difficult to distinguish from a pure amnestic disorder.

▼ APPROACH TO DIAGNOSIS

The first step in evaluating a patient with cognitive impairment of any kind is to determine the nature of the problem, which should initially be classified as affecting the level of consciousness (confusional state or coma) or the content of consciousness. **Table 5-2** lists key differences that may be useful in making this distinction. If the content (but not the level) of consciousness is impaired, a global cognitive disorder (dementia) must next be

Table 5-2. Differences Between Acute Confusional States and Dementia.

Feature	Acute Confusional State	Dementia
Level of consciousness	Impaired	Not impaired, except occasionally late in course
Course	Acute to subacute; fluctuating	Chronic; steadily progressive
Autonomic hyperactivity	Often present	Absent
Prognosis	Usually reversible	Usually irreversible[1]

[1]This is not an inherent feature of dementia but is currently the case.

distinguished from a more circumscribed deficit, such as amnesia or aphasia. This distinction is important because classification of the disorder determines the subsequent diagnostic approach.

In some cases, it may be difficult to distinguish dementia from a psychiatric disturbance (**pseudodementia**). Pseudodementia due to psychiatric disease is discussed later in this chapter.

The final step in the diagnosis of dementia or an amnestic syndrome is to identify the specific cause. The greatest emphasis should be on finding a treatable cause, but identification of untreatable causes can also be important, to provide the patient and family with prognostic information or genetic counseling, or to alert family members and medical personnel to the risk of a transmissible disease. At present, only approximately 10% of dementias are reversible, but the extent to which the quality and duration of life can be improved in these cases justifies the effort and expense required to detect them.

HISTORY

The general approach to obtaining a neurologic history is considered in Chapter 1, Neurologic History & Examination. Because dementia implies deterioration in cognitive ability, it is important to establish that the patient's level of functioning has declined. Data that can help to establish the cause of dementia include the time course of deterioration, associated symptoms (eg, headache, gait disturbance, or incontinence), family history of a similar condition, concurrent medical illnesses, and the use of therapeutic or recreational drugs (**Table 5-3**).

Table 5-3. Clinical Features Helpful in the Differential Diagnosis of Dementia.

Feature	Most Suggestive of
History	
Unprotected sexual intercourse, intravenous drug abuse, hemophilia, or blood transfusions	HIV-associated dementia
Family history	Huntington disease, Wilson disease
Headache	Brain tumor, chronic subdural hematoma
Vital signs	
Hypothermia	Hypothyroidism
Hypertension	Vascular dementia
Hypotension	Hypothyroidism
Bradycardia	Hypothyroidism
General examination	
Meningismus	Chronic meningitis
Jaundice	Acquired hepatocerebral degeneration, Wilson disease
Kayser–Fleischer rings	Wilson disease
Mental status examination	
Prominent memory loss	Alzheimer disease
Aphasia	Frontotemporal dementia (semantic dementia, progressive nonfluent aphasia)
Hallucinations	Lewy body disease
Cranial nerves	
Papilledema	Brain tumor, chronic subdural hematoma
Argyll Robertson pupils	Neurosyphilis
Ophthalmoplegia	Progressive supranuclear palsy
Pseudobulbar palsy	Vascular dementia, progressive supranuclear palsy

(Continued)

Table 5-3. Clinical Features Helpful in the Differential Diagnosis of Dementia. (*Continued*)

Feature	Most Suggestive of
Motor	
Limb apraxia	Corticobasal degeneration
Tremor	Lewy body disease, corticobasal degeneration, acquired hepatocerebral degeneration, Wilson disease, HIV-associated dementia
Asterixis	Acquired hepatocerebral degeneration, Wilson disease
Myoclonus	Creutzfeldt–Jakob disease, HIV-associated dementia
Rigidity	Lewy body disease, corticobasal degeneration, acquired hepatocerebral degeneration, Creutzfeldt–Jakob disease, progressive supranuclear palsy, Wilson disease
Chorea	Huntington disease, Wilson disease
Other	
Gait apraxia	Normal-pressure hydrocephalus
Hyporeflexia (from associated polyneuropathy)	Neurosyphilis, vitamin B_{12} deficiency, HIV-associated dementia

GENERAL PHYSICAL EXAMINATION

The general physical examination can contribute to etiologic diagnosis when it reveals signs of a systemic disease responsible for dementia. Particularly helpful signs are listed in Table 5-3.

MENTAL STATUS EXAMINATION

The mental status examination (**Table 5-4**) helps to determine whether the level or the content of consciousness is impaired and whether cognitive dysfunction is global or circumscribed. A disorder of the level of consciousness (eg, confusional state) is suggested by sleepiness, inattention, impairment of immediate recall, or disorientation regarding place or time. Abnormalities in these areas are unusual in dementia until the disorder is far advanced.

To determine if cognitive dysfunction is global or circumscribed, different spheres of cognition are tested in turn. These include memory, language, parietal lobe functions (eg, pictorial construction, right–left discrimination, localization of objects in space), and frontal lobe or diffuse cerebral cortical functions (eg, judgment, abstraction, thought content, ability to perform previously learned acts). Multiple areas of cognitive function are impaired in dementia. The Montreal Cognitive Assessment (**Table 5-5**) and Minimental Status Examination provide useful bedside screening when cognitive impairment is suspected.

Dementia from different causes may preferentially impair different spheres of cognition, and this can provide diagnostic clues. For example, Alzheimer disease affects memory disproportionately, whereas language function is often most impaired in frontotemporal dementia.

NEUROLOGIC EXAMINATION

Certain disorders that produce dementia also affect vision, coordination, or motor or sensory function. Detecting such associated neurologic abnormalities can help to establish an etiologic diagnosis. Neurologic signs suggesting causes of dementia are listed in Table 5-3.

LABORATORY INVESTIGATIONS

Laboratory studies that can help to identify the cause of dementia are listed in **Table 5-6**.

DEMENTIA

DIFFERENTIAL DIAGNOSIS

▶ Common Causes of Dementia

A wide variety of diseases can produce dementia, but only a few do so commonly. In its most typical presentation—with gradual cognitive decline in an elderly (≥65 years) patient—the most common causes of dementia are Alzheimer disease, vascular (formerly "multi-infarct") dementia, frontotemporal dementia, and Lewy body disease (**Figure 5-2**). Autopsy studies show that many elderly demented patients have histopathologic features of more than one such dementing process, such as Alzheimer disease and vascular disease (mixed dementia). In addition,

Table 5-4. Comprehensive Mental Status Examination.

Level of consciousness
Arousability
Orientation
Attention
Concentration

Language and speech
Comprehension
Repetition
Fluency
Naming
Reading
Writing
Calculation
Speech

Mood and behavior
Mood
Content of thought
Hallucinations
Delusions
Abstraction
Judgment

Memory
Immediate recall
Recent memory
Remote memory

Integrative sensory function
Astereognosis
Agraphesthesia
Two-point discrimination
Allesthesia
Extinction
Unilateral neglect and anosognosia
Disorders of spatial thought

Integrative motor function
Apraxia

Table 5-5. Montreal Cognitive Assessment (MOCA) Test for Dementia Screening.

Function	Tasks	Points
Visuospatial/ Executive	• Connect numbered/lettered dots in order	1
		1
	• Copy three-dimensional figure	3
	• Draw clockface showing given time	
Naming	• Name 3 pictured animals	3
Memory	• Recall 5 nouns after 5 minutes	0
Attention	• Repeat 5 digits forward and 3 digits backward	2
		1
	• Read list of letters and tap hand for each A	3
	• Serially subtract 7 from 100 to 65	
Language	• Repeat each of 2 sentences	2
	• Name ≥11 words beginning with given letter in 1 minute	1
Abstraction	• Explain similarity in each of two 2-item pairs	2
Delayed recall	• Recall 5 nouns tested before under "Memory" above	5
Orientation	• Give date, month, year, day, place, and city	6
Education	• (Add for ≤12 years of education)	(1)

Scores	
Total possible	30-(31)
Normal control (average)	27.4
Mild cognitive impairment (average)	22.1
Alzheimer disease (average)	16.2

vascular factors may influence the risk or progression of neurodegenerative disease. Patients who present with dementia before age 45 years are much less likely to have Alzheimer disease or vascular dementia; in these patients, a wider range of neurodegenerative (Huntington disease, corticobasal degeneration), inflammatory (multiple sclerosis, systemic lupus erythematosus, vasculitis), and infective (prion disease) causes must be entertained. Dementia that progresses rapidly over weeks to months results most often from prion (Creutzfeldt–Jakob) disease.

▶ Other Causes of Dementia

Reversible causes of dementia, such as normal-pressure hydrocephalus, intracranial mass lesions, vitamin B_{12}

deficiency, hypothyroidism, and neurosyphilis, are rare. However, they are important to diagnose because treatment can arrest or reverse intellectual decline.

Diagnosing dementia caused by Huntington disease or other heritable disorders allows patients and their families to benefit from genetic counseling. If Creutzfeldt–Jakob disease or HIV-associated dementia is diagnosed, precautions can be instituted against transmission, and HIV disease can be treated with antiretroviral drugs. Progressive multifocal leukoencephalopathy may indicate underlying immunosuppression from HIV infection, lymphoma, or leukemia and may thereby bring these disorders to attention.

Approximately 15% of patients referred for evaluation of possible dementia instead have other disorders (pseudodementias), such as depression. Depression in this setting is important to identify because it is readily treatable. Drug intoxication, often cited as a cause of dementia in the

Table 5-6. Laboratory Studies in Dementia.

Test	Most Useful in Diagnosis of
Blood	
Hematocrit, mean corpuscular volume (MCV), peripheral blood smear, vitamin B$_{12}$ level	Vitamin B$_{12}$ deficiency
Thyroid function tests	Hypothyroidism
Liver function tests	Acquired hepatocerebral degeneration, Wilson disease
Ceruloplasmin, copper	Wilson disease
FTA or MHA-TP	Neurosyphilis
Cerebrospinal fluid	
VDRL	Neurosyphilis
Cytology	Leptomeningeal metastases
Prion protein	Creutzfeldt–Jakob disease
Aβ42, tau, phospho-tau	Alzheimer disease
HIV mRNA	HIV-associated dementia
Other	
CT scan or MRI	Brain tumor, chronic subdural hematoma, vascular dementia, normal-pressure hydrocephalus, Alzheimer disease, frontotemporal dementia, Creutzfeldt–Jakob disease
PET scan	Alzheimer disease
EEG	Creutzfeldt–Jakob disease, dialysis dementia

elderly, actually produces an acute confusional state, rather than dementia.

NEURODEGENERATIVE PROTEINOPATHIES

In several neurodegenerative diseases, the production of **misfolded proteins** and their association to form **insoluble aggregates** appears to play an important role in pathogenesis (**Table 5-7**). These abnormal proteins can arise from either genetic or acquired modifications, and their pathologic effects may result from loss of normal protein function, gain of a toxic function, or a combination of these factors. Protein aggregation may be a mechanism for sequestering proteins that the cell's proteolytic machinery cannot process, but protein aggregates may also exert adverse effects on the cell, such as by interfering with axonal transport.

Except in rare inherited or infectious cases, the underlying cause of neurodegenerative proteinopathies is unknown. However, these diseases share several features. In addition to protein misfolding and aggregation, which sometimes produces characteristic histopathologic findings (see Table 5-7), these diseases may be associated with cell-to-cell **prionic transmission** (**Figure 5-3**), which allows them to spread through the nervous system to produce characteristic anatomic patterns of involvement. Disease spread is through the release of misfolded pathogenic proteins, alone or in vesicles, from affected neurons and subsequent uptake by neighboring neurons, or through direct transfer to adjacent cells in nanotubes.

At least two patterns of spread are observed in neurodegenerative proteinopathies: **contiguous propagation**, which affects anatomically adjacent areas and does not require synaptic connectivity, and **network propagation**, which involves synaptically (and therefore functionally) connected, and sometimes distant, regions. In Alzheimer disease, for example, β-amyloid pathology spreads centripetally from the cerebral cortex to subcortical regions, while tau pathology moves in the opposite direction, from the brainstem and entorhinal cortex to the neocortex. In Lewy body disease, α-synuclein deposits are seen first in the brainstem and olfactory bulb and ascend from there to the neocortex.

In addition to direct spread of pathogenic proteins, other mechanisms that may explain the spatial and temporal features of neurodegenerative proteinopathies include **differential susceptibility** of neuronal populations to proteotoxicity and different regional **thresholds** for symptomatic neuronal loss.

A given misfolded protein may also lead to divergent disease phenotypes. For example, tau is implicated in Alzheimer disease, frontotemporal dementia, progressive supranuclear palsy, and corticobasal degeneration, which have different clinical features. Molecular heterogeneity of abnormal prion proteins also corresponds to the clinically distinct Creutzfeldt–Jakob disease, variant Creutzfeldt–Jakob disease, fatal familial insomnia, and Gerstmann–Sträussler–Scheinker syndrome.

ALZHEIMER DISEASE

▶ Epidemiology

Alzheimer disease is the most common cause of dementia, accounting in whole or part for an estimated 60-70% of cases. Alzheimer disease affects approximately 15% of individuals of age 65 years or older and approximately 45% of those age 85 years or over. Its prevalence is >5 million cases in the United States and ~40 million cases worldwide. Men and women are affected with equal frequency, when adjusted for age. However, because women live longer, they account for approximately two-thirds of Alzheimer patients.

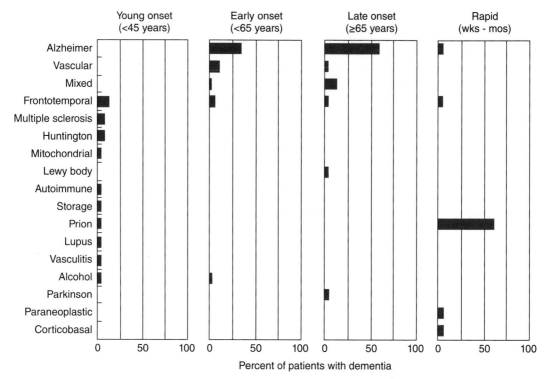

▲ **Figure 5-2.** Common causes of dementia based on age at presentation and rate of progression. "Mixed" refers to combined Alzheimer disease and vascular dementia. Totals of <100% reflect absence of an etiologic diagnosis in some cases. (Data from Kelley BJ, Boeve BF, Josephs KA. Young-onset dementia: demographic and etiologic characteristics of 235 patients. *Arch Neurol.* 2008;65:1502-1508. Garre-Olmo J, Genís Batlle D, del Mar Fernández M, et al. Incidence and subtypes of early-onset dementia in a geographically defined general population. *Neurology.* 2010;75:1249-1255. Geschwind MD, Shu H, Haman A, Sejvar JJ, Miller BL. Rapidly progressive dementia. *Ann Neurol.* 2008;64:97-108.)

Table 5-7. Neurodegenerative Proteinopathies.

Protein	Dementing Disease (s)	Transmission	Histopathologic Features
β-Amyloid (Aβ)	Alzheimer disease	Sporadic or inherited	Amyloid plaques, neurofibrillary tangles
Tau	Alzheimer disease Frontotemporal dementia Progressive supranuclear palsy Corticobasal degeneration	Sporadic or inherited	Neurofibrillary tangles or amorphous deposits (pretangles)
TDP-43	Frontotemporal dementia Frontotemporal dementia with motor neuron disease	Sporadic or inherited	TDP-43/ubiquitin-positive inclusions
Fused-in-sarcoma (FUS)	Frontotemporal dementia	Sporadic or inherited	FUS-positive inclusions
α-Synuclein	Parkinson disease Lewy body disease (Parkinson disease with dementia, dementia with Lewy bodies)	Sporadic or inherited	Lewy bodies
Huntingtin (Htt)	Huntington disease	Inherited	Polyglutamine inclusions
Prion protein (PrP)	Creutzfeldt–Jakob disease (CJD), Gerstmann–Sträussler–Scheinker syndrome (GSS), fatal familial insomnia, kuru	Sporadic, infectious, or inherited	PrP-positive plaques (variant CJD, GSS)

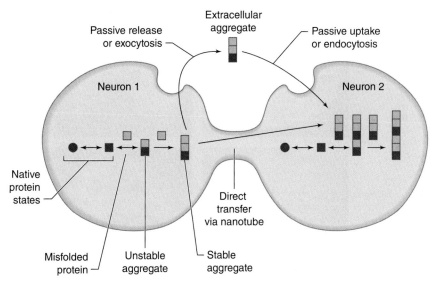

▲ **Figure 5-3.** Cell-to-cell (prionic) transmission of neurodegenerative proteinopathies. Abnormal proteins associated with neurodegenerative disease may misfold, leading to the formation of protein aggregates; misfolded proteins, protein aggregates, or both may be toxic and contribute to neuronal dysfunction. In addition, toxic protein aggregates may be transferred between cells to propagate the disease.

Pathology

Alzheimer disease is defined by characteristic histopathologic features, especially neuritic (senile) plaques and neurofibrillary tangles (**Figure 5-4**). **Neuritic plaques** are extracellular deposits that contain β-**amyloid (Aβ)** and other proteins, including presenilin 1, presenilin 2, α$_1$-antichymotrypsin, apolipoprotein E, α$_2$-macroglobulin, and ubiquitin. Plaques may also be found in cerebral and meningeal blood-vessel walls, producing **cerebral amyloid angiopathy**. **Neurofibrillary tangles** are intracellular deposits

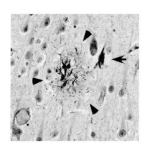
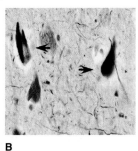

A **B**

▲ **Figure 5-4.** Characteristic extracellular neuritic plaque (arrowheads, **A**) and intracellular neurofibrillary tangles (arrows, **A** and **B**) in the brain of a patient with Alzheimer disease. (Used with permission of Shahriar Salamat, MD, PhD, University of Wisconsin School of Medicine and Public Health, Department of Pathology and Laboratory Medicine.)

containing hyperphosphorylated **tau** (a microtubule-associated protein) and ubiquitin. Gross inspection of the brain in Alzheimer disease shows cortical atrophy and associated ex vacuo hydrocephalus (**Figure 5-5**).

Etiology

Alzheimer disease is a progressive, degenerative disorder that is caused by a genetic defect in rare cases (see later), but is usually sporadic and of unknown cause. Abnormal metabolism, deposition, or clearance of two proteins—Aβ and tau—appears to be closely linked to pathogenesis.

Pathogenesis

1. **Genetics**—In ~1% of patients, Alzheimer disease is a familial disorder that results from a mutation in one of three functionally related membrane proteins (**Table 5-8**): β-**amyloid precursor protein (APP)**, **presenilin 1 (PS1)**, or **presenilin 2 (PS2)**. Onset of the disease in these patients is typically between the ages of 30 and 60 years. Patients with **Down syndrome (trisomy 21)** also develop early Alzheimer disease (mean onset at age 50 years), which is thought to be related to an extra copy of the *APP* gene, located on chromosome 21. Although the cause of sporadic Alzheimer disease is unknown, the gene defects in familial Alzheimer disease support possible roles for both APP, a protein with neurotrophic properties, and the presenilins, which are involved in APP metabolism.

   The risk of Alzheimer disease is also influenced by the inheritance pattern of **apolipoprotein E (*APOE*)**

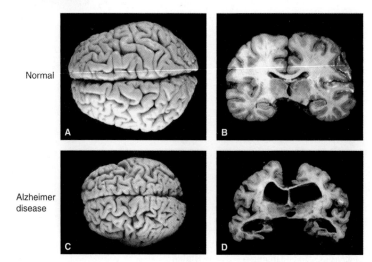

▲ **Figure 5-5.** Normal brain viewed from above (**A**) and in coronal section (**B**), compared with brain from a patient with Alzheimer disease, showing cortical atrophy (widened sulci, **C**) and ex vacuo hydrocephalus (enlarged ventricles, **D**). (Whole brain photos used with permission from Peter Anderson, D.V.M., PhD., PEIR Digital Library Image 15470. © University of Alabama at Birmingham, Department of Pathology. http://peir.net. Brain slice photos used with permission from A.C. McKee.)

gene isoforms ε2, ε3, and ε4. Risk increases from ~10-15% when all APOE genotypes are combined to ~20-30% with a single **apolipoprotein Eε4 (*APOE4*)** allele and to ~50% with two copies of *APOE4*; each copy of *APOE4* also lowers the age at onset by about 5 years. In contrast to *APOE4*, *APOE2* appears to confer relative protection from Alzheimer disease. The mechanism through which *APOE* genotype modifies susceptibility to Alzheimer disease is unknown, but may involve APOE binding to Aβ, impairing Aβ clearance, or acting as a transcription factor.

Polymorphisms at a number of other genetic loci appear to influence Alzheimer disease risk, but their effects are small. Nevertheless, the fact that they are involved in a wide variety of functions—including lipid metabolism, inflammation, intercellular signaling, and membrane transport—suggests that diverse processes may contribute to Alzheimer disease pathogenesis.

2. **Aβ and neuritic plaques**—Aβ is the principal constituent of neuritic plaques and is also deposited in cerebral and meningeal blood vessels in Alzheimer disease. Aβ is a 38- to 43-amino acid peptide produced by proteolytic cleavage of the transmembrane protein, APP (**Figure 5-6**). Normal processing of APP involves its cleavage by the enzyme α-**secretase**, which does not produce Aβ, and by β-**secretase** (**BACE;** β-site APP cleaving enzyme) and γ-**secretase**, yielding primarily a 40-amino acid fragment (**Aβ40**), which is secreted and cleared from the brain. In Alzheimer disease, a

Table 5-8. Principal Genes Implicated in Alzheimer Disease.

Gene	Gene Locus	Protein	Genotype	Phenotype
APP	21q21.3–q22.05	Amyloid β A4 precursor protein	Various missense mutations	Familial Alzheimer disease (autosomal dominant)
PS1	14q24.3	Presenilin 1	Various missense mutations	Familial Alzheimer disease (autosomal dominant) with early onset (age 35-55)
PS2	1q31–q42	Presenilin 2	Various missense mutations	Familial Alzheimer disease (autosomal dominant) in Volga Germans
APOE	19q13.2	Apolipoprotein E	*APOE4* polymorphism	Increased susceptibility to Alzheimer disease
Multiple	21	Unknown	Trisomy 21 or chromosome 21–14 or 21–21 translocation	Down syndrome (early-onset Alzheimer disease)

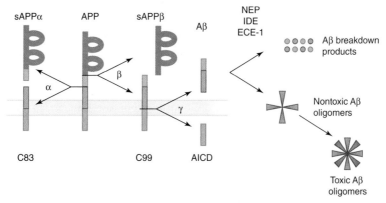

▲ **Figure 5-6.** Normal and pathologic (amyloidogenic) processing of APP and Aβ. APP, a membrane-spanning protein, is normally cleaved by α-secretase (α), or by β-secretase (β) and then γ-secretase (γ, a protein complex that includes presenilin 1 or 2, nicastrin, anterior pharynx defective 1 homolog [APH1], and presenilin enhancer 2 [PEN2]) to generate β-amyloid (Aβ), a secreted protein. APP mutations associated with familial Alzheimer disease shift Aβ production from a nontoxic 40-amino acid to a toxic (amyloidogenic) 42-amino acid form, which has a greater tendency to form amyloid deposits. Aβ normally undergoes enzymatic breakdown (by neprilysin [NEP], insulin-degrading enzyme [IDE], or endothelin-converging enzyme [ECE-1]) and clearance from the brain. However, it can also aggregate to form oligomers of increasing size, which are thought to be neurotoxic. AICD, APP intracellular domain; C83 and C99, C-terminal fragments of APP; sAPP, soluble APP.

disproportionate amount of **Aβ42**, a longer form of the molecule with an increased tendency to aggregate, is produced. Presenilins 1 and 2 contribute to γ-secretase activity.

Evidence for a causal role of Aβ in Alzheimer disease includes the involvement of APP mutations in some familial cases and the neurotoxicity of Aβ under some circumstances. However, there is a poor correlation between the extent of amyloid plaque deposition in the brain and the severity of dementia in Alzheimer disease. One explanation for this disparity is that soluble Aβ oligomers, rather than insoluble plaques, may be the toxic agent. Another possibility is that Aβ aggregation produces Alzheimer disease indirectly, such as by promoting the formation of tau-containing neurofibrillary tangles.

3. **Tau and neurofibrillary tangles**—Tau is a cytoplasmic protein that binds to tubulin and stabilizes microtubules, cytoskeletal structures that help maintain cell structure and facilitate intracellular transport. In Alzheimer disease and other **tauopathies**, tau becomes hyperphosphorylated and dissociates from microtubules; the microtubules disassemble, and hyperphosphorylated tau aggregates to form neurofibrillary tangles (**Figure 5-7**). How this leads to impaired neuronal function is unknown, but may involve a defect in axonal transport. A causal role for tau pathology in Alzheimer disease is supported by the observations that

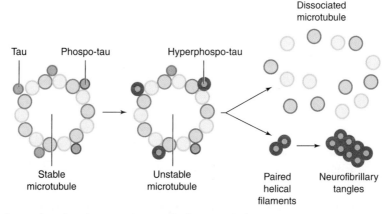

▲ **Figure 5-7.** Tau hyperphosphorylation and neurofibrillary tangle formation.

the abundance of neurofibrillary tangles correlates well with disease severity and that other tauopathies (eg, frontotemporal dementia), in which Aβ processing is normal, can also produce dementia.

4. **Synaptic and neuronal network dysfunction**—Alzheimer disease is accompanied by early changes in synaptic function, including altered excitatory activity, loss of dendritic spines, and ultimately loss of synapses. These changes, in turn, disrupt interneuronal connectivity and the function of brain circuits, such as the basal forebrain cholinergic, hypothalamic-hippocampal, and amygdala-hippocampal networks. Pathologic alterations at this level of brain organization may help explain memory loss and other cognitive defects in Alzheimer disease.

5. **Neuronal loss and brain atrophy**—Certain neuronal populations are preferentially lost in Alzheimer disease, including glutamatergic neurons in the entorhinal cortex and the CA1 sector of the hippocampus, as well as cholinergic neurons in the basal forebrain. Focal brain atrophy is seen in the affected areas.

6. **Vascular involvement**—The extent to which vascular pathology may contribute to Alzheimer disease is controversial. Evidence for such a connection includes the overlap between risk factors for vascular disease and Alzheimer disease (including *APOE* genotype), the involvement of blood vessels in amyloid pathology, and the frequent coexistence of Alzheimer and vascular histopathology.

▶ Risk Factors

The factors most conclusively associated with increased risk for Alzheimer disease are increasing age, female sex, and *APOE4* genotype. Other factors that have been implicated in some studies include family history of Alzheimer disease, depression, low educational level, smoking, diabetes, obesity, hypertension, and fatty diet. Besides *APOE4*, several other genes that modify risk have been identified, but the magnitude of their effects is small.

Some data suggest that cognitive engagement, physical activity, a low-fat and vegetable-rich diet, and light to moderate alcohol intake may favorably affect the risk of Alzheimer disease. However, no drugs have been shown to be effective in prevention. Estrogen administration does not appear to affect cognitive function in postmenopausal women after several years of follow-up, irrespective of when treatment is begun in relation to menopause.

▶ Clinical Findings

The clinical progression of Alzheimer disease is thought to comprise a presymptomatic phase of up to about 10 years characterized by the deposition of amyloid plaques, followed by a symptomatic phase of up to about 10 years, during which tangle formation occurs (**Figure 5-8**).

1. **Early manifestations**—The term **mild cognitive impairment (MCI)** is sometimes used to describe the early phase of cognitive decline observed in patients who later receive a diagnosis of Alzheimer disease. Impairment of recent memory is typically the first sign of Alzheimer disease and may be noticed only by family members. As the memory disorder progresses over months to several years, the patient becomes disoriented to time and then to place. Aphasia, anomia, and acalculia may develop, forcing the patient to leave work or give up the management of family finances. The depression apparent in the earlier stages of the disorder may give way to an agitated, restless state. Apraxias and visuospatial disorientation ensue, causing the patient to become lost easily. Primitive reflexes are commonly found. A frontal lobe gait disorder may become

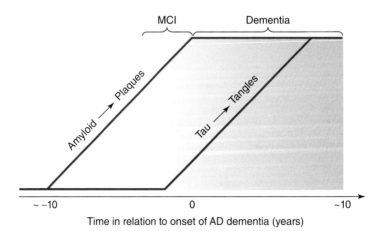

Figure 5-8. Relationship between plaques, tangles, and clinical progression of Alzheimer disease (AD). MCI, mild cognitive impairment.

apparent, with short, slow, shuffling steps, flexed posture, wide base, and difficulty in initiating walking.

2. **Late manifestations**—In the late stages, previously preserved social graces are lost, and psychiatric symptoms, including psychosis with paranoia, hallucinations, or delusions, may be prominent. Seizures occur in some cases. Examination at this stage may show rigidity and bradykinesia. Rare and usually late features of the disease include myoclonus, incontinence, spasticity, extensor plantar responses, and hemiparesis. Mutism, incontinence, and a bedridden state are terminal manifestations. Eating problems, febrile episodes, dyspnea, pneumonia, and pain are frequent complications in the final months of life, and death typically occurs from 5 to 10 years after the onset of symptoms.

3. **Atypical variants**—Several clinically atypical variants of autopsy-verified Alzheimer disease have been described in which memory is relatively preserved. These patients have early (<65 years of age) onset of symptoms, which correlate best with the density of neurofibrillary tangles. The **frontal variant** shows prominent behavioral and personality changes, including irritability, impulsivity, and disinhibition. The **posterior variant** is associated with visuospatial disorders, including Balint syndrome (optic ataxia, ocular apraxia, and simultanagnosia), Gerstmann syndrome (agraphia, acalculia, finger agnosia, and left-right disorientation), and visual agnosia. The **logopenic variant** exhibits anomia and impaired repetition.

Investigative Studies

Laboratory investigations should be undertaken to exclude other disorders, especially reversible or treatable conditions. Findings that may be useful in helping to establish a diagnosis of Alzheimer disease include CSF with reduced Aβ42 and increased tau and phospho-tau; MRI showing medial temporal lobe (including hippocampal) and often parietal greater than frontal lobe atrophy (**Figure 5-9**); positive amyloid positron emission tomography (PET) imaging; and ^{18}F-fluorodeoxyglucose PET demonstrating glucose hypometabolism in the temporal and parietal lobes.

Differential Diagnosis

Early Alzheimer disease may resemble depression or pure memory disorders such as the Korsakoff amnestic syndrome (see later discussion). More advanced Alzheimer disease must be distinguished from frontotemporal dementia, Lewy body disease, vascular dementia, Creutzfeldt–Jakob disease, and other dementing disorders, discussed later.

Treatment

No currently available treatment has been shown to reverse existing deficits or to arrest disease progression. However, **memantine** (**Table 5-9**), an NMDA-type glutamate receptor

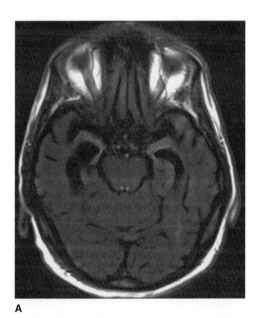
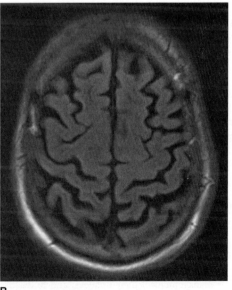

A   **B**

▲ **Figure 5-9.** Axial MRI in Alzheimer disease showing (**A**) bilateral hippocampal and (**B**) parietal (bottom) more than frontal (top) lobe atrophy. (Used with permission from Berkowitz AL. *Clinical Neurology and Neuroanatomy: A Location-Based Approach*. New York, NY: McGraw-Hill; 2017. Fig. 22-3.)

Table 5-9. Drugs Used in the Treatment of Alzheimer Disease.

Drug Class	Drug	Dose	Toxicity
Glutamate antagonist	Memantine	5 mg orally daily, increased by 5 mg each week to 10 mg orally twice daily	Dizziness, headache, constipation, confusion
Acetylcholinesterase inhibitor	Tacrine	10 mg orally 4 times daily; may be increased to 20 mg orally 4 times daily after 6 weeks	Abdominal cramps, nausea and vomiting, diarrhea, hepatocellular toxicity (liver enzymes should be monitored twice monthly for 4 months)
	Donepezil	5 mg orally at bedtime; may be increased to 10 mg orally at bedtime after 4-6 weeks	Nausea, diarrhea, vomiting, insomnia, fatigue, muscle cramps, anorexia
	Rivastigmine	1.5-6 mg orally twice daily	Nausea and vomiting, diarrhea, anorexia
	Galantamine	4-12 mg orally twice daily	Nausea and vomiting, dizziness, diarrhea, anorexia, weight loss
Combination	Memantine + Donepezil	28 mg/10 mg orally once daily	Same as for memantine and donepezil above

antagonist drug, may produce modest improvement in patients with moderate or severe Alzheimer disease.

Because cholinergic neuronal pathways degenerate and choline acetyltransferase is depleted in the brains of patients with Alzheimer disease, cholinergic replacement therapy has also been used for symptomatic treatment of cognitive dysfunction (see Table 5-9). **Acetylcholinesterase inhibitors**, including tacrine, donepezil, rivastigmine, and galantamine, have all been shown to produce small improvements in tests of cognitive function. Side effects include nausea and vomiting, diarrhea, and dizziness; tacrine also elevates serum transaminase levels. The better side-effect profile of donepezil and its once-daily dosage schedule are advantageous.

Experimental treatments under investigation include monoclonal antibodies directed against β-amyloid, secretase inhibitors, and tau aggregation inhibitors. Antipsychotic drugs, antidepressants, and anxiolytics may be useful in controlling behavioral disturbances associated with Alzheimer disease. However, evidence for their effectiveness is sparse, and in some cases (risperidone, olanzapine) their use is associated with an increased incidence of stroke in elderly patients.

Prognosis

Early in the course of the disease, patients can usually remain at home and continue social, recreational, and limited professional activities. Early diagnosis can allow patients time to plan orderly retirement from work, to arrange for management of their finances, and to discuss with physicians and family members the management of future medical problems. Patients in advanced stages of the disease may require care in a nursing facility and the use of psychoactive medications. These patients must be

protected and prevented from injuring themselves and their families by injudicious actions or decisions. Death from inanition or infection generally occurs 5 to 10 years after the first symptoms.

FRONTOTEMPORAL DEMENTIA

Frontotemporal dementia (FTD) comprises a genetically and clinically heterogeneous group of dementing disorders that produce frontal and temporal lobe degeneration and affect behavior and language preferentially. FTD differs in these respects from Alzheimer disease, which involves primarily the temporal and parietal lobes and causes prominent memory disturbance. Both FTD and Alzheimer disease exhibit tau-containing inclusions, but abnormal amyloid processing and plaques are seen only in Alzheimer disease.

Epidemiology

FTD is thought to be the third most common cause of dementia, after Alzheimer disease and vascular dementia. The average age at clinical onset is 50 to 60 years, which is younger than that for Alzheimer disease.

Pathology

FTD is characterized by atrophy of the frontal and temporal lobes. Histopathologic findings include neuronal loss, gliosis, and characteristic intracellular protein inclusions. **Tau inclusions** in FTD differ from those found in Alzheimer disease: The former are twisted, ribbon-like structures rather than paired helical filaments and include neurofibrillary tangles, amorphous deposits (pretangles), and, in some cases, Pick bodies. Inclusions are also sometimes found in the hippocampus, subcortical nuclei, brainstem, cerebellum, or spinal cord.

Etiology

In most cases, FTD is a sporadic neurodegenerative disease of unknown cause. However, 20% to 40% of patients report a family history of a neurodegenerative disorder, and approximately 10% appear to inherit frontotemporal dementia in an autosomal dominant fashion.

Pathogenesis

1. **Genetics**—Mutations in three genes—the **microtubule-associated protein tau (MAPT)**, **progranulin (GRN)**, and **chromosome 9 open reading frame 72 (C9ORF72)**—appear to be responsible for the majority of inherited cases. *MAPT* mutations are thought to produce disease largely by toxic gain of function, whereas *GRN* mutations cause loss of function through haploinsufficiency. *C9ORF72* mutations, which are the most common cause of familial FTD, take the form of expanded noncoding GGGCCC hexanucleotide repeats. Processing of the corresponding RNA is impaired, producing gain-of-function RNA transcripts that sequester RNA-binding proteins and give rise to non-canonically translated toxic dipeptide-repeat proteins; loss of normal C9ORF72 function may also contribute to pathogenesis. Less common mutations producing FTD affect genes for valosin-containing protein (*VCP*), charged multivesicular body protein 2B (*CHMP2B*), TAR-DNA binding protein (*TARDP*), or fused in sarcoma (*FUS*).

2. **Intracellular inclusions**—These include tau-containing inclusions (neurofibrillary tangles or amorphous deposits; see Figure 5-7) in patients with *MAPT* mutations; progranulin-, TDP-43-, and ubiquitin-positive inclusions in patients with *GRN* mutations; p62-, ubiquitin-, and unconventionally translated dipeptide repeat-positive inclusions in patients with *C9ORF72* mutations; and ubiquitin- and FUS-positive inclusions in patients with *FUS* mutations. In each case, the role of the inclusions in disease pathogenesis is uncertain.

3. **Neuronal dysfunction, neuronal loss, and brain atrophy**—It is unclear how much of the clinical picture in FTD results from abnormal neuronal function as opposed to neuronal loss. Eventually, however, there is marked brain atrophy affecting the frontal and anterior temporal lobes most prominently, together with neuronal loss and gliosis.

Clinical Findings

1. **Behavioral variant frontotemporal dementia** is characterized by prominent behavioral changes, including altered interpersonal interactions and personal conduct (eg, apathy and disinhibition), blunted emotions, and lack of insight. These behavioral abnormalities overshadow more modest cognitive defects, such as impaired judgment, inattention, or disorganization. This syndrome can be seen in patients with tau, TDP-43, C9ORF72, or FUS pathology.

2. **Semantic variant primary progressive aphasia** (semantic dementia) produces fluent (receptive) aphasia (see Chapter 1, Neurologic History & Examination) with word-finding difficulties, impaired comprehension, and anomia, and occurs with disease affecting the dominant temporal lobe. It is most common in patients with TDP-43 pathology.

3. **Nonfluent variant primary progressive aphasia** (progressive nonfluent aphasia) produces expressive aphasia (see Chapter 1) characterized by halting speech and agrammatism with preserved comprehension, and results from predominant involvement of the dominant frontal lobe. It is most common in patients with tau pathology.

4. **Overlap syndromes** occur in cases in which FTD is combined with features of parkinsonism (corticobasal degeneration [discussed later] or progressive supranuclear palsy [discussed later and in Chapter 11, Movement Disorders]) or motor neuron disease (amyotrophic lateral sclerosis [see Chapter 9, Motor Disorders]). Parkinsonian syndromes are seen most often in patients with tau pathology, whereas motor neuron involvement is associated with TDP-43 or C9ORF72 pathology.

Investigative Studies

MRI shows frontal and temporal lobe atrophy (**Figure 5-10**), and ^{18}F-fluorodeoxyglucose PET may show hypometabolism in these regions. In both cases, the abnormalities are often asymmetric, with right-sided atrophy predominating in behavioral and left-sided atrophy predominating in language variants. CSF levels of neurodegeneration-related proteins have been studied as potential markers of FTD, but so far, none are diagnostic. Genetic screening demonstrates mutations in some patients with a positive family history.

Differential Diagnosis

In contrast to Alzheimer disease, memory disturbance does not dominate the clinical picture in FTD, and onset typically occurs at an earlier age. The diagnosis is suggested by the onset of dementia before age 60 years, with behavioral disturbance or aphasia as the primary abnormality. FTD with altered behavior may be mistaken for a primary psychiatric disorder, and language variants can raise suspicion regarding stroke.

Treatment

Memantine and anticholinesterase drugs used to treat Alzheimer disease have not been shown to be effective in

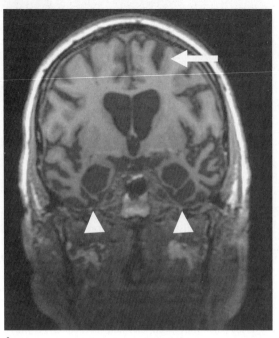 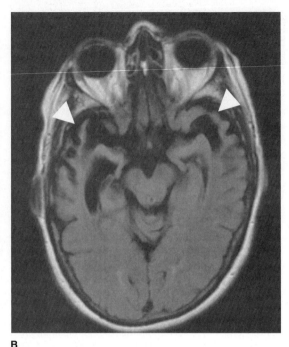

A   B

▲ **Figure 5-10.** Axial (**A**) and coronal (**B**) FLAIR MRI in frontotemporal dementia showing regional atrophy of the frontal (**arrow**) and temporal (**arrowheads**) lobes. (Used with permission from Jason Handwerker.)

FTD. Antidepressants, especially selective serotonin reuptake inhibitors and trazodone, may be useful for managing behavioral symptoms. Patients with parkinsonian features (corticobasal degeneration or progressive supranuclear palsy) may benefit from carbidopa/levodopa or dopamine receptor agonists (see Chapter 11, Movement Disorders).

▶ Prognosis

The duration of illness in FTD is typically 6-11 years from symptom onset and 2-5 years from clinical diagnosis.

CORTICOBASAL DEGENERATION

Corticobasal degeneration is a tauopathy related to FTD with tau pathology. It produces asymmetric frontoparietal cortical atrophy and depigmentation of the substantia nigra, with tau-positive neuronal and glial inclusions, ballooned neurons, and neuronal and glia cell loss. The classic **corticobasal syndrome** reflects involvement of both cerebral cortex and basal ganglia and consists of unilateral limb (usually arm) clumsiness and functional impairment due to some combination of apraxia, sensory loss, and myoclonus, together with extrapyramidal rigidity, bradykinesia, and postural tremor. Limb apraxia and sensory loss may produce the **alien-hand sign**, in which the limb moves seemingly of its own accord. Depression, apathy, irritability, and agitation are common psychiatric features. In

addition to corticobasal degeneration, the corticobasal syndrome can also be seen in progressive supranuclear palsy (see next section) and FTD. Rigidity and bradykinesia are typically unresponsive to antiparkinsonian medications.

PROGRESSIVE SUPRANUCLEAR PALSY

Progressive supranuclear palsy (**PSP**, or **Steele–Richardson–Olszewski syndrome**) is an idiopathic degenerative disorder that primarily affects the brainstem, subcortical gray matter, and cerebral cortex. Like tau-positive FTD and corticobasal degeneration, it is characterized pathologically by tau-positive intracellular inclusions. The classic clinical features are supranuclear ophthalmoplegia (especially affecting downgaze), pseudobulbar palsy, axial dystonia with or without extrapyramidal rigidity of the limbs, and dementia. Because PSP usually presents as a movement disorder with parkinsonian features, it is discussed further in Chapter 11, Movement Disorders.

LEWY BODY DISEASE

Parkinson disease (see Chapter 11, Movement Disorders) is accompanied by dementia in ~25% of cases. Patients who develop dementia at least 1 year after the onset of motor symptoms (tremor, rigidity, bradykinesia, postural instability) are classified as having **Parkinson disease with** dementia, whereas those in whom dementia has its onset prior to or within 1 year of the first motor symptoms are given the diagnosis of **dementia with Lewy bodies**. However, these two diagnoses cannot be distinguished pathologically, and the term **Lewy body disease** is sometimes used to encompass both.

Lewy body disease is characterized histopathologically by round, eosinophilic, intracytoplasmic neuronal inclusions (**Lewy bodies**) in the brainstem and cerebral cortex. These inclusions contain α-**synuclein**, a protein that is also found in Lewy bodies in Parkinson disease without dementia, and both Lewy body disease and Parkinson disease are, therefore, classified as **synucleinopathies**.

Lewy body disease causes cognitive decline without prominent early memory impairment. Features include fluctuating cognitive ability, well-formed visual hallucinations, and signs of parkinsonism, especially rigidity and bradykinesia.

Motor manifestations of Lewy body disease are treated with antiparkinsonian medications (see Chapter 11); some studies suggest that memantine or anticholinesterase drugs used to treat Alzheimer disease (see Table 5-9) may also be beneficial in dementia associated with Lewy body disease.

HUNTINGTON DISEASE

Huntington disease is an autosomal dominant neurodegenerative disorder characterized by chorea, psychiatric symptoms, and dementia. The cause is an expanded CAG trinucleotide repeat coding for a polyglutamine tract in the huntingtin (Htt) gene. The brain shows atrophy affecting the caudate nucleus, putamen, and cerebral cortex, with Htt aggregation in cytoplasmic and nuclear inclusions. Dementia usually becomes apparent after chorea and psychiatric symptoms have been present for a few years but precedes chorea in approximately one-fourth of cases. Impaired executive function (eg, judgment) and memory are prominent features, whereas language tends to be spared until late in the course. Huntington disease is discussed further in Chapter 11, Movement Disorders.

CREUTZFELDT–JAKOB (PRION) DISEASE

Creutzfeldt-Jakob disease (**CJD**) produces rapidly progressive dementia with variable focal degeneration of the cerebral cortex, basal ganglia, cerebellum, brainstem, and spinal cord. It is caused by a proteinaceous infectious particle (**prion**) and may be sporadic (approximately 85% of cases), genetic, or infectious. In the latter case, CJD can be transmitted via prion-contaminated tissue or surgical instruments (iatrogenic CJD) or by consumption of contaminated beef (variant CJD). Documented human-to-human transmission (by corneal transplantation, cortical electrode implantation, or administration of human growth hormone) is rare. The infectious agent is present in the brain, spinal cord, eyes, lungs, lymph nodes, kidneys, spleen, liver, and CSF, but not other body fluids.

The annual incidence is approximately 1 case per million. The sporadic disease has a peak age at onset of 55-75 years, whereas the genetically acquired disease usually begins earlier. More than one member of a family is affected in only 5-10% of cases, and conjugal cases are rare.

▶ Pathogenesis

Familial CJD is an autosomal dominant disorder caused by a mutation in the *PRNP* gene, which codes for the prion protein cellular isoform (PrP^C), a protein of unknown function. In sporadic CJD, PrP^C undergoes a conformational change to produce an abnormal prion protein (scrapie isoform, or PrP^{Sc}). PrP^{Sc} then serves as a template on which PrP^C is converted to additional PrP^{Sc}. In infectious CJD, PrP^{Sc} is introduced into the brain from an external source. In each case, the result is accumulation of abnormal PrP^{Sc} prions in brain tissue. The ability of PrP^{Sc} to induce the PrP^{Sc} conformation in PrP^C prions enables it to replicate without nucleic acids.

Prions have also been implicated in diseases of animals and in three other rare human disorders (**Table 5-10**)—**kuru**, a dementing disease of Fore-speaking tribes of New Guinea (apparently spread by cannibalism); **Gerstmann–Sträussler–Scheinker syndrome**, a familial disorder characterized by dementia and ataxia; and **fatal familial insomnia**, which produces disturbances of sleep and of autonomic, motor, and endocrine function.

▶ Clinical Findings

The clinical picture may be that of a diffuse central nervous system (CNS) disorder or of more localized dysfunction (**Table 5-11**). Dementia is present in virtually all cases and may begin as mild global cognitive impairment or a focal

Table 5-10. Prion Diseases.

Human diseases
Creutzfeldt–Jakob disease (familial, sporadic, iatrogenic, new variant)
Fatal familial insomnia
Gerstmann-Sträussler-Scheinker disease
Kuru

Animal diseases
Bovine spongiform encephalopathy
Feline spongiform encephalopathy
Scrapie (sheep and goats)
Transmissible mink encephalopathy
Wasting disease of deer and elk
Transmissible spongiform encephalopathy of captive wild ruminants

Adapted from Johnson RT, Gibbs CJ. Creutzfeldt-Jakob disease and related transmissible spongiform encephalopathies. *N Engl J Med.* 1998;339:1994-2004.

Table 5-11. Clinical Features of Sporadic Creutzfeldt–Jakob Disease.

Feature	Percentage
Cognitive	
Memory loss	100
Behavioral abnormalities	57
Other	73
Motor	
Myoclonus	78
Cerebellar ataxia	71
Pyramidal signs	62
Extrapyramidal signs	56
Lower motor neuron signs	12
Visual disturbances	42
Periodic EEG complexes	60

Data from Brown P, Gibbs CJ Jr, Rodgers-Johnson P, et al. Human spongiform encephalopathy: the National Institutes of Health series of 300 cases of experimentally transmitted disease. *Ann Neurol.* 1994;35:513.

cortical disorder such as aphasia, apraxia, or agnosia. Progression to akinetic mutism or coma typically ensues over a period of months. Psychiatric symptoms including anxiety, euphoria, depression, labile affect, delusions, hallucinations, and changes in personality or behavior may be prominent. Fever is absent.

Aside from cognitive abnormalities, the most frequent clinical manifestations are myoclonus (often induced by a startle), extrapyramidal signs (rigidity, bradykinesia, tremor, dystonia, chorea, or athetosis), cerebellar signs, and pyramidal signs. Visual field defects, cranial nerve palsies, and seizures occur less often.

A distinct variant of CJD results from the transmission of **bovine spongiform encephalopathy ("mad cow disease")** to humans. This variant is characterized by earlier onset (typically in the teens or young adulthood), invariable cerebellar involvement, prominent early psychiatric abnormalities, and diffuse amyloid plaques.

▶ Investigative Studies

The most sensitive and specific tests are diffusion-weighted MRI and apparent diffusion coefficient MRI, which show hyperintense signals in the basal ganglia and cortical ribbon (**Figure 5-11**), and detection of PrP^Sc amplified by real-time quaking-induced conversion in cerebrospinal fluid or brain-biopsy tissue. The electroencephalogram (EEG) may show periodic sharp waves or spikes (**Figure 5-12**), which are absent in the variant form described previously, and CSF protein may be elevated (≤100 mg/dL). In familial cases, mutant prions may be detectable in DNA from lymphocytes.

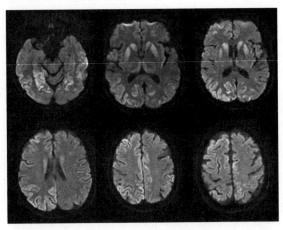

▲ **Figure 5-11.** Diffusion-weighted image of the brain in Creutzfeldt–Jakob disease, showing characteristic hyperintensities (**white**) in the basal ganglia and cortical ribbon. (Used with permission from J. Biller M.D.)

▶ Differential Diagnosis

A variety of other disorders must be distinguished from CJD. Alzheimer disease is often a consideration, especially in patients with a less fulminant course and a paucity of cerebellar and extrapyramidal signs. Where subcortical involvement is prominent, Parkinson disease, cerebellar degeneration, or progressive supranuclear palsy may be suspected. Striking focal signs raise the possibility of an intracerebral mass lesion. Acute metabolic disorders that produce altered mentation and myoclonus (eg, sedative drug withdrawal) can mimic CJD.

▶ Prognosis

No treatment is currently available. The disease is usually relentlessly progressive and invariably fatal. In most sporadic cases, death occurs within 1 year after the onset of symptoms. Depending on the specific mutation present, familial forms of the disease may have a longer course (1-5 years).

CEREBROVASCULAR DISEASE

VASCULAR DEMENTIA

Vascular disease is generally considered the second most common cause of dementia, after Alzheimer disease, and many patients have features of both diseases. Patients with this diagnosis may have multiple large (>1 cm in diameter) cortical infarcts; strategic infarcts involving hippocampus or thalamus; multiple small (eg, lacunar) infarcts affecting subcortical white matter, basal ganglia, or thalamus; diffuse ischemic lesions of subcortical white matter (**Binswanger disease**); intracerebral hemorrhages

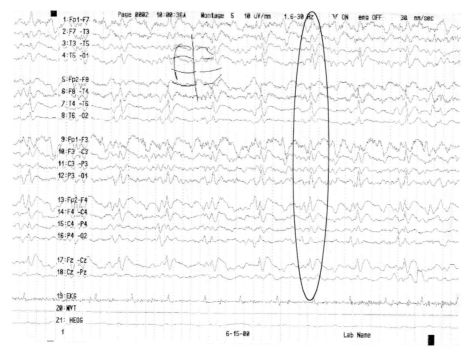

▲ **Figure 5-12.** EEG in Creutzfeldt-Jakob disease with typical triphasic waves in all leads, which occur repetitively about once every second.

(eg, **cerebral amyloid angiopathy**); or combinations of these.

Although vascular dementia is usually sporadic, genetic causes are also recognized. These include autosomal dominant cerebral amyloid angiopathy (usually due to mutations in the gene for amyloid precursor protein) and cerebral arteriopathy with subcortical infarcts and leukoencephalopathy (CADASIL, due to mutations in *NOTCH3*).

▶ Clinical Findings

The most classic presentation of patients with vascular dementia includes a history of hypertension, a stepwise progression of deficits, a more or less abrupt onset of dementia, and focal neurologic symptoms or signs. A history of clinically apparent stroke may be absent. The neurologic examination may show pseudobulbar palsy with dysarthria, dysphagia, and pathologic emotionality (**pseudobulbar affect**); focal motor and sensory deficits; ataxia; gait apraxia; hyperreflexia; and extensor plantar responses. Memory disturbance is typically less prominent than in Alzheimer disease. Instead, impaired attention, information processing, and executive function, as well as depression and apathy, are common. Patients with large or strategically located infarcts may present more acutely (**early-onset poststroke dementia**).

▶ Investigative Studies

The MRI (**Figure 5-13**) may show multiple large infarcts, multiple small (lacunar) infarcts, areas of low density in subcortical white matter, or combinations of these findings and is more sensitive than CT scan for detecting these abnormalities.

Additional laboratory studies should be performed to exclude cardiac emboli, polycythemia, thrombocytosis, cerebral vasculitis, and meningovascular syphilis as underlying causes, particularly in younger patients and those without a history of hypertension.

▶ Treatment and Prognosis

Hypertension, when present, should be treated to reduce the incidence of subsequent infarction and to prevent other end-organ diseases. Neither antiplatelet agents nor statins have been shown to reduce the incidence or progression of vascular dementia, but may be indicated to reduce the risk of other adverse effects of thromboembolic disease or hyperlipidemia. Mean survival is 3-5 years after diagnosis.

CHRONIC SUBDURAL HEMATOMA

Chronic subdural hematoma usually affects patients aged 50 to 70 years, often after minor head trauma. Other risk factors include alcoholism, cerebral atrophy, epilepsy,

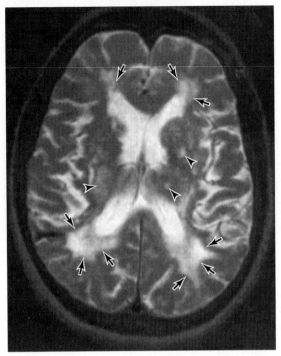

▲ **Figure 5-13.** T2-weighted MRI in vascular dementia, showing foci of abnormal high signal intensity adjacent to the lateral ventricles (**arrows**) and within the basal ganglia (**arrowheads**).

anticoagulation, ventricular shunts, and long-term hemodialysis. The onset of symptoms may be delayed for months after trauma. Hematomas are bilateral in approximately one-sixth of cases.

▶ Clinical Findings

Headache is the initial symptom in most patients; confusion, vomiting, and hemiparesis may follow, with dementia a later development. The most frequent signs are cognitive disturbance, hemiparesis, papilledema, and extensor plantar responses. Aphasia, visual field defects, and seizures are uncommon.

The hematoma can usually be seen on CT scan (**Figure 5-14**) as an extra-axial, crescent-shaped area of decreased density, with ipsilateral obliteration of cortical sulci and, often, ventricular compression. The scan should be carefully reviewed for evidence of bilateral subdural collections. Isodense collections may become more apparent after contrast infusion.

▶ Treatment

Unless contraindicated by medical problems or spontaneous improvement, symptomatic hematomas should be

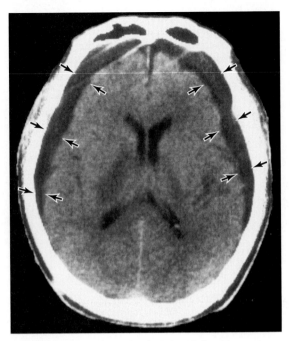

▲ **Figure 5-14.** CT scan in chronic subdural hematoma, showing bilateral low-density collections between the inner table of the skull and the cerebral hemispheres (**arrows**).

surgically evacuated. Approaches include craniotomy and burr-hole or twist-drill craniostomy. Neither corticosteroid nor prophylactic anticonvulsant treatment has been shown to be beneficial.

OTHER CEREBRAL DISORDERS

NORMAL-PRESSURE HYDROCEPHALUS

Normal-pressure hydrocephalus (NPH), a potentially reversible cause of dementia, is characterized by the clinical triad of gait disorder, dementia, and urinary dysfunction. It may be idiopathic or secondary to conditions that interfere with CSF absorption, such as subarachnoid hemorrhage, traumatic brain injury, or meningitis. The mean age at onset is ~70 years. Those affected have an increased incidence of vascular risk factors, including hyperlipidemia, diabetes, obesity, and physical inactivity, and NPH often coexists with subcortical small-vessel cerebrovascular disease.

▶ Pathophysiology

NPH is characterized by ventricular enlargement, with or without cerebral cortical atrophy, which affects the sylvian fissures out of proportion to cortical sulci. NPH is a form of **communicating hydrocephalus** (because the lateral, third, and fourth ventricles remain in communication) or **nonobstructive hydrocephalus** (because the flow of CSF between the ventricles is not impaired). In contrast, **noncommunicating** or **obstructive hydrocephalus** is caused by blockade of CSF circulation *within* the ventricular system (eg, by an intraventricular cyst or tumor) and is associated with increased CSF pressure and often with headache and papilledema.

NPH has been attributed to impaired absorption of CSF from the subarachnoid space over the cerebral hemispheres, through arachnoid villi, and into the venous circulation (**Figure 5-15**), or increased intracranial pressure pulsatility. In either case, ventricular enlargement may exert pressure on corticospinal axons mediating leg movement and urination, as well as on periventricular end arteries supplying frontal regions involved in cognition.

▶ Clinical Findings

Normal-pressure hydrocephalus usually develops over months, and gait disorder is typically the initial manifestation. This typically takes the form of **gait apraxia**, characterized by difficulty in standing and initiating walking (magnetic gait), shuffling gait, unstable turns, and a tendency to fall forward (anteropulsion) or backward (retropulsion). The patient can perform the leg movements associated with walking, bicycling, or kicking a ball and can trace figures with the feet while lying or sitting but is unable to do so with the legs bearing weight. Motor perseveration (the inappropriate repetition of motor activity) and grasp reflexes in the hands and feet may occur. The gait disorder is bilaterally symmetric, there is no weakness or ataxia, and pyramidal signs (spasticity, hyperreflexia,

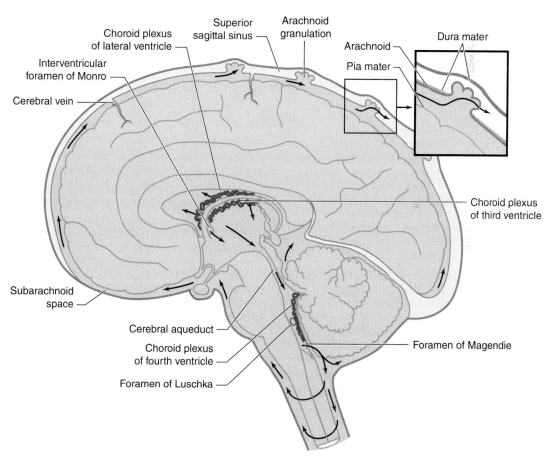

▲ **Figure 5-15.** Circulation of cerebrospinal fluid (CSF). CSF is produced by the choroid plexus (red), which consists of specialized secretory tissue located within the cerebral ventricles. It flows from the lateral and third ventricles through the cerebral aqueduct and fourth ventricle and exits the ventricular system through two laterally situated foramina of Luschka and a single, medially located foramen of Magendie. CSF then enters and circulates through the subarachnoid space surrounding the brain and spinal cord. It is ultimately absorbed through arachnoid granulations into the venous circulation.

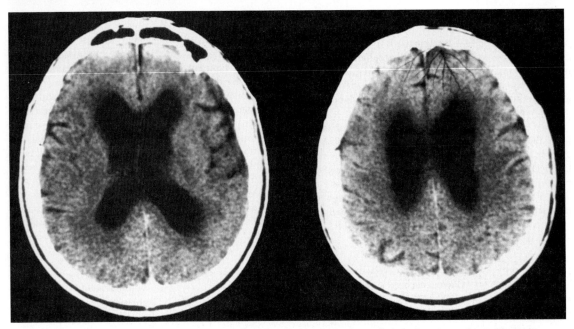

▲ **Figure 5-16.** CT scan at two transverse levels in normal-pressure hydrocephalus, showing enlarged lateral ventricles without enlargement of the cortical sulci.

and extensor plantar responses) are rarely present. Dementia is manifested by executive dysfunction and memory impairment, and may be accompanied by depression. Urinary symptoms include urgency and frequency, with or without incontinence, and tend to have their onset after the gait disorder and dementia are established. Fecal incontinence is uncommon.

▶ Investigative Studies

Lumbar puncture reveals normal or low opening pressure. The CT scan or, preferably, MRI shows enlarged lateral ventricles without increased prominence of cortical sulci (**Figure 5-16**). Periventricular white matter lesions may be seen. The likelihood of a favorable response to treatment is best predicted by transient improvement, most often in gait, following removal of 30-50 mL of CSF by lumbar puncture (**tap test**). Gait should be tested immediately before and 2-4 hours after CSF removal.

▶ Differential Diagnosis

The gait disorder, which usually appears first, may resemble that associated with Parkinson disease or other causes of parkinsonism (see Chapter 11, Movement Disorders). If both gait disorder and dementia are present, Alzheimer disease and vascular dementia must also be considered. MRI and CSF tap test should distinguish NPH from these conditions. However, it is important to note that many patients with NPH, including those who can benefit from

treatment, may have more than one disorder. In particular, vascular lesions on MRI should not necessarily exclude patients from eligibility for shunting, although the extent of concurrent disease may influence post-shunt prognosis.

▶ Treatment

Treatment of NPH involves shunting of CSF, usually by the ventriculoperitoneal (VP) route. From 60-90% of patients with idiopathic NPH benefit from this procedure, and gait disorder, dementia, and urinary dysfunction can all improve. Ventricular size should be monitored for several months by serial imaging studies to confirm effective shunting. Complications of shunting include postural headache and subdural effusion (from overdrainage), shunt obstruction (which occurs in ~30% of cases and may require shunt revision), and bacterial meningitis.

BRAIN TUMOR & WHOLE-BRAIN RADIOTHERAPY

Brain tumors (see Chapter 6, Headache & Facial Pain) produce dementia and related syndromes by a combination of local and diffuse effects, including edema, compression of adjacent brain structures, increased intracranial pressure, impairment of cerebral blood flow, and disruption of neuronal connectivity. Cognitive function in patients with brain tumor can also be impaired by radiotherapy or chemotherapy. The tumors most likely to produce generalized cerebral syndromes are gliomas arising in the frontal or

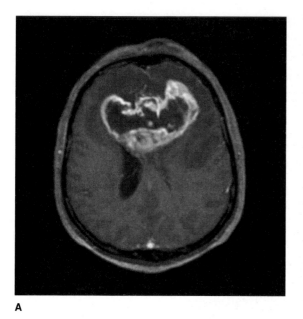 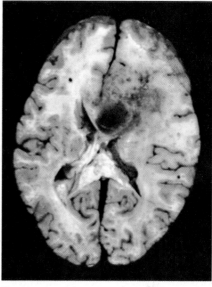

A   B

▲ **Figure 5-17.** Brain MRI (**A**) and postmortem horizontal brain slice (**B**) showing infiltrating glioblastoma multiforme crossing the corpus callosum to affect the frontal lobes of both cerebral hemispheres (butterfly glioma). (Used with permission from Reisner HM. *Pathology: A Modern Case Study.* New York, NY: McGraw-Hill; 2015. Fig 21-27.)

temporal lobes or the corpus callosum (**Figure 5-17**). Although such lesions tend to infiltrate subcortical white matter extensively, they may initially give rise to few focal neurologic signs.

The dementia associated with brain tumor is characterized by prominent mental slowness, apathy, impaired concentration, and subtle alterations in personality. Depending on the areas of involvement, memory disorder, aphasia, or agnosia may be seen. Brain tumors ultimately produce headache, seizures, or focal sensorimotor disturbances.

Meningeal neoplasia, discussed in Chapter 4 as a cause of confusional states, may also produce dementia, which is commonly associated with headache, as well as symptoms and signs of dysfunction at multiple sites in the nervous system. The diagnosis is established by cytologic studies of the CSF.

Whole-brain radiotherapy, used to treat various tumors of the head and neck, is associated with an increased incidence of dementia, especially in patients ≤65 years of age. Factors that may be involved in pathogenesis include direct injury to brain tissue or blood vessels and inhibition of angiogenesis or neurogenesis.

CHRONIC TRAUMATIC ENCEPHALOPATHY

Severe or repetitive, concussive or subconcussive head injury may cause progressive cognitive dysfunction, sometimes leading to dementia. Histopathologic features include neurofibrillary tangles containing hyperphosphorylated tau, β-amyloid deposits in diffuse or neuritic plaques or in blood vessels, and α-synuclein-positive Lewy bodies. Although classically described in boxers (**punch-drunk syndrome** or **dementia pugilistica**), this condition is recognized increasingly in other athletes and military veterans subject to head trauma. Early features include headache and impaired attention and concentration, followed by depression, explosive behavior, and short-term memory deficits. Executive dysfunction and other cognitive impairments ensue, leading to dementia with word-finding difficulty and aggressive behavior. Suicidality is common. Associated features include dysarthria, tremor, spasticity, ataxia, and gait disturbance. Neuroimaging studies may show cortical or hippocampal atrophy, enlarged ventricles, and signs of diffuse axonal injury. Evidence of an additional neurodegenerative disease, such as motor neuron disease, Alzheimer disease, Lewy body disease, or frontotemporal dementia, is present at autopsy in about one-third of cases.

SYSTEMIC DISORDERS

INFECTION

▶ **HIV-Associated Neurocognitive Disorders**

Human immunodeficiency virus (HIV-1) infection of the brain can produce a range of HIV-associated neurocognitive disorders (**HAND**), which occur in 15-55%

of HIV-infected individuals. These syndromes include **asymptomatic neurocognitive impairment** (demonstrable only by cognitive testing), **minor neurocognitive disorder** (mild to moderate cognitive and functional impairment), and **HIV-associated dementia** (moderate to severe cognitive and functional impairment). Combination antiretroviral therapy of HIV infection has reduced the prevalence of HIV-associated dementia, but increased the prevalence of milder forms of HAND, as patients live longer. Thus, asymptomatic neurocognitive impairment now accounts for about 70% of HAND. Cardiovascular risk factors, advanced age, and drug abuse increase the risk of HAND.

A. Pathogenesis

HIV-1 invades the brain in blood-borne macrophages early in the course of systemic infection and infects brain macrophages, microglia, and astrocytes, but not neurons. Neurologic, including cognitive, symptoms are thought to result from neurotoxic effects of viral proteins or of cytokines, chemokines, and other soluble factors released by inflammatory cells. Combination antiretroviral therapy inhibits viral replication, but persistent chronic inflammation and latent HIV-1 infection may continue to impair brain function in treated individuals.

B. Pathology

Prior to the introduction of effective treatment, the brain in HIV-1-associated dementia typically showed perivascular infiltration by macrophages, multinucleated giant cells, astrogliosis, and neuronal loss, affecting the basal ganglia, subcortical white matter, thalamus, and brainstem. With combination antiretroviral therapy, histopathologic abnormalities are generally less marked. However, microglial activation is a prominent feature, and inflammation is most pronounced in the hippocampus and entorhinal and temporal cortex. Deposits of β-amyloid and hyperphosphorylated tau are also observed.

C. Clinical Findings

HAND usually has an insidious onset and can produce cognitive, behavioral, and motor deficits. Asymptomatic neurocognitive impairment is characterized by abnormalities on neuropsychological testing without evident functional decline. Mild neurocognitive disorder impairs memory, learning, or executive function to some degree, but typically allows the patient to continue self-care and often employment. Gait disorder, tremor, and defects in fine motor performance may occur. HIV-associated dementia is more severe, with increased memory loss and executive dysfunction, and precludes independence. Parkinsonian features (bradykinesia, postural instability) and postural or intention tremor (see Chapter 11, Movement Disorders) are sometimes present. Depression is common.

D. Investigative Studies

There is no definitive laboratory test for HAND. CSF may show mild to moderate elevation of protein (≤200 mg/dL); modest, usually mononuclear pleocytosis (≤50 cells/μL); and oligoclonal bands. MRI shows cortical and subcortical atrophy with diffuse signal abnormalities in subcortical white matter (**Figure 5-18**) and is useful for excluding other HIV-related neuropathologic processes, such as opportunistic infection. Neuropsychological testing is useful for detecting asymptomatic neurocognitive impairment and mild neurocognitive disorder.

E. Treatment

Patients with HAND should receive combination antiretroviral therapy as described for HIV-1 meningitis in Chapter 4, Confusional States, and at https://aidsinfo.nih.gov/guidelines. Parkinsonian features may respond to antiparkinsonian drugs (see Chapter 10, Movement Disorders).

F. Prognosis

The course may be relatively static, steadily progressive, or acutely exacerbated by concurrent disease or antiretroviral treatment (immune reconstitution inflammatory syndrome; see *Organ Transplantation* in Chapter 4, Confusional States). Combination antiretroviral therapy can

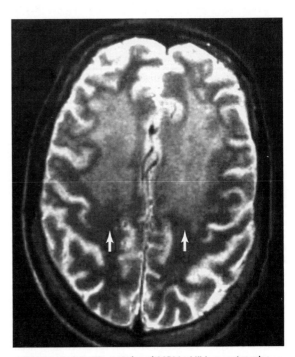

▲ **Figure 5-18.** T2-weighted MRI in HIV-associated dementia, showing increased signal intensity (**arrows**) in subcortical white matter.

arrest but not reverse HAND-related deficits, and has extended median survival from months to years.

▶ Neurosyphilis

Syphilis is caused by *Treponema pallidum* and transmitted by sexual contact, which results in infection in approximately one-third of encounters with infected individuals. The incidence of syphilis is especially high in patients with HIV infection. Treponemes invade the CNS in about 40% of those infected and persist in about 12%. Dementia from neurosyphilis (**general paresis**), a late manifestation of neurosyphilis (**Figure 5-19**), was common in the prepenicillin era but is now rare.

A. Clinical Findings

1. **Primary syphilis** is characterized by local skin lesions (chancres) that usually appear within 1 month of exposure. Hematogenous spread of *T. pallidum* produces symptoms and signs of **secondary syphilis**, including fever, skin rash, alopecia, anogenital skin lesions, and ulceration of mucous membranes, within 1 to 6 months. Neurologic symptoms are uncommon.

2. **Early neurosyphilis** may be asymptomatic. Alternatively, it may manifest as **meningeal syphilis**, which occurs 2-12 months after primary infection and causes headache, stiff neck, nausea and vomiting, and cranial nerve (especially II, VII, or VIII) involvement, or **meningovascular syphilis**, which is seen 4-7 years into the course and usually presents with transient ischemic attacks or stroke (see Chapter 13, Stroke).

3. **Late (parenchymatous) neurosyphilis** produces the syndromes of general paresis and tabes dorsalis, which can occur separately or together (taboparesis); either

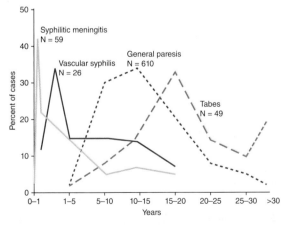

▲ **Figure 5-19.** Interval between primary syphilitic infection and neurosyphilis syndromes. (Reproduced, with permission, from Simon RP. Neurosyphilis. *Arch Neurol.* 1985;42:606-613. Copyright © 1985. American Medical Association. All rights reserved.)

one can occur in combination with optic atrophy. **General paresis** is a chronic meningoencephalitis caused by active spirochetal infection. Onset is with gradual memory loss or altered affect, personality, or behavior. This is followed by global intellectual deterioration with grandiosity, depression, psychosis, and focal weakness. Terminal features include incontinence, seizures, or strokes. Neurologic examination may show tremor of the face and tongue, paucity of facial expression, dysarthria, and pyramidal signs. **Taboparesis** is the coexistence of **tabes dorsalis** (see Chapter 10, Sensory Disorders) with general paresis. Signs and symptoms of tabes dorsalis include Argyll Robertson pupils (see Chapter 7, Neuro-Ophthalmic Disorders), lancinating (stabbing) pains, areflexia, posterior column sensory deficits with sensory ataxia and Romberg sign, incontinence, impotence, Charcot (hypertrophic) joints, and genu recurvatum (hyperextended knees).

B. Investigative Studies

Treponemal serologic blood tests (fluorescent treponemal antibody absorbed [FTA-ABS] or microhemagglutination-*Treponema pallidum* [MHATP]) are reactive in almost all patients with active neurosyphilis, but non-treponemal blood tests (Venereal Disease Research Laboratory [VDRL] or rapid plasma reagin [RPR]) can be negative; therefore, a treponemal blood test should be obtained in all suspected cases. If this is nonreactive, neurosyphilis is effectively excluded; if it is reactive, lumbar puncture should be performed to confirm the diagnosis of neurosyphilis and provide a baseline CSF profile against which to gauge the efficacy of subsequent treatment. The CSF in active neurosyphilis usually shows a lymphocytic pleocytosis and reactive non-treponemal CSF serology (eg, VDRL), except in early meningeal and meningovascular syphilis, isolated intracranial granuloma (**gumma**), and end-stage tabes dorsalis. Other CSF abnormalities include protein elevation, increased γ-globulin, and the presence of oligoclonal bands. The MRI in general paresis may show meninges-based mass lesions (gummas) or unilateral or bilateral medial temporal lobe T2 high-intensity abnormalities, with or without associated atrophy.

C. Treatment

General paresis is treated as described earlier for syphilitic meningitis (see Chapter 4, Confusional States). Transient fever, tachycardia, hypotension, and leukocytosis may occur within hours after therapy is started (**Jarisch–Herxheimer reaction**). Failure of the CSF to return to normal within 6 months after treatment of neurosyphilis requires retreatment.

D. Prognosis

General paresis may improve or stabilize after treatment, but in some cases it continues to worsen. Patients with persistently reactive CSF serologic tests but no pleocytosis are unlikely to respond to penicillin therapy but are usually treated nevertheless.

Progressive Multifocal Leukoencephalopathy

Progressive multifocal leukoencephalopathy (**PML**) results from reactivation of **JC polyoma virus** infection, which is usually asymptomatic, in immunosuppressed patients. These include individuals with lymphoma, leukemia, or HIV infection and those treated with immunomodulatory drugs for multiple sclerosis or Crohn disease (eg, natalizumab) or for psoriasis (eg, dimethyl fumarate). The disease targets oligodendrocytes, leading to diffuse and patchy demyelination of the cerebral hemispheres, brainstem, and cerebellum.

The course is typically subacute and progressive, leading to death in approximately 50% of patients within 3 to 6 months, although mortality is lower (approximately 20%) in patients on natalizumab. PML associated with natalizumab does not occur until years after treatment. Fever and systemic symptoms are absent. Dementia and focal cortical dysfunction are prominent. Signs include hemiparesis, visual deficits, aphasia, dysarthria, and sensory impairment. Ataxia and headache are uncommon, and seizures do not occur.

The CSF is usually normal but may show a mild increase in pressure, white cell count, or protein. The CT scan or MRI shows multifocal white matter abnormalities, typically without enhancement or mass effect (**Figure 5-20**).

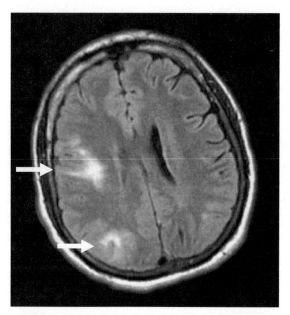

▲ **Figure 5-20.** Axial FLAIR MRI in progressive multifocal leukoencephalopathy, showing abnormally high signal intensity (**arrows**) in white matter of the right parietal and occipital lobes.

Diagnosis is by detection of JC virus DNA in CSF or brain biopsy using the polymerase chain reaction.

Treatment of PML is with combination antiretroviral therapy for patients with HIV infection and discontinuation of the drug for patients receiving natalizumab. Plasma exchange is also used in the latter group but its benefit is uncertain.

METABOLIC & NUTRITIONAL DISORDERS

Alcoholism

Certain complications of alcoholism can cause dementia. These include acquired hepatocerebral degeneration from alcoholic liver disease (see *Non-Wilsonian Hepatocerebral Degeneration* later in this chapter), chronic subdural hematoma (discussed earlier in this chapter), and nutritional deficiency states. A dementia caused by direct toxic effects of ethanol on the brain has been proposed, but no distinctive abnormalities have been identified in the brains of demented alcoholics. Dementia in alcoholics is more likely to be explained by misdiagnosis of Korsakoff syndrome (see later in this chapter), or by the metabolic, traumatic, or nutritional complications of alcoholism mentioned previously. The latter include the following:

1. **Pellagra**, caused by deficiency of **niacin**, injures neurons in the cerebral cortex, basal ganglia, brainstem, cerebellum, and anterior horns of the spinal cord. Systemic involvement is manifested by diarrhea, glossitis, anemia, and erythematous skin lesions. Neurologic involvement may produce dementia; psychosis; confusional states; pyramidal, extrapyramidal, and cerebellar signs; polyneuropathy; and optic neuropathy. Treatment is with nicotinamide, 10-150 mg orally daily, but neurologic deficits may persist.

2. **Marchiafava–Bignami syndrome** is characterized by necrosis of the corpus callosum and subcortical white matter and occurs most often in malnourished alcoholics. The course can be acute, subacute, or chronic. Clinical features include dementia, spasticity, dysarthria, gait disorder, and coma. The diagnosis can sometimes be made by CT scan or MRI. No specific treatment is available, but cessation of drinking and improvement of nutrition are advised. The outcome is variable: patients may die, survive with dementia, or recover.

Hypothyroidism

Hypothyroidism (myxedema) can produce a reversible dementia or chronic organic psychosis. The dementia is characterized by mental slowness, memory loss, and irritability, without focal cortical deficits. Psychiatric manifestations are typically prominent and include depression, paranoia, visual and auditory hallucinations, mania, and suicidal behavior.

Patients with myxedema may complain of headache, hearing loss, tinnitus, vertigo, weakness, or paresthesia. Examination may show deafness, dysarthria, or cerebellar ataxia. The most suggestive finding is delayed relaxation of the tendon reflexes. Diagnosis and treatment are discussed in Chapter 4, Confusional States. Cognitive dysfunction is usually reversible with treatment.

▶ Vitamin B$_{12}$ Deficiency

Vitamin B$_{12}$ deficiency is a rare cause of reversible dementia and organic psychosis, which can occur with or without hematologic and other neurologic manifestations. The dementia consists of global cognitive dysfunction with mental slowness, impaired concentration, and memory disturbance; aphasia and other focal cortical disorders do not occur. Diminished vibration and position sense in the lower extremities is common. Psychiatric manifestations are often prominent and include depression, mania, and paranoid psychosis with visual and auditory hallucinations. Laboratory findings, CNS imaging, and treatment are discussed in Chapter 4, Confusional States.

ORGAN FAILURE

▶ Dialysis Dementia

This is a rare disorder in patients receiving chronic hemodialysis. Clinical features include personality changes, hallucinations, dysarthria, dysphagia, asterixis, myoclonus, and seizures. The EEG shows paroxysmal high-voltage slowing with intermixed spikes and slow waves. Removing aluminum from the dialysate has decreased the syndrome's incidence.

▶ Acquired Hepatocerebral Degeneration

Acquired (non-Wilsonian) hepatocerebral degeneration is an uncommon complication of chronic hepatic cirrhosis with spontaneous or surgical portosystemic shunting. Symptoms may be related to failure of the liver to detoxify ammonia. Neurologic symptoms precede hepatic symptoms in approximately one-sixth of patients.

A. Clinical Findings

Systemic manifestations of chronic liver disease are usually present. The neurologic syndrome is fluctuating but progressive over years and may be punctuated by episodes of acute hepatic encephalopathy. Dementia, dysarthria, and cerebellar, extrapyramidal, and pyramidal signs are common. Dementia is marked by mental slowness, apathy, impaired attention and concentration, and memory disturbance. Cerebellar signs include gait and limb ataxia and dysarthria; nystagmus is rare. Extrapyramidal involvement may produce rigidity, resting tremor, dystonia, chorea, or athetosis. Asterixis, myoclonus, hyperreflexia, and extensor plantar responses are common; paraparesis is rare.

Laboratory studies show abnormal hepatic blood chemistries and elevated blood ammonia, but the degree of abnormality may not correspond to the severity of neurologic symptoms. MRI may show lesions in the basal ganglia and subcortical white matter. The CSF is normal except for increased glutamine and occasional mild elevation of protein.

B. Differential Diagnosis

Wilson disease can be distinguished by its earlier onset, Kayser-Fleischer rings, and abnormal copper metabolism. Alcoholic cerebellar degeneration primarily affects gait and is not accompanied by extrapyramidal or pyramidal signs.

C. Treatment & Prognosis

Treatment is as described for hepatic encephalopathy (see Chapter 4, Confusional States). Death results from progressive liver failure or variceal bleeding.

▶ Wilson Disease

Wilson disease (hepatolenticular degeneration) is a rare but treatable autosomal recessive hereditary disorder of copper metabolism that produces dementia and extrapyramidal symptoms (see Chapter 11, Movement Disorders). The disease results from homozygous or compound heterozygous mutations in *ATP7B*, a gene coding for the β polypeptide of a copper-transporting ATPase.

PSEUDODEMENTIA

The term "pseudodementia" is sometimes used to describe disorders that can be mistaken for dementia, especially depression. However, other conditions can mimic dementia as well. Because depression and other dementia mimics are common and often treatable, identifying them is important.

DEPRESSION

Both dementia and depression can be characterized by mental slowness, apathy, self-neglect, withdrawal, irritability, difficulty with memory and concentration, and changes in behavior and personality. Moreover, depression and other psychiatric disturbances can be a feature of dementing illnesses (**Table 5-12**), depression and dementia may coexist as independent disorders, and late-life depression may be a harbinger of subsequent dementia. Clinical features that help in the differentiation are listed in **Table 5-13**. When depression is being considered, psychiatric consultation should be obtained. If not correctable by treatment of an underlying medical disease or by a change in medication, depression should be treated directly. Treatments include cognitive behavioral therapy, antidepressant drugs, exercise,

Table 5-12. Psychiatric Features of Selected Dementias.

Disease	Psychiatric features
Alzheimer disease	Apathy, depression, anxiety, delusions
Frontotemporal dementia (behavioral variant)	Disinhibition, impulsivity, gluttony
Progressive supranuclear palsy	Apathy, depression
Lewy body disease	Illusions, hallucinations, paranoia
Huntington disease	Apathy, irritability, depression, anxiety
Creutzfeldt-Jakob (prion) disease	Agitation, depression
Vascular dementia	Apathy, depression, anxiety
Brain tumor	Apathy, personality change
Chronic traumatic encephalopathy	Depression, explosive behavior
HIV-associated neurocognitive disorders	Apathy
Neurosyphilis	Grandiosity, depression, illusions, hallucinations
Hypothyroidism	Depression, paranoia, hallucinations
Vitamin B$_{12}$ deficiency	Depression, mania, paranoia, hallucinations

Table 5-13. Dementia versus Pseudodementia of Depression: Distinguishing Features.

Dementia	Depression
Insidious onset	Abrupt onset
Progressive deterioration	Plateau of dysfunction
No history of depression	History of depression may exist
Patient typically unaware of extent of deficits and does not complain of memory loss	Patient aware of and may exaggerate deficits and frequently complains of memory loss
Somatic complaints uncommon	Somatic complaints common
Variable affect	Depressed affect
Few vegetative symptoms	Prominent vegetative symptoms
Impairment often worse at night	Impairment usually not worse at night
Neurologic examination and laboratory studies may be abnormal	Neurologic examination and laboratory studies normal

transcranial magnetic stimulation, and electroconvulsive therapy.

FUNCTIONAL COGNITIVE DISORDER

Patients with this condition complain of recurrent cognitive symptoms, despite an absence of objectively verifiable cognitive defects. Examples include name- or other word-finding difficulties, misplacing keys or other objects, and losing track of conversations or ongoing tasks. Forgotten items can often be recalled later (mnestic block). Those affected are typically of working age, well-educated, and socially and economically successful. They may have a history of anxiety or depression and recently increased psychological stress. Despite the perceived deficits, work performance has not objectively declined, friends and family members are unaware that a problem exists, and symptoms are not verifiably progressive. Neuropsychological testing (eg, Montreal Cognitive Assessment) should be performed and repeated after ~1 year to document any deterioration in function. Treatment includes reassurance, measures to reduce stress, and correction of other possible contributing factors (discussed next).

SLEEP DISORDERS

Sleep disorders associated with reduced sleep time or sleep fragmentation (obstructive sleep apnea, insomnia) can impair cognitive function by interfering with memory consolidation and, in the case of obstructive sleep apnea, causing apnea-related cerebral hypoxia. Because both obstructive sleep apnea and insomnia are more prevalent at older ages, they often affect the same population at increased risk for dementia; moreover, obstructive sleep apnea may itself increase dementia risk. Sleep-related cognitive deficits are important to identify because they are often treatable and reversible.

Obstructive sleep apnea affects ~40% of men and ~20% of women over age 40. It is caused by upper airway collapse and leads to sleep fragmentation, hypoxia, elevated blood pressure, and sympathetic hyperactivity. Associated symptoms include snoring, nocturia, and daytime sleepiness. Adverse cognitive effects include impaired attention, verbal memory, and executive function. Diagnosis is by overnight polysomnography, and treatment is with a continuous positive airway pressure (CPAP) device for ≥4-6 hours per night during sleep, which may improve cognitive deficits over several months. Obstructive sleep apnea is a risk factor for hypertension, atrial fibrillation, and stroke.

Insomnia affects up to 10% of the general population and can be caused by a wide variety of medical and psychiatric conditions, alcohol and other recreational or therapeutic drugs, and poor sleep hygiene. Patients with insomnia may experience defective verbal memory. Treatment or correction of the underlying factors listed above may improve insomnia and associated cognitive deficits.

DISORDERS OF VISION & HEARING

Sensory deficits are common in the elderly population at high risk for dementia and can interfere with both cognitive function and cognitive testing. Social isolation and depression are likely contributing factors. Visual impairment may result from presbyopia, cataract, glaucoma, or macular degeneration, and treatment (eg, cataract surgery) can improve cognition. Hearing impairment (presbyacusis) may be amenable to therapeutic cerumen disempaction, hearing aids, or cochlear implants.

DRUG SIDE EFFECTS

The aged population most at risk for dementia is also highly susceptible to adverse drug effects, including effects on cognitive function that can be mistaken for dementia. Factors involved include the frequency of multiple medical problems (and, therefore, polypharmacy) in this population, age-related changes in pharmacokinetics (including drug distribution volume, metabolism, and clearance), and attenuation of physiologic homeostatic mechanisms. Drugs especially likely to cause confusional states that may be misdiagnosed as dementia include benzodiazepines and other sedative-hypnotics, opiate analgesics, and anticholinergics (see Chapter 4, Confusional States).

AMNESTIC SYNDROMES

A disorder of memory (**amnestic syndrome**) may occur as one feature of an acute confusional state or dementia, or as an isolated abnormality. The latter condition is discussed in this section.

Memory is a complex function that can be viewed as having different components with different anatomic bases (**Figure 5-21**). **Declarative** (explicit or conscious) **memory** includes **working memory**, which permits acute manipulation of newly presented information, as well as longer-term **semantic** (factual) and **episodic** (personal) **memory**. **Nondeclarative** (implicit or unconscious) **memory** includes **procedural memory** required to carry out well-learned and seemingly automatic tasks and **emotional memory** that attaches affective significance to objects or events.

Memory can also be seen as comprising the phases of **registration, storage**, and **retrieval of information**. Autopsy and imaging studies suggest that the hippocampus, parahippocampal region of the medial temporal lobe, and neocortical association areas are among the anatomic structures important in memory processing (**Figure 5-22**). Bilateral damage to these regions results in impairment of **short-term memory**, which is manifested clinically by the inability to form new memories. **Long-term memory**, which involves retrieval of previously learned information, is relatively preserved, perhaps because these memories are strengthened by activity-dependent synaptic plasticity,

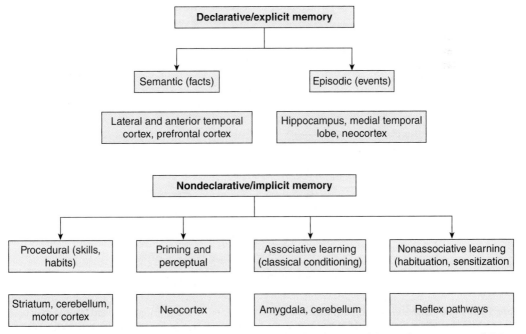

▲ **Figure 5-21.** Forms of memory and their anatomic bases. (Modified from Kandel ER, Schwartz JH, Jessell TM [editors]: *Principles of Neural Science*; 4th ed. New York, NY: McGraw-Hill; 2000.)

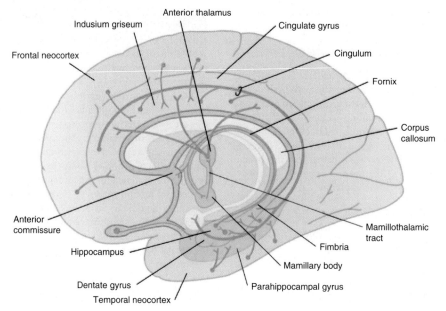

▲ **Figure 5-22.** Anatomic structures involved in memory processing. These include the hippocampus, parahippo-campal gyrus, and neocortical association areas. (Used with permission from Waxman SG. *Clinical Neuroanatomy.* 28th ed. New York, NY: McGraw-Hill, 2017. Fig 19-11.)

stored more diffusely, or both. Some patients with amnestic syndromes may attempt to fill in gaps in memory with false recollections (**confabulation**), which can take the form of elaborate contrivances or of genuine memories misplaced in time. The longest-standing and most deeply ingrained memories, however, such as one's own name, are almost always spared in organic memory disturbances. In contrast, such personal memories may be prominently or exclusively impaired in **dissociative (psychogenic) amnesia**.

ACUTE AMNESIA

HEAD TRAUMA

Head injuries resulting in loss of consciousness are invariably associated with an amnestic syndrome. Patients seen shortly after such an injury exhibit a confusional state in which they are unable to incorporate new memories (**anterograde, or posttraumatic amnesia; Figure 5-23**),

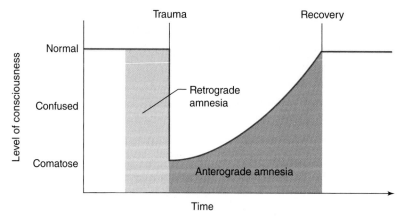

▲ **Figure 5-23.** Retrograde and anterograde amnesia in posttraumatic memory disorders. Head trauma may produce transient coma, followed by a confusional state during which the patient is unable to form new memories. With recovery, this ability is restored, but there is persistent amnesia for the period of coma and confusion (**anterograde amnesia**) and for a variable period preceding the trauma (**retrograde amnesia**); the latter deficit may improve with time.

although they may behave in an apparently normal automatic fashion. In addition, **retrograde amnesia** is present, covering a variable period prior to the trauma.

As full consciousness returns, the ability to form new memories is restored. Events occurring in the confusional interval tend to be permanently lost to memory, however. Exceptions are islands of memory for a lucid interval between trauma and unconsciousness, or for periods of lesser impairment in the course of a fluctuating posttraumatic confusional state. The period of retrograde amnesia begins to shrink, with the most remote memories the first to return. The severity of the injury tends to correlate with the duration of confusion and with the extent of permanent retrograde and posttraumatic amnesia.

HYPOXIA OR ISCHEMIA

Global cerebral hypoxia or ischemia, such as occurs in cardiac arrest, can produce an amnestic syndrome due to the selective vulnerability of hippocampal neurons involved in memory formation to these insults. Amnesia after cardiac arrest tends to occur with coma lasting ≥12 hours. There is severe impairment of the ability to incorporate new memories, with relative preservation of registration and remote memory, producing an isolated disorder of short-term memory. Retrograde amnesia for the period preceding the insult may occur. Patients exhibit a lack of concern about their impairment and sometimes confabulate. Amnesia after cardiac arrest may be the sole manifestation of neurologic dysfunction, or it may coexist with cerebral watershed syndromes, such as bibrachial paresis, cortical blindness, or visual agnosia (see Chapter 13, Stroke). Recovery often occurs within several days, although deficits may persist.

Carbon monoxide poisoning may be associated with a delayed amnestic syndrome, occurring days to weeks after acute intoxication, that is frequently accompanied by affective disturbances and focal cortical or extrapyramidal dysfunction. Brain injury results from a combination of hypoxia (from competition between carbon monoxide and oxygen for binding to hemoglobin), ischemia (from myocardial hypoxia leading to hypotension), demyelination (from oligodendrocyte toxicity), and inflammation. Acute carbon monoxide poisoning is suggested by cherry-red coloration of the skin and mucous membranes, elevated carboxyhemoglobin levels, or cardiac arrhythmia. CT scan or MRI may show lesions in the basal ganglia, especially the globus pallidus. Treatment consists of the administration of normo- or hyperbaric oxygen.

BILATERAL POSTERIOR CEREBRAL ARTERY OCCLUSION

The posterior cerebral artery supplies the medial temporal lobe, thalamus, posterior internal capsule, and occipital cortex (**Figure 5-24**). Ischemia or infarction in this

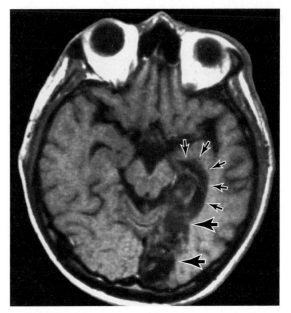

▲ **Figure 5-24.** T1-weighted MRI in a patient with an old left posterior cerebral artery occlusion, showing tissue loss in the medial temporal (**small arrows**) and occipital (**large arrows**) lobes and associated dilation of the temporal and occipital horns of the lateral ventricle. (Used with permission from A. Gean.)

territory, typically when bilateral, may produce a transient or permanent amnestic syndrome. Emboli in the vertebrobasilar system (see Chapter 13, Stroke) are a frequent cause.

The amnestic syndrome is usually associated with unilateral or bilateral hemianopia and sometimes with visual agnosia, alexia without agraphia, anomia, sensory disturbances, or signs of upper midbrain dysfunction (especially impaired pupillary light reflex). Recent memory tends to be selectively impaired, with relative preservation of remote memory and registration.

The CT scan or MRI shows infarction in any combination of the previously mentioned regions. Evaluation and treatment are described in Chapter 13, Stroke.

TRANSIENT GLOBAL AMNESIA

Transient global amnesia is a syndrome of unknown cause that tends to occur in middle-aged or elderly patients. It is characterized by the acute onset of anterograde and sometimes also retrograde memory loss, which lasts for ≤24 (usually 4-6) hours, without impairment of other cognitive functions. Patients appear agitated and perplexed and may repeatedly inquire about their whereabouts, the time, and the nature of what they are experiencing. Knowledge of personal identity is preserved, as are remote memories and registration, but new memories cannot be formed, which accounts for the patient's repetitive questions. The patient's obvious concern distinguishes transient global amnesia from most other amnestic syndromes, in which there is lack of awareness of the deficit. EEG and CT scans are normal, although abnormal hippocampal signals are sometimes observed with MRI. Full recovery is the rule but recurrence is reported in 3-24% of patients.

ALCOHOLIC BLACKOUTS

Short-term consumption of large amounts of ethanol by alcoholic or nonalcoholic individuals may lead to "blackouts"—transient amnestic episodes that are not caused by global confusion, seizures, head trauma, or the Wernicke-Korsakoff syndrome. These spells are characterized by an inability to form new memories, without impairment of long-term memory or immediate recall. The disorder is self-limited, and no specific treatment is required, but reduction of ethanol intake should be recommended, and thiamine should be given to treat possible Wernicke encephalopathy (see Chapter 4, Confusional States).

WERNICKE ENCEPHALOPATHY

Wernicke encephalopathy is caused by thiamine deficiency and classically produces an acute confusional state, ataxia, and ophthalmoplegia. Amnesia may be the major or sole cognitive disturbance, however, especially after thiamine treatment is begun and other cognitive abnormalities improve. Because patients with Wernicke encephalopathy usually present with global confusion rather than isolated amnesia, the disorder is discussed more fully in Chapter 4, Confusional States.

DISSOCIATIVE (PSYCHOGENIC) AMNESIA

Amnesia may be a manifestation of a dissociative disorder. In such patients, a prior psychiatric history, additional psychiatric symptoms, or a precipitating emotional stress can often be identified. Dissociative amnesia is characterized by an isolated or a disproportionate loss of traumatic or stressful personal memories. Dissociative amnesia is usually localized in time to the immediate aftermath of a traumatic experience or selective for some but not other events during such a period. Less frequent patterns include amnesia restricted to certain categories of information, continuous amnesia for events from some time in the past up to and including the present, and generalized amnesia. In some cases, patients may be unable to remember even their own name, an exceedingly rare finding in organic amnesia. Despite such disorientation to person, orientation to place and time may be preserved. In addition, recent memories may be less affected than remote memories; the reverse of the pattern customarily seen in amnesia is caused by organic disease. Psychiatric consultation should be obtained regarding treatment.

CHRONIC AMNESIA

ALCOHOLIC KORSAKOFF AMNESTIC SYNDROME

The Korsakoff amnestic syndrome, which occurs in chronic alcoholism and other malnutrition states, is thought to result from thiamine deficiency leading to bilateral degeneration of the dorsomedial thalamic nuclei. It is usually preceded by one or more episodes of Wernicke encephalopathy (see Chapter 4, Confusional States), and is often associated with other residua of Wernicke encephalopathy, such as nystagmus, gait ataxia, or polyneuropathy. The essential defect is an inability to form new memories, resulting in significant impairment of short-term memory. Long-term memory is also frequently affected, although to a lesser extent, and registration is intact. Patients are typically apathetic and lack insight into their disorder. They may attempt to reassure the physician that no impairment exists and try to explain away their obvious inability to remember. **Confabulation** is often, but not invariably, a feature.

Korsakoff syndrome can be prevented by prompt administration of thiamine to patients with Wernicke encephalopathy. Patients with established Korsakoff syndrome should also receive thiamine to prevent the progression of deficits, although existing deficits are unlikely to be reversed.

POSTENCEPHALITIC AMNESIA

Patients who recover from acute viral encephalitis (see Chapter 4, Confusional States), particularly that caused by **herpes simplex virus**, may be left with a permanent and static amnestic syndrome. The syndrome is similar to that produced by chronic alcoholism in that an inability to form new memories is its outstanding feature. Remote memories are affected to a lesser extent than are recent ones, and registration is intact. Confabulation may occur. Often there is total amnesia for the period of the acute encephalitis.

Patients may also exhibit other symptoms of limbic system disease. These include docility, indifference, flatness of mood and affect, inappropriate jocularity and sexual allusions, hyperphagia, impotence, repetitive stereotyped motor activity, and the absence of goal-oriented activity. Complex partial seizures, with or without secondary generalization, may occur.

BRAIN TUMOR

Brain tumor is a rare cause of an amnestic syndrome. Tumors that can present in this manner include those that are located in or compress the third ventricle. The amnestic syndrome closely resembles Korsakoff syndrome and may be accompanied by lethargy, headache, endocrine disturbances, visual field defects, or papilledema. Surgery, cranial irradiation, or chemotherapy for brain tumor may also impair memory (see *Brain Tumor & Whole-Brain Radiotherapy* earlier in this chapter). The diagnosis of brain tumor is made by CT scan or MRI. Treatment consists of surgery or irradiation or both, depending on the type of tumor and its location.

AUTOIMMUNE LIMBIC ENCEPHALITIS

Autoimmune inflammation and degeneration of gray matter regions of the CNS can occur in the presence (**paraneoplastic syndromes**) or absence of systemic cancer. When limbic structures are predominantly affected, an amnestic syndrome is a prominent feature (**limbic encephalitis**). In many patients, limbic encephalitis is associated with the production of autoantibodies directed against either intracellular or cell-surface (including synaptic) neuronal antigens (**Table 5-14**). Neuronal loss in autoimmune limbic encephalitis involving intracellular antigens is thought to be mediated by cytotoxic T cells, whereas that involving neuronal cell-surface antigens is likely to be antibody-mediated.

Paraneoplastic limbic encephalitis may be associated with small-cell cancer of the lung, testicular seminoma, or thymoma, and symptoms often precede diagnosis of the underlying cancer. Histopathologic findings include neuronal loss, reactive gliosis, microglial proliferation, and perivascular lymphocytic cuffing affecting gray matter of the hippocampus, cingulum, piriform cortex, inferior frontal lobes, insula, and amygdala. Symptoms develop over several weeks. There is profound impairment of recent

Table 5-14. Autoimmune Limbic Encephalitis.

Antibody	Associated neoplasm
Against intracellular antigens	
Anti-Hu	Small cell lung carcinoma
Anti-Ma2	Testicular seminoma
Anti-glutamic acid decarboxylase (GAD)	Thymoma, small cell lung carcinoma
Against cell surface antigens	
Anti-AMPA receptor	Thymoma, small cell lung carcinoma
Anti-GABA$_B$ receptor	Small cell lung carcinoma
Anti-leucine-rich glioma inactivated 1 (LGI1)	Thymoma
Anti-contactin–associated protein 2 (CASPR2)	Thymoma
Anti-adenylate kinase 5 (AK5)	—

Data from Graus F et al. A clinical approach to diagnosis of autoimmune encephalitis. *Lancet Neurol.* 2016;15:391–404 and McKeon A. Autoimmune encephalopathies and dementias. *Continuum.* 2016;22:538–558.

memory, with less involvement of remote memory and sparing of registration; confabulation occurs in some cases. Mood disorders, delusions, hallucinations, sleep

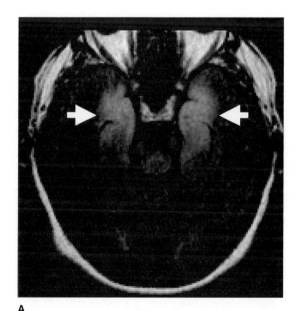

A

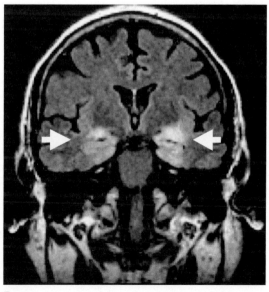

B

▲ **Figure 5-25.** FLAIR MRI with axial (**A**) and coronal (**B**) views in limbic encephalitis, showing increased signal (**arrows**) in the medial temporal lobes.

disturbance, complex partial or generalized seizures, and dementia may develop. Depending on the extent to which gray matter regions outside the limbic system are involved, cerebellar, pyramidal, bulbar, and peripheral nerve disturbances may also occur.

The CSF usually show a modest mononuclear pleocytosis (≤100 cells/µL)) and mildly elevated protein; the IgG index may be increased and oligoclonal bands may be present. Diffuse slowing or bitemporal slow waves and spikes are sometimes seen on EEG. MRI may reveal abnormal signal intensity in the medial temporal lobes (**Figure 5-25**).

Other, especially treatable, disorders (eg, herpes simplex virus encephalitis) should be excluded. Korsakoff syndrome should be considered because patients with cancer are susceptible to nutritional deficiency, and thiamine administration may prevent worsening.

Acute treatment is with methylprednisolone (1 g intravenously daily for 3-5 days, then weekly for 6-8 weeks), intravenous immunoglobulin (0.4 g/kg intravenously daily for 3-5 days, then weekly for 6-8 weeks), or plasma exchange. Chronic treatment for patients who respond acutely includes tapering intravenous or oral corticosteroids over 4-6 months, oral azathioprine or mycophenolate mofetil, or intravenous rituximab. Treatment of any underlying malignancy may also have a beneficial effect on autoimmune limbic encephalitis. The response to treatment depends partly on the antigen against which autoimmunity is directed, with cell-surface antigens affording a better prognosis.

Headache & Facial Pain

6

Table 6-1. Causes of Headache and Facial Pain.

Acute onset
Common causes
Subarachnoid hemorrhage
Other cerebrovascular diseases
Meningitis or encephalitis
Ophthalmic disorders (glaucoma, acute iritis)
Less common causes
Seizures
Lumbar puncture
Hypertensive encephalopathy
Coitus
Subacute onset
Giant cell (temporal) arteritis
Intracranial mass (tumor, subdural hematoma, abscess)
Pseudotumor cerebri (idiopathic intracranial hypertension)
Trigeminal neuralgia (tic douloureux)
Glossopharyngeal neuralgia
Postherpetic neuralgia
Persistent idiopathic facial pain
Chronic
Migraine
Medication overuse headache
Cluster headache and trigeminal autonomic cephalalgias
Tension-type headache
Icepick-like pain
Cervical spine disease
Sinusitis
Dental disease

Headache occurs in all age groups and accounts for 1% to 2% of emergency department evaluations and up to 4% of medical office visits; the causes are myriad (**Table 6-1**). Although most often a benign condition (especially when chronic and recurrent), headache of new onset may be the earliest or the principal manifestation of serious systemic or intracranial disease and therefore requires thorough and systematic evaluation.

An etiologic diagnosis of headache is based on understanding the pathophysiology of head pain; obtaining a history, with characterization of the pain as acute, subacute, or chronic; performing a careful physical examination; and formulating a differential diagnosis.

▼ APPROACH TO DIAGNOSIS

PATHOPHYSIOLOGY OF HEADACHE & FACIAL PAIN

PAIN-SENSITIVE STRUCTURES

Headache is caused by traction, displacement, inflammation, or distention of the pain-sensitive structures in the head or neck. Isolated involvement of the bony skull, most

of the dura, or most regions of brain parenchyma does not produce pain.

A. Pain-Sensitive Structures Within the Cranial Vault

These include the venous sinuses (eg, sagittal sinus); anterior and middle meningeal arteries; dura at the base of the skull; trigeminal (V), glossopharyngeal (IX), and vagus (X) nerves; proximal portions of the internal carotid artery and its branches near the circle of Willis; brainstem periaqueductal gray matter; and sensory nuclei of the thalamus.

B. Extracranial Pain-Sensitive Structures

These include periosteum of the skull; skin; subcutaneous tissues, muscles, and arteries; neck muscles; second (C2) and third (C3) cervical nerves; eyes, ears, teeth, sinuses, and oropharynx; and mucous membranes of the nasal cavity.

RADIATION OR PROJECTION OF PAIN

A. The **trigeminal (V) nerve** carries sensation from intracranial structures in the anterior and middle fossae of the skull (above the cerebellar tentorium). Discrete intracranial lesions in these locations can produce pain that radiates in the trigeminal nerve distribution (**Figure 6-1**).

B. The **glossopharyngeal (IX) and vagus (X) nerves** convey sensation from part of the posterior fossa; pain originating in this area may also be referred to the ear or throat, as in glossopharyngeal neuralgia.

C. The **upper cervical (C2-C3) nerves** transmit stimuli from infratentorial and cervical structures; therefore, pain from posterior fossa lesions often projects to the second and third cervical dermatomes (see Figure 6-1).

HISTORY

CLASSIFICATION & APPROACH TO THE DIFFERENTIAL DIAGNOSIS

A. Acute Headache & Facial Pain

Headaches that are new in onset or clearly different from any the patient has experienced previously are commonly a symptom of serious illness and demand prompt evaluation. The sudden onset of "the worst headache I've ever had in my life" (classically due to subarachnoid hemorrhage), neck and facial pain (cervical arterial dissection), diffuse headache with neck stiffness and fever (meningitis), and head pain centered about one eye (acute glaucoma) are striking examples. Acute headaches may also accompany more benign processes such as systemic viral infections or other febrile illnesses.

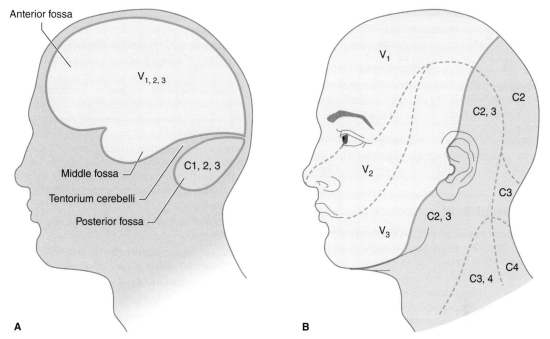

▲ **Figure 6-1.** Innervation of pain-sensitive intracranial compartments (**A**) and corresponding extracranial sites of pain radiation (**B**). The trigeminal (V) nerve, especially its ophthalmic (V1) division, innervates the anterior and middle cranial fossae; lesions in these areas can produce frontal headache. The upper cervical nerve roots (especially C2) innervate the posterior fossa; lesions here can cause occipital headache.

B. Subacute Headache & Facial Pain

Subacute headaches are those that persist or recur over weeks to months. Such headaches may also signify serious medical disorders, especially when the pain is progressive or when it occurs in elderly patients. Patients with subacute headache should be asked about recent head trauma (subdural hematoma or postconcussive syndrome); malaise, fever, or neck stiffness (subacute meningitis); focal neurologic abnormalities or weight loss (primary or metastatic brain tumor); visual changes (giant cell arteritis, idiopathic intracranial hypertension); or medications predisposing to headache (nitrates).

C. Chronic Headache & Facial Pain

Headaches that have recurred over years (eg, migraine or tension-type headaches) usually have a benign cause, although each acute attack may be profoundly disabling. When treating these patients, it is important to determine whether the present headache is similar to those suffered previously or is new—and thus represents a different process.

PRECIPITATING FACTORS

Precipitating factors can provide a guide to the cause of chronic headache. Such factors include: dental surgery; acute exacerbation of chronic sinusitis or hay fever; systemic

viral infection; psychologic tension, emotional stress, or fatigue; menses; hunger; fasting; consumption of ice cream or foods containing nitrite (hot dogs, salami, ham, and most sausage), phenylethylamine (chocolate), or tyramine (cheddar cheese); and exposure to bright lights. Precipitation of headache by alcohol is especially typical of cluster headache. Chewing and eating commonly trigger pain associated with glossopharyngeal neuralgia and tic douloureux; jaw claudication is associated with giant cell arteritis or temporomandibular joint dysfunction. Oral contraceptive agents and nitrates may precipitate or exacerbate migraine. Headache may also be provoked by coughing or sneezing, especially in patients with structural lesions in the posterior fossa. Posttraumatic headaches begin within a week of head trauma and are most often migrainous in nature.

PRODROMAL SYMPTOMS (AURAS)

Prodromal symptoms or auras, such as scintillating scotomas or other visual changes, often occur with migraine; they may also occur in patients with seizure disorders and postictal headaches.

CHARACTERISTICS OF PAIN

Headache or facial pain may be described in a variety of ways. **Pulsating or throbbing** pain is characteristic of migraine. A steady sensation of **tightness or pressure** is commonly seen with tension-type headache. Neck discomfort may occur in migraine due to the convergence of trigeminal and cervical pain pathways within the brainstem. The pain produced by intracranial mass lesions is typically **dull and steady. Sharp, lancinating** (stabbing) pain suggests a neuritic cause such as trigeminal neuralgia. **Icepick-like** pain may be described also by patients with migraine, cluster headache, or giant cell arteritis.

Headache of virtually any description can occur in patients with migraine or brain tumors; therefore, the character of the pain alone does not provide a reliable etiologic guide.

LOCATION OF PAIN

A. **Unilateral** headache is an invariable feature of cluster headache and occurs in the majority of migraine attacks; most patients with tension-type headache report bilateral pain.

B. **Ocular** or **retro-orbital** pain suggests a primary ophthalmic disorder such as acute iritis or glaucoma, optic (II) nerve disease (eg, optic neuritis), or retro-orbital inflammation (eg, Tolosa–Hunt syndrome). It is also common in migraine or cluster headache.

C. **Paranasal** pain localized to one or several sinuses, often associated with tenderness of the overlying periosteum and skin, occurs with acute sinus infection or outlet obstruction.

D. **Focal** headache may result from intracranial mass lesions, but even in such cases it is replaced by bioccipital and bifrontal pain when the intracranial pressure becomes elevated.

E. **Bandlike** or **occipital** discomfort is commonly associated with tension-type headache. Occipital localization can also occur with meningeal irritation from infection or hemorrhage and with disorders of the joints, muscles, or ligaments of the upper cervical spine.

F. Pain within the **first (V1) division of the trigeminal nerve**, characteristically described as burning in quality, is a common feature of postherpetic neuralgia.

G. Lancinating pain localized to the **second (V2)** or **third (V3) division of the trigeminal (V) nerve** suggests trigeminal neuralgia (tic douloureux).

H. The **pharynx** and **external auditory meatus** are the most frequent sites of pain caused by glossopharyngeal neuralgia.

ASSOCIATED SYMPTOMS

Manifestations of underlying systemic disease can aid in the etiologic diagnosis of headache and should always be sought.

A. **Recent weight loss** may accompany cancer, giant cell arteritis, or depression.

B. **Fever** or **chills** may indicate systemic infection or meningitis.

C. **Dyspnea** or other symptoms of heart disease raise the possibility of subacute infective endocarditis and resultant brain abscess.

D. **Visual disturbances** suggest an ocular disorder (eg, glaucoma), migraine, or an intracranial process involving the optic nerve (optic neuritis) or tract or central visual pathways.

E. **Nausea** and **vomiting** are common in migraine and posttraumatic headache and can also be seen with intracranial mass lesions. Some patients with migraine report that diarrhea or other gastrointestinal symptoms accompany attacks.

F. **Photophobia** may be prominent in migraine, acute meningitis, or subarachnoid hemorrhage.

G. **Myalgias** often accompany tension-type headache, systemic viral infections, and giant cell arteritis.

H. **Ipsilateral rhinorrhea** and **lacrimation** during attacks typify cluster headache.

I. **Transient loss of consciousness** may be seen in both migraine (basilar migraine) and glossopharyngeal neuralgia (due to cardiac syncope; Chapter 12, Seizures & Syncope).

OTHER FEATURES OF HEADACHE

A. Temporal Pattern of Headache

Headaches from mass lesions are commonly increased by bending over, as are sinus headaches. Headaches from mass lesions, however, increase in severity over time. Cluster headaches frequently awaken patients from sleep; they often recur at the same time each day or night. Tension-type headaches can develop whenever stressful situations occur and are often maximal at the end of a workday. Migraine headaches are episodic and may be worse during menses (**Figure 6-2**).

B. Conditions Relieving Headache

Migraine headaches are frequently relieved by darkness, sleep, vomiting, or pressing on the ipsilateral temporal artery, and their frequency may diminish during pregnancy. Post-lumbar-puncture and low-pressure headaches are typically relieved by recumbency, whereas headaches caused by intracranial mass lesions may be less severe with the patient standing.

C. Conditions Exacerbating Headache

Discomfort exacerbated by rapid changes in head position such as bending over or by events that transiently raise intracranial pressure, such as coughing and sneezing, is often associated with an intracranial mass but can also occur in migraine. Anger, excitement, or irritation can

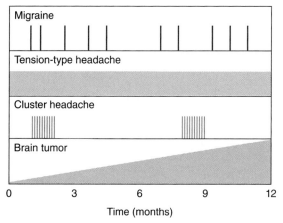

▲ **Figure 6-2.** Temporal patterns of headache. Migraine headache is episodic and may occur at varying intervals. Tension-type headache may be present every day. Cluster headache occurs in bouts separated by symptom-free periods. Headache caused by brain tumor often increases in severity with time.

precipitate or worsen both migraine and tension-type headaches. Stooping, bending forward, sneezing, or blowing the nose characteristically worsens the pain of sinusitis. **Postural headache** (maximal when upright, nearly absent when lying down) occurs with low cerebrospinal fluid (CSF) pressure caused by lumbar puncture, head injury, or spontaneous spinal fluid leak. Fluctuations in intensity and duration of the headache with no obvious cause, especially when associated with similar fluctuations in mental status, are seen with subdural hematoma.

D. History of Headache

The characteristics of the present headache should be compared with those of previous occurrences, because headache with features different from those previously experienced calls for especially careful investigation.

PHYSICAL EXAMINATION

A general physical examination is mandatory, because headache is a nonspecific accompaniment of many systemic disorders. If possible, the patient should be observed during an episode of headache or facial pain.

VITAL SIGNS

A. Temperature

Although fever suggests a viral syndrome, meningitis, encephalitis, or brain abscess, headache from these causes can also occur without fever. Moreover, headache can accompany many systemic infections.

B. Pulse

Tachycardia can occur in a tense, anxious patient with a tension-type headache or accompany any severe pain. Paroxysmal headache associated with tachycardia and perspiration is characteristic of pheochromocytoma.

C. Blood Pressure

Hypertension per se rarely causes headache unless the blood pressure elevation is acute, as with pheochromocytoma, or very high, as with hypertensive encephalopathy. Chronic hypertension, however, is the major risk factor for hemorrhagic or ischemic stroke, which can be associated with acute headache. Subarachnoid hemorrhage is commonly followed by marked acute elevation of blood pressure.

D. Respiration

Hypercapnia from respiratory insufficiency of any cause can elevate intracranial pressure and produce headache.

GENERAL PHYSICAL EXAMINATION

A. Weight Loss

Weight loss or cachexia in a patient with headache suggests cancer or chronic infection. Polymyalgia rheumatica and giant cell arteritis can also be accompanied by weight loss.

B. Skin

Focal inflammation (cellulitis) of the face or overlying the skull indicates local infection, which may be the source of intracranial abscess or cause venous sinus thrombosis. Cutaneous abnormalities elsewhere may suggest vasculitis (including that from meningococcemia), endocarditis, or cancer. The neurofibromas or café-au-lait spots of von Recklinghausen disease (neurofibromatosis) may be associated with benign or malignant intracranial tumors that can produce headache. Cutaneous angiomas sometimes accompany arteriovenous malformations (AVMs) of the central nervous system, which may be associated with chronic headache—or acute headache if they bleed. Herpes zoster that affects the face and head most often involves the eye and the skin around the periorbital tissue, causing facial pain.

C. Scalp, Face, & Head

Scalp tenderness is characteristic of migraine headache, subdural hematoma, giant cell arteritis, and postherpetic neuralgia. Nodularity, erythema, or tenderness over the temporal artery suggests giant cell arteritis. Localized tenderness of the superficial temporal artery also accompanies acute migraine. Recent head trauma or a mass lesion can cause a localized area of tenderness. Trauma causes characteristic ecchymosis (see Figure 1-4).

Paget disease, myeloma, or metastatic cancer of the skull may produce head pain that is boring in quality and associated with skull tenderness. In Paget disease, arteriovenous shunting within bone may make the scalp feel warm.

Disorders of the eyes, ears, or teeth may cause headache. Tooth percussion may reveal periodontal abscess. Sinus tenderness may indicate sinusitis. A bruit over the orbit or skull suggests an intracranial AVM, carotid artery-cavernous sinus fistula, aneurysm, or meningioma. Lacerations of the tongue raise the possibility of postictal headache. Ipsilateral conjunctival injection, lacrimation, Horner syndrome (see Chapter 7, Neuro-Ophthalmic Disorders), and rhinorrhea occur with cluster headache. Temporomandibular joint disease is accompanied by local tenderness and crepitus over the joint. Jaw claudication is characteristic of temporal arteritis.

D. Neck

Cervical muscle spasm occurs with tension-type and migraine headaches, cervical spine injuries, cervical arthritis, or meningitis. Carotid bruits may be associated with cerebrovascular disease.

Meningeal signs must be sought carefully, especially if headache is of recent onset. Meningeal irritation causes **nuchal** (neck) **rigidity** mainly in the anteroposterior direction, whereas cervical spine disorders restrict movement in all directions. Discomfort or hip and knee flexion during neck flexion (**Brudzinski sign**) indicates meningeal irritation (see Figure 1-5). Meningeal signs may be absent or difficult to demonstrate in the early stages of subacute (eg, tuberculous) meningitis, in the first few hours after subarachnoid hemorrhage, and in comatose patients.

E. Heart & Lungs

Brain abscess may be associated with congenital heart disease, which may be evidenced by heart murmur or cyanosis. Lung abscess may also be a source of brain abscess.

NEUROLOGIC EXAMINATION

A. Mental Status Examination

During the mental status examination, patients with acute headache may be confused, as is commonly seen with subarachnoid hemorrhage and meningitis. Headache with symptoms of dementia may be indicative of intracranial tumor, particularly one in the frontal lobe or infiltrating across the corpus callosum.

B. Cranial Nerve Examination

Cranial nerve abnormalities can suggest and localize an intracranial tumor or other mass lesion. **Papilledema**, the hallmark of increased intracranial pressure, may be seen with space-occupying intracranial lesions, carotid

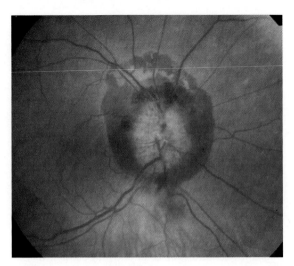

▲ **Figure 6-3.** Disc edema and a large peripapillary subhyaloid hemorrhage in the right eye of a patient with aneurysmal rupture and subarachnoid hemorrhage. (Used with permission from Biousse V, Newman NJ. *Neuro-Ophthalmology Illustrated.* 2nd ed. New York, NY: Thieme; 2016; 571. Copyright © 2016 Thieme Medical Publishers, Inc.)

artery-cavernous sinus fistula, pseudotumor cerebri, or hypertensive encephalopathy. Superficial retinal hemorrhages (**subhyaloid hemorrhages**) are characteristic of subarachnoid hemorrhage in adults (**Figure 6-3**). Ischemic retinopathy may be found in patients with vasculitis.

Progressive oculomotor (III) nerve palsy, especially when it causes pupillary dilatation, may be the presenting sign of an expanding posterior communicating artery aneurysm; alternatively, it may reflect increasing intracranial pressure and incipient brain herniation. Decreased pupillary reactivity to light occurs in optic neuritis. Extraocular muscle palsies occur in Tolosa–Hunt syndrome (see Chapter 7, Neuro-Ophthalmic Disorders). Proptosis suggests an orbital mass lesion or carotid artery-cavernous sinus fistula.

Decreased sensation over the site of facial pain—most commonly the first (V1) division of the trigeminal (V) nerve—is found in postherpetic neuralgia. Trigger areas on the face and pharynx suggest trigeminal and glossopharyngeal neuralgia, respectively.

C. Motor Examination

Asymmetric motor function or gait ataxia in a patient with a history of subacute headache demands complete evaluation to exclude intracranial mass lesions.

D. Sensory Examination

Focal or segmental sensory impairment or diminished corneal sensation (corneal reflex) is strong evidence against a benign cause of pain.

ACUTE HEADACHE

Sudden onset of a new headache may be a symptom of serious intracranial or systemic disease; it must be investigated promptly and thoroughly.

SUBARACHNOID HEMORRHAGE

Spontaneous (nontraumatic) subarachnoid hemorrhage (bleeding into the subarachnoid space) is usually the result of a ruptured cerebral arterial aneurysm or an AVM.

Rupture of a **saccular (berry) aneurysm** accounts for approximately 75% of cases of subarachnoid hemorrhage, with an annual incidence of 6 per 100,000. Most arise sporadically, but some are familial. Families with two or more affected persons should have all members screened. Both autosomal and recessive patterns of inheritance occur.

Rupture occurs most often during the fifth and sixth decades; sex distribution is approximately equal. The risk of rupture of an intracranial aneurysm varies with the patient's age and the site and size of the aneurysm; approximately 5% of autopsied individuals have cerebral aneurysms, and most have never experienced symptoms. Hypertension has not been conclusively demonstrated to predispose to the development of aneurysms, but acute elevation of blood pressure (eg, at orgasm) may be responsible for aneurysm rupture.

Fusiform aneurysms result from circumferential dilation of a cerebral arterial trunk. In contrast to saccular aneurysms, they are thought to be caused by atherosclerosis or dissection, affect the vertebrobasilar system preferentially, and can present with symptoms of ischemia or mass effect, in addition to rupture.

Intracranial AVMs, a less frequent cause of subarachnoid hemorrhage (10%), occur twice as often in men as in women, and usually bleed in the second to fourth decades, although a significant incidence extends into the sixties. Blood in the subarachnoid space can also result from intracerebral hemorrhage, embolic stroke, and trauma.

PATHOLOGY

Cerebral arterial aneurysms are usually congenital and result from developmental weakness of the vessel wall, especially at sites of branching. They typically arise from intracranial arteries about the circle of Willis at the base of the brain (**Figure 6-4**), occur in 2% of patients, and are multiple in approximately 20% of cases. Other congenital abnormalities, such as polycystic kidney disease or coarctation of the aorta, may be associated with berry aneurysms.

Occasionally, systemic infections such as infective endocarditis disseminate to a cerebral artery and cause aneurysm formation; such **mycotic aneurysms** account for 2% to 3% of aneurysmal ruptures. Mycotic aneurysms are

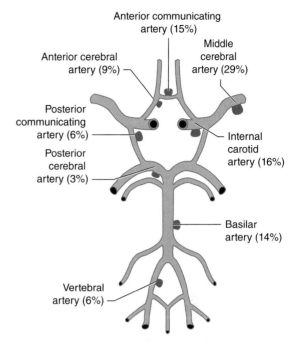

▲ **Figure 6-4.** Frequency distribution of intracranial aneurysms.

usually more distal along the course of cerebral arteries than are berry aneurysms.

AVMs consist of abnormal vascular communications that permit arterial blood to enter the venous system without passing through a capillary bed. They are most common in the middle cerebral artery distribution.

PATHOPHYSIOLOGY

Rupture of an intracranial artery elevates intracranial pressure and distorts pain-sensitive structures, producing headache. Intracranial pressure may reach systemic perfusion pressure and acutely decrease cerebral blood flow; together with the concussive effect of the rupture, this is thought to cause the loss of consciousness that occurs at the onset in approximately 50% of patients. Rapid elevation of intracranial pressure can also produce subhyaloid retinal hemorrhages (see Figure 6-3).

CLINICAL FINDINGS

A. Symptoms & Signs

The classic (but not invariable) presentation of subarachnoid hemorrhage is with the sudden onset of an unusually severe generalized headache, classically described as the worst headache the patient has ever experienced. However, among patients presenting with the abrupt onset of an unusually severe headache, only 8% to 10% will have subarachnoid hemorrhage (see also reversible cerebral vasoconstriction syndrome characterized by recurrent thunderclap headache in Chapter 13). Abrupt onset to maximal intensity is the essential feature of subarachnoid hemorrhage headache. The absence of headache essentially excludes the diagnosis. One-third of patients present with headache alone. In the remainder, loss of consciousness is frequent at onset, as are vomiting and neck stiffness. Symptoms may begin at any time of day and during either rest or exertion.

The most significant feature of the headache is that it is new. Milder but otherwise similar headache (**sentinel headache**) may have occurred in the weeks prior to the acute event and probably represent small prodromal hemorrhages or aneurysmal stretch.

The headache is not always severe, especially if hemorrhage is from a ruptured AVM rather than an aneurysm. Although the duration of the hemorrhage is brief, the intensity of the headache may remain unchanged for several days and may subside slowly over approximately 2 weeks. Recurrence of the headache usually signifies **rebleeding**.

Blood pressure frequently rises precipitously as a result of the hemorrhage. Meningeal irritation may induce temperature elevations up to 39°C (102.2°F) during the first 2 weeks. There is frequently associated confusion, stupor, or coma. Nuchal rigidity and other evidence of meningeal irritation (see Figure 1-5) are common, but may not occur

for several hours after the onset of headache. Preretinal globular subhyaloid hemorrhages (found in 20%-40% of cases; see Figure 6-3) are most suggestive of the diagnosis.

With aneurysmal rupture, bleeding occurs mainly in the subarachnoid space rather than within brain parenchyma. Therefore, prominent focal neurologic signs are uncommon, and even when present, they may bear no relationship to the site of the aneurysm. An exception is oculomotor (III) nerve palsy from compression of the nerve ipsilateral to a posterior communicating artery aneurysm. Bilateral extensor plantar responses and abducens (VI) nerve palsy are frequent nonlocalizing signs that result from increased intracranial pressure.

Ruptured AVMs tend to occur within brain tissue and accordingly produce focal neurologic signs, such as hemiparesis, aphasia, or visual field defects.

B. Laboratory Findings

Patients presenting with subarachnoid hemorrhage are investigated first by computed tomography (CT) scanning (**Figure 6-5**), which confirms the hemorrhage in more than 90% of patients with aneurysmal rupture and can help identify a focal source. The test is most sensitive in the first six hours after bleeding occurs, when sensitivity approaches 100%. Complications, including intracerebral

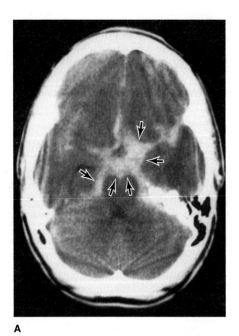
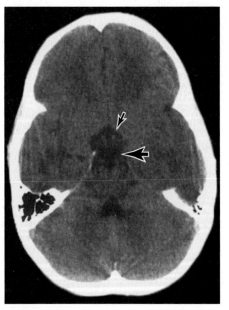

A   B

▲ **Figure 6-5.** (**A**) Nonenhanced brain CT scan from a patient with an acute aneurysmal subarachnoid hemorrhage. Areas of high density (arrows) represent blood in the subarachnoid space at the base of the brain (most aneurysms occur in this region about the circle of Willis; see Figure 6-4). (Used with permission from H. Yonas.) (**B**) A normal nonenhanced brain CT scan of the same region. Interpeduncular cistern, large arrow; suprasellar cistern, small arrow. (Used with permission from C. Jungreis.)

or intraventricular extension of blood, hydrocephalus, and infarction, can also be identified. Aneurysms themselves may not be evident on CT, but most AVMs can be seen after administration of contrast material. Magnetic resonance imaging (MRI) is especially useful for detecting small AVMs in the brainstem, which are poorly seen on CT scan.

In patients with a normal neurologic examination, a normal CT scan within 6 hours of symptom onset is held by many authorities to exclude subarachnoid hemorrhage. CT scans that are technically inadequate or delayed, or that otherwise fail to confirm the diagnosis of subarachnoid hemorrhage, necessitate lumbar puncture (see Chapter 2, Investigative Studies). The CSF in subarachnoid hemorrhage usually has a markedly elevated opening pressure and is grossly bloody, containing 100,000 to >1 million/μL red blood cells. As heme from these cells is degraded, first (by heme oxygenase) to the green pigment, biliverdin, and then (by biliverdin reductase) to the yellow pigment, bilirubin, the supernatant of the centrifuged CSF becomes yellow-tinged (**xanthochromic**) within 12 hours after hemorrhage. The pigment can be detected spectrophotometrically. White blood cells are initially present in the CSF in the same proportion to red cells as in the peripheral blood. However, **chemical meningitis** caused by blood in the subarachnoid space may produce a pleocytosis of several thousand white blood cells during the first 48 hours and a reduction in CSF glucose 4 to 8 days after hemorrhage. In the absence of pleocytosis, CSF glucose after subarachnoid hemorrhage is normal. The peripheral white blood cell count is often modestly elevated but rarely exceeds 15,000/μL.

The electrocardiogram (ECG) may reveal a host of abnormalities, including peaked or deeply inverted T waves, a short PR interval, or tall U waves.

Once the diagnosis of subarachnoid hemorrhage is confirmed by CT or lumbar puncture, four-vessel cerebral arteriography is undertaken. Both the carotid and vertebral arteries should be studied to visualize the entire cerebral vascular anatomy, as multiple aneurysms occur in 20% of patients and AVMs are frequently supplied from multiple vessels. Angiography should be performed at the earliest convenient time, and is a prerequisite to the rational planning of surgical treatment. It is therefore not necessary for patients who are not surgical candidates, such as those who are deeply comatose. CT and magnetic resonance angiography do not yet have the resolution needed to replace conventional catheter angiography.

DIFFERENTIAL DIAGNOSIS

The sudden onset of severe headache, with confusion or obtundation, nuchal rigidity, absence of focal neurologic deficits, and bloody spinal fluid is highly specific for subarachnoid hemorrhage.

Other disorders can also produce obtundation and bloody spinal fluid, but are distinguished by additional findings, such as prominent focal neurologic deficits (hypertensive intracerebral hemorrhage) or signs of endocarditis (ruptured mycotic aneurysm) or a presenting history of head trauma.

Traumatic lumbar puncture can be excluded as the cause of bloody CSF by comparing red blood cell counts in the first and last tubes of CSF obtained and by examination of the centrifuged CSF specimen. Blood clears as fluid is removed after a traumatic tap, but not after subarachnoid hemorrhage. Because blood introduced by traumatic lumbar puncture does not have time to undergo enzymatic breakdown to bilirubin, centrifugation of the specimen reveals a colorless supernatant.

Bacterial meningitis is excluded by the presence of blood in the CSF or on CT scan.

COMPLICATIONS & SEQUELAE

A. Recurrence of Hemorrhage

Recurrence of aneurysmal hemorrhage occurs in approximately 20% of patients over 10 to 14 days. It is the major acute complication and roughly doubles the mortality rate. Acute recurrence of hemorrhage from AVM is less common.

B. Intraparenchymal Extension of Hemorrhage

Although hemorrhages from an AVM commonly involve the brain parenchyma, this is far less common with aneurysmal hemorrhage. However, rupture of an aneurysm of the anterior cerebral or middle cerebral artery may direct a jet of blood into the brain with resultant intracerebral hematoma producing hemiparesis, aphasia, and sometimes transtentorial herniation.

C. Arterial Vasospasm

Delayed arterial narrowing (**vasospasm**) occurs in vessels surrounded by subarachnoid blood and is associated with ischemic neurologic deficits in more than one-third of cases. Clinical ischemia typically does not appear before day 4 after the hemorrhage, peaks at day 7 to 8, and then resolves spontaneously. The diagnosis can be confirmed by transcranial Doppler or cerebral angiography (see Chapter 2, Investigative Studies). The severity of vasospasm is related to the amount of subarachnoid blood, and vasospasm is less common when less blood is present, such as after traumatic subarachnoid hemorrhage or rupture of an AVM. Vasospasm appears to be only one element in the genesis of delayed ischemic neurologic deficits following subarachnoid hemorrhage, as one-third of patients with delayed ischemia clinically do not have demonstrable vasospasm.

D. Acute or Subacute Hydrocephalus

Acute or subacute hydrocephalus may develop during the first three days—or after several weeks—as a result of impaired CSF absorption in the subarachnoid space. Progressive somnolence, nonfocal findings, and impaired upgaze due to downward pressure on the midbrain should suggest the diagnosis.

E. Seizures

Seizures occur in fewer than 10% of cases and only after damage to the cerebral cortex. Decorticate or decerebrate posturing is common acutely and may be mistaken for seizures.

F. Other Complications

Although inappropriate secretion of antidiuretic hormone and resultant diabetes insipidus can occur, they are uncommon.

TREATMENT

A. Medical Treatment

Medical treatment is directed toward preventing elevation of arterial or intracranial pressure that might re-rupture the aneurysm or AVM. Typical measures include absolute bed rest with the head of the bed elevated 15 to 20 degrees, mild sedation, and analgesics for headache (antiplatelet drugs should be avoided). Because patients who are hypertensive on admission have increased mortality, reducing blood pressure (to approximately 160/100 mm Hg) is prudent, but bed rest and mild sedation are often adequate in this regard.

Fever is common and worsens outcome. Induced normothermia is essential (infusion of 4° C NaCl is suggested). Hypotension should be prevented to ensure adequate cerebral perfusion, but intravenous fluids should be isosmotic (normal saline) and should be administered with care, as overhydration can exacerbate cerebral swelling. Hyponatremia is frequently seen and should be managed by oral administration of NaCl, or intravenous 3% normal saline, rather than by fluid restriction.

Following definitive surgical treatment of the ruptured aneurysm and in the absence of other aneurysms, vasospasm can be treated by induced hypertension with phenylephrine or dopamine. The calcium channel antagonist nimodipine, 60 mg orally (or by nasogastric tube) every 4 hours for 21 days, reduces delayed ischemic neurologic deficits in patients with a ruptured aneurysm through neuroprotective mechanisms rather than by a direct effect on vasospasm. Seizures are uncommon after aneurysmal rupture, but the hypertension accompanying an acute seizure increases the risk of re-rupture. Accordingly, prophylactic administration of an anticonvulsant (eg, phenytoin, 300 mg/d) is recommended in the perioperative period and then is discontinued following definite treatment.

B. Surgical Treatment

1. **Aneurysm**—Definitive surgical therapy of a **ruptured aneurysm** consists of clipping the neck of the aneurysm or endovascular placement of a coil to induce clotting.

    The neurologic examination is used to grade the patient's surgical candidacy (**Table 6-2**). In patients who are fully alert (Hunt and Hess grades I and II) or only mildly confused (grade III), surgery has been shown to improve the clinical outcome. In contrast, stuporous (grade IV) or comatose (grade V) patients do not appear to benefit.

    As rebleeding is maximal within the first 24 hours following aneurysmal rupture, early surgical intervention is indicated. This approach reduces the period at risk for rebleeding and permits aggressive treatment of vasospasm with volume expansion and pharmacologic elevation of blood pressure.

    Treatment of associated **unruptured aneurysms** is individualized. Surgery is favored by young age, previous rupture, family history of aneurysmal rupture, observed aneurysm growth, and low operative risk. Decreased life expectancy and asymptomatic small (<7-mm diameter) aneurysms favor conservative management.

2. **AVM**—Surgically accessible AVMs may be removed by en-bloc resection or obliterated by ligation of feeding vessels or by embolization with a local intra-arterial catheter. Because the risk of an early second hemorrhage

Table 6-2. Clinical Grading of Patients With Aneurysmal Subarachnoid Hemorrhage.

Grade	Level of Consciousness	Associated Clinical Features	Surgical Candidate
I	Normal	None or mild headache and stiff neck	Yes
II	Normal	Moderate headache and stiff neck; minimal neurologic deficit (eg, cranial nerve palsy) in some cases	Yes
III	Confusional state	Focal neurologic deficits in some cases	Yes
IV	Stupor	Focal neurologic deficits in some cases	No
V	Coma	Decerebrate posturing in some cases	No

is much less with AVMs than with aneurysms, surgical treatment can be undertaken electively at a convenient time after the bleeding episode.

PROGNOSIS

The mortality rate from aneurysmal subarachnoid hemorrhage is high. Approximately 20% of patients die before reaching a hospital, 25% die subsequently from the initial hemorrhage or its complications, and 20% die from rebleeding prior to surgical correction. Most deaths occur in the first few days after the hemorrhage.

The probability of survival after aneurysmal rupture is related to the patient's state of consciousness and the time elapsed since rupture. On day 1, the probability of survival is 60% for symptom-free and 30% for somnolent patients; at 1 month, these groups have survival probabilities of 90% and 60%, respectively. Among survivors of aneurysmal subarachnoid hemorrhage, approximately one-half have permanent brain injury.

Nearly 90% of patients recover after subarachnoid hemorrhage from ruptured AVM. Although recurrent hemorrhage remains a danger, conservative management compares favorably with surgery.

OTHER CEREBROVASCULAR DISORDERS

INTRACEREBRAL HEMORRHAGE

Intracerebral hemorrhage commonly presents with headache, vomiting, altered consciousness, and focal neurologic deficits. Headache in this setting results from compression of pain-sensitive structures by the hematoma. The most common cause of nontraumatic intracerebral hemorrhage is hypertension, but AVMs and bleeding into tumors can present in a similar manner. The CT scan shows a hematoma, which is usually located in the basal ganglia, thalamus, cerebellum, pons, or subcortical white matter. Intracerebral hemorrhage is discussed in more detail in Chapter 13, Stroke.

CEREBRAL ISCHEMIA

Headache occurs at onset of stroke or TIA in one-third of patients and may persist for hours to several days. The association of headache is independent of stroke etiology (thrombotic, embolic, lacunar), stroke severity, or hypertension. Headache is more common with younger age, female gender, cerebellar location, and a history of migraine.

Headaches associated with **ischemic stroke** are typically mild to moderate in intensity, and nonthrobbing in character. Their location is determined by the pain projection sites of the involved arteries and is most often, but not invariably, ipsilateral to the ischemic hemisphere. Carotid lesions usually produce frontal (trigeminal distribution) pain, whereas posterior fossa strokes usually present with occipital headache. Headache accompanying **retinal artery embolism** or **posterior cerebral artery spasm or occlusion** may be erroneously diagnosed as migraine because of the associated visual impairment.

Headache also occurs as part of the cerebral hyperperfusion syndrome after **carotid endarterectomy** and may be associated with hypertension, focal sensory or motor signs, seizures, and altered consciousness. This syndrome occurs on the second or third postoperative day and typically produces intense throbbing anterior headache on the operated side, often associated with nausea. The cause is thought to be impaired autoregulation of cerebral blood flow.

Headache associated with cerebral infarction may require analgesics for symptomatic relief.

Cerebral ischemia is discussed in more detail in Chapter 13, Stroke.

MENINGITIS OR ENCEPHALITIS

Patients with infection of the meningeal covering of the brain (meningitis) present with a combination of new headache (87%), neck stiffness (83%), fever (77%), and altered mental state (69%). Infection involving brain parenchyma (encephalitis) presents similarly with headache (81%), fever (90%), and altered consciousness (97%), but seizures are frequent (67% in encephalitis while only 5% in meningitis).

Headache is a prominent feature of inflammation of the brain (encephalitis) or its meningeal coverings (meningitis) caused by bacterial, viral, or other infections, as well as granulomatous processes, neoplasms, or chemical irritants. The pain is caused by inflammation of intracranial pain-sensitive structures, including blood vessels at the base of the brain.

The headache is commonly throbbing in character, bilateral, and occipital or nuchal in location. Its severity is increased by sitting upright, moving the head, compressing the jugular vein, or performing other maneuvers (eg, sneezing, coughing) that transiently increase intracranial pressure. Photophobia may be prominent. The headache rarely presents suddenly, developing instead over hours to days.

Neck stiffness and other signs of meningeal irritation (see Figure 1-5) must be sought with care, as they may not be obvious early in the course or in encephalitis. Fever and lethargy or confusion are often, but not always, prominent features.

Mental status abnormalities accompany most cases of bacterial but few cases of aseptic meningitis. Changes may evolve rapidly and vary in severity from mild confusion to coma. Their duration at presentation is less than 24 hours in about 50% of cases of bacterial meningitis. The clinical and laboratory findings in bacterial meningitis are summarized in Table 4-8.

The diagnosis of bacterial meningitis is suggested by a CSF examination that shows an increased white blood cell count (**pleocytosis**) and low glucose concentration (**hypoglycorrhachia**) (see Table 4-9). Bacterial, syphilitic, tuberculous, viral, fungal, and parasitic infections may be distinguished by CSF glucose, Gram stain, acid-fast stain, India ink preparation, cryptococcal antibody assays, Venereal Disease Research Laboratory (VDRL), and cultures (see Table 4-5). Treatment of meningitis and encephalitis is discussed in detail in Chapter 4, Confusional States.

BRAIN ABSCESS

Encapsulated pus from contiguous or hematogenous sources produces an expanding mass resulting in headache, change in mental status, focal neurologic defects, and fever. Seizures are the presenting event in 20% to 25% of cases. Headache is a frequent presentation (see Table 3-7) but the classic triad of headache with fever and focal neurologic signs occurs in less than 20%. Progression is rapid with a mean interval of 8.3 days between symptom onset and hospital admission. MRI and CT scanning differentiate abscess from primary or metastatic cancers. Etiology, clinical findings, evaluation, and treatment are discussed in Chapter 3, Coma.

OTHER CAUSES OF ACUTE HEADACHE

SEIZURES

Preictal, ictal, and postictal headaches occur but only the latter are common; they are associated most often with generalized tonic-clonic seizures but also occur following seizures of simple and complex partial phenomenology. Migrainous features (throbbing, nausea and vomiting, photophobia, phonophobia) are common and similar to patients' non-ictal headaches. It may be important to differentiate these headaches from those of subarachnoid hemorrhage or meningitis. If doubt exists about the cause, lumbar puncture can be undertaken: seizures may produce a mild CSF pleocytosis (up to approximately 10 cells/μL after single seizures or up to approximately 100 cells/μL after status epilepticus), but CSF glucose content is normal.

LUMBAR PUNCTURE

Post-lumbar-puncture headache is diagnosed by a history of a dural puncture (eg, spinal tap, spinal anesthesia) and is characteristically a **postural headache**, with marked increase in pain in the upright position and relief with recumbency. The pain is typically occipital, comes on within 48 to 72 hours after the procedure, and lasts 1 to 2 days. Nausea and vomiting may occur. Headache is caused by persistent leak of CSF from the spinal subarachnoid space, with resultant traction on pain-sensitive structures at the base of the brain.

The risk of this complication can be reduced by using a small-gauge needle (22 gauge or smaller) for the puncture. Lying flat afterward, for any length of time, does not lessen the risk.

Low-pressure headache syndromes are usually self-limited. When this is not the case, they may respond to the administration of caffeine sodium benzoate, 500 mg intravenously, which can be repeated after 45 minutes if headache persists or recurs upon standing. In persistent cases, the subarachnoid rent can be sealed by injection of autologous blood into the epidural space at the site of the puncture; this requires an experienced anesthesiologist.

Spontaneous intracranial hypotension can produce headache similar in character to that caused by lumbar puncture. T1-weighted, gadolinium-enhanced MRI may show smooth enhancement of the pachymeninges and a "sagging brain" (**Figure 6-6**); the enhancement may be confused with that associated with meningitis. Low CSF pressure can produce the same MRI picture in the absence of headache. Autologous blood patch injection may produce immediate relief.

HYPERTENSIVE ENCEPHALOPATHY

Headache may be due to a sudden elevation in blood pressure caused by pheochromocytoma, sexual intercourse, the combination of monoamine oxidase inhibitors and tyramine-containing foods such as cheddar cheese, or—the most important cause—malignant hypertension. Blood pressures of 250/150 mm Hg or higher—characteristic of malignant hypertension—produce cerebral edema and displace pain-sensitive structures. The induced pain is described as severe and throbbing. Other signs of diffuse or focal central nervous system dysfunction are also present, such as lethargy, hemiparesis, or focal seizures; on CT or MRI, posterior white matter changes may be seen (see Figure 4-21). Treatment is with antihypertensive drugs (see Chapter 4, Confusional States), but care must be taken to avoid hypotension, which can produce cerebral ischemia and cause stroke.

COITUS

Most coital headaches are benign. Men are more often affected than women. The pain may be either a dull, bilateral pain occurring during sexual excitement or a severe, sudden headache occurring at the time of orgasm, presumably caused by a marked increase in systemic blood pressure. Persistent headache after orgasm—worse in the upright posture—has also been described, is reminiscent of post-lumbar-puncture headache, and is associated with low opening pressures at lumbar puncture. Each of these headaches is benign and subsides over minutes to days.

Patients reporting severe headache in association with orgasm should be evaluated for possible subarachnoid hemorrhage (see earlier discussion). If no hemorrhage is

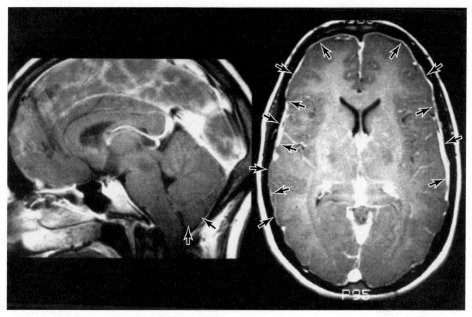

▲ **Figure 6-6.** Spontaneous intracranial hypotension in a 27-year-old woman presenting with severe postural headaches. Sagittal and axial T1-weighted images obtained after gadolinium injections show features of "sagging brain": downward displacement of the cerebellar tonsils into the foramen magnum (arrows, left image), effacement of the brainstem cisterns (left image; compare with normal sagittal MRI in Figure 2-6), and diffuse dural enhancement (arrows, right image). MRI abnormalities and symptoms reversed following an epidural blood patch. (Used with permission from H.A. Rowley.)

found, prophylactic treatment with indomethacin, 50 to 100 mg orally 30 to 60 minutes prior to intercourse, may be effective.

OPHTHALMIC DISORDERS

Pain about the eye may occur in migraine and cluster headache and is also the presenting feature of iritis and glaucoma. **Acute iritis** produces extreme eye pain with photophobia. The diagnosis is confirmed by slit lamp examination; acute management involves pharmacologic dilatation of the pupil. **Angle-closure glaucoma** produces pain within the globe that radiates to the forehead. When it occurs after middle age, such a pain syndrome should prompt diagnostic tonometry.

SUBACUTE HEADACHE

GIANT CELL ARTERITIS

Giant cell arteritis, also known as **temporal arteritis**, is a systemic vasculitis that affects medium-sized and large arteries, especially branches of the external carotid artery. It is characterized pathologically by subacute granulomatous inflammation (consisting of lymphocytes, neutrophils, and giant cells). Inflammation of the pain-sensitive arterial wall produces headache, and arterial stenosis leads to ischemia.

Giant cell arteritis affects Caucasians most often, women twice as frequently as men, and is uncommon before 60 years of age. It is frequently associated with malaise, myalgia, weight loss, arthralgia, and fever (**polymyalgia rheumatica** complex) due to periarticular inflammation. The most common symptom is a new, nonspecific headache, which can be unilateral or bilateral and is often fairly severe and boring in quality. It is characteristically localized to the scalp, especially over the temporal arteries. Scalp tenderness may be especially apparent when lying with the head on a pillow or brushing the hair. Pain or stiffness in the jaw during chewing (**jaw claudication**) is highly suggestive of giant cell arteritis and is due to arterial ischemia in the muscles of mastication (the tongue may also be affected). **Ocular involvement** can manifest as transient visual obscurations in one or both eyes lasting minutes to a few hours. Diplopia from ischemia to cranial nerves or extra ocular muscles may be a presenting feature. Anterior ischemic optic neuropathy, characterized by pallid disk edema in one or both eyes, results in permanent visual loss. Involvement of the **ophthalmic artery** may lead to sudden visual loss, as is discussed in Chapter 7, Neuro-Ophthalmic Disorders.

The erythrocyte sedimentation rate (ESR) is elevated, but not invariably. The mean Westergren ESR is approximately 100 mm/h in giant cell arteritis (range, 29-144 mm/h) and polymyalgia rheumatica (range, 58-160 mm/h); the normal upper limit of the Westergren ESR in elderly patients is reported to be as high as 40 mm/h. Elevated ESR, C-reactive protein level >2.45 mg/dL, and thrombocytosis (>400,000 platelets/µL) each make the diagnosis more likely.

The diagnosis is made by biopsy of an affected temporal artery, which is characteristically thickened, nonpulsatile, dilated, and tender. The arteries may be affected in a patchy manner, and serial sections may be necessary to demonstrate histologic vasculitis.

Possible giant cell arteritis requires prompt evaluation to avoid visual loss, but therapy should not be withheld pending biopsy diagnosis and should be continued despite negative biopsy findings if the diagnosis can be made with confidence on clinical grounds. Initial therapy is with prednisone 60 to 100 mg/d orally. The dose is decreased, usually after 1 to 2 months, depending on the clinical response. Alternatively, treatment can be started with intravenous methylprednisolone (500-1,000 mg every 12 hours for 2 days), with prednisone substituted thereafter. The sedimentation rate returns rapidly toward normal with prednisone therapy and must be maintained within normal limits as the drug dose is tapered over 1 to 2 years. Although dramatic improvement in headache may occur within 2 to 3 days after institution of therapy, associated blindness is usually irreversible.

INTRACRANIAL MASS

The new onset of headache in middle or late life should always raise concern about a mass lesion, such as a **brain tumor** (**Table 6-3**), **subdural hematoma**, or **brain abscess** (see Chapter 3, Coma), although mass lesions may or may not produce headache, depending on proximity to pain-sensitive intracranial structures or the ventricular system. Only about one-half of patients with brain tumor complain of headache (**Table 6-4**), although symptoms vary to some extent with tumor type and are more common with metastatic than primary brain tumors.

Headaches associated with brain tumors are most often nonspecific in character, mild to moderate in severity, dull and steady in nature, and intermittent. The pain is characteristically bifrontal, worse ipsilaterally, and aggravated by a change in position or by maneuvers that increase intracranial pressure, such as coughing, sneezing, and straining at stool. Headache is worse with bending over. Both tension or migraine type features may be found. Evidence of lateralized features on exam are most suggestive of a mass. The classic brain tumor headache (severe, early morning, and associated with nausea and vomiting) is uncommon; nausea and vomiting occur in less than half of brain tumor patients. The occurrence of headaches in brain tumor is

Table 6-3. Relative Incidence of Primary Central Nervous System Tumors.

Tumor Type	Incidence (%)
Meningioma	34.4
Glioblastoma	16.7
Pituitary	13.1
Nerve sheath[1]	8.6
Astrocytoma	7.0
Other neuroepithelial	5.1
Lymphoma	2.4
Oligodendroglioma	2.0
Ependymoma	1.8
Embryonal[2]	1.0
Craniopharyngioma	0.7
Germ cell tumor	0.5
Other	6.6

[1]Includes acoustic neuroma.
[2]Includes medulloblastoma.
Data for 2004-2007 from Central Brain Tumor Registry of the United States (www.cbtrus.org).

proportional to tumor size and midline shift. Subdural hematoma frequently presents with conspicuous headache, because its large size increases the likelihood of impinging upon pain-sensitive structures.

An uncommon type of headache that suggests brain tumor is characterized by a sudden onset of severe pain that reaches maximal intensity within seconds, persists for minutes to hours, and subsides rapidly. This may be associated with altered consciousness or "drop attacks." Although classically associated with **third ventricular colloid cysts**, these paroxysmal headaches can be produced by tumors at

Table 6-4. Symptoms of Brain Tumors.

Symptom	Percent With Symptom		
	Low-Grade Glioma	Malignant Glioma	Meningioma (Benign)
Headache	40	50	36
Seizure	65-95	15-25	40
Hemiparesis	5-15	30-50	22
Altered mental status	10	40-60	21

Data from De Angelis LM. Brain tumors. *N Engl J Med.* 2001; 344:114.

many different intracranial sites. Trigeminal autonomic cephalalgia type headaches (see below) may be the presenting feature of pituitary tumors.

Suspicion of an intracranial mass lesion demands prompt evaluation by CT scan or MRI. Brain tumor is excluded by a normal contrast-enhanced brain MRI scan. Tumor treatment depends on the histologic type (benign or malignant, primary or metastatic, pathologic grade), but may include surgical excision, radiation, and chemotherapy. Prognosis also varies with tumor characteristics, as well as age, biomarkers, and gene polymorphisms.

IDIOPATHIC INTRACRANIAL HYPERTENSION

Idiopathic intracranial hypertension (**pseudotumor cerebri**) is the result of a diffuse increase in intracranial pressure that can cause headache of diffuse but variable character, papilledema, pulsatile tinnitus, visual loss, and diplopia (from abducens [VI] nerve palsy). Impaired CSF absorption due to venous outflow obstruction may be involved in pathogenesis. Intracranial hypertension can also be symptomatic of a variety of disorders (**Table 6-5**), but these are less common than the idiopathic form.

Women are affected much more commonly than men, with a peak incidence in the third decade. Most patients are obese. Diffuse headache is almost always a presenting symptom. The headaches are daily in occurrence, pulsatile or pressing, moderate in intensity, and aggravated by coughing or straining. Transient (seconds-long) visual obscurations and visual blurring also occur in most cases. Visual acuity is normal in most patients at presentation, but moderate to severe papilledema is seen in almost all. Visual loss can develop from increased intracranial pressure, which leads to optic (II) nerve atrophy. Like visual loss from glaucoma, that due to idiopathic intracranial hypertension is characterized by gradually constricting visual fields with late loss of central acuity. Associated pulsatile tinnitus is common.

Table 6-5. Disorders Associated With Intracranial Hypertension.

Intracranial venous drainage obstruction (eg, venous sinus thrombosis, head trauma, polycythemia, thrombocytosis)

Endocrine dysfunction (eg, obesity, withdrawal from steroid therapy, Addison disease, hypoparathyroidism)

Vitamin and drug therapy (eg, hypervitaminosis A and 13 cis-retinoic acid in children and adolescents, tetracycline, minocycline, nalidixic acid)

Other (eg, chronic hypercapnia, severe right heart failure, chronic meningitis, hypertensive encephalopathy, severe iron deficiency anemia)

Idiopathic

Symptoms of idiopathic intracranial hypertension are generally self-limited over several months and papilledema may disappear, but CSF pressure remains elevated for years, and recurrent symptomatic episodes occur in 10%. Using MRI or CT brain scanning, lumbar puncture, and laboratory studies, idiopathic intracranial hypertension must be differentiated from intracerebral mass lesions and from the disorders listed in Table 6-5. Imaging studies may show small ("slit-like") ventricles and demonstrate an empty sella turcica in 70% of instances. The optic nerve sheath is characteristically dilated, and the back of the globe is flattened. Elevated intracranial pressure (CSF opening pressure >250 mm H_2O) is documented by lumbar puncture, and removal of 20 to 40 mL of CSF may transiently relieve headache. Cells, glucose, and protein content of the CSF are normal. However, it should be noted that obese individuals without idiopathic intracranial hypertension may have opening pressures as high as 250 mm H_2O.

If other causes (see Table 6-5) are identified, specific treatment should be given. Cerebral venous thrombosis must be excluded by imaging. Treatment of idiopathic cases is with acetazolamide (1000-1250 mg/d); topiramate may also be effective for headache treatment. Corticosteroids are effective, but have untoward side effects, and papilledema tends to rebound when they are discontinued. Obese patients should be encouraged to lose weight. In cases refractory to medical treatment, optic nerve sheath fenestration or lumboperitoneal or ventriculoperitoneal shunting may be needed to preserve vision and decrease headache.

TRIGEMINAL NEURALGIA

Trigeminal neuralgia (**tic douloureux**) is a facial pain syndrome that develops in middle to late life and is more common in women than men.

Pain is unilateral and typically confined to the area supplied by the second (V2) and third (V3) divisions of the trigeminal (V) nerve (**Figure 6-7**). Involvement of the first division or bilateral disease occurs in less than 5% of cases. Pain occurs as lightning-like, momentary (>1 second to approximately 2 minutes) jabs of excruciating pain that spontaneously abate, and attacks are stereotypic in a given patient. Occurrence during sleep is uncommon. Pain-free intervals may last for minutes to weeks, but long-term spontaneous remission is rare. Stimulation of trigger zones about the cheek, nose, or mouth by touch, cold, wind, talking, or chewing can precipitate the pain. In classical trigeminal neuralgia, physical examination discloses no abnormalities; trigeminal sensory deficits or abnormal trigeminal (eg, corneal or jaw jerk) reflexes exclude an idiopathic diagnosis. Rarely, similar pain may occur in multiple sclerosis or with brainstem tumors, which should be considered in young patients, in those with ophthalmic division pain, and in all patients who show neurologic described for trigeminal neuralgia, or more continuous and burning or aching in quality. Rarely, cardiac syncope due to bradyarrhythmia (Chapter 12, Seizures & Syncope) accompanies the pain. Trigger areas are usually around the tonsillar pillars, so symptoms are initiated by swallowing or talking. Paroxysms of pain can occur many times daily.

Women are affected more frequently than men. Symptoms begin at a somewhat younger age than in trigeminal neuralgia. The diagnosis is established by the history and by reproducing pain through stimulation of peritonsillar trigger zones. There are no abnormal neurologic signs. Bilateral symptoms, abnormal signs, or other atypical features should prompt a search for disorders that can mimic glossopharyngeal neuralgia, such as multiple sclerosis, cerebellopontine angle tumor, and nasopharyngeal carcinoma.

As in trigeminal neuralgia, conventional imaging techniques show no abnormalities, but high-resolution MRI techniques may reveal microvascular or space occupying lesions compressing the glossopharyngeal (IX) nerve.

Carbamazepine or phenytoin (as described earlier for trigeminal neuralgia) usually produces dramatic relief; microvascular decompression has been used in drug-resistant cases.

HERPETIC & POSTHERPETIC NEURALGIA

Varicella-zoster virus infection produces a febrile illness with a disseminated vesicular rash (chickenpox). After the primary infection, the virus remains dormant in sensory ganglia but may reactivate, particularly with age or immunosuppression, resulting in a unilateral vesicular eruption termed **shingles**. These eruptions, which occur in a dermatomal distribution (most commonly thoracic, 50%; ophthalmic distribution of the trigeminal nerve, 25%), are associated with sharp, lancinating, localized radicular pain with dysesthesia. In patients over 50, pain may persist beyond six weeks. This constitutes **postherpetic neuralgia**.

The syndrome does not occur before age 50 years and becomes increasingly common with advancing age, in immunocompromised patients, and in those with leukemia or lymphoma.

Postherpetic neuralgia is characterized by constant, severe, stabbing or burning, dysesthetic pain. In the head, the first division (V1) of the trigeminal (V) nerve is most commonly affected, so pain localized to the forehead on one side is usually the presenting feature (**Figure 6-8**). Scarring, resulting from healing of the vesicular rash, may be present in the distribution of pain. Careful testing of the painful area reveals decreased cutaneous sensitivity to pinprick. The other major complication of herpes zoster in the trigeminal distribution is decreased corneal sensation with impaired blink reflex, which can lead to corneal abrasion, scarring, and ultimately loss of vision.

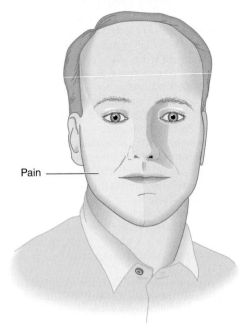
Pain

Figure 6-7. Distribution of symptoms in trigeminal neuralgia.

abnormalities on examination or who experience bilateral symptoms.

CT scan, conventional MRI, and arteriography are normal. Although high-resolution MRI techniques may show microvascular nerve compression, no standard technique has been identified to document symptomatic vascular compression.

Treatment with carbamazepine 400 to 1200 mg/d orally in three divided doses produces remission of pain within 24 hours in a high percentage of cases. Rarely, blood dyscrasia occurs as an adverse reaction to carbamazepine. Oxcarbazepine (600-1,800 mg/d in two divided doses) appears equally effective, without risk of blood dyscrasia. Intravenous administration of phenytoin 250 mg will abort an acute attack, and phenytoin 200 to 400 mg/d orally may be effective alone or in combination with carbamazepine if a second drug is necessary. Lamotrigine (400 mg/d) or baclofen (10 mg three times daily to 20 mg four times daily) can be used in refractory cases. Posterior fossa microvascular decompression surgery is used in patients who fail or cease to respond to drugs. The superior cerebellar artery is the most commonly implicated.

GLOSSOPHARYNGEAL NEURALGIA

Glossopharyngeal neuralgia is a rare syndrome mainly characterized by unilateral pain localized to the oropharynx, tonsillar pillars, base of the tongue, or auditory meatus. Pain may be paroxysmal, resembling that

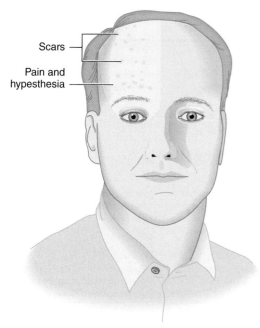

Scars

Pain and
hypesthesia

Figure 6-8. Distribution of symptoms and signs in postherpetic neuralgia.

The intensity and duration of the cutaneous eruption and the acute pain of herpes zoster can be reduced by acute treatment for 7 to 10 days with acyclovir (800 mg five times daily), famciclovir, or valacyclovir, but these treatments have not been shown to lessen the likelihood of postherpetic neuralgia, although the duration of the postherpetic pain may be attenuated. Corticosteroids (60 mg/d prednisone, orally for 2 weeks, with rapid tapering) taken during the acute herpetic eruption may reduce acute herpetic pain, but not the development of postherpetic neuralgia.

Once the postherpetic pain syndrome is established, the most useful treatment has been tricyclic antidepressants such as amitriptyline, 25 to 150 mg/d orally, which are thought to act directly on central nervous system pain-integration pathways, rather than via an antidepressant effect; nortriptyline or desipramine may be better tolerated. Tricyclic antidepressant drugs may be more effective when combined with a phenothiazine (perphenazine). The anticonvulsants gabapentin (1,800-3,600 mg/d) and pregabalin (600 mg/d) have shown some benefit.

Lidocaine-prilocaine (2.5% cream) or lidocaine (5% gel or cutaneous patch) is an effective topical therapy. Topical capsaicin (0.075% cream or 8% patch) can also be helpful, but may cause local skin irritation. Capsaicin acts as a transient receptor potential cation channel (TRPV1) antagonist to deplete pain-mediating peptides (substance P, calcitonin gene-related peptide) from peripheral sensory neurons. In otherwise intractable cases, weekly intrathecal administration of methylprednisolone may reduce pain.

PERSISTENT IDIOPATHIC FACIAL PAIN

Constant, boring, mainly unilateral, lower facial pain for which no cause can be found is referred to as persistent idiopathic or **atypical facial pain**. Unlike trigeminal neuralgia, it is not confined to the trigeminal nerve distribution and is not paroxysmal. Neurologic and neuroradiographic examinations are normal. This idiopathic disorder must be distinguished from similar pain syndromes related to nasopharyngeal carcinoma, intracranial extension of squamous cell carcinoma of the face, or infection at the site of a tooth extraction. Treatment is with amitriptyline 20 to 250 mg/d orally, alone or in combination with phenelzine 30 to 75 mg/d orally. Phenytoin can be an effective alternative, especially if a tricyclic antidepressant is poorly tolerated.

CHRONIC HEADACHE

MIGRAINE

Migraine is common (prevalence 12%) and is manifested by recurrent headache. The migraine attack begins with visual or other neurologic (usually sensory) symptoms in approximately 15% to 30% of patients (**migraine with aura**, or **classic migraine**), followed by the headache phase. In most cases, however, no aura occurs (**migraine without aura**, or **common migraine**). Before puberty, males and females are equally affected. After puberty, two-thirds to three-quarters of migraine cases occur in women. Onset is early in life—approximately 25% begin during the first decade, 55% by age 20, and more than 90% before age 40.

GENETICS

Although candidate genes remain uncertain, a family history of migraine in at least one first-degree relative is present in most cases, and twin studies demonstrate the involvement of both inheritance and environmental factors. For those with affected relatives, the risk of migraine is enhanced three times. Autosomal dominant inheritance occurs in several well-recognized migraine syndromes, including **familial hemiplegic migraine** and cerebral autosomal dominant arteriopathy with subcortical infarcts (**CADASIL**). Hemiplegic migraine also occurs in families. Mutations in genes encoding membrane ion channels have been implicated in this syndrome (**Table 6-6**).

STRUCTURAL FEATURES

Migraine is associated with an increase in MRI-detected white matter lesions, infarct-like lesions, and volumetric changes in cerebral gray and white matter. Women may be affected more frequently, as may patients with aura. No clear association with headache frequency is firmly established.

Table 6-6. Autosomal Dominant and Hereditary Disorders Associated With Migraine.

Gene	Protein	Disease	Features
CACNA1A	α$_1$ subunit of neuronal Ca$_v$2.1 (P/Q-type) voltage-gated calcium channel	Familial hemiplegic migraine (FHM1); (50% of identified families have CACNA1A mutations)	Hemiplegic migraine, cerebellar ataxia, seizures
ATP1A2	α$_2$ subunit of sodium-potassium pump	Familial hemiplegic migraine (FHM2); (20% of identified families have ATP1A2 mutations)	Hemiplegic migraine, seizures
SCN1A	α subunit of Na$_v$1.1 voltage-gated sodium channel	Familial hemiplegic migraine (FHM3)	Hemiplegic migraine, seizures
MTTL1	mtDNA A-to-G transition at nucleotide 3243	Mitochondrial encephalopathy with lactic acidosis and stroke-like episodes (MELAS)	Migraine, seizures, hemiparesis, hemianopsia, cortical blindness, and episodic vomiting
NOTCH3	Notch3 (transmembrane receptor)	Cerebral autosomal dominant arteriopathy with subcortical infarcts (CADASIL)	Migraine with aura, stroke, dementia
TREX1	3' repair exonuclease 1 (DNA repair enzyme)	Retinal vasculopathy with cerebral leukodystrophy (RVCL)	Migraine, blindness, stroke, dementia, Raynaud phenomenon, nephropathy, cirrhosis

The clinical significance of these MRI finding is uncertain; cognitive consequences have not been found.

PRECIPITATING FACTORS

In many patients, migraine attacks are heralded by prodromal fatigue or cognitive, affective, or gastrointestinal symptoms, which can last for up to 1 day. The basis for this **premonitory phase** is poorly understood, but it may reflect altered hypothalamic or brainstem functions. Migraine attacks can be precipitated by certain foods (tyramine-containing cheeses; meat, such as hot dogs or bacon, with nitrite preservatives; chocolate containing phenylethylamine but not chocolate alone) and by food additives such as monosodium glutamate, a commonly used flavor enhancer. Lifestyle issues such as fasting, emotion, menses, drugs (especially oral contraceptive agents and vasodilators such as nitroglycerin), weather changes, sleep disturbances, and bright lights may also trigger attacks.

PATHOGENESIS

Based on the efficacy of vasoconstrictive ergot alkaloids (eg, ergotamine) in aborting the acute migraine attack and of vasodilators such as amyl nitrite in abolishing the migraine aura, intracranial vasoconstriction and extracranial vasodilation were long held to be the respective causes of the aura and headache phases of migraine. However, more recent studies support cortical spreading depression as responsible for both the aura and headache (**Figure 6-9**). Resultant sensitization (increased neuronal responsiveness to painful and non-painful stimuli) results in many of the migrainous symptoms, including cutaneous allodynia (pain produced from an innocuous stimulus).

Functional MRI during migraine headache demonstrates cerebral blood flow changes in the dorsal pons and the cingulate, visual, and auditory cortices. These signals propagate with characteristics similar to cortical spreading depression. At the onset of the **aura phase** (occurring in up to 30% of patients), a decrease in cerebral blood flow in the occipital cortex spreads anteriorly across the cortex according to cytoarchitectural rather than vascular boundaries (see Figure 6-9). In this respect, and in its rate of propagation (2-5 mm/minute), it resembles the phenomenon of **spreading depression**, in which a slow wave of neuronal and glial depolarization decreases blood flow and inhibits neuronal activity in its wake. However, the areas of decreased blood flow do not correspond to the cortical regions responsible for a particular aura, the extent of decrease is insufficient to cause ischemic symptoms, blood flow may remain depressed after aura symptoms have resolved and headache has begun, and headache may begin during the aural phase as well. Inhibiting spreading depression can prevent the migraine aura (but not the subsequent headache). These findings suggest that changes in neuronal activity, rather than ischemia, produce the aura. However, what initiates spreading depression is poorly understood.

Two principal mechanisms have been proposed to explain the **headache phase**. According to one theory, pain is triggered peripherally in primary sensory trigeminal neurons innervating the meninges and blood vessels, perhaps as a result of sterile inflammation (see Figure 6-9). These neurons project to the nucleus caudalis in

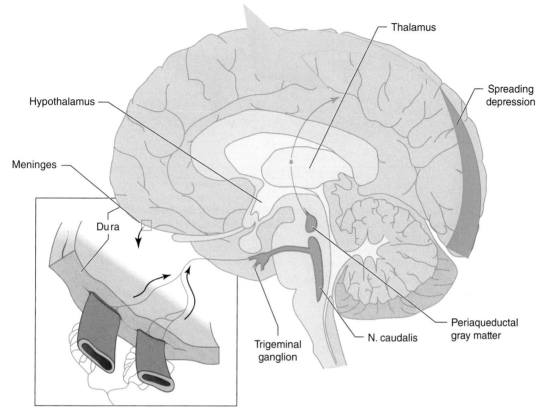

Figure 6-9. Central and peripheral nervous system sites proposed to be involved in migraine pathogenesis. During the aura phase, a reduction in cortical blood flow spreads anteriorly from the occipital cortex (large arrow), which is thought to be due to spreading depression. During the headache phase, sterile inflammation in the meninges may activate trigeminal (V) nerve sensory fibers that project to the nucleus caudalis, periaqueductal gray, sensory thalamic nuclei, and primary somatosensory cortex (small arrows). Alternatively, this central sensory pathway may convey normal afferent signals that are interpreted as noxious.

the brainstem, and from there to the periaqueductal gray, sensory thalamic nuclei, and somatosensory cortex. Another theory holds that a primary disturbance of central pain pathways produces sensitization, so that normally innocuous sensory input is misinterpreted as signaling pain, a phenomenon termed **allodynia.**

CLINICAL FINDINGS

A. Migraine With Aura (Classic Migraine)

In 30% of migraine patients, headache is preceded by transient neurologic symptoms (aura) lasting less than one hour. Auras may be visual, sensory (affecting limb, face, or tongue), vertebrobasilar, or motor. The most common auras are visual alterations, particularly hemianopic field defects and scotomas (blind spots) and scintillations (flickerings) that enlarge and spread peripherally (**Figure 6-10**).

A throbbing unilateral headache ensues (**Figure 6-11**). The frequency of headache varies, but more than 50% of patients experience no more than one attack per week. The duration of episodes is greater than 2 hours and less than 1 day in most patients. Remissions are common during the second and third trimesters of pregnancy and after menopause.

Although hemicranial pain is a hallmark of classic migraine, headaches can also be bilateral or occipital in location—characteristics commonly attributed to tension-type headache, which likely represents trigeminal and upper cervical afferent pathways converging in the brainstem.

During the headache, prominent associated symptoms include nausea, vomiting, photophobia, phonophobia, irritability, osmophobia, and lassitude. Vasomotor and autonomic symptoms are also common. Lightheadedness, vertigo, impaired hearing, diplopia, dysarthria, tinnitus,

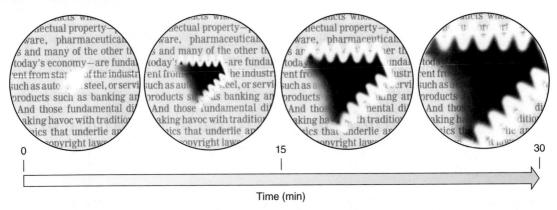

▲ **Figure 6-10.** Successive maps of scintillating scotoma (blind spot) to show the evolution of fortification figures (jagged edges) and associated scotoma in a patient with classic migraine. As the fortification moves laterally, a region of transient blindness remains.

ataxia, or altered consciousness may occur with **basilar migraine**. Migrainous aura occasionally produces neurologic deficits that persist into or beyond the pain phase (eg, **hemiplegic migraine**) and may rarely cause stroke. Motor manifestations of migraine can be distinguished from stroke by both the gradual onset ("migrainous march") and spontaneous resolution of symptoms.

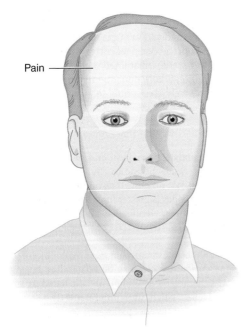

Pain

▲ **Figure 6-11.** Distribution of pain in migraine. Hemicranial pain (the pattern shown) is most common, but the pain can also be holocephalic, bifrontal, or unilateral frontal in distribution or, less commonly, localized to the occiput or the vertex of the skull.

Especially after 50 years of age, the aura may occur without headache (late-life **migraine equivalents**). Symptoms include visual disturbance, hemiparesis, hemisensory loss, dysarthria, or aphasia and usually last for 15 to 60 minutes (the gradual, non-stroke-like, "migrainous march" of sensory–motor symptoms is diagnostically helpful).

Other migraine subtypes include retinal migraine (headache with monocular scotoma), vestibular migraine, and menstrual migraine.

B. Migraine Without Aura (Common Migraine)

Migraine without aura is much more common than migraine with aura and produces headache that is most often unilateral in location, pulsating in quality, and moderate to severe in intensity. Nausea, vomiting, photophobia, and phonophobia are common. As the pain persists, associated cervical muscle contraction can compound the symptoms. Scalp tenderness is often present during the episode. If untreated, headache usually persists for 4 to 72 hours and is occasionally terminated by vomiting. In both common and classic migraine, compressing the ipsilateral carotid or superficial temporal artery during headache may reduce its severity.

C. Chronic (Transformed) Migraine and Medication Overuse Headache

Episodic migraine can change its clinical features over months to years, evolving into a chronic headache syndrome with nearly daily pain. The headache often loses its classic migrainous features. Obesity, prior headache frequency, and caffeine use are associated risk factors. A common subgroup of chronic migraine is that of headache from medication overuse.

Overuse of medications used to treat migraine or other forms of headache can lead to a chronic daily headache. Most patients have migraine as their underlying problem and have overused simple analgesics or triptans, but patients with other types of headache and those using other classes of drugs are also susceptible. Most patients are women. Headache is characteristically present at least 15 days per month for at least 3 months. Treatment involves tapering or withdrawal of the offending medications and beginning prophylactic therapy (see Table 6-8). Corticosteroids may be useful for "bridge therapy" to attenuate exacerbation of headache by drug withdrawal.

THE MIGRAINE POSTDROME

Following cessation of a migraine episode, migraine symptoms may reoccur with sudden head movement. A feeling of exhaustion (or rarely elation/euphoria) also may also be experienced.

TREATMENT

Tables 6-7 and **6-8** summarize treatment options in migraine. Addressing lifestyle issues pertaining to regularity of habits can be helpful (see precipitating factors). Pharmacologic treatment can be divided into measures used to abort attacks in progress (abortive) and to prevent future episodes (prophylactic).

Acute migraine attacks often respond to simple analgesics or, if these are ineffective, to migraine-specific therapies: serotonin 5-HT$_{1B/D}$ receptor agonists (triptans) or ergot alkaloids (eg, dihydroergotamine). A new class of antimigraine drugs—calcitonin gene-related peptide receptor antagonists (eg, telcagepant, olcegepant, and CGRP monoclonal antibodies)—may prove to be useful for this purpose. Drugs for acute (abortive) treatment (Table 6-7) must be taken at the onset of symptoms to be maximally effective. Rapidly absorbed parenteral formulations are superior to oral preparations. Nausea, a prominent feature of migraine, is also a common side effect of some antimigraine drugs, so that administration by other than the oral route or concomitant administration of an antiemetic (Table 6-7) may be necessary. Ergot alkaloids and triptans are felt by many to be contraindicated in patients with hypertension or other cardiovascular disease but the mechanism of action of these drugs is not via vasoconstriction.

Prophylactic treatment should be used in patients with two or more headaches per week or those in whom abortive treatment is inadequate. Tricyclic antidepressants, β-blockers, anticonvulsants, and calcium channel blockers can be tried in that order, unless concurrent illnesses or medications dictate differently (see Table 6-8). Chronic migraine (greater than 15 days/month), unresponsive to pharmacotherapeutics, has been treated, in specialized centers, with botulinum toxin injections.

For migraine during **pregnancy**, women can expect a decrease in headache frequency in the second and third trimesters and a return to prepregnancy frequency after delivery. For acute headache treatment, acetaminophen is safe for mild to moderate pain. More severe headaches can be treated with narcotic analgesics; sumatriptan appears safe even in the first trimester. Prochlorperazine (oral or suppository) is safe for both nausea and headache. See **Table 6-9** for recommended agents. Other antimigraine drugs may be teratogenic or cause complications in pregnancy.

CLUSTER HEADACHE & TRIGEMINAL AUTONOMIC CEPHALALGIAS (TACs)

CLINICAL FINDINGS

Cluster headache presents as repetitive episodes (clusters) of brief (15-180 minutes), very severe, unilateral, constant, nonthrobbing headaches. Episodes may be precipitated by alcohol or vasodilating drugs, especially if used during a cluster siege. The headache may begin as a burning sensation over the lateral aspect of the nose or as pressure behind the eye (**Figure 6-12**). The headache is associated with ipsilateral conjunctival injection, lacrimation, nasal stuffiness, or Horner syndrome (**Figure 6-13**).

Cluster headaches are always unilateral and usually recur on the same side in a given patient. They occur most often at night, awakening the patient from sleep; patients may pace restlessly during attacks. Headaches are recurrent (daily to multiple times daily), occurring often at nearly the same time of day (circadian periodicity) and for a cluster period of weeks to a few months; seasonal recurrences also occur. Between clusters, the patient may be free from headaches for months or years. The cause is unknown, but functional MRI during attacks has shown posterior inferior hypothalamic gray matter activation homolateral to the headache.

Cluster headache occurs much more frequently in men than in women (3:1) and typically begins at a somewhat later age than migraine (mean onset at 25 years). There is occasionally a family history.

TREATMENT

At the onset of a headache cluster, treatment involves measures both to abort the acute attack and to prevent subsequent ones.

A. Acute Treatment

Prompt relief of pain is achieved by inhalation of 100% oxygen (7-12 L/min for 15-20 minutes) or subcutaneous administration of sumatriptan (6 mg, repeated once per attack if necessary) (see Table 6-7). Alternative abortive treatments include intranasal sumatriptan, zolmitriptan, or lidocaine; subcutaneous octreotide; intravenous, intramuscular, subcutaneous, or intranasal dihydroergotamine; and oral zolmitriptan.

Table 6-7. Acute (Abortive) Treatment of Migraine Headache.

Drug	Route[1]	Strength	Recommended Dose	Comments
Simple analgesics (limited to 14 days/month)				
Aspirin	PO	325 mg	650 mg q4h	May cause gastric pain or bleeding
Naproxen sodium	PO	250, 375, 500 mg	500-1,000 mg at onset, then 250-500 prn after 1 hour	
Ibuprofen	PO	200, 400, 600, 800 mg	800-1,200 mg at onset, then 600-800 mg q4-8h	
Ketoprofen	PO	25, 50, 75, 100, 150, 200 mg	75-150 mg q6h	
Acetaminophen	PO PR	325, 500 mg	650-1,000 mg at onset, then q4h	Acetaminophen/isometheptene/dichloralphenazone is marketed as Midrin.
Combination analgesics (limited to nine days per month)				
Midrin	PO	Two capsules followed by one every four hours as needed, max five in twelve hours		Acetaminophen/dichloralphenazone/isometheptene
Excedrin	PO	Two capsules, repeat every six hours as needed, max eight in twenty-four hours		Acetaminophen/aspirin/caffeine
(If analgesics ineffective, switch to migraine-specific agents for next headache)				
Triptans				
Sumatriptan**	NS PO SC	20 mg/spray 25, 50, 100 mg 6 mg	20 mg 50-100 mg 6 mg	May repeat once after 2 hours for partial response. May cause nausea and vomiting; contraindicated in pregnancy, coronary or peripheral vascular disease, concurrent treatment with monoamine oxidase inhibitors, and possibly hemiplegic or basilar migraine. Common side effects: chest tightness, extremity paresthesias
Rizatriptan*	PO	5, 10 mg	10 mg	
Zolmitriptan**	PO NS	2.5, 5 mg 5 mg/spray	2.5-5 mg 5 mg	
Almotriptan**	PO	6.25, 12.5 mg	6.25-12.5 mg	*Onset of effect 30 minutes
Eletriptan*	PO	20, 40 mg	40 mg	**Onset of effect 45-60 minutes
Frovatriptan***	PO	2.5 mg	2.5 mg	*** Require 4 hours for effect but are long acting
Naratriptan***	PO	1, 2.5 mg	2.5 mg	Triptan response rate 60-80%. Faster-acting triptans have more frequent headache recurrence which can be attenuated by NSAID co-administration.
Ergot alkaloids (not to be combined with triptans)				
Ergotamine/caffeine (Cafergot)	PR	2 mg/100 mg	1/4-2 suppositories, up to 5 per week	May cause nausea and vomiting; contraindicated in pregnancy and coronary or peripheral vascular disease
Dihydroergotamine (DHE)	NS	0.5 mg/spray	1 spray to each nostril, up to 5 times per week	Repeat after 15 minutes. May cause nausea and vomiting; contraindicated in pregnancy and coronary or peripheral vascular disease
	SC	1 mg/mL	1-2 mg	Repeat 1 mg q12h, up to 6 mg
	IV		0.75-1.25 mg IV	

(Continued)

Table 6-7. Acute (Abortive) Treatment of Migraine Headache. (*Continued*)

Drug	Route[1]	Strength	Recommended Dose	Comments
Narcotic analgesics (associated with increased frequency of migraine episodes; should be avoided)				
Codeine/aspirin	PO	15, 30, 60/325 mg	30-120 mg codeine	
Meperidine	PO, IM	50, 100 mg	50-200 mg	
Butorphanol	NS	10 mg/mL (1 mg/spray)	1 spray every 3-4 hours as needed	
Antiemetics				
Prochlorperazine	PO	5, 10, 15 mg	25 mg q6h	Adjunctive treatment to reduce nausea and improve enteric absorption of antimigraine drugs. Extrapyramidal side effects may occur.
	PR	2.5, 5, 25 mg	25 mg q12h	
	IM, IV	5 mg/mL	10 mg (with 10 mg diphenhydramine)	
Chlorpromazine	IM	25 mg/mL	50 mg	
	IV	25 mg/mL	0.1 mg/kg drip over 20 minutes	
Promethazine	PO, PR	12.5, 25, 50 mg	25-50 mg q6h	
Metoclopramide	PO	5, 10 mg	5-20 mg tid	

[1]bid, twice daily; hs, at bedtime; IM, intramuscular; IV, intravenous; NS, nasal spray; PO, oral; PR, rectal; prn, as needed; q, every; qd, every day; qod, every other day; SC, subcutaneous; tid, three times daily.

Table 6-8. Prophylactic Treatment of Migraine Headache (Slow Titration Attenuates Side Effects).

Drug	Route[1]	Strength	Recommended Dose	Comments
Anti-inflammatory agents				
Aspirin	PO	325 mg	325 mg qod	May cause gastric pain or bleeding
Naproxen sodium	PO	275, 550 mg	550-825 mg bid	Sumatriptan and naproxen more effective than either alone (combined in Treximet)
Antidepressants				
Amitriptyline	PO	10, 25, 50, 75, 100, 150 mg	10-300 mg hs	May cause dry mouth or urinary retention. Begin with lowest dose and increase slowly. Adding an anticonvulsant may increase efficacy.
Nortriptyline	PO	10, 25, 50, 75 mg	10-150 mg hs	
Desipramine	PO	10, 25, 50, 75, 100 mg	25-300 mg qhs	
Protriptyline	PO	5, 10 mg	15-40 md/d in 3-4 doses	Protriptyline is less sedating than other tricyclics but dry mouth, and constipation may be problematic.
Venlafaxine	PO	25, 37.5, 50, 75 mg	75-150 mg daily	A serotonin-norepinephrine reuptake inhibitor

(*Continued*)

Table 6-8. Prophylactic Treatment of Migraine Headache (Slow Titration Attenuates Side Effects). (*Continued*)

Drug	Route[1]	Strength	Recommended Dose	Comments
β-Receptor antagonists				
Propranolol*	PO PO (long acting)	10, 20, 40, 60, 80, 90 mg 60, 80, 120, 160 mg	20-120 mg bid 60-320 mg qd	Listed in descending order of efficacy. Adverse effects include fatigue and exacerbation of depression. Symptomatic bradycardia may occur at high doses. Contraindicated in asthma and congestive heart failure and in patients on calcium channel blockers. To discontinue, taper over 1-2 weeks. *Most effective
Timolol*	PO	10, 20 mg	10-30 mg qd	
Metoprolol*	PO	50, 100 mg	100-200 mg qd	
Nadolol	PO	40, 80, 120, 160 mg	40-240 mg qd	
Atenolol	PO	50, 100 mg	50-200 mg qd	
Anticonvulsants				
Valproic acid	PO	125, 250, 500 mg; 500 mg extended release	250-500 mg bid or 1,000 mg qhs as single dose with extended release	Begin with lowest dose. Contraindicated in women of childbearing age
Topiramate	PO	25, 50, 100, 200 mg	25-200 mg qd	Start 25 mg hs and increase by 25 mg/d every 7 days as tolerated. Optimal dose 100 mg/d. Paresthesias in 50%. Altered mental state may require lowering dose. Rare: nephrolithiasis, angle-closure glaucoma
Gabapentin	PO	100, 300, 400, 600, 800 mg	1800-2,400 mg qd	Less effective than other anticonvulsants. Sedating
Calcium channel antagonists				
Verapamil	PO	40, 80, 120 mg	80-160 mg tid	Contraindicated by severe left ventricular dysfunction, hypotension, sick sinus syndrome without artificial pacemaker, and second- or third-degree AV nodal block and in patients on β-blockers. Constipation is most common side effect. Verapamil is ineffective in migraine without aura.
Flunarizine	PO (long acting) PO	240 mg 5, 10 mg	240 mg qd-bid 5-15 mg/day	
Other agents[2]				
Riboflavin (vitamin B2)	PO	Various	400 mg/d	May require 4-8 weeks for onset and increased effect over 3-6 months. Urine turns dark.
Onabotulinum toxin A	IM	100 units/vial	100-250 units	Not effective in episodic but very effective in chronic migraine. Injected into head and neck muscles
Candesartan	PO	4, 8, 16, 32 mg	16 mg daily (in one dose)	Fatigue, dizziness; teratogenic. Hypotension (an angiotensin II inhibitor)

[1]bid, twice daily; hs, at bedtime; IM, intramuscular; IV, intravenous; NS, nasal spray; PO, oral; PR, rectal; prn, as needed; q, every; qd, every day; qod, every other day; SC, subcutaneous; tid, three times daily.
[2]Other agents reported as effective include magnesium 200-1200 mg/d, coenzyme Q10 150 mg tid, feverfew 6.25 mg tid, butterbur 75 mg bid, and memantine 5-20 mg tid.

Table 6-9. Migraine Treatment in Pregnancy and Lactation.

Acute (abortive) treatment of migraine headache
Acetaminophen
Sumatriptan
Meperidine
Nausea
Ondansetron
Headache and nausea
Prochlorperazine oral or suppository
Prophylactic treatment of migraine headache
Propranolol
Memantine
Cyproheptadine (not during lactation)
During lactation
Sumatriptan
Ibuprofen
Diclofenac

B. Maintenance Prophylaxis

Several drugs used in the treatment of migraine (see Table 6-8) are also useful for preventing recurrent

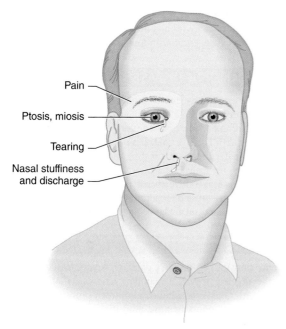

▲ **Figure 6-12.** Distribution of symptoms and signs in cluster headache.

Labels on figure: Pain — Ptosis, miosis — Tearing — Nasal stuffiness and discharge

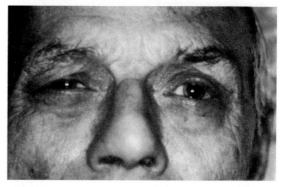

▲ **Figure 6-13.** Ptosis of the right eye during acute cluster headache. Other components of Horner syndrome (pupillary miosis and regional anhidrosis) may also occur.

symptoms during an active bout of cluster headache (maintenance prophylaxis). The most widely used drug is verapamil (80 mg three times daily or sustained-release 240 mg/d; doses of 720 mg/d may be required). Anticonvulsants such as valproic acid (500-2,000 mg/d), gabapentin (300-3,600 mg/d), and topiramate (50-200 mg/d) (often used in combination with verapamil) are second-line agents. Melatonin (10 mg/d) can also be helpful. Botulinum toxin is not effective. Drugs used for maintenance prophylaxis are discontinued at the end of the cluster.

C. Transitional Prophylaxis

Administration of prednisone at the beginning of a cluster cycle can be abortive, when given as 40 to 80 mg/d orally for 1 week, and then discontinued by tapering the dose over the following week. Intravenous methylprednisolone or dihydroergotamine may be useful as well.

D. Cluster Headache Variants

Chronic rather than episodic cluster headaches may occur. **Hypnic headache,** a bilateral nocturnal syndrome, lacks the autonomic components of cluster headache and occurs in the elderly. Suppressive therapy includes lithium or indomethacin. **Paroxysmal hemicrania** headaches occur in groups with daily attacks of 2-3 minutes and respond dramatically to indomethacin 25 to 50 mg three times daily.

    Hemicrania continua describes continuous pain with exacerbations of hours to days. It is also indomethacin responsive. A syndrome of hemicrania continua (continual pain with exacerbations) has been described as a presenting feature of **pituitary tumors**. Further, short-lasting, unilateral syndromes with conjunctival injection and tearing occur (attacks of 1-600 seconds); they respond to lamotrigine or topiramate.

E. Invasive Treatment

Invasive treatments are reserved for patients who fail to respond to medications; these include greater occipital nerve block, radiofrequency trigeminal ganglion ablation, or trigeminal rhizotomy.

TENSION-TYPE HEADACHE

Tension-type headache is the term used to describe chronic or recurrent headache of unapparent cause that lacks features of migraine or other headache syndromes. The underlying pathophysiologic mechanism is unknown, and "tension" is unlikely to be primarily responsible. Contraction of neck and scalp muscles has not been demonstrated by electromyography and, if present, is probably a secondary phenomenon.

In its classic form (**Figure 6-14**), tension-type headache is a chronic disorder that begins after age 20 years. It is characterized by attacks of nonthrobbing, bilateral occipital head pain that is not associated with nausea, vomiting, or prodromal visual disturbance. Headache duration is from hours to days. The pain is sometimes likened to a tight band around the head.

Women are more commonly affected than men. Although tension-type headache and migraine have been traditionally considered distinct disorders, many patients have headaches that exhibit features of both. Thus, occasional patients who are classified as having tension-type headaches experience throbbing headaches, unilateral head pain, or nausea with attacks. In consequence, it may be more

accurate to view tension-type headache and migraine as representing opposite poles of a single clinical spectrum.

Drugs used in the treatment of tension-type headache include some of the same agents used for migraine (see Tables 6-7 and 6-8). Acute attacks may respond to aspirin, other nonsteroidal anti-inflammatory drugs, or acetaminophen. Tension-type headache in migraineurs may respond to triptans. For prophylactic treatment, amitriptyline, nortriptyline, or imipramine is often effective. Trials of botulinum toxin mostly show that it is unhelpful. Massage, physical therapy, and relaxation techniques can provide additional benefit in selected cases.

ICEPICK-LIKE PAIN

Very brief, sharp, severe pain located in the scalp, occurring mainly in the V1 trigeminal distribution (Figure 6-1), is called "icepick-like pain." Women are more commonly affected. Paroxysms of pain are single or repetitive or occur in clusters, either at a single point or scattered over the scalp. Pain is experienced as an electric-like jab that reaches maximal intensity in less than 1 second, resolves rapidly, and is severe enough to cause involuntary flinching. Icepick-like pain is more common in those with migraine or cluster headache, but may occur in individuals who are otherwise headache-free. Patients frequently seek medical attention because of the intensity of the pain. If the bouts of pain are recurrent, treatment may be indicated. The syndrome responds to indomethacin (25-50 mg three times daily); gabapentin (400 mg twice daily) and melatonin (3-12 mg at bedtime) have also been reported as effective. Lancinating exacerbations of highly localized regional (mainly parietal) oval areas of pain are termed **nummular headaches**. Treatment is with gabapentin or indomethacin.

CERVICAL SPINE DISEASE

Injury or degenerative disease processes involving the upper neck can produce pain in the occiput or orbital regions. The most important source of discomfort is irritation of the second cervical (C2) nerve root. Disk disease or abnormalities of the articular processes affecting the lower cervical spine refer pain to the ipsilateral arm or shoulder, not to the head, although cervical muscle spasm may occur. Acute pain of cervical origin is treated with immobilization of the neck (eg, with a soft collar) and analgesic or anti-inflammatory drugs.

SINUSITIS

Acute sinusitis can produce pain and tenderness localized to the affected frontal or maxillary sinuses. Inflammation in the ethmoidal or sphenoidal sinuses produces a deep midline pain behind the nose. Sinusitis pain is increased by bending forward and by coughing or sneezing. Percussion over the frontal or maxillary area produces tenderness and accentuation of pain.

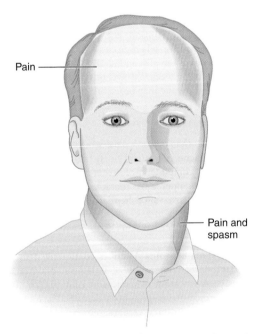

Pain

Pain and spasm

▲ **Figure 6-14.** Distribution of symptoms and signs in tension-type headache.

Sinusitis is treated with vasoconstrictor nose drops (eg, phenylephrine, 0.25%, instilled every 2-3 hours), antihistamines, and antibiotics. In refractory cases, surgical sinus drainage may be necessary.

Patients who complain of chronic "sinus" headache rarely have recurrent inflammation of the sinuses; they are much more likely to have a primary headache syndrome.

DENTAL DISEASE

Temporomandibular joint dysfunction is a poorly defined syndrome characterized by preauricular facial pain, limitation of jaw movement, tenderness of the muscles of mastication, and "clicking" of the jaw with movement. Symptoms are often associated with malocclusion, bruxism, or clenching of the teeth and may result from spasm of the masticatory muscles. Some patients benefit from local application of heat, jaw exercises, nocturnal use of a bite guard, or nonsteroidal anti-inflammatory drugs.

Infected tooth extraction sites can also give rise to pain, which is characteristically constant, unilateral, and aching or burning in character. Acute dental pain rarely crosses the midline. Although radiologic studies may be normal, injection of a local anesthetic at the extraction site relieves the symptoms. Treatment is with jawbone curettage and antibiotics.

7

Neuro-Ophthalmic Disorders

APPROACH TO DIAGNOSIS

Disorders that affect the ocular muscles, ocular motor (III, IV, and VI) cranial nerves, or visual or ocular motor pathways in the brain produce a wide variety of neuro-ophthalmic disturbances. Because the anatomic pathways of the visual and ocular motor systems traverse major portions of the brainstem and cerebral hemispheres, neuro-ophthalmic symptoms and signs are often valuable in the anatomic localization and diagnosis of neurologic disease.

FUNCTIONAL ANATOMY OF THE VISUAL SYSTEM

VISUAL INPUT

Visual information enters the nervous system when light, refracted and focused by the **lens**, creates a visual image on the **retina** at the back of the eye (**Figure 7-1**). The action of the lens causes this image to be reversed in the horizontal and vertical planes. Thus, the superior portion of the visual image falls on the inferior retina and vice versa, and the temporal (lateral) and nasal (medial) fields are likewise reversed (**Figure 7-2**). The center of the visual field is focused at the **fovea**, where the retina's perceptual sensitivity is greatest. Within the retina, photoreceptor cells (**rods** and **cones**) transduce incident light into neuronal impulses, which are transmitted by retinal neurons to the **optic (II) nerve**. At this and all other levels of the visual system, the topographic relations of the visual field are preserved.

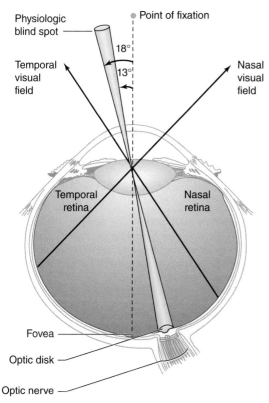

Figure 7-1. Representation of the visual field at the level of the retina: the point of fixation is focused on the fovea, the physiologic blind spot on the optic disk, the temporal half of the visual field on the nasal side of the retina, and the nasal half of the visual field on the temporal side of the retina.

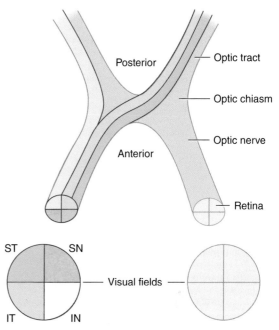

Figure 7-2. Representation of the visual field at the level of the optic nerve, chiasm, and optic tract. Quadrants of the visual field are designated ST (superior temporal), IT (inferior temporal), SN (superior nasal), and IN (inferior nasal).

PERIPHERAL VISUAL PATHWAYS

Each **optic nerve** contains fibers from one eye, but the nasal (medial) fibers, conveying information from the temporal (lateral) visual fields, cross in the **optic chiasm** (see Figures 1-13 and 7-2). As a result, each **optic tract** contains fibers not from one eye, but from one-half of the visual fields of both eyes. Because of this arrangement, **prechiasmal lesions** affect vision in the ipsilateral eye and **retrochiasmal lesions** produce defects in the contralateral half of the visual field of *both* eyes (see Figure 1-13).

CENTRAL VISUAL PATHWAYS

The optic tracts terminate in the **lateral geniculate nuclei**, synapsing on neurons that project through the **optic radiations** to the primary visual or **calcarine cortex** (area 17), located near the posterior poles of the occipital lobes, and visual association areas (areas 18 and 19). Here, too, the visual image is represented in such a way that its topographic organization is preserved (**Figure 7-3**). The central region of the visual field (**macula**) is represented in the most posterior portion of the visual cortex, whereas the inferior and superior parts of the field (superior and inferior retina) are represented above and below the calcarine fissure, respectively.

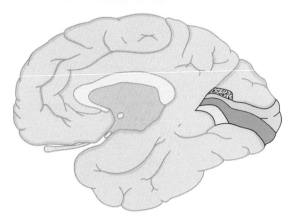

Upper peripheral quadrant of retina

Upper quadrant of macula

Lower quadrant of macula

Lower peripheral quadrant of retina

▲ **Figure 7-3.** Representation of the visual field at the level of the primary visual cortex, midsagittal view, shows the medial surface of the right occipital lobe, which receives visual input from the left side of the visual field of both eyes.

VASCULAR SUPPLY OF VISUAL PATHWAYS

The vascular supply of the visual system is derived from the ophthalmic, middle cerebral, and posterior cerebral arteries (**Figure 7-4**); ischemia or infarction in the territory of any of these vessels can produce visual field defects.

1. **Retina**—The retina is supplied by the central retinal artery, a branch of the ophthalmic artery, which is itself a branch of the internal carotid artery. Because the central retinal artery subsequently divides into superior and inferior retinal branches, vascular disease of the retina tends to produce altitudinal (ie, superior or inferior) visual field deficits.

2. **Optic nerve**—The optic nerve receives arterial blood primarily from the ophthalmic artery and its branches.

3. **Optic radiations**—As the optic radiations course backward toward the visual cortex, they are supplied by branches of the middle cerebral artery. Ischemia or infarction in the distribution of the middle cerebral artery may thus cause loss of vision in the contralateral visual field (see Figure 7-7).

4. **Primary visual cortex**—The primary visual cortex is supplied principally by the posterior cerebral artery. Occlusion of one posterior cerebral artery produces blindness in the contralateral visual field, although the dual (middle and posterior cerebral) arterial supply to the macular region of the visual cortex may spare central (macular) vision.

Because the left and right posterior cerebral arteries arise together from the basilar artery, occlusion at the tip of the basilar artery can cause bilateral occipital infarction (see figure 7-4) and complete cortical blindness—although, in some cases, macular vision is spared.

FUNCTIONAL ANATOMY OF THE OCULAR MOTOR SYSTEM

EXTRAOCULAR MUSCLES

Movement of the eyes is accomplished by the action of six muscles attached to each globe (**Figure 7-5**). These muscles act to move the eye into each of six cardinal positions of gaze. Equal and opposed actions of these six muscles in the resting state place the eye in mid- or primary position, that is, looking directly forward. When the function of one extraocular muscle is disrupted, the eye is unable to move in the direction of action of the affected muscle (**ophthalmoplegia**) and may deviate in the opposite direction because of the unopposed action of other extraocular muscles. When the eyes are thus misaligned, visual images of perceived objects fall on a different region of each retina, creating the illusion of double vision, or **diplopia**.

CRANIAL NERVES

The extraocular muscles are innervated by the oculomotor (III), trochlear (IV), and abducens (VI) nerves. Because of this differential innervation of the ocular muscles, the pattern of their involvement in pathologic conditions can help to distinguish a disorder of the ocular muscles from a disorder that affects a cranial nerve. Cranial nerves that control eye movement traverse long distances to pass from the brainstem to the eye; they are thereby rendered vulnerable to injury by a variety of pathologic processes.

1. **Oculomotor (III) nerve**—The oculomotor nerve supplies the medial rectus, superior and inferior rectus, and inferior oblique muscles and carries fibers to the levator palpebrae (which raises the eyelid). It also supplies the parasympathetic fibers responsible for pupillary constriction. With a complete nerve III lesion, the eye is partially abducted, and cannot be adducted elevated, and depressed; the eyelid droops (ptosis), and the pupil is nonreactive.

2. **Trochlear (IV) nerve**—The trochlear nerve innervates the superior oblique muscle. Lesions of this nerve result in defective depression of the adducted eye.

3. **Abducens (VI) nerve**—Lesions of the abducens nerve cause lateral rectus palsy, with impaired abduction of the affected eye.

CRANIAL NERVE NUCLEI

The nuclei of the oculomotor (III) and trochlear (IV) nerves are located in the dorsal midbrain, ventral to the cerebral aqueduct (of Sylvius), whereas the abducens (VI)

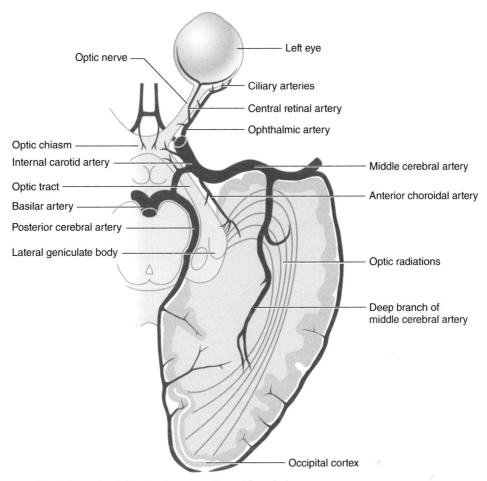

Figure 7-4. Arterial supply of the visual system, viewed from below.

nerve nucleus occupies a similarly dorsal and periventricular position in the pons. Lesions involving these nuclei give rise to clinical abnormalities similar to those produced by involvement of their respective cranial nerves; in some cases, nuclear and nerve lesions can be distinguished.

1. **Oculomotor (III) nerve nucleus**—Although each oculomotor nerve supplies muscles of the ipsilateral eye only, fibers to the superior rectus originate in the contralateral oculomotor nerve nucleus, and the levator palpebrae receives bilateral nuclear innervation. Thus, ophthalmoplegia affecting only one eye with ipsilateral ptosis or superior rectus palsy suggests oculomotor nerve disease, whereas ophthalmoplegia with bilateral ptosis or contralateral superior rectus palsy is probably due to a nuclear lesion.

2. **Trochlear (IV) nerve nucleus**—It is not possible to distinguish clinically between lesions of the trochlear nerve (see earlier) and those of its nucleus.

3. **Abducens (VI) nerve nucleus**—In disorders affecting the abducens nerve nucleus (rather than the nerve itself), lateral rectus paresis is often associated with facial weakness, paresis of ipsilateral conjugate gaze, or a depressed level of consciousness. This is because of the proximity of the abducens nerve nucleus to the facial (VII) nerve fasciculus, pontine lateral gaze center, and ascending reticular activating system, respectively. When a Horner syndrome (miosis of the pupil, ptosis, and sometimes segmental anhidrosis) accompanies an abducens nerve palsy, the lesion is in the cavernous sinus.

SUPRANUCLEAR CONTROL OF EYE MOVEMENTS

Supranuclear control of eye movements enables the two eyes to act in concert to produce **version (conjugate gaze)** or **vergence (convergence and divergence)** movements.

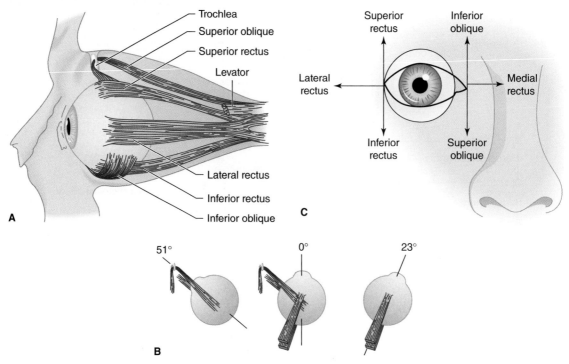

A

B

C

▲ **Figure 7-5.** Anatomy and function of extraocular muscles. (**A**) Extraocular muscles in the left orbit (lateral view). (**B**) An illustration of the right eye viewed from above in the primary position (**center figure**) showing the angle of attachment of the superior and inferior rectus muscles and the superior and inferior oblique muscles. With the eye directed to the right, the superior and inferior rectus muscles can now be examined as pure elevators and depressors of the globe (**right image**), and with the eye deviated to the left, the oblique muscles can now be examined as pure elevators and depressors of the globe as illustrated in C. (**C**) The six cardinal positions of gaze for testing eye movement. The eye is adducted by the medial rectus and abducted by the lateral rectus. The adducted eye is elevated by the inferior oblique and depressed by the superior oblique; the abducted eye is elevated by the superior rectus and depressed by the inferior rectus.

1. **Brainstem gaze centers**—Centers that control horizontal (lateral) and vertical gaze are located in the pons and pretectal region of the midbrain, respectively, and receive descending inputs from the cerebral cortex that allow voluntary control of gaze (**Figure 7-6**). Each lateral gaze center, located in the paramedian pontine reticular formation (PPRF) adjacent to the abducens nerve nucleus, mediates ipsilateral, conjugate, horizontal gaze via its connections to the ipsilateral abducens (VI) and contralateral oculomotor (III) nerve nucleus. A lesion in the pons affecting the PPRF therefore produces a gaze preference away from the side of the lesion and toward the side of an associated hemiparesis, if present. Disorders of vertical gaze, typically impaired upgaze, may result from mass lesions that exert downward pressure on the dorsal midbrain, such as pineal tumors (Parinaud syndrome).

2. **Cortical input**—The PPRF receives cortical input from the contralateral frontal lobe, which regulates rapid eye movements (saccades), and from the ipsilateral parietooccipital lobe, which regulates slow eye movements (pursuits). Therefore, a destructive lesion affecting the frontal cortex interferes with the mechanism for contralateral horizontal gaze and may result in a gaze preference toward the side of the lesion (and away from the side of associated hemiparesis). By contrast, an irritative (seizure) focus in the frontal lobe may cause gaze away from the side of the focus.

HISTORY

NATURE OF COMPLAINT

The first step is to obtain a clear description of the complaint. Patients may only complain of vague symptoms, such as blurred vision, which provide little diagnostic information. Therefore, it is important to determine

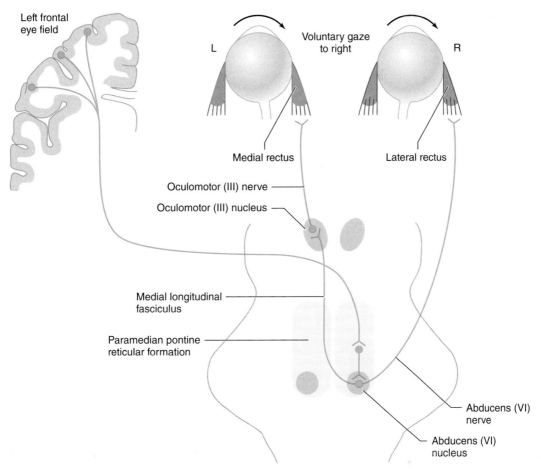

Left frontal
eye field

Voluntary gaze
to right

L

R

Medial rectus

Lateral rectus

Oculomotor (III) nerve

Oculomotor (III) nucleus

Medial longitudinal
fasciculus

Paramedian pontine
reticular formation

Abducens (VI)
nerve

Abducens (VI)
nucleus

▲ **Figure 7-6.** Neuronal pathways involved in horizontal gaze.

whether the patient means to describe decreased visual acuity in one or both eyes, loss of vision in part of the visual field, diplopia, an unstable visual image, pain in or about the eye, or some other problem.

TEMPORAL PATTERN OF SYMPTOMS

Once the nature of the complaint has been established, inquiries regarding its temporal pattern can provide clues to the underlying pathologic process:

1. **Sudden onset**—Vascular disorders that affect the eye or its connections in the brain tend to produce symptoms of sudden onset.
2. **Slow onset**—With inflammatory or neoplastic disease, symptoms usually evolve over a longer period.
3. **Transient, recurrent symptoms**—Transient and recurrent symptoms suggest a select group of pathologic processes, including intermittent ischemia, multiple sclerosis, and myasthenia gravis.

ASSOCIATED NEUROLOGIC ABNORMALITIES

The nature of any associated neurologic abnormalities, such as impaired facial sensation, weakness, ataxia, or aphasia, can help in localizing the site of involvement.

MEDICAL HISTORY

The history should be scrutinized for conditions that predispose the patient to neuro-ophthalmic problems as follows:

1. **Multiple sclerosis** often involves the optic nerve or brainstem, leading to a variety of neuro-ophthalmic disorders. A history of disturbances that also involve other parts of the central nervous system should suggest this diagnosis.
2. **Atherosclerosis, hypertension,** and **diabetes** can be complicated by vascular disorders of the eye, cranial nerves, or visual or ocular motor pathways in the brain.
3. **Endocrine disorders** (eg, hyperthyroidism) can cause ocular myopathy.

4. **Connective tissue disease** and **systemic cancer** can affect the visual and ocular motor systems at a variety of sites in the brain or subarachnoid space.

5. **Nutritional deficiencies** may present with neuro-ophthalmic symptoms, as in the amblyopia (decreased visual acuity) associated with malnutrition and the ophthalmoplegia of Wernicke encephalopathy (thiamine deficiency).

6. **Drugs** (eg, ethambutol, isoniazid, digitalis, clioquinol) may be toxic to the visual system, and others (sedative drugs, anticonvulsants) commonly produce ocular motor disorders.

NEURO-OPHTHALMIC EXAMINATION

VISUAL ACUITY

▶ Assessment

To identify neuro-ophthalmic problems, vision should be tested under conditions that eliminate refractive errors. Therefore, patients should be examined wearing their spectacles (a pinhole can be substituted if the corrective lenses usually worn are not available at the time of testing). Visual acuity must be assessed for each eye separately. Distant vision is tested using a Snellen eye chart, with the patient 6 m (20 ft) away. Near vision is tested with a Rosenbaum pocket eye chart held approximately 36 cm (14 in) from the patient. In each case, the smallest line of print that can be read is noted.

▶ Recording

Visual acuity is expressed as a fraction (eg, 20/20, 20/40, 20/200). The numerator is the distance (in feet) from the test figures at which the examination is performed, and the denominator is the distance (in feet) at which figures of a given size can be correctly identified by persons with normal vision. For example, if a patient standing 20 ft away from the eye chart is unable to identify figures that can normally be seen from that distance but can identify the larger figures that would be visible 40 ft away with normal acuity, the visual acuity is recorded as 20/40. If the patient can read most of a given line but makes some errors, acuity may be recorded as 20/40–1, for example, indicating that all but one letter on the 20/40 line were correctly identified. When visual acuity is markedly reduced, it can still be quantified, though less precisely, by the distance at which the patient can count fingers (CF), discern hand movement (HM), or perceive light. If an eye is totally blind, the examination will reveal no light perception (NLP).

▶ Red–Green Color Vision

Red–green color vision is often disproportionately impaired in optic nerve lesions and can be tested with colored objects such as pens or hatpins or with color vision plates.

VISUAL FIELDS

Evaluating the visual fields can be a lengthy and tedious procedure if conducted in an undirected fashion. Familiarity with the common types of visual field defects is important if testing is to be reasonably rapid and yield useful information. The most common visual field abnormalities are illustrated in **Figure 7-7**.

▶ Extent of Visual Fields

The normal monocular visual field subtends an angle of approximately 160 degrees in the horizontal plane and approximately 135 degrees in the vertical plane. With binocular vision, the horizontal range of vision exceeds 180 degrees.

▶ Physiologic Blind Spot

Within the normal field of each eye is a 5-degree blind spot, corresponding to the optic disk, which lacks receptor cells. The blind spot is located 15 degrees temporal to fixation in each eye.

▶ Measurement Techniques

Like visual acuity, the visual field must be examined separately for each eye as described below:

1. **Confrontation (Figure 7-8)** is the simplest method for visual field testing. The examiner stands at about arm's length from the patient, with the eyes of both patient and examiner aligned in the horizontal plane. The eye not being tested is covered by the patient's hand or an eye patch. The examiner closes the eye opposite the patient's covered eye, and the patient is instructed to fix on the examiner's open eye. Now the monocular fields of patient and examiner are superimposed, which allows comparison of the patient's field with the examiner's presumably normal field. The examiner uses the index fingers of either hand to locate the boundaries of the patient's field, moving them slowly inward from the periphery in all directions until the patient detects them. The boundaries are then defined more carefully by determining the farthest peripheral sites at which the patient can detect slight movements of the fingertips or the white head of a pin. The patient's blind spot can be located in the region of the examiner's own blind spot, and the sizes of these spots can be compared using a pin with a white head as the target. The procedure is then repeated for the other eye.

2. Subtle field defects may be detected by asking the patient to compare the brightness of colored objects presented at different sites in the field or by measuring the fields using a pin with a red head as the target.

3. In young children, the fields may be assessed by standing behind the child and bringing an attention-getting object, such as a toy, forward around the child's head in various directions until it is first noticed.

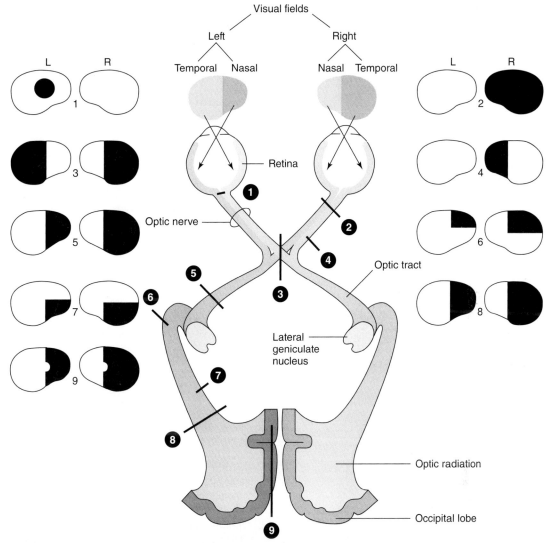

▲ **Figure 7-7.** Common visual field defects and their anatomic bases. 1. **Central scotoma** caused by inflammation of the optic disk (optic neuritis) or optic nerve (retrobulbar neuritis). 2. **Total blindness of the right eye** from a complete lesion of the right optic nerve. 3. **Bitemporal hemianopia** caused by pressure exerted on the optic chiasm by (for example) a pituitary tumor. 4. **Right nasal hemianopia** caused by a perichiasmal lesion (eg, calcified internal carotid artery). 5. **Right homonymous hemianopia** from a lesion of the left optic tract. 6. **Right homonymous superior quadrantanopia** caused by partial involvement of the optic radiation by a lesion in the left temporal lobe (Meyer loop). 7. **Right homonymous inferior quadrantanopia** caused by partial involvement of the optic radiation by a lesion in the left parietal lobe. 8. **Right homonymous hemianopia** from a complete lesion of the left optic radiation. (A similar defect may also result from lesion 9.) 9. **Right homonymous hemianopia (with macular sparing)** resulting from posterior cerebral artery occlusion.

4. A gross indication of visual field abnormalities may be obtained in obtunded patients by determining whether they blink in response to a visual threat—typically the examiner's finger—brought toward the patient's eye in various regions of the field.

5. Although many visual field deficits are detectable by these screening procedures, more precise mapping of the fields requires the use of standard tangent screen testing or automated perimetry techniques.

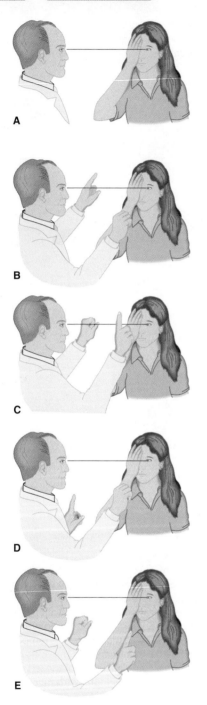

Figure 7-8. Confrontation testing of the visual field. (A) The left eye of the patient and the right eye of the examiner are aligned. (B) Testing the superior nasal quadrant. (C) Testing the superior temporal quadrant. (D) Testing the inferior nasal quadrant. (E) Testing the inferior temporal quadrant. The procedure is then repeated for the patient's other eye.

OPHTHALMOSCOPY

Ophthalmoscopy of the optic fundus is particularly important for evaluating disorders that affect the retina or optic disk and examining patients with a suspected increase in intracranial pressure.

▶ Preparation of the Patient

The examination should be conducted in a dark room so that the pupils are dilated; in some patients, the use of mydriatic (sympathomimetic or anticholinergic) eye drops is necessary. In the latter case, visual acuity and pupillary reflexes should be assessed before instilling the drops. Mydriatic agents should be avoided in patients with untreated closed-angle glaucoma, and in situations—such as impending or ongoing transtentorial herniation—in which the state of pupillary reactivity is an important guide to management.

▶ Examination of the Fundus

Familiarity with the normal appearance of the optic fundus (see Figure 1-10) is necessary if abnormalities are to be appreciated.

A. Optic Disk

1. **Normal appearance**—The optic disk is usually easily recognizable as a yellowish, slightly oval structure situated nasally at the posterior pole of the eye (Figure 1-10). The temporal side of the disk is often paler than the nasal side. The disk margins should be sharply demarcated, though the nasal edge is commonly less distinct than the temporal edge. The disk is normally in the same plane as the surrounding retina. Blood vessels crossing the border of the optic disk are distinct and pulsatile and become obscured when the disk swells.

2. **Optic disk swelling**—Optic nerve swelling due to papilledema implies increased intracranial pressure and must be differentiated from swelling due to other causes, such as local inflammation (papillitis) and ischemic optic neuropathy. Papilledema is almost always bilateral, does not typically impair vision (except for enlargement of the blind spot), and is not associated with eye pain. Papilledema can be simulated by disk abnormalities such as drusen (colloid or hyaline bodies).

   Increased intracranial pressure is thought to cause papilledema by blocking axonal transport in the optic nerve. Because the optic nerve sheath communicates with the subarachnoid space, disorders associated with increased intracranial pressure that also obstruct the subarachnoid space, such as meningitis, are less likely to cause papilledema. The ophthalmoscopic changes in papilledema typically develop over days or weeks but may become apparent within hours after a sudden increase in intracranial pressure—as, for example, after intracranial hemorrhage. In early papilledema (see Figure 1-11), the retinal veins appear engorged and spontaneous venous pulsations are absent. The disk may be hyperemic, and linear hemorrhages may be seen at its borders. The disk margins become blurred, with the temporal edge last to be affected. In fully developed papilledema, the optic disk is elevated above the plane of the retina, and blood vessels crossing the border of the disk become obscured.

3. **Optic disk pallor**—Optic disk pallor with impaired visual acuity, visual field defects, or loss of pupillary reactivity is associated with a wide variety of disorders that affect the optic nerve, including inflammatory conditions, nutritional deficiencies, and degenerative diseases. A pale optic disk with normal visual function can also occur as a congenital variant, and an optic disk may appear artificially pale if a cataract has been removed.

B. Arteries & Veins

The caliber of the retinal arteries and veins should be observed where they arise from the disk and pass over its edges onto the retina. Features to note include whether these vessels are easily visible throughout their course, whether they appear engorged, and whether spontaneous venous pulsations (which indicate normal intracranial pressure) are present. The remainder of the visible retina is inspected, noting the presence of hemorrhages, exudates, or other abnormalities.

C. Macula

The macula, a somewhat paler area than the rest of the retina, is located approximately two disk diameters temporal to the temporal margin of the optic disk. It can be visualized quickly by having the patient look at the light from the ophthalmoscope. Ophthalmoscopic examination of the macula can reveal abnormalities related to visual loss from age-related macular degeneration, macular holes, or hereditary cerebromacular degenerations.

PUPILS

Size

The size and reactivity of the pupils reflect the integrity of neuronal pathways from the optic nerve to the midbrain (**Figure 7-9**). The normal pupil is round, regular, and centered within the iris; its size varies with age and with the intensity of ambient light. In a brightly illuminated room, the diameter of normal pupils is approximately 3 mm in adults, smaller in the elderly, and greater than or equal to 5 mm in children. Pupil size may be asymmetric in up to 20% of people (physiologic **anisocoria**), but the difference is less than or equal to 1 mm. Symmetrically rapid

constriction of the pupils in bright light indicates that pupillary function is normal and excludes oculomotor (III) nerve compression.

Reaction to Light

Direct (ipsilateral) and **consensual (contralateral)** pupillary constriction in response to a bright light shone in one eye demonstrates the integrity of the pathways shown in Figure 7-9. Normally, the direct response to light is slightly brisker and more pronounced than the consensual response.

Reaction to Accommodation

When the eyes converge to focus on a nearer object (**accommodation**), the pupils normally constrict. This reaction is tested by having the patient focus alternately on a distant object and a finger held just in front of the nose.

Pupillary Abnormalities

A. Nonreactive Pupils

Unilateral disorders of pupillary constriction are seen with local disease of the iris (trauma, iritis, glaucoma), oculomotor (III) nerve compression (tumor, aneurysm), administration of a mydriatic agent, and optic nerve disorders (optic neuritis, multiple sclerosis).

B. Light-Near Dissociation

Impaired pupillary reactivity to light with preserved constriction during accommodation (light-near dissociation) is usually bilateral and may result from neurosyphilis, diabetes, optic nerve disorders, and tumors compressing the midbrain tectum.

C. Argyll Robertson Pupils

These pupils are small, poorly reactive to light, often irregular in shape, and frequently unequal in size; they show light-near dissociation. Neurosyphilis is the classic cause, but other lesions in the region of the Edinger-Westphal nucleus (eg, multiple sclerosis) are now more common (**Table 7-1**).

D. Tonic Pupil

The tonic (**Adie**) pupil (Table 7-1) is larger than the contralateral unaffected pupil and reacts sluggishly to changes in both illumination and accommodation. Because the tonic pupil does eventually react, anisocoria becomes less marked during the examination. This abnormality is most commonly a manifestation of a benign, often familial disorder that frequently affects young women (**Holmes–Adie syndrome**) and may be associated with depressed deep tendon reflexes (especially in the legs), segmental anhidrosis (localized lack of

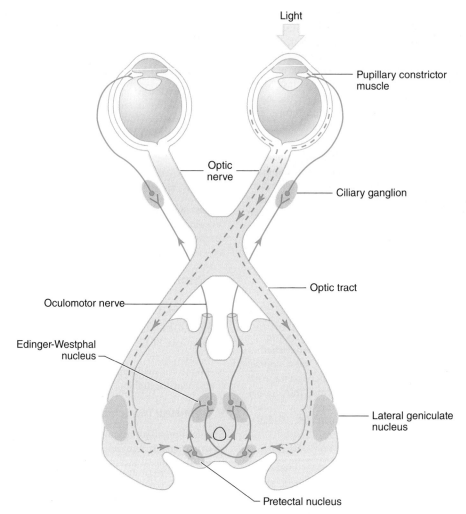

Figure 7-9. Anatomic basis of the pupillary light reflex. The afferent visual pathways from the retina to the pretectal nuclei of the midbrain are represented by dashed lines and the efferent pupilloconstrictor pathways from the midbrain to the pupillary constrictor muscles by solid lines. Note that illumination of one eye results in bilateral pupillary constriction.

sweating), orthostatic hypotension, or cardiovascular autonomic instability. Adie pupils may be bilateral. The pupillary abnormality may be caused by degeneration of the ciliary ganglion, followed by aberrant reinnervation of the pupilloconstrictor muscles.

E. Horner Syndrome

Horner syndrome (Tables 7-1 and **7-2**) results from a lesion of the central or peripheral sympathetic nervous system and consists of a small (miotic) pupil associated with mild ptosis (**Figure 7-10**) and sometimes loss of sweating (**anhidrosis**).

1. **Oculosympathetic pathways**—The sympathetic pathway controlling pupillary dilation consists of an uncrossed three-neuron arc: **hypothalamic neurons**, which descend through the brainstem to the intermediolateral column of the spinal cord at the T1 level, **preganglionic sympathetic neurons** projecting from the spinal cord to the superior cervical ganglion, and **postganglionic sympathetic neurons** that originate in the superior cervical ganglion, ascend in the neck along the internal carotid artery, and enter the orbit with the first (ophthalmic) division of the trigeminal (V) nerve. Horner syndrome is caused by interruption of these pathways at any site (Figure 7-10).

Table 7-1. Common Pupillary Abnormalities.

	Appearance	Response	Differential Diagnosis
Tonic (Adie) pupil	Unilateral (rarely bilateral) dilated pupil	Reacts sluggishly and only to persistent bright light or 0.125% pilocarpine eye drops; accommodation less affected	Holmes–Adie syndrome, ocular trauma, autonomic neuropathy
Horner syndrome	Unilateral small pupil and slight ptosis	Normal response to light and accommodation	Lateral medullary infarcts, cervical cord lesions, pulmonary apical or mediastinal tumors, neck trauma or masses, carotid artery dissection or thrombosis, intrapartum brachial plexus injury, cluster headache
Argyll Robertson pupil	Unequal irregular pupils <3 mm in diameter (usually bilateral)	Poorly reactive to light; more responsive to accommodation	Neurosyphilis; mimicked by diabetes, pineal region tumors, multiple sclerosis

2. **Clinical features**—The lesions and resulting pupillary abnormality are usually unilateral. The pupil diameter on the involved side is typically reduced by 0.5 to 1 mm compared with the normal side. This inequality is most marked in dim illumination. The pupillary abnormality is accompanied by mild to moderate ptosis (see later) of the upper lid (as opposed to the pronounced ptosis seen with oculomotor nerve lesions), often associated with elevation of the lower lid (lower lid ptosis). When Horner syndrome has been present since infancy, the ipsilateral iris is lighter and blue (**heterochromia iridis**).

Table 7-2. Causes of Horner Syndrome.

Central (first) neuron Brainstem infarction* Hypothalamic region tumor, hemorrhage or infarction Multiple sclerosis Syrinx Transverse myelopathy	28%
Preganglionic (second) neuron Thoracic or neck tumor (Pancoast tumor, schwannoma, neuroblastoma, thyroid) Trauma or surgery (neck, thorax) Vascular (jugular ectasia, subclavian artery aneurysm)	44%
Postganglionic (third) neuron Base of skull, parasellar, orbital, or cavernous sinus* mass Vascular (fibromuscular dysplasia, carotid dissection*) Cluster headache	28%
Unknown cause	15%

*Most common.

Percentages from Almog Y, Gepstein R, Kesler A. Diagnostic value of imaging in Horner syndrome in adults. *J Neuro-Ophthalmol.* 2010;30:7-11. Etiologies from Reede D, Garcon E, Smoker WRK, Kardon R. Horner's syndrome: clinical and radiographic evaluation. *Neuroimag Clin N Am,* 2008;18:369-385.

Deficits in the pattern of sweating, which are most prominent in acute-onset Horner syndrome, can help localize the lesion. If sweating is decreased on an entire half of the body and face, the lesion is in the central nervous system. Cervical lesions produce anhidrosis of the face, neck, and arm only. Sweating is unimpaired if the lesion is above the bifurcation of the carotid artery. The differential diagnosis of Horner syndrome is presented in Table 7-2.

F. Relative Afferent Pupillary Defect (Marcus Gunn Pupil)

The involved pupil constricts less markedly in response to direct illumination than to illumination of the contralateral pupil, whereas normally the direct response is greater than the consensual response. The abnormality is detected by rapidly moving a bright flashlight back and forth between the eyes while continuously observing the suspect pupil (**Gunn pupillary test**). Relative afferent pupillary defect is commonly associated with disorders of the ipsilateral optic nerve, which interrupt the afferent limb and affect the pupillary light reflex (see Figure 7-9). Such disorders also commonly impair vision (especially color vision) in the involved eye.

OPTOKINETIC RESPONSE

Optokinetic nystagmus consists of eye movements elicited by sequential fixation on a series of targets passing in front of a patient's eyes, such as telephone poles seen from a moving train. For clinical testing, a revolving drum with vertical stripes or a vertically striped strip of cloth is moved across the visual field to generate these movements. Testing produces a slow following phase in the direction of the target's movement, followed by a rapid return jerk in the opposite direction. The slow (pursuit) phase tests parieto-occipital and the rapid return (saccadic) movement tests frontal lobe function in the hemisphere toward which the stimulus is moved. The presence of an optokinetic response reflects the ability to perceive movement or contour and is

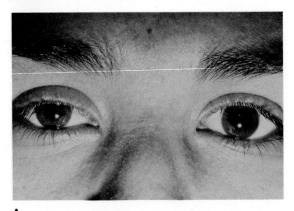

A

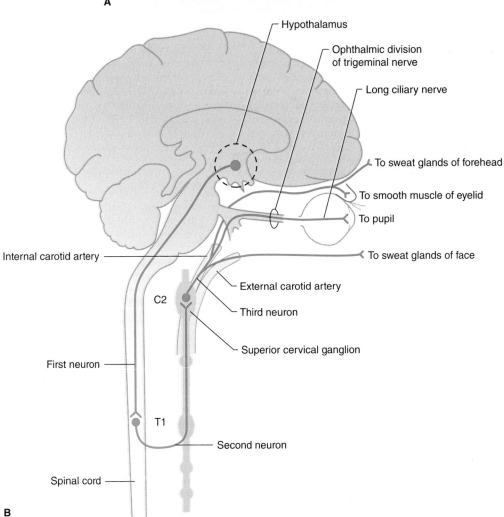

B

▲ **Figure 7-10.** (**A**) Right Horner syndrome after direct carotid puncture for arterial injection. (**B**) Oculosympathetic pathway involved in Horner syndrome. This three-neuron pathway projects from the hypothalamus to the intermediolateral column of the spinal cord, then to the superior cervical (sympathetic) ganglion, and finally to the pupil, smooth muscle of the eyelid, and sweat glands of the forehead and face.

sometimes useful for documenting visual perception in newborns or in psychogenic blindness. Visual acuity required to produce the optokinetic response is minimal, however (20/400, or finger counting at 3 to 5 ft). Unilateral impairment of the optokinetic response may be found when targets are moved toward the side of a parietal lobe lesion.

EYELIDS

The eyelids (**palpebrae**) should be examined with the patient's eyes open. The distance between the upper and lower lids (interpalpebral fissure) is usually approximately 10 mm and equal in both eyes, though physiologic asymmetries do occur. The position of the inferior margin of the upper lid relative to the superior border of the iris should be noted in order to detect drooping (**ptosis**) or abnormal elevation of the eyelid (**lid retraction**). The upper lid normally covers 1 to 2 mm of the iris.

Unilateral ptosis is seen with paralysis of the levator palpebrae muscle itself, lesions of the oculomotor (III) nerve or its superior branch, and Horner syndrome. In the last condition, ptosis is customarily associated with miosis and may be momentarily overcome by effortful eye opening.

Bilateral ptosis suggests a disorder affecting the oculomotor (III) nerve nucleus, neuromuscular junction (eg, myasthenia gravis), or muscle (eg, myotonic, ocular, or oculopharyngeal dystrophy).

Lid retraction (abnormal elevation of the upper lid) is seen in hyperthyroidism and in **Parinaud syndrome** caused by tumors in the pineal region (see later).

EXOPHTHALMOS

Abnormal protrusion of the eye from the orbit (**exophthalmos or proptosis**) is best detected by standing behind the seated patient and looking down at the eyes from above. Causes include hyperthyroidism (Graves disease, **Figure 7-11**), orbital tumor or pseudotumor, and carotid artery-cavernous sinus fistula. A bruit may be audible on auscultation over the proptotic eye in patients with carotid artery-cavernous sinus fistula or other vascular anomalies.

EYE MOVEMENTS

▶ Ocular Excursion & Gaze

Ocular palsies and gaze palsies are detected by having the patient gaze in each of the six cardinal positions (see Figure 7-5). If voluntary eye movement is impaired or the patient is unable to cooperate with the examination (eg, is stuporous or comatose), reflex eye movements can be induced by **doll's head (oculocephalic)** or **cold-water caloric (oculovestibular)** testing (see Chapter 3, Coma). If limitations in eye movement are observed, the muscles involved are noted, and the nature of the abnormality is determined according to the following scheme.

A. Ocular Palsy

Weakness of one or more eye muscles results from nuclear or infranuclear (nerve, neuromuscular junction, or muscle) lesions. An ocular palsy cannot be overcome by caloric stimulation of reflex eye movement. Nerve lesions produce distinctive patterns of ocular muscle involvement.

1. **Oculomotor (III) nerve palsy**—A complete lesion of the oculomotor nerve produces closure of the affected eye because of impaired levator function. Passively elevating the paralyzed lid (**Figure 7-12**) shows the involved eye to be laterally deviated because of the unopposed action of the lateral rectus muscle, which is not innervated by the oculomotor nerve. Diplopia is present in all directions of gaze except for lateral gaze toward the side of involvement. Pupil function may be normal (pupillary sparing) or impaired (as illustrated).

2. **Trochlear (IV) nerve palsy**—With trochlear nerve lesions, which paralyze the superior oblique muscle, the involved eye is elevated during primary (forward) gaze; the extent of elevation increases during adduction and decreases during abduction. Elevation is greatest when the head is

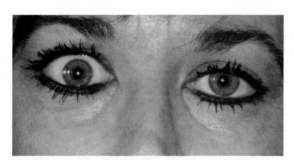

▲ **Figure 7-11.** Graves ophthalmopathy in a 41-year-old woman. Note the protrusion of the right globe.

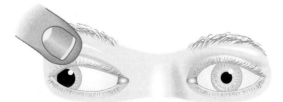

▲ **Figure 7-12.** Clinical findings with oculomotor (III) nerve lesion. With the ptotic lid passively elevated, the affected (right) eye is abducted; it cannot adduct. On attempted downgaze, the unaffected superior oblique muscle, which is innervated by the trochlear (IV) nerve, will cause the eye to turn inward.

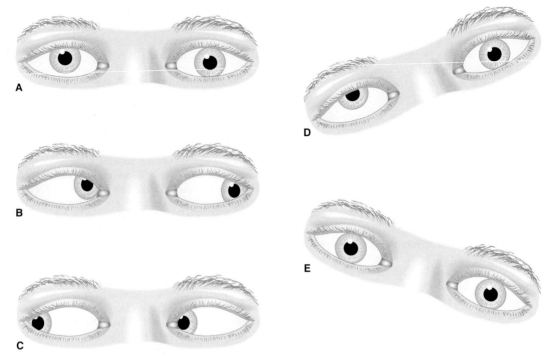

▲ **Figure 7-13.** Clinical findings with trochlear (IV) nerve lesion. The affected (right) eye is elevated on forward gaze (**A**). The extent of elevation is increased with adduction (**B**) and decreased with abduction (**C**). Elevation increases with head tilting to the affected side (**D**) and decreases with head tilting in the opposite direction (**E**).

tilted toward the side of the involved eye and abolished by tilt in the opposite direction (Bielschowsky head-tilt test; **Figure 7-13**). Diplopia is most pronounced when the patient looks downward with the affected eye adducted (as in looking at the end of one's nose). Spontaneous head tilting, intended to decrease or correct the diplopia, is present in approximately one-half of patients with unilateral palsies and in a greater number with bilateral palsies.

3. **Abducens (VI) nerve palsy**—An abducens nerve lesion causes paralysis of the lateral rectus muscle, resulting in adduction of the involved eye at rest (due to the uninvolved oculomotor nerve) and failure of attempted abduction (**Figure 7-14**). Diplopia occurs on lateral gaze to the side of the affected eye.

B. Gaze Palsy

Gaze palsy is the diminished ability of a pair of yoked muscles (muscles that operate in concert to move the two eyes in a given direction) to move the eyes in voluntary gaze; it is caused by supranuclear lesions in the brainstem or cerebral hemisphere. Gaze palsy, unlike ocular palsies, affects both eyes and usually can be overcome by caloric stimulation. Its pathophysiology and causes are discussed more fully in the section that follows on binocular

disorders of eye movement. Mild impairment of upgaze is not uncommon in normal elderly subjects.

C. Internuclear Ophthalmoplegia

Internuclear ophthalmoplegia (INO) results from a lesion of the medial longitudinal fasciculus, an ascending pathway in

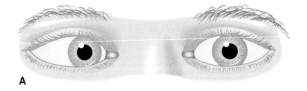

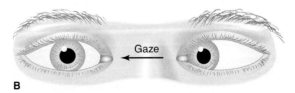

▲ **Figure 7-14.** Clinical findings with abducens (VI) nerve lesion. The affected (right) eye is adducted at rest (**A**) and cannot be abducted (**B**).

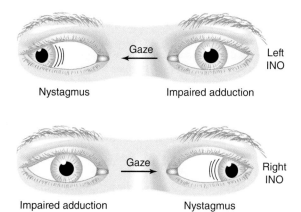

Nystagmus   Impaired adduction   Gaze ←   Left INO

Impaired adduction   Nystagmus   Gaze →   Right INO

▲ **Figure 7-15.** Eye movements in internuclear ophthalmoplegia (INO) resulting from a bilateral lesion of the medial longitudinal fasciculus.

the brainstem that projects from the abducens (VI) to the contralateral oculomotor (III) nerve nucleus (see Figure 7-6). As a consequence of INO, the actions of the abducens (VI) and oculomotor (III) nerves during voluntary gaze or caloric-induced movement are uncoupled. Excursion of the abducting eye is full, but adduction of the contralateral eye is impaired (**Figure 7-15**). INO cannot be overcome by caloric stimulation, but can be distinguished from oculomotor (III) nerve palsy by noting preserved adduction with convergence. It is usually caused by multiple sclerosis or brainstem stroke.

D. One-and-a-Half Syndrome

A pontine lesion affecting both the medial longitudinal fasciculus and the ipsilateral paramedian pontine reticular formation (lateral gaze center) produces a syndrome that combines internuclear ophthalmoplegia with an inability to gaze toward the side of the lesion (**Figure 7-16**).

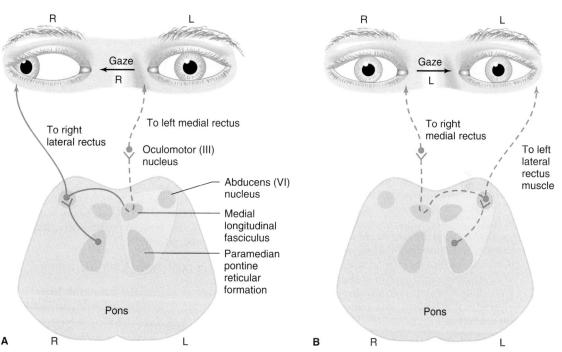

▲ **Figure 7-16.** One-and-a-half syndrome. This results from a pontine lesion (blue area) involving the paramedian pontine reticular formation (lateral gaze center), medial longitudinal fasciculus, and sometimes also the abducens (VI) nucleus, and affecting the neuronal pathways indicated by dotted lines. Attempted gaze away from the lesion (**A**) activates the uninvolved right lateral gaze center and abducens (VI) nucleus; the right lateral rectus muscle contracts, and the right eye abducts normally. Involvement of the medial longitudinal fasciculus interrupts the pathway to the left oculomotor (III) nucleus, and the left eye fails to adduct. On attempted gaze toward the lesion (**B**), the left lateral gaze center cannot be activated, and the eyes do not move. There is a complete (bilateral) gaze palsy in one direction (toward the lesion) and one-half (unilateral) gaze palsy in the other direction (away from the lesion), accounting for the name of the syndrome.

The ipsilateral eye is immobile in the horizontal plane, and movement of the contralateral eye is restricted to abduction, which may be associated with nystagmus. The causes include pontine infarct, multiple sclerosis, and pontine hemorrhage.

Diplopia Testing

When the patient complains of double vision (**diplopia**), eye movements should be tested to determine its anatomic basis. The patient is asked to fix vision on an object, such as a flashlight, in each of the six cardinal positions of gaze (see Figure 7-5). With normal conjugate gaze, light from the flashlight falls at the same spot on both corneas; a lack of such congruency confirms that gaze is disconjugate. When the patient notes diplopia in a given direction of gaze, each eye should be covered in turn and the patient asked to report which of the two images disappears. The image displaced farther in the direction of gaze is always referable to the weak eye, because that image will not fall on the fovea. A variation of this procedure is the **red glass test**, in which one eye is covered with translucent red glass, plastic, or cellophane; this allows the eye responsible for each image to be identified.

Nystagmus

Nystagmus is rhythmic oscillation of the eyes. **Pendular nystagmus**, which usually has its onset in infancy, occurs with equal velocity in both directions. **Jerk nystagmus** is characterized by a slow phase of movement in one direction, followed by a fast phase in the opposite direction; the direction of jerk nystagmus is specified by stating the direction of the fast phase (eg, leftward-beating nystagmus). Jerk nystagmus usually increases in amplitude with gaze in the direction of the fast phase (Alexander law).

Nystagmus can occur at the extremes of voluntary gaze in normal subjects and is also a normal component of both the optokinetic response and the response to caloric stimulation of reflex eye movements. In other settings, however, it may be due to anticonvulsant or sedative drugs or disease in the peripheral vestibular apparatus, central vestibular pathways, or cerebellum.

To detect nystagmus, the eyes should be observed in the primary position and in each of the cardinal positions of gaze (see Figure 7-5). Nystagmus is described in terms of the position of gaze in which it occurs, its direction and amplitude, precipitating factors such as changes in head position, and associated symptoms, such as vertigo.

Many forms of nystagmus and related ocular oscillations have been described, but two syndromes of acquired **pathologic jerk nystagmus** are by far the most common.

A. Gaze-Evoked Nystagmus

Gaze-evoked nystagmus occurs when the patient attempts to gaze in one or more directions away from the primary position. The fast phase of nystagmus is in the direction of gaze. Nystagmus evoked by gaze in a single direction is a common sign of early or mild residual ocular palsy. Multidirectional gaze-evoked nystagmus is most often an effect of anticonvulsant or sedative drugs, but can also result from cerebellar or central vestibular dysfunction.

B. Vestibular Nystagmus

Nystagmus caused by a lesion of the **peripheral vestibular** apparatus is characteristically unidirectional, horizontal, or both horizontal and rotatory oscillations, as is associated with severe vertigo. Its amplitude increases with gaze toward the fast phase. In contrast, **central vestibular nystagmus** may be bidirectional and purely horizontal, vertical, or rotatory, and the accompanying vertigo is typically mild. **Positional nystagmus**, elicited by changes in head position, can occur with either peripheral or central vestibular lesions. The most helpful distinguishing features are the presence of hearing loss or tinnitus with peripheral lesions and of corticospinal tract or additional cranial nerve abnormalities with central lesions.

DISORDERS OF THE VISUAL SYSTEM

MONOCULAR DISORDERS

Common syndromes of monocular visual loss include two reversible and two irreversible disorders. **Transient monocular blindness** caused by optic nerve or retinal ischemia is sudden in onset and resolves rapidly. **Optic neuritis** produces subacute, painful, unilateral visual loss with partial resolution. Less reversible visual loss of sudden onset occurs in idiopathic **ischemic optic neuropathy** and in **giant cell (temporal) arteritis**.

TRANSIENT MONOCULAR BLINDNESS

Transient monocular blindness (**amaurosis fugax**) is characterized by typically painless, unilateral transient diminution or loss of vision that develops over seconds, remains maximal for 1 to 5 minutes, and resolves over 10 to 20 minutes. Although the cause of these episodes often remain uncertain, most cases result from transient ischemia of the optic nerve or retina. Both embolic and nonembolic etiologies are known. Most cases result from transient ischemia of the optic nerve or retina. The presence of what appears to be embolic material in retinal arteries during episodes suggests that emboli are a frequent cause. The risk of subsequent hemispheric stroke is increased, but this risk is unrelated to the frequency or duration of these episodes.

Diagnostic evaluation and treatment of patients with transient monocular blindness resemble that for patients with hemispheric transient ischemic attacks (TIAs) (see Chapter 13, Stroke.)

AUTOIMMUNE OPTIC NEURITIS

Inflammation of the optic nerve produces the syndrome of optic neuritis. The most common cause is demyelination (acute demyelinating optic neuritis). Less common causes include parameningeal, meningeal, or intraocular inflammation associated with viral infections or postviral syndromes. Rare causes include toxins (eg, methanol, ethambutol), neurosyphilis, and vitamin B_{12} deficiency. Unilateral impairment of visual acuity occurs over hours to days, becoming maximal within 2 weeks. Visual loss is associated with headache, globe tenderness, or eye pain in more than 90% of patients; the pain is typically exacerbated by eye movement.

Visual field testing demonstrates a central scotoma (blind spot) associated with decreased visual acuity. Examination of the fundus shows unilateral disk swelling when the nerve head is involved, but is normal when the inflammatory process is posterior to the optic disk (retrobulbar neuritis), as is most common in demyelinating disease. The pupils are equal in size but show less pronounced constriction in response to illumination of the affected eye (relative afferent pupillary defect; Marcus Gunn pupil). Recovery of vision begins in a few weeks and may progresses for a year. Normal vision returns in the majority of cases.

Optic neuritis is the first manifestation of multiple sclerosis in 25% of cases and occurs in 70% of multiple sclerosis patients at some point. Diffuse gadolinium enhancement of the optic nerve on MRI is typical of acute demyelinating optic neuritis, and T2-hyperintense lesions are also seen in the brain in 50% to 70% of these patients. In North America, with 15-year follow-up, 72% of optic neuritis patients with one or more T2 lesions in brain, but only approximately 25% without T2 lesions, develop multiple sclerosis.

Intravenous methylprednisolone, 1 g/d for 3 to 5 days, with or without an oral prednisone taper, from 1 mg/kg/d over 11 days, can hasten recovery but does not alter the final visual outcome or the likelihood of developing multiple sclerosis. Evolving data support immunomodulatory treatment for optic neuritis as presumed multiple sclerosis if demyelinating lesions are seen on brain MRI (see Figure 9-4).

Bilateral spontaneous optic neuritis and transverse myelitis occur in neuromyelitis optica (NMO) spectrum disorder, formerly called Devic disease. The presence of aquaporin-4 antibodies (APQ4) is diagnostic and represents an evolving group of autoimmune demyelinating diseases. Such autoimmune aquaporin-4 channelopathy disorders now include lesions beyond the cord, around the third and fourth ventricles and the aqueduct of Sylvius, and processes beyond the CNS (skeletal muscle). Immunosuppressive therapies are evolving. Further details are provided in Chapter 9, Motor Disorders.

NONARTERITIC ANTERIOR ISCHEMIC OPTIC NEUROPATHY

Ischemic infarction of the anterior portion of the optic nerve is a major cause of visual loss beginning in middle age. Risk factors include hypertension and diabetes. Visual loss is sudden in onset, painless, always monocular, and without premonitory ocular symptoms. The visual deficit is usually maximal at onset and frequently subtotal; the pattern of visual loss varies between patients. In some cases, the course is stuttering or progressive.

Examination reveals ipsilateral disk swelling, often with peripapillary hemorrhages. A relative afferent pupillary defect will be present. Although ischemic optic neuropathy is often assumed to be atherosclerotic in origin, presentation of symptoms on awaking is a common feature suggesting nocturnal arterial hypotension, often from antihypertensive medications, may be causative. Patients with anterior ischemic optic neuropathy have a structurally smaller than normal disk (observable in the uninvolved eye), and 15% to 25% of patients will go on to have the contralateral eye affected within 3 to 5 years. Modification of vascular risk factors is indicated.

Spontaneous improvement of vision occurs over 6 months. As disk swelling resolves, ophthalmoscopic evaluation shows optic atrophy. MRI imaging of the optic nerve is normal. Treatment with corticosteroids during the first 2 weeks may enhance recovery (prednisone 80 mg daily for 14 days then tapered over a month). Aspirin is ineffective.

ARTERITIC ANTERIOR ISCHEMIC OPTIC NEUROPATHY: GIANT CELL (TEMPORAL) ARTERITIS

Arteritic infarction of the anterior portion of the optic nerve is the most devastating complication of giant cell, or temporal, arteritis. This disorder is usually accompanied by systemic symptoms such as fever, malaise, night sweats, weight loss, and headache (see Chapter 6, Headache & Facial Pain) and often by **polymyalgia rheumatica** (see Chapter 9, Motor Disorders). Scalp tenderness and jaw claudication may occur. The visual loss is usually sudden and often total, but transient visual obscurations may precede optic nerve infarction. On examination, the optic disk appears swollen and pale. The erythrocyte sedimentation rate and C-reactive protein are typically increased. Definitive diagnosis is by temporal artery biopsy.

Patients should be treated immediately with corticosteroids (methylprednisolone 1,000 mg/d intravenously for at least 3 days, followed by prednisone 60-80 mg/d orally) to protect what vision remains and to preclude involvement, over the next days to weeks, of the contralateral eye (occurring in 50% of untreated patients). Prednisone may be gradually reduced over many months while monitoring the erythrocyte sedimentation rate.

Because giant cell arteritis is treatable, it is most important to distinguish it from idiopathic or nonarteritic anterior ischemic optic neuropathy as the cause of monocular visual loss. Patients with giant cell arteritis tend to be older (aged 70-80 years) and may have premonitory symptoms. Very helpful differential features are the erythrocyte sedimentation rate, exceeding 50 mm/h (Westergren) in most patients with giant cell arteritis, and an elevated C-reactive protein.

BINOCULAR DISORDERS

PAPILLEDEMA

Papilledema is painless, passive, typically bilateral disk swelling associated with increased intracranial pressure. Transient visual obscurations may precede frank disk swelling. Associated nonspecific symptoms of raised intracranial pressure include headache, nausea, vomiting, and diplopia occurring mainly from abducens (VI) nerve palsy.

The speed with which papilledema develops depends on the underlying cause. When intracranial pressure increases suddenly, as in subarachnoid or intracerebral hemorrhage, disk swelling may be seen within hours, but it most often evolves over days. Papilledema may require 2 to 3 months to resolve after restoration of normal intracranial pressure.

Funduscopic examination (see Figure 1-11) reveals (in order from onset) blurring of the nerve fiber layer, absence of venous pulsations (signifying intracranial pressure greater than approximately 200 mm Hg), hemorrhages in the nerve fiber layer, elevation of the disk surface with blurring of the margins, and disk hyperemia. Papilledema requires urgent evaluation to search for an intracranial mass and to exclude papillitis from, for example, meningeal carcinoma, sarcoidosis, or syphilis, which may produce a similar ophthalmoscopic appearance. A diagnosis of **idiopathic intracranial hypertension (pseudotumor cerebri)** is established by exclusion when cerebrospinal fluid (CSF) pressure is elevated, but an intracranial mass lesion and other disorders associated with intracranial hypertension (see Table 6-5) are excluded by history, laboratory, computed tomography (CT) scanning, or MRI with contrast enhancement, and meningeal inflammation is excluded by CSF examination. This idiopathic form, which is the most common, occurs most often in obese women during the childbearing years. Although it is usually self-limited, prolonged elevation of intracranial pressure with papilledema can lead to permanent visual loss (discussed further in Chapter 6, Headache & Facial Pain).

Less common causes of papilledema include congenital cyanotic heart disease and disorders associated with increased CSF protein content, such as spinal cord tumor and idiopathic inflammatory polyneuropathy (Guillain–Barré syndrome).

CHIASMAL LESIONS

Visual impairment is the most frequent symptom of a chiasmal lesion. The major lesions are tumors, especially those of pituitary origin (which can be associated with headache, acromegaly, amenorrhea, galactorrhea, and Cushing syndrome). Other causes include trauma, multiple sclerosis, and berry aneurysms. The classic pattern of chiasmal visual deficits is **bitemporal hemianopia** (see Figure 7-7). Except with **pituitary apoplexy** due to acute intrapituitary hemorrhage, chiasmal visual loss is gradual in onset with impairment in depth perception preceding lateral visual field loss. Associated involvement of the oculomotor (III), trochlear (IV), trigeminal (V), or abducens (VI) nerve suggests tumor expansion laterally into the cavernous sinus (discussed later).

Headache, endocrine abnormalities, and occasionally blurred or double vision may occur in patients with an enlarged sella turcica, in whom neither tumor nor increased intracranial pressure is found. This **empty sella syndrome** is most common in women who have had multiple pregnancies and occurs mainly between the fourth and seventh decades of life. Anterior pituitary deficiency occurs in a quarter of such women.

RETROCHIASMAL LESIONS

▶ Optic Tract & Lateral Geniculate Body

Lesions of the optic tract and lateral geniculate body are usually due to infarction. The resulting visual field abnormality is typically a **noncongruous homonymous hemianopia**; that is, the field defect is not the same in the two eyes. Associated hemisensory loss may occur with thalamic lesions.

▶ Optic Radiations

Lesions of the optic radiations produce a **congruous** (bilaterally symmetric) **homonymous hemianopia**. Visual acuity is normal in the unaffected portion of the field. With lesions in the **temporal lobe**, where tumors are the most common cause, the field deficit is denser superiorly than inferiorly, resulting in a **superior quadrantanopia** ("pie in the sky" deficit; see Figure 7-7).

Lesions affecting the optic radiations in the **parietal lobe** may be due to tumor or vascular disease and are usually associated with contralateral weakness and sensory loss. A gaze preference is common in the acute phase, with the eyes conjugately deviated to the side of the parietal lesion. The visual field abnormality is either complete homonymous hemianopia or **inferior quadrantanopia** (see Figure 7-7). The optokinetic response to a visual stimulus moved toward the side of the lesion is impaired, which is not the case with pure temporal or occipital lobe lesions.

Occipital Cortex

Lesions in the occipital cortex usually produce **homonymous hemianopia** affecting the contralateral visual field. The patient may be unaware of the visual deficit. Because the region of the occipital cortex in which the macula is represented is often supplied by branches of both the posterior and middle cerebral arteries (see Figure 7-4), visual field abnormalities of the occipital lobe, caused by vascular lesions, may show **sparing of macular vision** (see Figure 7-7). Such "macular sparing" may also result from bilateral cortical representation of the macular region of the visual field.

The most common cause of visual impairment in the occipital lobe is infarction in the posterior cerebral artery territory. Occipital lobe arteriovenous malformations (AVMs), vertebral angiography, and watershed infarction after cardiac arrest (Figure 13-22) are less common causes. Additional symptoms and signs of basilar artery ischemia may be seen. Tumors and occipital lobe AVMs are often associated with unformed visual hallucinations that are typically unilateral, stationary or moving, and brief or flickering; they can be colored or not colored.

Bilateral occipital lobe involvement produces **cortical blindness**. Pupillary reactions are normal, and bilateral macular sparing may preserve central (tunnel) vision. With more extensive lesions, denial of blindness may occur (**Anton syndrome**).

DISORDERS OF EYE MOVEMENT

GAZE PALSIES

Lesions in the cortex or brainstem may impair conjugate (yoked) movement of the eyes, producing gaze disorders. In milder gaze palsies, the eyes may move fully, but the speed or the amplitude of the fast eye movements is reduced.

HEMISPHERIC LESIONS

Acute hemispheric lesions produce tonic deviation of both eyes toward the side of the lesion and away from the side of the hemiparesis (**Figure 7-17A**). This gaze deviation may last for several days in alert patients (somewhat longer in comatose patients). Seizure discharges involving the frontal gaze centers can also produce gaze deviation by driving the eyes away from the discharging focus. When the ipsilateral motor cortex is

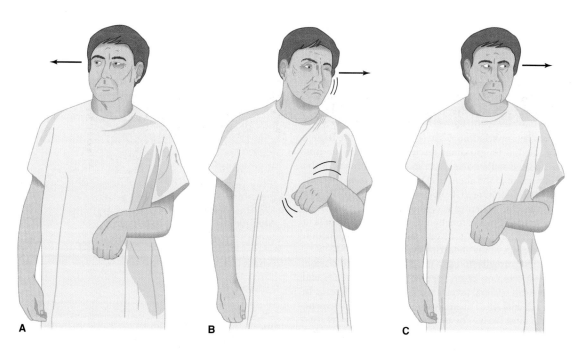

A   **B**   **C**

▲ **Figure 7-17.** Disorders of gaze associated with hemispheric and brainstem lesions. (**A**) Destructive lesion in the frontal lobe of the right cerebral hemisphere. (**B**) Seizure arising from the frontal lobe of the right cerebral hemisphere. (**C**) Destructive lesion in the right pons. Arrows indicate the direction of gaze preference (away from the hemiparetic side in [**A**] and toward the convulsing or hemiparetic side in [**B**] and [**C**]).

also involved, producing focal motor seizures, the patient gazes toward the side of the seizure-induced motor activity (**Figure 7-17B**).

MIDBRAIN LESIONS

Lesions of the dorsal midbrain affect the center responsible for voluntary upward gaze and may therefore produce upgaze paralysis. In addition, all or some of the features of **Parinaud syndrome** may occur: preserved reflex vertical eye movements with the doll's head maneuver or Bell phenomenon (elevation of the eye upon eyelid closure), nystagmus (especially on downward gaze and typically associated with retraction of the eyes), paralysis of accommodation, midsized pupils, and light-near dissociation.

PONTINE LESIONS

The pontine gaze center is in the region of the paramedian pontine reticular formation (see Figure 7-6). Brainstem lesions at the level of the pontine gaze centers produce disorders of conjugate horizontal gaze but, unlike hemispheric lesions, cause eye deviation toward, rather than away from, the side of the hemiparesis (**Figure 7-17C**). This occurs because the corticobulbar pathways that regulate gaze have crossed at this level, but the descending (pyramidal) motor pathways have not. Brainstem gaze palsies are characteristically far more resistant to attempts to move the eyes (via the doll's head maneuver or caloric stimulation) than are hemispheric gaze pareses. In addition, gaze palsies from brainstem lesions are commonly associated with abducens (VI) nerve palsies because of the proximity of the abducens nucleus to the pontine gaze center.

INTERNUCLEAR OPHTHALMOPLEGIA

Internuclear ophthalmoplegia (INO) results from lesions of the **medial longitudinal fasciculus** between the mid pons and the oculomotor nerve nucleus that result in the disconnection of the abducens (VI) nucleus from the contralateral oculomotor (III) nucleus (see Figure 7-6). The site of the INO is named according to the side on which oculomotor (III) nerve function is impaired. INO results in a characteristic disconjugate gaze with impaired adduction and nystagmus of the abducting eye (see Figure 7-15).

An INO usually implies intrinsic brainstem disease. The most common cause, especially in young adults and patients with bilateral involvement, is multiple sclerosis. In older patients and those with unilateral involvement, stroke is most likely. These two causes encompass at least 80% of all cases. Rarer causes include brainstem encephalitis, intrinsic brainstem tumors, syringobulbia, sedative drug intoxication, and Wernicke encephalopathy. Because oculomotor muscle weakness of myasthenia gravis can mimic a lesion of the medial longitudinal fasciculus, it must be ruled out in patients with isolated INO.

OCULAR NERVE PALSIES

OCULOMOTOR (III) NERVE LESIONS

Lesions of the oculomotor (III) nerve can occur at any of several levels. The most common causes are listed in **Table 7-3**; oculomotor disorders resulting from diabetes are discussed separately later.

▶ Brainstem

Within the brainstem, other neurologic signs permit localization of the lesion; associated contralateral hemiplegia (Weber syndrome) and contralateral ataxia (Benedikt syndrome) are the most common vascular syndromes.

▶ Subarachnoid Space

As the oculomotor (III) nerve exits the brainstem in the interpeduncular space, it is susceptible to injury from trauma and from aneurysms of the posterior communicating artery. Such compressive lesions typically impair the pupillary light reflex, which tends to be spared with ischemic (eg, diabetic) lesions.

▶ Cavernous Sinus

In the cavernous sinus (**Figure 7-18**), the oculomotor (III) nerve is usually involved together with the trochlear (IV) and abducens (VI) nerves and the first (V1) and

Table 7-3. Causes of Oculomotor (III), Trochlear (IV), and Abducens (VI) Nerve Lesions.[1]

Cause	Nerve III	Nerve IV	Nerve VI	Multiple
	Percent of cases			
Unknown	24	32	26	12
Vasculopathy[2]	20	18	12	4
Aneurysm	16	1	4	8
Trauma	15	29	5	18
Neoplasm	13	5	22	36
Other[3]	12	15	21	22

[1]Percent of all cases by nerve: III, 25%; IV, 12%; VI, 43%; multiple, 13%.
[2]Includes diabetes.
[3]Includes (in order of frequency) congenital, neurosurgical, multiple sclerosis, stroke, meningitis or encephalitis, carotid cavernous fistula, myasthenia, ophthalmoplegic migraine, hydrocephalus, subarachnoid hemorrhage, arteriovenous malformation, spinocerebellar atrophy, sinus disease, radiation, chemotherapy, and herpes zoster.
Data from Richards BW, Jones FR Jr, Younge BR. Causes and prognosis in 4,278 cases of paralysis of the oculomotor, trochlear, and abducens cranial nerves. *Am J Ophthalmol.* 1992;113:489-496.

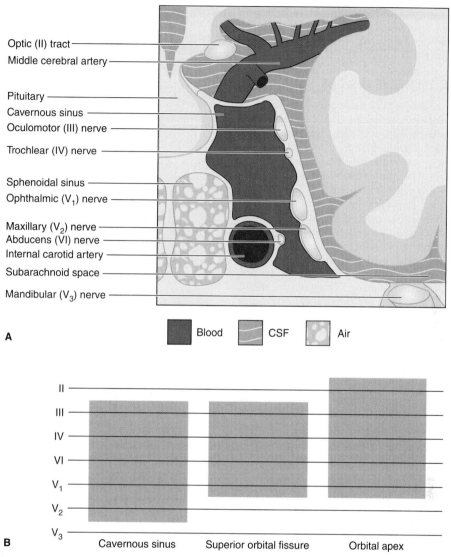

Figure 7-18. Position of cranial nerves in the cavernous sinus and adjacent structures. **(A)** Coronal view through the cavernous sinus, with the midline at left and the temporal lobe at right. **(B)** Location of cranial nerves as they course anteriorly (left to right) in relation to the cavernous sinus, superior orbital fissure, and orbital apex. Note that a lesion in the cavernous sinus spares the optic (II) and mandibular (V₃) nerves, a lesion in the superior orbital fissure additionally spares the maxillary (V₂) nerve, and a lesion in the orbital apex spares both V_2 and V_3 but may involve II.

sometimes the second (V2) division of the trigeminal nerve. Horner syndrome may occur. Oculomotor (III) nerve lesions in the cavernous sinus tend to produce partial deficits that may or may not spare the pupil.

▶ Orbit

Unlike cavernous sinus lesions, orbital lesions that affect the oculomotor (III) nerve are often associated with optic (II) nerve involvement and exophthalmos; however,

disorders of the orbit and cavernous sinus may be clinically indistinguishable except by CT scanning or MRI.

TROCHLEAR (IV) NERVE LESIONS

Head trauma, often minor, is a common cause of an isolated trochlear (IV) nerve palsy (Table 7-3). Although trochlear palsies in middle-aged and elderly patients are frequently attributed to vascular disease or diabetes, they often occur without obvious cause. For patients with isolated nontraumatic trochlear (IV) nerve palsies in whom diabetes, myasthenia, thyroid disease, and orbital mass lesions have been excluded, observation is the appropriate clinical approach.

ABDUCENS (VI) NERVE LESIONS

Patients with abducens (VI) nerve lesions complain of horizontal diplopia due to weakness of the lateral rectus muscle. Lateral rectus palsies can occur as a result of disorders of either the muscle itself or the abducens (VI) nerve, and each of these possibilities should be investigated. The causes of abducens (VI) nerve lesions are summarized in Table 7-3. In elderly patients, abducens (VI) nerve involvement is most often idiopathic or caused by vascular disease or diabetes, but the erythrocyte sedimentation rate should be determined to exclude a rare presentation of giant cell arteritis. Imaging of the base of the skull is indicated to exclude nasopharyngeal carcinoma or other tumors. In painless abducens palsy, when the above studies are normal, other systemic and neurologic symptoms are absent, and intracranial pressure is not elevated, patients can be followed conservatively. A trial of prednisone (60 mg/d orally for 5 days) may produce dramatic relief in painful abducens (VI) nerve palsy, giving support to a tentative diagnosis of idiopathic inflammation of the superior orbital fissure (**superior orbital fissure syndrome**) or cavernous sinus (**Tolosa–Hunt syndrome**). Persistent pain despite treatment with corticosteroids should prompt investigation of the cavernous sinus by CT scanning or MRI, followed, in some cases, by angiography. The presence of a concurrent Horner syndrome localizes the underlying lesion to the cavernous sinus.

DIABETIC OPHTHALMOPLEGIAS

An isolated oculomotor (III), trochlear (IV), or abducens (VI) nerve lesion may occur in patients with diabetes mellitus; noninvasive imaging procedures (CT scanning or MRI) reveal no abnormality. Diabetic oculomotor (III) nerve lesions are characterized by **pupillary sparing**, which is commonly attributed to infarction of the central portion of the nerve with sparing of the more peripherally situated fibers that mediate pupillary constriction. Pupil-sparing oculomotor palsies also can be seen with compressive, infiltrative, or inflammatory lesions of the oculomotor (III) nerve or with infarcts, hemorrhages, or tumors that affect the oculomotor (III) nucleus or fascicle within the midbrain. Pain, when present, may be severe enough to suggest aneurysmal expansion as a likely diagnosis.

In known diabetics, painful ophthalmoplegia with exophthalmos and metabolic acidosis requires urgent attention to determine the possibility of fungal infection in the paranasal sinus, orbit, or cavernous sinus by **mucormycosis**. The diagnosis is usually made by biopsy of the nasal

Table 7-4. Causes of Painful Ophthalmoplegia.

Orbit
Orbital pseudotumor
Sinusitis
Tumor (primary or metastatic)
Infection (bacterial or fungal)
Cavernous sinus
Tolosa–Hunt syndrome (idiopathic granulomatous inflammation)
Tumor (primary or metastatic)
Carotid artery-cavernous sinus fistula or thrombosis
Aneurysm
Sella and posterior fossa
Pituitary tumor or apoplexy
Aneurysm
Metastatic tumor
Other
Diabetes
Migraine
Giant cell arteritis

mucosa. Urgent treatment with amphotericin B and surgical debridement of necrotic tissue is required.

PAINFUL OPHTHALMOPLEGIAS

Dysfunction of one or more of the ocular motor nerves with accompanying pain may be produced by lesions located anywhere from the posterior fossa to the orbit (**Table 7-4**). An evaluation should consist of careful documentation of the clinical course, inspection and palpation of the globe for proptosis (localizing the process to the orbit or anterior cavernous sinus), auscultation over the globe to detect a bruit (supporting a diagnosis of carotid artery-cavernous sinus fistula or another vascular anomaly), and evaluation for diabetes. Useful laboratory studies include blood glucose, orbital CT scan or MRI, carotid arteriography, and orbital venography.

Therapy for these disorders is dictated by the specific diagnosis. Idiopathic inflammation of the orbit (**orbital pseudotumor**) or cavernous sinus (**Tolosa–Hunt syndrome**) responds dramatically to corticosteroids (prednisone 60-100 mg/d orally). However, the pain and ocular signs associated with some neoplasms may also improve transiently during corticosteroid therapy so that a specific etiologic diagnosis may depend on biopsy.

MYASTHENIA GRAVIS

Myasthenia eventually involves the ocular muscles in approximately 90% of patients; more than 60% present with ocular muscle involvement. The syndrome is painless, pupillary responses are always normal, and there are no sensory abnormalities. The diagnosis is confirmed by a positive response to intravenous edrophonium (Tensilon). Details of this disorder are discussed in Chapter 9, Motor Disorders. The classic disorder is associated with observable fatigue of eyelid elevation during sustained upgaze for 60 seconds.

OCULAR MYOPATHIES

Ocular myopathies are painless syndromes that spare pupillary function and are usually bilateral. The most common is the myopathy of **hyperthyroidism**, a cause of double vision beginning in midlife or later. Many patients are otherwise clinically euthyroid at the time of diagnosis. Double vision on attempted elevation of the globe is the most common symptom, but in mild cases there is lid retraction during staring or lid lag during rapid up-and-down movements of the eye. Exophthalmos is a characteristic finding, especially in advanced cases (see Figure 7-11). The diagnosis can be confirmed by the forced duction test, which detects mechanical resistance to forced movement of the anesthetized globe in the orbit. This restrictive ocular myopathy is usually self-limited. The patient should be referred for testing of thyroid function and treated for hyperthyroidism as appropriate.

The progressive external ophthalmoplegias (PEO) are a group of syndromes characterized by slowly progressive, symmetric impairment of ocular movement that cannot be overcome by caloric stimulation. Pupillary function is spared, and there is no pain; ptosis may be prominent. This clinical picture can be produced by **ocular** or **oculopharyngeal muscular dystrophy**. High-resolution T1-weighted orbital MRI show "spongiform" signal abnormalities in ocular muscles. Progressive external ophthalmoplegia associated with myotonic contraction on percussion of muscle groups (classically, the thenar group in the palm) suggests the diagnosis of **myotonic dystrophy**. In **Kearns–Sayre–Daroff syndrome**, which has been associated with deletions in muscle mitochondrial DNA, progressive external ophthalmoplegia is accompanied by pigmentary degeneration of the retina, cardiac conduction defects, cerebellar ataxia, and elevated CSF protein levels. The muscle biopsy shows ragged red fibers that reflect the presence of abnormal mitochondria. These PEO syndromes with associated extra orbital co-morbidities are referred to as "ophthalmoplegia plus" syndromes. Disorders that simulate progressive external ophthalmoplegia include progressive supranuclear palsy and Parkinson disease, but in these conditions the impairment of (usually vertical) eye movements can be overcome by oculocephalic or caloric stimulation.

Disorders of Equilibrium

(Continued on Next Page)

APPROACH TO DIAGNOSIS

Equilibrium is the ability to maintain orientation of the body and its parts in relation to external space. It depends on continuous visual, labyrinthine, and proprioceptive somatosensory input and its integration in the brainstem and cerebellum. Disorders of equilibrium result from diseases that affect central or peripheral vestibular pathways, the cerebellum, or sensory pathways involved in proprioception. Such disorders usually present with one of two clinical problems: **vertigo** or **ataxia**.

VERTIGO

Vertigo is the illusion of movement of the body or the environment. It may be associated with other symptoms, such as **impulsion** (a sensation that the body is being hurled or pulled in space), **oscillopsia** (a visual illusion of moving back and forth), nausea, vomiting, or gait ataxia.

Vertigo must be distinguished from nonvertiginous **dizziness**, which includes sensations of light-headedness, faintness, or giddiness not associated with an illusion of movement. In contrast to vertigo, these sensations are produced by conditions that deprive the brain of blood, oxygen, or glucose (eg, excessive vagal stimulation, orthostatic hypotension, cardiac arrhythmia, myocardial ischemia, hypoxia, or hypoglycemia) and may culminate in loss of consciousness (**syncope**; see Chapter 12, Seizures & Syncope).

The first step in the differential diagnosis of vertigo is to localize the pathologic process to the peripheral or central vestibular pathways (**Figure 8-1**). Certain characteristics of vertigo, including the presence of any associated abnormalities, can help differentiate between peripheral and central causes (**Table 8-1**).

PERIPHERAL VERTIGO

Peripheral vestibular lesions affect the **labyrinth** of the inner ear or the vestibular division of the **vestibulocochlear (VIII) nerve**. Vertigo from peripheral lesions tends to be intermittent, lasts for briefer periods, and produces more distress than vertigo of central origin (see next section). **Nystagmus** (rhythmic oscillation of the eyes) is always present with peripheral vertigo; in this setting it is usually unidirectional and never vertical. Peripheral lesions commonly produce additional symptoms of inner ear or vestibulocochlear (VIII) nerve dysfunction, such as **hearing loss** and **tinnitus** (the illusion of hearing a nonexistent sound, such as ringing in the ears).

CENTRAL VERTIGO

Vertigo of central nervous system origin usually results from lesions that affect the brainstem **vestibular nuclei** or their connections; rarely, vertigo is produced by a cerebral cortical lesion, such as when it occurs as a symptom of complex partial seizures (see Chapter 12, Seizures & Syncope).

Central vertigo may occur with or without **nystagmus**; if nystagmus is present, it can be vertical, unidirectional, or multidirectional and may differ in character in the two eyes. (Vertical nystagmus is oscillation in a vertical plane; nystagmus produced by upgaze or downgaze is not necessarily in the vertical plane.) Vertigo from central lesions may be accompanied by intrinsic brainstem or cerebellar signs, such as **motor or sensory deficits**, **hyperreflexia**, **extensor plantar responses**, **dysarthria**, or **limb ataxia**.

ATAXIA

Ataxia is incoordination or clumsiness of movement that is not the result of muscle weakness. It can be caused by vestibular, cerebellar, or sensory (proprioceptive) disorders. Ataxia can affect eye movement, speech (producing dysarthria), individual limbs, the trunk, stance, or gait (**Table 8-2**).

VESTIBULAR ATAXIA

The same central and peripheral lesions that cause peripheral or central vertigo can also produce vestibular ataxia. **Nystagmus** is frequently present and is typically unilateral

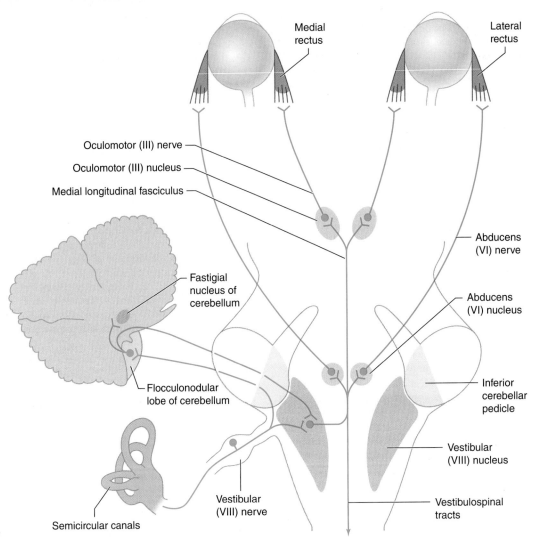

Figure 8-1. Peripheral and central vestibular pathways. The vestibular (VIII) nerve terminates in the vestibular (VIII) nucleus in the brainstem and midline cerebellar structures that project to the vestibular nucleus. From here, bilateral pathways in the medial longitudinal fasciculus ascend to the abducens (VI) and oculomotor (III) nuclei and descend to the spinal cord (vestibulospinal tracts).

and most pronounced on gaze away from the side of vestibular involvement. Dysarthria is not a component of vestibular ataxia. Vestibular ataxia is **gravity-dependent**: Incoordination of the limbs becomes apparent only when the patient attempts to stand or walk.

CEREBELLAR ATAXIA

Cerebellar ataxia is produced by lesions of the **cerebellum** or its afferent or efferent connections in the **cerebellar peduncles**, **red nucleus**, **pons**, or **spinal cord**. Because of the crossed connection between the frontal cerebral cortex

and the cerebellum, unilateral frontal disease can also occasionally mimic a disorder of the contralateral cerebellar hemisphere. The clinical manifestations of cerebellar ataxia consist of irregularities in the rate, rhythm, amplitude, and force of voluntary movements.

▶ Hypotonia

Cerebellar ataxia is commonly associated with reduced muscle tone (hypotonia), which results in defective posture maintenance. Limbs are easily displaced by a relatively small force and, when shaken by the examiner, exhibit an

Table 8-1. Characteristics of Peripheral and Central Vertigo.

	Peripheral	Central
Vertigo	Often intermittent; severe	Often constant; usually less severe
Nystagmus	Always present, unidirectional, never vertical	May be absent, uni- or bidirectional, may be vertical
Hearing loss or tinnitus	Often present	Rarely present
Intrinsic brainstem or cerebellar signs[1]	Absent	Typically present

[1]Motor or sensory deficits, hyperreflexia, extensor plantar responses, dysarthria, or limb ataxia.

increased range of excursion. The range of arm swing during walking may be similarly increased. Tendon reflexes take on a **pendular** quality, so that several oscillations of the limb may occur after the reflex is elicited. When muscles are contracted against resistance that is then removed, the antagonist muscle fails to **check** the movement and compensatory muscular relaxation does not occur promptly. This results in **rebound** movement of the limb.

▶ Incoordination

In addition to hypotonia, cerebellar ataxia is associated with incoordination of voluntary movements. Simple movements are delayed in onset, and their rates of acceleration and deceleration are decreased. The rate, rhythm, amplitude, and force of movements fluctuate, so they appear jerky. Clinical manifestations include **terminal**

dysmetria, or "overshoot" when the limb is directed at a target, and terminal **intention tremor** as the limb approaches the target. More complex movements may be decomposed into a succession of individual movements rather than a single smooth act (**asynergia**). Movements that involve rapid changes in direction or greater physiologic complexity, such as walking, are most affected.

▶ Eye Movement Abnormalities

Because the cerebellum has a prominent role in controlling eye movements, ocular abnormalities are common in cerebellar disease. These include **nystagmus** and related ocular oscillations, **gaze paresis**, and defective saccadic and pursuit movements.

▶ Anatomic Basis of Clinical Signs

Various anatomic regions of the cerebellum (**Figure 8-2**) have distinct functions, corresponding to the somatotopic organization of their motor, sensory, visual, and auditory connections (**Figure 8-3**).

1. **Midline lesions**—The middle zone of the cerebellum—the vermis and flocculonodular lobe and their associated subcortical (fastigial) nuclei—is involved in the control of axial functions, including eye movements, head and trunk posture, stance, and gait. Midline cerebellar disease results in a clinical syndrome characterized by **nystagmus** and other disorders of ocular motility, **dysarthria**, oscillation of the head and trunk (**titubation**), instability of stance, and **gait ataxia** (**Table 8-3**). Selective involvement of the superior cerebellar vermis, as in alcoholic cerebellar degeneration, produces exclusively or primarily gait ataxia, as predicted by the somatotopic map of the cerebellum (see Figure 8-3).

2. **Hemispheric lesions**—The lateral cerebellum (cerebellar hemispheres) helps coordinate movements and maintain tone in the ipsilateral limbs. The hemispheres

Table 8-2. Characteristics of Vestibular, Cerebellar, and Sensory Ataxia.

	Vestibular	Cerebellar	Sensory
Vertigo	Present	May be present	Absent
Nystagmus	Present	Often present	Absent
Dysarthria	Absent	May be present	Absent
Limb ataxia	Absent	Usually present (one limb, unilateral, legs only, or all limbs)	Present (typically legs)
Stance	May be able to stand with feet together; typically worse with eyes closed	Unable to stand with feet together and eyes either open or closed	Often able to stand with feet together and eyes open but not with eyes closed (Romberg sign)
Vibration and position sense	Normal	Normal	Impaired
Ankle reflexes	Normal	Normal	Depressed or absent

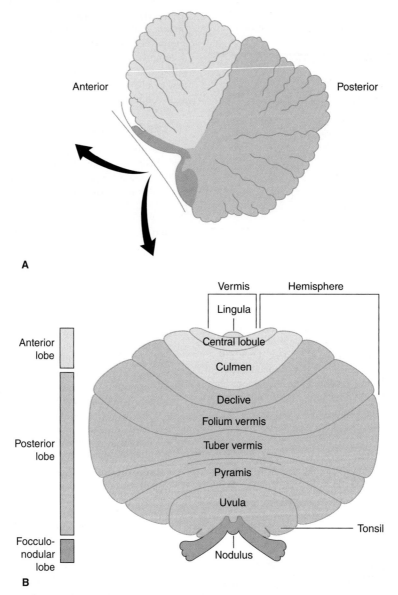

Anterior   Posterior

A

Vermis   Hemisphere

Lingula

Anterior
lobe   Central lobule

Culmen

Declive

Folium vermis

Posterior
lobe   Tuber vermis

Pyramis

Uvula

Tonsil

Focculo-
nodular   Nodulus
lobe

B

▲ **Figure 8-2.** Anatomic divisions of the cerebellum, shown in midsagittal view (**A**), or unfolded (**arrows**) and viewed from behind (**B**).

also regulate ipsilateral gaze. Disorders affecting one cerebellar hemisphere cause **ipsilateral hemiataxia** and limb hypotonia as well as nystagmus and transient **ipsilateral gaze paresis** (inability to look voluntarily toward the affected side). Involvement of the medial (paravermian) portion of either cerebellar hemisphere can also produce **dysarthria**.

3. **Diffuse disease**—Many cerebellar disorders—typically toxic, metabolic, and degenerative conditions—affect the cerebellum diffusely. The clinical picture in such states combines the features of midline and bilateral hemisphere disease.

SENSORY ATAXIA

Sensory ataxia results from disorders that affect the proprioceptive pathways in peripheral sensory nerves, sensory roots, posterior columns of the spinal cord, or medial lemnisci. Thalamic and parietal lobe lesions are rare causes of contralateral sensory hemiataxia.

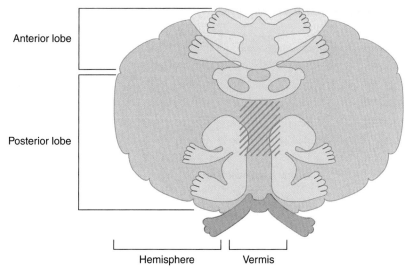

Anterior lobe

Posterior lobe

Hemisphere   Vermis

▲ **Figure 8-3.** Functional organization of the cerebellum. The view is similar to that in Figure 8-2B but is of a monkey rather than a human cerebellum. The three cerebellar homunculi represent areas to which proprioceptive and tactile stimuli project, and the stripes represent areas to which auditory and visual stimuli project.

Sensations of joint position and movement (**kinesthesis**) originate in pacinian corpuscles and unencapsulated nerve endings in joint capsules, ligaments, muscle, and periosteum. These sensations are transmitted via heavily myelinated A fibers of primary afferent neurons, which enter the dorsal horn of the spinal cord and ascend uncrossed in the posterior columns (**Figure 8-4**). Proprioceptive information from the legs is conveyed in the medially located fasciculus gracilis, and information from the arms is conveyed in the more laterally situated fasciculus cuneatus. These tracts synapse on second-order sensory neurons in the nucleus gracilis and nucleus cuneatus in the lower medulla. The second-order neurons decussate as internal arcuate fibers and ascend in the contralateral medial lemniscus. They terminate in the ventral posterior nucleus of the thalamus, from which third-order sensory neurons project to the parietal cortex.

Sensory ataxia from polyneuropathy or posterior column lesions typically affects the gait and legs in symmetric fashion; the arms are involved to a lesser extent or are spared entirely. Examination reveals impaired sensation of **joint position** in the affected limbs, and **vibration sense** is also commonly disturbed. Vertigo, nystagmus, and dysarthria are characteristically absent.

Table 8-3. Clinical Patterns of Cerebellar Ataxia.

Pattern of Involvement	Signs	Causes
Midline	Nystagmus, dysarthria, head and trunk titubation, gait ataxia	Tumor, multiple sclerosis
Superior vermis	Gait ataxia	Wernicke encephalopathy, alcoholic cerebellar degeneration, tumor, multiple sclerosis
Cerebellar hemisphere	Nystagmus, ipsilateral gaze paresis, dysarthria, ipsilateral hypotonia, ipsilateral limb ataxia, gait ataxia, falling to side of lesion	Infarction, hemorrhage, tumor, multiple sclerosis
Pancerebellar	Nystagmus, bilateral gaze paresis, dysarthria, bilateral hypotonia, bilateral limb ataxia, gait ataxia	Sedative drug intoxication, hypothyroidism, autosomal dominant spinocerebellar ataxias, paraneoplastic cerebellar degeneration, Wilson disease, infectious and parainfectious encephalomyelitis, Creutzfeldt–Jakob disease, multiple sclerosis

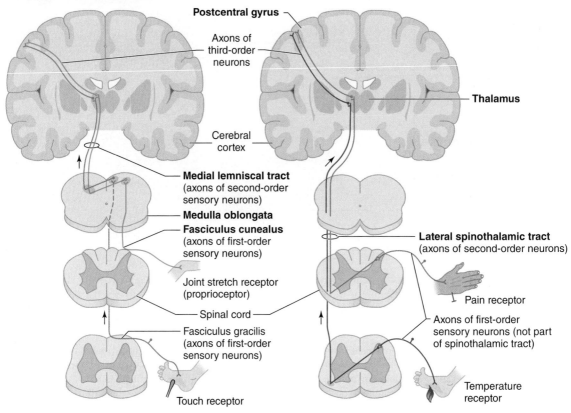

Figure 8-4. Pathways mediating proprioception (left, light blue) and other somatic sensory modalities (touch, left and pain and temperature, right). (Used with permission from Fox SI. *Human Physiology.* 10th ed. Boston, MA: McGraw-Hill; 2008.)

HISTORY

SYMPTOMS & SIGNS

▶ Vertigo

True vertigo must be distinguished from a light-headed or presyncopal sensation. Vertigo is typically described as spinning, rotating, or moving. When the description is vague, the patient should be asked specifically if the symptom is associated with a **sense of movement**, of either the patient or the environment.

The circumstances under which symptoms occur may also be diagnostically helpful. Vertigo is often brought on by changes in head position. In contrast, symptoms that occur upon arising after prolonged recumbency suggest orthostatic hypotension, and may be relieved immediately by sitting or lying down. Orthostatic hypotension and other cerebral hypoperfusion states can also lead to loss of consciousness, which is rarely associated with true vertigo.

Symptoms associated with vertigo may help to localize the site of the causal lesion. Hearing loss or tinnitus strongly suggests a disorder of the peripheral vestibular apparatus (labyrinth or vestibulocochlear [VIII] nerve). Dysarthria, dysphagia, diplopia, or focal weakness or sensory loss affecting the face or limbs points to a likely central (brainstem) lesion.

▶ Ataxia

Ataxia associated with vertigo suggests a vestibular disorder, whereas ataxia with numbness or tingling in the legs is common in patients with sensory ataxia. Because proprioceptive deficits may be partly compensated for by other sensory cues, patients with sensory ataxia may report that their balance is improved by watching their feet when they walk or by using a cane or the arm of a companion for support. Thus, they may be less steady in the dark and have more difficulty descending than ascending stairs.

ONSET & TIME COURSE

The mode of onset and time course may help to identify the cause of a disorder of equilibrium.

▶ Sudden

Sudden onset of disequilibrium, without a prior history of such events, occurs with infarcts and hemorrhages in the brainstem or cerebellum (eg, lateral medullary syndrome, cerebellar hemorrhage or infarction).

▶ Episodic

Episodic disequilibrium of acute onset suggests transient ischemic attacks in the basilar artery distribution, benign positional vertigo, Ménière disease, or vestibular migraine. Disequilibrium from transient ischemic attacks is usually accompanied by cranial nerve deficits, neurologic signs in the limbs, or both. Ménière disease is usually associated with progressive hearing loss and tinnitus as well as vertigo. Vestibular migraine produces headache or other migrainous symptoms (see Chapter 6, Headache & Facial Pain).

▶ Chronic & Progressive

Chronic, progressive disequilibrium evolving over weeks to months is most suggestive of a toxic, nutritional, immune-mediated, or neoplastic disorder. Evolution over months to years is characteristic of an inherited spinocerebellar degeneration.

MEDICAL HISTORY

The medical history should be scrutinized for diseases that affect the sensory pathways (vitamin B_{12} deficiency, syphilis), cerebellum (hypothyroidism), or both (multiple sclerosis, tumors, paraneoplastic syndromes) and for drugs that impair vestibular or cerebellar function (ethanol, sedative drugs, phenytoin, aminoglycoside antibiotics, quinine, salicylates).

FAMILY HISTORY

A hereditary degenerative disorder may be the cause of chronic, progressive cerebellar ataxia. Such disorders include spinocerebellar degenerations, Friedreich ataxia, ataxia-telangiectasia, and Wilson disease.

GENERAL PHYSICAL EXAMINATION

Several features of the general physical examination may provide clues to the underlying disorder.

1. **Orthostatic hypotension** is associated with tabes dorsalis, polyneuropathies, and spinocerebellar degenerations.
2. **Skin** may show oculocutaneous telangiectasia (ataxia-telangiectasia), or it may be dry with brittle hair (hypothyroidism) or have a lemon-yellow coloration (vitamin B_{12} deficiency).
3. **Pigmented corneal (Kayser–Fleischer) rings** are seen in Wilson disease (see Chapter 11, Movement Disorders).

4. **Skeletal abnormalities** include kyphoscoliosis in Friedreich ataxia, hypertrophic or hyperextensible joints in tabes dorsalis, and pes cavus in certain hereditary neuropathies. Abnormalities at the craniocervical junction may be associated with Arnold–Chiari malformation or other congenital anomalies involving the posterior fossa.

NEUROLOGIC EXAMINATION

MENTAL STATUS EXAMINATION

Acute confusional state with ataxia suggests ethanol or sedative drug intoxication or Wernicke encephalopathy. **Dementia** with cerebellar ataxia is seen in Wilson disease, prion diseases (Creutzfeldt–Jakob disease and Gerstmann–Sträussler–Scheinker syndrome), hypothyroidism, paraneoplastic syndromes, and some spinocerebellar degenerations. Dementia with sensory ataxia suggests syphilitic taboparesis or vitamin B_{12} deficiency. **Amnesia** and cerebellar ataxia are associated with chronic alcoholism (**Korsakoff amnestic syndrome**, see Chapter 5, Dementia & Amnestic Disorders).

STANCE & GAIT

Observation of stance and gait is helpful for distinguishing among vestibular, cerebellar, and sensory ataxia. Ataxia from any cause can produce a wide-based and unsteady stance and gait, often associated with reeling or lurching movements.

▶ Stance

An ataxic patient asked to stand with the feet together may be reluctant or unable to do so. With urging, the patient may gradually move the feet closer together but will typically leave some space between them.

1. Patients with **sensory ataxia** and some with **vestibular ataxia** may be able to stand with the feet together and eyes open, using vision to compensate for the loss of proprioceptive or labyrinthine input. When the eyes are closed, eliminating visual cues, there is increased unsteadiness and sometimes falling (**Romberg sign**). With a vestibular lesion, the tendency is to fall toward the side of the lesion.
2. Patients with **cerebellar ataxia** cannot compensate for their deficit using visual input, and are unstable on their feet whether the eyes are open or closed.

▶ Gait

1. The gait in **cerebellar ataxia** is wide-based, often with a staggering quality that can suggest drunkenness. Oscillation of the head or trunk (**titubation**) may be present. With a unilateral cerebellar hemisphere lesion, there is a tendency to deviate toward the side of the lesion when the patient tries to walk in a straight line or circle or marches in place with eyes closed. **Tandem** (heel-to-toe)

gait, which requires walking with an especially narrow base, is always impaired in cerebellar ataxia.

2. In **sensory ataxia**, the gait is also wide-based, and tandem gait is poor. In addition, the feet are typically lifted high off the ground and slapped down heavily (**steppage gait**) to enhance proprioceptive input. Stability may be dramatically improved by letting the patient use a cane or lightly rest a hand on the examiner's arm for support. If the patient attempts to walk in the dark or with eyes closed, gait is much more impaired.

3. Gait ataxia may also be a manifestation of **conversion disorder** or **malingering**. The most helpful observation in identifying factitious gait ataxia is that such patients may exhibit wildly reeling or lurching movements from which they are able to recover without falling, whereas recovery from such awkward positions actually requires excellent equilibrium.

CRANIAL NERVES

Abnormalities of extraocular (III, IV, and VI) and vestibulocochlear (VIII) nerve function are typically present with vestibular disease and often present with lesions of the cerebellum.

▶ Eye Movements

1. The eyes are examined in the primary position of gaze (looking directly forward) to detect misalignment in the horizontal or vertical plane.

2. The patient is asked to turn the eyes in each of the cardinal directions of gaze (see Chapter 1, Neurologic History & Examination) to detect ocular nerve palsy or **gaze paresis** (inability to move the two eyes coordinately in any of the cardinal directions of gaze).

3. **Nystagmus**—an involuntary oscillation of the eyes—is characterized in terms of the positions of gaze in which it occurs (**gaze-evoked nystagmus**), its amplitude, and the direction of its fast phase. **Pendular nystagmus**, usually due to visual impairment beginning in infancy, has the same velocity in both directions, whereas **jerk nystagmus** has fast (vestibular-induced) and slow (cortical) phases. The direction of jerk nystagmus is defined by the direction of the fast component.

4. Fast voluntary eye movements (**saccades**) are elicited by having the patient rapidly shift gaze between targets in different regions of the visual field. Slow voluntary eye movements (**pursuits**) are assessed by having the patient track a slowly moving target such as the examiner's finger.

5. **Peripheral** vestibular disorders produce unidirectional horizontal jerk nystagmus that is maximal on gaze away from the involved side.

6. **Central** vestibular disorders can cause unidirectional or bidirectional horizontal nystagmus, vertical nystagmus, or gaze paresis.

Table 8-4. Assessment of Hearing Loss.

	Weber Test	**Rinne Test**
Normal	Sound perceived as coming from midline	Air conduction > bone conduction
Sensorineural hearing loss	Sound perceived as coming from normal ear	Air conduction > bone conduction
Conductive hearing loss	Sound perceived as coming from affected ear	Bone conduction > air conduction on affected side

7. **Cerebellar** lesions are associated with a wide range of ocular abnormalities, including gaze paresis, defective saccades or pursuits, nystagmus in any or all directions, and **ocular dysmetria** (overshoot of visual targets during saccadic eye movement).

▶ Hearing

Preliminary examination of the vestibulocochlear (VIII) nerve should include otoscopic inspection of the auditory canals and tympanic membranes, assessment of auditory acuity in each ear, and Weber and Rinne tests (**Table 8-4**) performed with a 256-Hz tuning fork.

1. In the **Weber test**, unilateral **sensorineural** hearing loss (from lesions of the cochlea or vestibulocochlear nerve) causes the patient to perceive the sound produced by a vibrating tuning fork placed at the vertex of the skull as coming from the normal ear. With a **conductive** (external or middle ear) disorder, sound is localized to the abnormal ear.

2. The **Rinne test** may also distinguish between sensorineural and conductive defects in the affected ear. Air conduction (tested by holding the vibrating tuning fork next to the external auditory canal) normally produces a louder sound than does bone conduction (tested by placing the base of the tuning fork over the mastoid bone). This also occurs with **sensorineural** hearing loss due to vestibulocochlear nerve lesions but is reversed in **conductive** hearing loss.

▶ Positional Vertigo Testing

When vertigo occurs with a change in position, the Nylen–Bárány or Dix–Hallpike maneuver (**Figure 8-5**) is used to try to reproduce the precipitating circumstance. The head is rapidly lowered 30 degrees below horizontal and the eyes are observed for nystagmus, while the patient is asked to note the onset, severity, and cessation of vertigo. This is repeated with the head and eyes turned first to the right and then to the left.

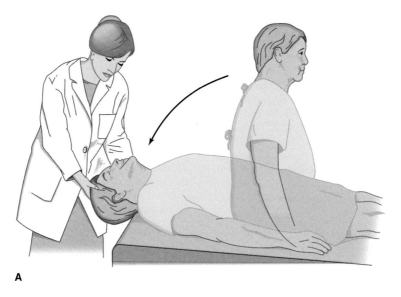

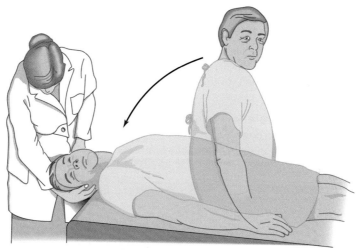

▲ **Figure 8-5.** Test for positional vertigo and nystagmus. The patient is seated on a table with the head and eyes directed forward (**A**) and is then quickly lowered to a supine position with the head over the table edge, 45 degrees below horizontal. The patient's eyes are then observed for nystagmus, and the patient is asked to report any vertigo. The test is repeated with the patient's head and eyes turned 45 degrees to the right (**B**), and again with the head and eyes turned 45 degrees to the left (not shown).

Positional nystagmus and **vertigo** are usually associated with peripheral vestibular lesions and are most often a feature of **benign positional vertigo.** This is typically characterized by severe distress, a **latency** of several seconds between assumption of the position and the onset of vertigo and nystagmus, a tendency for the response to remit spontaneously (**fatigue**) as the position is maintained, and attenuation of the response (**habituation**) as the offending position is repeatedly assumed (**Table 8-5**).

Table 8-5. Characteristics of Positional Nystagmus.

Feature	Peripheral Lesion	Central Lesion
Vertigo	Severe	Mild
Latency	2-40 s	No
Fatigability	Yes	No
Habituation	Yes	No

Positional vertigo can also occur with central vestibular disease.

Caloric Testing

Disorders of the vestibuloocular pathways can be detected by caloric testing. Caloric testing should be preceded by careful otoscopic examination and should not be undertaken if the tympanic membrane is perforated. The patient is placed supine with the head elevated 30 degrees to bring the superficially situated lateral semicircular canal into the upright position. Each ear canal is irrigated in turn with cold (~33°C) or warm (~44°C) water for 40 seconds, with at least 5 minutes between tests. Warm water tends to produce less discomfort than cold.

1. In the **normal, awake patient**, cold-water caloric stimulation produces nystagmus with the slow phase toward and the fast phase away from the irrigated ear. Warm water irrigation produces the opposite response and is generally better tolerated.

2. In patients with **unilateral labyrinthine, vestibulocochlear (VIII) nerve, or vestibular nuclear dysfunction**, irrigation of the affected side fails to cause nystagmus or elicits nystagmus that is later in onset or briefer in duration than on the normal side.

Other Cranial Nerves

Papilledema associated with disequilibrium suggests an intracranial mass lesion, usually in the posterior fossa, causing increased intracranial pressure. Optic atrophy may be present in multiple sclerosis, neurosyphilis, or vitamin B_{12} deficiency. A depressed corneal reflex or facial palsy ipsilateral to the lesion (and the ataxia) can accompany

cerebellopontine angle tumor. Weakness of the tongue or palate, hoarseness, or dysphagia results from lower brainstem disease.

MOTOR SYSTEM

Examination of motor function in a patient with a disorder of equilibrium should disclose the pattern and severity of ataxia and any associated pyramidal, extrapyramidal, or lower motor neuron involvement that might suggest a cause. The clinical features that help distinguish cerebellar disease from disease involving these other motor systems are summarized in **Table 8-6**.

Muscle Tone

1. **Hypotonia** is characteristic of cerebellar disorders; with unilateral cerebellar hemispheric lesions, the ipsilateral limbs are hypotonic.

2. Extrapyramidal hypertonia (**rigidity**) may occur in disorders that affect both the cerebellum and basal ganglia (eg, Wilson disease, acquired hepatocerebral degeneration, and some spinocerebellar ataxias).

3. Ataxia with **spasticity** may be seen in conditions that affect both the cerebellum and upper motor neuron pathways (eg, multiple sclerosis, posterior fossa tumors or congenital anomalies, vertebrobasilar infarction, some spinocerebellar ataxias, Friedreich ataxia, and vitamin B_{12} deficiency).

Coordination

1. Truncal stability is assessed by examining gait (discussed earlier) and by observing the seated, unsupported patient. In addition to gait ataxia, patients may show

Table 8-6. Clinical Features Distinguishing Cerebellar from Other Motor Systems Disorders.

	Cerebellar	Upper Motor Neuron	Lower Motor Neuron	Extrapyramidal
Strength	Normal	Decreased	Decreased	Normal
Tone	Decreased	Increased (spastic)[1]	Normal	Increased (rigid)[1] or decreased
Tendon reflexes	Normal	Increased[1]	Decreased[1]	Normal
Plantar responses	Flexor	Extensor[1]	Flexor	Flexor
Atrophy	Absent	Absent	Present[1] or absent	Absent
Fasciculations	Absent	Absent	Present[1] or absent	Absent
Tremor	Intention tremor[1] or absent	Absent	Absent	Resting tremor[1] or absent
Chorea or athetosis	Absent	Absent	Absent	Present[1] or absent
Akinesia	Absent	Absent	Absent	Present[1] or absent
Ataxia	Present[1]	Absent	Absent	Absent

[1]Most helpful diagnostic features.

oscillation of the head or trunk (**titubation**) and **truncal ataxia** while seated, causing a tendency to fall (toward the affected side with a lateralized cerebellar lesion).

2. Movement of the arm is observed as the patient's finger tracks back and forth between his or her own nose or chin and the examiner's finger. With cerebellar ataxia, an **intention tremor** characteristically appears near the beginning and end of each such movement, and the patient may overshoot the target.
3. When the patient is asked to raise the arms rapidly to a given height—or when the extended and outstretched arms are displaced by a sudden force—there may be overshoot (**rebound**). Impaired ability to check the force of muscle contractions can also be demonstrated by having the patient flex the arm at the elbow against resistance, and then suddenly removing the resistance. If the limb is ataxic, continued contraction without resistance may cause the hand to strike the patient (whose head should be turned to the side to avoid being hit in the face).
4. **Ataxia of the legs** is demonstrated by the supine patient's inability to run the heel of the foot smoothly up and down the opposite shin.
5. **Ataxia of any limb** is reflected by irregularity in the rate, rhythm, amplitude, and force of rapid successive tapping movements.

Weakness

1. Pure vestibular, cerebellar, or sensory disorders do not cause weakness, but weakness may occur in disorders that also affect motor pathways.
2. **Distal weakness** can be seen in disorders that produce sensory ataxia, such as polyneuropathies and Friedreich ataxia.
3. **Paraparesis** may be superimposed on ataxia in vitamin B_{12} deficiency, multiple sclerosis, foramen magnum lesions, or spinal cord tumors.
4. **Ataxic quadriparesis, hemiataxia with contralateral hemiparesis**, or **ataxic hemiparesis** suggests a brainstem lesion.

Abnormal Involuntary Movements

1. **Chorea** or **parkinsonism** (see Chapter 11, Movement Disorders) may accompany cerebellar signs in multiple system atrophy, Wilson disease, acquired hepatocerebral degeneration, certain autosomal dominant spinocerebellar ataxias (eg, SCA3 or Machado–Joseph disease), dentatorubral-pallidoluysian atrophy, and ataxia-telangiectasia.
2. **Myoclonus** is a prominent manifestation of Creutzfeldt–Jakob disease and dentatorubral-pallidoluysian atrophy, both of which may also produce ataxia.

SENSORY SYSTEM

Joint Position Sense

In sensory ataxia, joint position sense is always impaired in the legs and may be defective in the arms. Joint position sense is tested by asking the patient to detect passive movement of the joints, beginning distally and moving proximally, to establish the upper level of any deficit in each limb. With normal joint position sense, it should be possible to detect even the smallest displacement of a joint by the examiner. Abnormal position sense also can be demonstrated by positioning a limb and having the patient, with eyes closed, place the opposite limb in the same position.

Vibration Sense

Vibration sense is also frequently impaired in sensory ataxia. The patient is asked to detect vibration of a 128-Hz tuning fork placed on a bony prominence. Successively more proximal sites are tested to determine the upper level of the deficit in each limb. The patient's threshold for detecting vibration is compared with the examiner's ability to detect it in the hand that holds the tuning fork.

REFLEXES

1. Tendon reflexes are typically **hypoactive**, with a **pendular** quality, in cerebellar disorders; unilateral cerebellar lesions produce ipsilateral hyporeflexia.
2. **Hyporeflexia of the legs** is a prominent manifestation of Friedreich ataxia, tabes dorsalis, and polyneuropathies that cause sensory ataxia.
3. **Hyperactive reflexes** and **extensor plantar responses** may accompany ataxia caused by multiple sclerosis, vitamin B_{12} deficiency, focal brainstem lesions, and certain autosomal dominant spinocerebellar ataxias.

INVESTIGATIVE STUDIES

BLOOD TESTS

Blood studies may disclose low vitamin B_{12} levels and hematologic abnormalities (macrocytic anemia, leukopenia with hypersegmented neutrophils, thrombocytopenia with giant platelets) in vitamin B_{12} deficiency, decreased levels of thyroid hormones in hypothyroidism, elevated hepatic enzymes and low ceruloplasmin and copper concentrations in Wilson disease, immunoglobulin deficiency and elevated α-fetoprotein in ataxia-telangiectasia, or autoantibodies in autoimmune (including paraneoplastic) cerebellar degenerations.

DNA TESTING

Blood, saliva, and other sources can be tested for gene defects associated with a variety of disorders that cause disorders of equilibrium. These include certain autosomal dominant spinocerebellar ataxias, dentatoru-bral-pallidoluysian atrophy, ataxia-telangiectasia, fragile X-associated tremor/ataxia syndrome, and Friedreich ataxia.

CEREBROSPINAL FLUID

The cerebrospinal fluid (CSF) shows elevated protein with cerebellopontine angle, brainstem, or spinal cord tumors; hypothyroidism; and some polyneuropathies. Increased protein concentration with pleocytosis is found in infectious or parainfectious encephalitis, paraneoplastic cerebellar degeneration, and neurosyphilis. Elevated pressure and bloody CSF characterize cerebellar hemorrhage, but lumbar puncture is contraindicated if cerebellar hemorrhage is suspected. CSF VDRL is reactive in tabes dorsalis, and oligoclonal immunoglobulin G (IgG) bands may be present in multiple sclerosis or other inflammatory disorders.

CT & MR IMAGING

Computed tomography (CT) can demonstrate posterior fossa tumors or malformations, cerebellar infarction or hemorrhage, and cerebellar or brainstem atrophy associated with degenerative disorders (eg, spinocerebellar ataxias). **Magnetic resonance imaging (MRI)** provides better visualization of posterior fossa lesions, including cerebellopontine angle tumors, and is superior to CT for detecting lesions of multiple sclerosis. MRI can also detect endolymphatic hydrops in the inner ear in Ménière disease.

EVOKED POTENTIALS

Visual evoked potentials may be helpful in evaluating patients with suspected multiple sclerosis. Brainstem auditory evoked potentials can localize disease to peripheral vestibular pathways and help identify cerebellopontine angle tumors.

CHEST X-RAY & ECHOCARDIOGRAPHY

The chest X-ray may reveal a lung tumor in paraneoplastic cerebellar degeneration, and the chest X-ray or echocardiogram may provide evidence of cardiomyopathy associated with Friedreich ataxia.

AUDIOMETRY

This is useful in vestibular disorders associated with auditory impairment and can distinguish conductive, labyrinthine, vestibulocochlear (VIII) nerve, and brainstem disease. Tests of pure tone hearing are abnormal when sounds are transmitted through air with conductive hearing loss and when transmitted through either air or bone with labyrinthine or vestibulocochlear (VIII) nerve disorders. Speech discrimination is markedly impaired with vestibulocochlear (VIII) nerve lesions, less impaired in labyrinthine disorders, and normal with conductive hearing loss or brainstem disease.

ELECTRONYSTAGMOGRAPHY

This can detect and characterize nystagmus, including that elicited by caloric stimulation.

▼ PERIPHERAL VESTIBULAR DISORDERS

Table 8-7 provides a list of peripheral vestibular disorders and features helpful in their differential diagnosis.

BENIGN POSITIONAL VERTIGO

Positional vertigo is vertigo that occurs upon changing head position. It is usually associated with peripheral vestibular lesions, but also may be due to central (brainstem or cerebellar) disease.

PATHOGENESIS

Benign positional vertigo is the most common cause of vertigo of peripheral origin. It results from **canalolithiasis**, in which debris (otoconia) floating in the endolymph stimulates a semicircular canal, most often the posterior canal. Benign positional vertigo may follow head trauma, but in most instances, no precipitating factor can be determined. When head trauma is the cause, the labyrinth is the usual site of injury. However, fractures of the petrosal bone may lacerate the vestibulocochlear (VIII) nerve, producing vertigo and hearing loss; hemotympanum or CSF otorrhea suggests such a fracture.

CLINICAL FINDINGS

The syndrome is characterized by brief (seconds to minutes) episodes of severe vertigo and nystagmus, which may be accompanied by nausea and vomiting. Symptoms may occur with any change in head position but are usually most severe in the lateral decubitus position with the affected ear down. Episodic vertigo typically continues for several weeks and then resolves spontaneously; in some cases, it is recurrent. Hearing loss is not a feature.

Peripheral and central causes of positional vertigo usually can be distinguished by the Nylen–Bárány or Dix–Hallpike maneuver (see Figure 8-5). Vertigo evoked by this maneuver is always accompanied by positional nystagmus when the underlying cause is peripheral, and is typically unidirectional, rotatory, and delayed in onset by several seconds after assumption of the precipitating head position. If the position is maintained, nystagmus and vertigo resolve within seconds to minutes. If the maneuver is repeated, the response is attenuated. In contrast, positional vertigo of central origin tends to be less severe, and positional nystagmus may be absent. In contrast,

Table 8-7. Differential Diagnosis of Peripheral Vestibular Disorders.

Disorder	Laterality	Hearing Loss		Other Cranial Nerve Palsies
		Conductive	Sensorineural	
Benign positional vertigo[1,2]	Unilateral	–	–	–
Ménière disease[1]	Unilateral or bilateral	–	+	–
Acute peripheral vestibulopathy[1]	Unilateral	–	–	–
Otosclerosis	Bilateral	+	+	–
Cerebellopontine angle tumor	Unilateral[3]	–	+	±
Toxic vestibulopathy				
Alcohol	Bilateral	–	–	–
Aminoglycosides	Bilateral	–	+	–
Salicylates	Bilateral	–	+	–
Quinine & quinidine	Bilateral	–	+	–
Cisplatin	Bilateral	–	+	–
Vestibulocochlear (VIII) neuropathy				
Basilar meningitis	Unilateral or bilateral	–	+	±
Hypothyroidism	Bilateral	–	+	–
Diabetes	Bilateral	–	+	±
Paget disease of the skull (osteitis deformans)	Bilateral	–	+	±

[1]Most common causes.
[2]When due to head trauma, may be accompanied by hearing loss and other cranial nerve palsies.
[3]Bilateral in neurofibromatosis 2

there is no latency, fatigue, or habituation in central positional vertigo.

When benign positional vertigo is documented in this manner, no additional diagnostic investigation (eg, auditory or vestibular testing or imaging) is required.

TREATMENT

The mainstay of treatment is **repositioning (Epley) maneuvers**, which use gravity to move endolymphatic debris out of the semicircular canal and into the vestibule, where it can be reabsorbed. In one such maneuver (**Figure 8-6**), the head is turned 45 degrees in the direction of the affected ear (determined clinically, as described earlier), and the patient reclines to a supine position, with the head (still turned 45 degrees) hanging down over the end of the examining table. The head, still hanging down, is then turned 90 degrees in the opposite direction, to 45 degrees toward the opposite ear. Next, the patient rolls to a lateral decubitus position with the affected ear up, and the head still turned 45 degrees toward the unaffected ear and hanging down. Finally, the patient turns to a prone position and sits up.

Vestibulo-suppressant drugs (**Table 8-8**) may also be useful in the acute period. Vestibular rehabilitation, which promotes compensation for vestibular dysfunction through the recruitment of other sensory modalities, may also be helpful.

MÉNIÈRE DISEASE

Ménière disease is characterized by repeated episodes of **vertigo** lasting from ~20 minutes to ~12 hours, accompanied by **tinnitus** and progressive, low- to medium-frequency sensorineural **hearing loss**. It is thought to be the second most common peripheral cause of vertigo, after benign positional vertigo.

PATHOGENESIS

Most cases are sporadic, but up to ~10% cluster in families. Onset is usually between ages 20 and 50 years, and men are affected more often than women. Symptoms are thought to result from an increase in the volume of labyrinthine endolymph (**endolymphatic hydrops**), which results in distension of the endolymphatic space and its encroachment on the perilymphatic space. The cochlear duct and saccule are

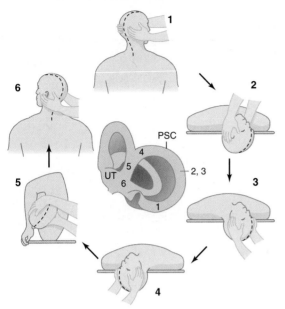

▲ **Figure 8-6.** Repositioning treatment for benign positional vertigo resulting from canalolithiasis. In the example shown, repositioning maneuvers are used to move endolymphatic debris out of the posterior semicircular canal (PSC) of the right ear and into the utricle (UT), the larger of two membranous sacs in the vestibule of the labyrinth, where this debris can be reabsorbed. The numbers (1-6) refer to both the position of the patient and the corresponding location of debris within the labyrinth. The patient is seated, and the head is turned 45 degrees to the right (1). The head is lowered rapidly to below the horizontal (2); the examiner shifts position (3); and the head is rotated rapidly 90 degrees in the opposite direction, so it now points 45 degrees to the left, where it remains for 30 seconds (4). The patient then rolls onto the left side without turning the head in relation to the body and maintains this position for another 30 seconds (5) before sitting up (6). This maneuver may need to be repeated until nystagmus is abolished. The patient must then avoid the supine position for at least 2 days. Used with permission from Robert W. Baloh and Martin Allen Samuels. From Samuels MA, Feske SK, eds. *Office Practice of Neurology.* New York, NY: Churchill Livingstone; 1995.

affected most often. The cause of endolymphatic hydrops is unknown, but immune mechanisms may be involved.

CLINICAL FINDINGS

At the time of the first acute attack, patients already may have noted the insidious onset of tinnitus, hearing loss, and a sensation of fullness in the ear. Acute attacks are characterized by vertigo, nausea, and vomiting and recur at intervals ranging from weeks to years. Hearing deteriorates in a

Table 8-8. Drugs Used in the Treatment of Vertigo.

Drug	Dosage
Antihistamines	
Meclizine	25 mg PO q4-6h
Promethazine	25-50 mg PO, IM, or PR q4-6h
Dimenhydrinate	50 mg PO or IM q4-6h or 100 mg PR q8h
Anticholinergics	
Scopolamine	0.5 mg transdermally q3d
Benzodiazepines	
Diazepam	5-10 mg IM q4-6h
Sympathomimetics	
Amphetamine	5-10 mg PO q4-6h
Ephedrine	25 mg PO q4-6h

IM, intramuscularly; PO, orally; PR, rectally.
Data from Baloh RW, Honrubia V, Kerber KA. *Baloh and Honrubia's Clinical Neurophysiology of the Vestibular System.* 4th ed. New York, NY: Oxford University Press; 2010.

stepwise fashion, with bilateral involvement in ~15% to ~50% of patients. As hearing loss increases, vertigo tends to become less severe.

Physical examination during an acute episode shows spontaneous horizontal or rotatory nystagmus (or both) that may change direction. Although spontaneous nystagmus is characteristically absent between attacks, caloric testing usually reveals impaired vestibular function. The hearing deficit is not always sufficiently advanced to be detectable at the bedside. Audiometry shows low-frequency pure-tone hearing loss that fluctuates in severity, impaired speech discrimination, and increased sensitivity to loud sounds. Endolymphatic hydrops can be demonstrated by MRI.

TREATMENT

Symptomatic management of acute attacks is with antihistamines, benzodiazepines, or other drugs listed in Table 8-8. Between episodes, patients may be treated with a low-salt diet and diuretics, such as hydrochlorothiazide (50 mg orally daily) plus triamterene (25 mg orally daily), or with the histamine H_3 receptor antagonist betahistine (16-48 mg orally three times daily). In persistent, disabling cases, vestibular ablation by intratympanic gentamicin, vestibular (VIII) nerve section, or labyrinthectomy may be beneficial.

ACUTE PERIPHERAL VESTIBULOPATHY

This term is used to describe a spontaneous attack of vertigo of inapparent cause that resolves spontaneously and is not accompanied by hearing loss or central nervous system dysfunction. It includes disorders diagnosed as **acute labyrinthitis** or **vestibular neuronitis** and may follow a febrile illness. Acute peripheral vestibulopathy may result from viral infection (eg, reactivation of latent herpes simplex virus in vestibular ganglia), but this association has never been proven. Acute peripheral vestibulopathy is considered the third most common cause of peripheral vertigo, after benign positional vertigo and Ménière disease.

The disorder is characterized by the acute onset of vertigo, nausea, and vomiting, typically lasting up to 2 weeks. Symptoms may recur, and some degree of vestibular dysfunction may be permanent. During an attack, the patient appears acutely ill, typically lies on one side with the affected ear upward, and is reluctant to move the head. Nystagmus with the fast phase away from the affected ear is always present. The vestibular response to caloric testing is defective in one or both ears but auditory acuity is normal.

Acute peripheral vestibulopathy must be distinguished from central causes of acute vertigo; the latter are suggested by vertical nystagmus, altered consciousness, motor or sensory deficit, or dysarthria.

Treatment of acute peripheral vestibulopathy is with a 10- to 14-day course of prednisone (20 mg orally twice daily), the drugs listed in Table 8-8, or both.

OTOSCLEROSIS

Otosclerosis is caused by immobility of the stapes. Its most distinctive feature is bilateral conductive hearing loss, but sensorineural hearing loss and recurrent episodic vertigo may also occur, whereas tinnitus is infrequent. Auditory symptoms usually begin before 30 years of age, and familial occurrence is common. Imaging studies may be diagnostically useful. Sodium fluoride, vitamin D, intratympanic dexamethasone, and surgical stapedectomy are recognized treatments.

CEREBELLOPONTINE ANGLE TUMOR

PATHOGENESIS

The most common tumor in the cerebellopontine angle—a triangular region in the posterior fossa bordered by the cerebellum, lateral pons, and petrous ridge—is the histologically benign **acoustic neuroma**. Also termed **neurilemoma**, **neurinoma**, or **schwannoma**, it typically arises from the neurilemmal sheath of the vestibular portion of the vestibulocochlear (VIII) nerve in the internal auditory canal. Less common tumors at this site include meningiomas, epidermoid tumors, and lipomas.

Acoustic neuromas usually occur as isolated lesions in patients 30 to 60 years old, but may also be a manifestation of neurofibromatosis. **Neurofibromatosis 1 (von Recklinghausen disease)** is a common autosomal dominant disorder arising from mutations in the gene for **neurofibromin 1** (*NF1*). Characterized by *unilateral* acoustic neuromas, neurofibromatosis 1 is associated with café-au-lait spots on the skin, cutaneous neurofibromas, axillary or inguinal freckles, optic gliomas, iris hamartomas, and dysplastic bony lesions. **Neurofibromatosis 2** is a rare autosomal dominant disorder caused by mutations in the gene for **merlin** (*NF2*). Its hallmark is *bilateral* acoustic neuromas, which may be accompanied by other central or peripheral nervous system tumors, including neurofibromas, meningiomas, gliomas, and schwannomas.

PATHOPHYSIOLOGY

Cerebellopontine angle tumors produce symptoms by compressing or displacing the cranial nerves, brainstem, and cerebellum and by obstructing CSF flow. Because of their anatomic relationship to the vestibulocochlear (VIII) nerve, the trigeminal (V) and facial (VII) nerves are often affected.

CLINICAL FINDINGS

▶ Symptoms & Signs

Insidious hearing loss is usually the initial symptom. Less often, patients present with headache, vertigo, gait ataxia, facial pain, tinnitus, a sensation of fullness in the ear, or facial weakness. Vertigo ultimately develops in 20% to 30% of patients, but nonspecific unsteadiness is more common. Symptoms may be stable or progress over months or years.

Unilateral sensorineural hearing loss is the most common finding on examination. Other frequent findings are ipsilateral facial palsy, depressed or absent corneal reflex, and sensory loss over the face. Ataxia, spontaneous nystagmus, other lower cranial nerve palsies, and signs of increased intracranial pressure are less common. Unilateral vestibular dysfunction can usually be demonstrated with caloric testing.

▶ Laboratory Findings

Audiometry shows a sensorineural deficit with high-frequency pure-tone hearing loss, poor speech discrimination, and marked tone decay. CSF protein is elevated in approximately 70% of patients, usually in the range of 50 to 200 mg/dL. The most useful imaging study is MRI of the cerebellopontine angle. Acoustic neuromas may cause abnormal brainstem auditory evoked potentials.

DIFFERENTIAL DIAGNOSIS

Meningioma should be considered in patients who present with more than isolated vestibulocochlear (VIII) nerve disease. Cholesteatoma is suggested by conductive hearing loss, early facial weakness, or facial twitching, with normal CSF protein. Metastatic carcinoma may also present as a lesion in the cerebellopontine angle.

TREATMENT

Treatment is complete surgical excision. Patients with acoustic neuroma and neurofibromatosis 2 may benefit from bevacizumab, a monoclonal antibody against vascular endothelial growth factor (VEGFA). In untreated cases, severe complications can result from brainstem compression or hydrocephalus.

TOXIC VESTIBULOPATHIES

ALCOHOL

Alcohol can cause acute positional vertigo beginning as early as ~30 minutes after ingesting amounts sufficient to produce blood levels ≥40 mg/dL. Alcohol diffuses into the cupula, then into the endolymph, leaves the cupula, and finally leaves the endolymph. Because alcohol is less dense than endolymph, this renders the peripheral vestibular system gravity-sensitive, resulting in two phases of vertigo that together last up to ~12 hours. During the first phase, the cupula is lighter than endolymph, and vertigo is accompanied by nystagmus that beats toward the lower ear with the patient in the lateral recumbent position. About 3.5-5 hours after this phase resolves, as endolymph becomes heavier than the cupula, vertigo returns, with nystagmus that beats toward the upper ear in lateral recumbency.

AMINOGLYCOSIDES

Aminoglycoside antibiotics are widely recognized ototoxins that can produce both vestibular and auditory symptoms. Streptomycin, gentamicin, and tobramycin are the agents most likely to cause **vestibular toxicity**, and amikacin, kanamycin, and tobramycin are associated with **hearing loss**. Aminoglycosides concentrate in the perilymph and endolymph and exert their ototoxic effects by destroying sensory hair cells. The risk of toxicity is related to drug dosage, plasma concentration, duration of therapy, conditions—such as renal failure—that impair drug clearance, preexisting vestibular or cochlear dysfunction, and concomitant administration of other ototoxic agents.

Symptoms of vertigo, nausea, vomiting, and gait ataxia may begin acutely; physical findings include spontaneous nystagmus and the Romberg sign. The acute phase typically lasts 1 to 2 weeks and is followed by gradual improvement. Prolonged or repeated aminoglycoside therapy may be associated with chronic, progressive vestibular dysfunction.

SALICYLATES

Salicylates, when used chronically and in high doses, can cause vertigo, tinnitus, and sensorineural hearing loss—all usually reversible when the drug is discontinued. Symptoms result from cochlear and vestibular end-organ damage. **Salicylism** is characterized by headache, tinnitus, hearing loss, vertigo, nausea, vomiting, thirst,

hyperventilation, and sometimes a confusional state. Severe intoxication may be associated with fever, skin rash, hemorrhage, dehydration, seizures, psychosis, or coma. Laboratory findings include a high plasma salicylate level (≥0.35 mg/mL) and combined metabolic acidosis and respiratory alkalosis. Treatments include gastric lavage, activated charcoal, forced diuresis, peritoneal dialysis or hemodialysis, and hemoperfusion.

QUININE & QUINIDINE

Quinine and quinidine can produce **cinchonism**, which resembles salicylate intoxication in many respects. Manifestations include tinnitus, impaired hearing, vertigo, visual deficits (including disordered color vision), nausea, vomiting, abdominal pain, hot flushed skin, and sweating. Fever, encephalopathy, coma, and death can occur. Symptoms usually result from overdosage, but can also be due to idiosyncratic reactions to therapeutic doses.

CISPLATIN

Cisplatin is an antineoplastic drug used to treat solid tumors of the ovary, testis, uterine cervix, lung, head and neck, bladder, and other tissues. It causes ototoxicity, which is commonly bilateral and irreversible, in a high percentage of patients. Tinnitus, hearing loss, and vestibular dysfunction may all occur.

VESTIBULOCOCHLEAR NEUROPATHY

Involvement of the vestibulocochlear (VIII) nerve by systemic disease is an uncommon cause of vertigo. **Basilar meningitis** from bacterial, syphilitic, or tuberculous infection or sarcoidosis can compress the vestibulocochlear and other cranial nerves, but hearing loss is a more common consequence than vertigo. Metabolic disorders associated with vestibulocochlear neuropathy include **hypothyroidism, diabetes**, and **Paget disease**.

CEREBELLAR & CENTRAL VESTIBULAR DISORDERS

Many disorders can produce acute or chronic cerebellar dysfunction (**Table 8-9**). Some of these may also involve central vestibular pathways (eg, Wernicke encephalopathy, vertebrobasilar ischemia or infarction, multiple sclerosis, and posterior fossa tumors). For this reason, cerebellar and central vestibular disorders are considered together here.

ACUTE DISORDERS

DRUG INTOXICATION

Pancerebellar dysfunction—manifested by nystagmus, dysarthria, and limb and gait ataxia—is a prominent feature of intoxication with ethanol, sedative-hypnotics,

Table 8-9. Causes of Acute or Chronic Cerebellar Ataxia.

Acute
Drug intoxications: ethanol, sedative-hypnotics, anticonvulsants, hallucinogens
Wernicke encephalopathy
Vertebrobasilar ischemia or infarction
Cerebellar hemorrhage
Inflammatory disorders

Chronic
Multiple sclerosis
Alcoholic cerebellar degeneration
Toxin-induced cerebellar degeneration
Hypothyroidism
Autoimmune cerebellar degeneration
Autosomal dominant spinocerebellar ataxias
Dentatorubral-pallidoluysian atrophy
Ataxia-telangiectasia
Fragile X-associated tremor/ataxia syndrome
Multiple system atrophy
Hepatocerebral degeneration
Prion diseases
Posterior fossa tumors
Posterior fossa malformations

anticonvulsants, and some hallucinogens. The severity of symptoms is dose-related; therapeutic doses of sedatives or anticonvulsants commonly produce nystagmus, but other cerebellar signs imply toxicity. Because drug-induced cerebellar ataxia is often associated with altered consciousness, drug intoxication is discussed in detail in Chapter 4, Confusional States.

WERNICKE ENCEPHALOPATHY

Pathogenesis

Wernicke encephalopathy (discussed in more detail in Chapter 4, Confusional States) is an acute disorder comprising the clinical triad of **ataxia**, **ophthalmoplegia**, and **confusion**. It is caused by **thiamine (vitamin B_1)** deficiency and is most common in chronic alcoholics, but may occur as a consequence of malnutrition from any cause.

Clinical Findings

Cerebellar and vestibular involvement both contribute to ataxia, which affects gait primarily or exclusively; the legs are ataxic in only about 20% of patients, and the arms in 10%. Dysarthria is rare. Other findings include an amnestic syndrome or global confusional state, horizontal or combined horizontal and vertical nystagmus, bilateral lateral rectus palsy, and absent ankle reflexes. Caloric testing shows bilateral or unilateral vestibular dysfunction.

Conjugate gaze palsy, pupillary abnormalities, and hypothermia can occur.

Diagnosis & Treatment

The diagnosis should be suspected in alcoholic and other malnourished patients and is confirmed by the clinical response to **thiamine**. Ocular palsies improve within hours and ataxia, nystagmus, and confusion within a few days. Horizontal nystagmus may persist. Ataxia is fully reversible in only approximately 40% of patients, in whom recovery takes weeks to months.

VERTEBROBASILAR ISCHEMIA & INFARCTION

Transient ischemic attacks and strokes in the vertebrobasilar system (see also Chapter 13, Stroke) are often associated with ataxia or vertigo.

Internal Auditory Artery Occlusion

The internal auditory (labyrinthine) artery originates from the anterior inferior cerebellar (or, less commonly, basilar) artery (**Figure 8-7**) and supplies the vestibulocochlear (VIII) nerve. Isolated occlusion of this vessel causes vertigo and nystagmus, with the fast phase directed away from the involved side, and unilateral sensorineural hearing loss.

Lateral Medullary Infarction

Lateral medullary infarction, which is caused by occlusion of the proximal vertebral artery and, less often, the posterior inferior cerebellar artery, produces **Wallenberg syndrome (Figure 8-8)**. Clinical manifestations vary, but the most common are listed here, together with their likely anatomic correlates.

1. **Vertigo**, **nausea**, **vomiting**, and **nystagmus** (vestibular nucleus)
2. **Loss of pain and temperature sense over the contralateral limbs and trunk** (lateral spinothalamic tract)
3. **Loss of pain and temperature sense over the ipsilateral face** (spinal trigeminal nucleus and tract)
4. **Truncal and gait ataxia** (vestibular nucleus and inferior cerebellar peduncle)
5. **Ipsilateral limb ataxia** (inferior cerebellar peduncle)
6. **Ipsilateral Horner syndrome** (descending sympathetic tract)
7. **Dysphagia, dysarthria, hoarseness,** and **ipsilateral palatal paralysis** (nucleus ambiguus)

Cerebellar Infarction

The cerebellum is supplied by the superior cerebellar, anterior inferior cerebellar, and posterior inferior cerebellar arteries. The territory supplied by each of these vessels is highly variable, but the superior, middle, and inferior

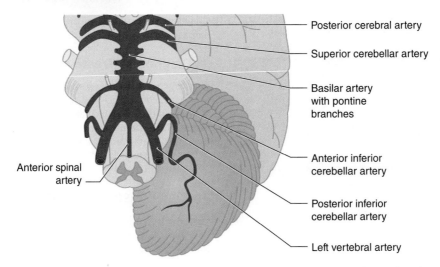

▲ **Figure 8-7.** Principal arteries of the posterior fossa. (Used with permission from Waxman SG. *Clinical Neuroanatomy.* 26th ed. New York, NY: McGraw-Hill; 2010.)

cerebellar peduncles are typically supplied by the superior, anterior inferior, and posterior inferior cerebellar arteries, respectively.

Signs of cerebellar infarction include **ipsilateral limb ataxia**, **lateropulsion** (falling toward or, less commonly, away from the side of the lesion), and **hypotonia**. Headache, nausea, vomiting, vertigo, nystagmus, dysarthria, ocular or gaze palsies, facial weakness or sensory loss, and contralateral hemiparesis or hemisensory deficit may

also occur. Occlusions of the superior cerebellar, anterior inferior cerebellar, and posterior inferior cerebellar arteries may be clinically indistinguishable, but associated brainstem findings can help in this regard. Thus, midbrain, pontine, and medullary signs may suggest infarction in the superior cerebellar, anterior inferior cerebellar, and posterior inferior cerebellar territories, respectively. Brainstem infarction or compression by cerebellar edema can result in coma and death.

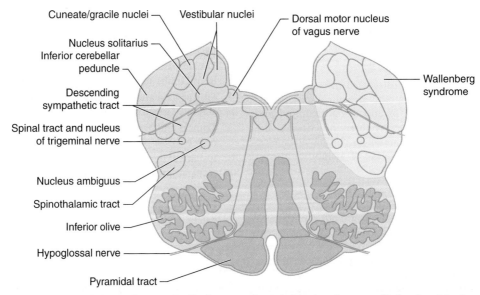

▲ **Figure 8-8.** Lateral medullary infarction (Wallenberg syndrome) showing the area of infarction (blue) and anatomic structures affected.

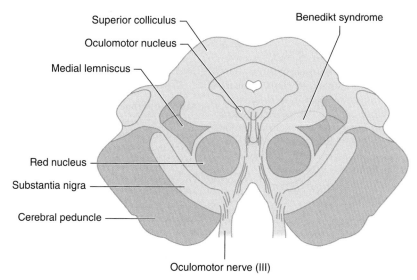

Superior colliculus

Oculomotor nucleus

Medial lemniscus

Benedikt syndrome

Red nucleus

Substantia nigra

Cerebral peduncle

Oculomotor nerve (III)

▲ **Figure 8-9.** Paramedian midbrain infarction (Benedikt syndrome). The area of infarction is indicated in blue.

Diagnosis is by CT or MRI, which differentiates between infarction and hemorrhage and should be obtained promptly. Brainstem compression is an indication for surgical decompression and resection of infarcted tissue, which can be lifesaving.

▶ Paramedian Midbrain Infarction

Paramedian midbrain infarction, caused by occlusion of the paramedian penetrating branches of the basilar artery, affects the oculomotor (III) nerve root fibers and red nucleus (**Figure 8-9**). The result (**Benedikt syndrome**) is ipsilateral oculomotor (III) nerve involvement (producing medial rectus palsy with a fixed dilated pupil) and contralateral limb ataxia (typically affecting only the arm). Cerebellar signs result from involvement of the red nucleus, which receives a crossed projection from the cerebellum in the ascending limb of the superior cerebellar peduncle.

CEREBELLAR HEMORRHAGE

▶ Pathogenesis

Cerebellar hemorrhage (see also Chapter 13, Stroke) is usually due to hypertensive vascular disease; less common causes include anticoagulation, arteriovenous malformation, blood dyscrasia, tumor, and trauma. Hypertensive cerebellar hemorrhages are usually located in the deep white matter of the cerebellum and commonly extend into the fourth ventricle.

▶ Clinical Findings

Hypertensive cerebellar hemorrhage causes the sudden onset of **headache**, which may be accompanied by **nausea**,

vomiting, and **vertigo**, followed by **gait ataxia** and **impaired consciousness**, usually evolving over hours.

At presentation, patients can be fully alert, confused, or comatose. The blood pressure is typically elevated, and nuchal rigidity may be present. The pupils are often small and sluggishly reactive. Ipsilateral gaze palsy (with gaze preference away from the side of hemorrhage) and ipsilateral peripheral facial palsy are common. The gaze palsy cannot be overcome by cold-water caloric stimulation. Nystagmus may be present, and the ipsilateral corneal reflex may be depressed. The patient, if alert, exhibits ataxia of stance and gait; limb ataxia is less common. In the late stage of brainstem compression, there is spasticity in the legs and extensor plantar responses.

▶ Diagnosis & Treatment

The diagnosis of cerebellar hemorrhage can be missed or delayed, and death result, if gait is not tested promptly in every patient with hypertension and either acute headache or depressed consciousness. This is because gait ataxia is often the earliest neurologic sign in this condition.

The CSF is frequently bloody, but lumbar puncture should be avoided if cerebellar hemorrhage is suspected, because it may lead to brain herniation. Diagnosis is by CT. Treatment consists of surgical evacuation of the hematoma, which can be lifesaving.

INFLAMMATORY DISORDERS

▶ Viral Infection

Cerebellar ataxia can result from cerebellitis due to a variety of viral infections. Among these, varicella-zoster is most common in children, and reactivation of varicella-zoster or Ebstein–Barr virus is most common in adults. Less frequent causes include coxsackie virus, echo virus, influenza virus, and parvovirus B19. Truncal ataxia is usually the most prominent sign of cerebellar involvement and may be accompanied by headache, nausea, vomiting, and altered consciousness. Viral cerebellitis is usually self-limited and recovery is good, especially in children.

JC polyoma virus, which causes progressive multifocal leukoencephalopathy, can infect the cerebellum of immunocompromised patients. Progressive multifocal leukoencephalopathy is discussed in more detail in Chapter 5, Dementia & Amnestic Disorders.

Bacterial Infection

Bacterial infection is an uncommon cause of cerebellar ataxia, but 10% to 20% of brain abscesses are located in the cerebellum, and ataxia may be a feature of encephalitis due to *Listeria monocytogenes*. *Listeria* typically affects healthy adults who consume tainted foods, such as cheese, meat, or fruit. A prodromal flulike illness is followed by a neurologic disorder that involves the brainstem and cerebellum. Signs include ataxia, cranial nerve (especially V, VI, VII, IX, and X) palsies, hemiparesis, altered consciousness, and meningismus. MRI shows diffuse and focal, abscess-like lesions and CSF shows pleocytosis. Treatment is with ampicillin (2 g IV every 4 hours), often together with gentamicin (1.5 mg/kg IV loading followed by 1-2 mg/kg IV every 8 hours).

Fungal Infection

Fungal infection of the cerebellum is rare but may occur in immunocompromised patients or following neurosurgical procedures or epidural injections. Organisms involved include *Aspergillus*.

Prion Infection

Prion diseases (Creutzfeldt–Jakob and Gerstmann–Sträussler–Scheinker syndrome) can produce cerebellar ataxia associated with dementia. These are discussed in more detail in Chapter 5, Dementia & Amnestic Disorders.

Acute Postinfectious Cerebellar Ataxia of Childhood

Acute postinfectious cerebellar ataxia of childhood is the most common cause of acute ataxia in children. It usually affects children aged 1-6 years and follows a viral illness or vaccination. Gait ataxia is the most prominent clinical feature. MRI is typically normal; CSF may show mild pleocytosis. Most patients recover completely within one month.

Acute Disseminated Encephalomyelitis

Acute disseminated encephalomyelitis, a monophasic illness caused by immune-mediated demyelination of CNS white matter, may affect the cerebellum, producing ataxia.

Other common features include impaired consciousness, seizures, focal neurologic signs, and myelopathy (see Chapter 9, Motor Disorders).

Fisher Variant of Guillain–Barré Syndrome

Ataxia, **ophthalmoplegia**, and **areflexia** characterize this variant of Guillain–Barré syndrome (see Chapter 9, Motor Disorders). Incomplete forms of the Fisher variant and forms that overlap with classic Guillain–Barré syndrome also occur. Symptoms develop over days and are thought to be caused by autoantibodies against GQ1b ganglioside located on ocular motor and dorsal root ganglion nerves. Ataxia primarily affects the gait and trunk, with lesser involvement of the individual limbs; dysarthria is uncommon. Ophthalmoplegia can involve the pupils as well as extraocular muscles. CSF protein may be elevated and anti-GQ1b antibodies may be detected in the blood. Respiratory insufficiency is rare, and the usual course is a gradual and often complete recovery over weeks to months.

EPISODIC DISORDERS

MOTION SICKNESS

Motion sickness affects up to 30% of the general population, with susceptibility influenced by genetics, age (peak ~9 years), and concurrent disorders (eg, migraine). Symptoms are triggered by real or perceived movement of the affected individual or of his or her environment, as occurs during vehicular travel, watching 3D movies, or using virtual reality devices. Features include nausea, vomiting, vertigo, headache, pallor, sweating, salivation, anorexia, osmophobia, and a sensation of warmth. Motion sickness may be prevented by lying supine or viewing the horizon while traveling, and habituation therapy may be effective in the long term. Muscarinic anticholinergic drugs (eg, scopolamine, 1.5 mg transdermally) and H1 antihistamines (eg, dimenhydrinate, 50 mg orally) are useful for acute attacks, but dopamine D_2 and serotonin 5-HT$_3$ receptor antagonist anti-emetics are not.

VESTIBULAR MIGRAINE

Vestibular migraine is characterized by episodic vertigo accompanied by other features of migraine attacks, such as headache, photophobia, phonophobia, or visual aura. Treatment includes vestibular rehabilitation training and drugs used for other forms of migraine, as discussed in detail in Chapter 6, Headache & Facial Pain.

AUTOSOMAL DOMINANT EPISODIC ATAXIAS

Episodic ataxias are autosomal dominant disorders characterized by transient attacks of cerebellar ataxia that may be precipitated by physical or emotional stress. Episodic ataxia 1 (**EA1**) results from mutations in *KCNA1*, which codes for the Kv1.1 voltage-gated potassium channel. Attacks last from seconds to minutes and may occur many times per day; myokymia—a quivering, involuntary movement of muscle—commonly occurs between episodes.

EA2 is caused by mutations in *CACNA1A*, which codes for the α_{1A} subunit of the P/Q-type voltage-gated calcium channel; this gene is also affected in spinocerebellar ataxia 6 (SCA6; discussed later in this chapter) and familial hemiplegic migraine (see Chapter 6, Headache & Facial Pain). Attacks are more prolonged than in EA1, typically lasting for hours, and nystagmus and slowly progressive ataxia persist between acute episodes. **Acetazolamide** (500 mg orally four times daily) can often prevent or relieve acute symptoms in EA2.

EA5 likewise affects voltage-gated calcium channels, but in this case the mutation is in *CACNB4*, which encodes the β subunit. **EA6** is due to mutations in *SLC1A3*, which encodes the EAAT1 glial glutamate transporter. Glutamate uptake is reduced, leading to enhanced excitatory input onto cerebellar Purkinje cells. EA1 and EA6 are thought to impair channel function through dominant negative effects, whereas EA2 involves haploinsufficiency; the mechanism in EA5 is uncertain.

CHRONIC DISORDERS

MULTIPLE SCLEROSIS

▶ Pathogenesis

Multiple sclerosis (see also Chapter 9, Motor Disorders) is characterized clinically by remitting and relapsing neurologic dysfunction at multiple sites in the central nervous system. Because these include vestibular, cerebellar, and sensory pathways, multiple sclerosis can produce disorders of equilibrium. Symptoms and signs are associated with **demyelination** and **axonal loss**, which primarily affect white matter.

▶ Clinical Findings

Cerebellar signs are present in approximately one-third of patients on initial examination and ultimately develop in twice that number. **Nystagmus, dysarthria,** and **limb ataxia** are common, but **vertigo** is less so. **Gait ataxia** is a presenting complaint in 10-15% of patients and is usually due to cerebellar involvement.

▶ Diagnosis

The diagnosis relies on a history of multiple episodes of neurologic dysfunction separated in both time and space. Subclinical lesions may be evident from physical findings such as optic neuritis, internuclear ophthalmoplegia, or pyramidal signs, or from laboratory investigations. CSF analysis may reveal oligoclonal bands, elevated IgG,

increased protein, or a mild lymphocytic pleocytosis. Visual, auditory, or somatosensory evoked response recording (see Chapter 2, Investigative Studies) can also document subclinical sites of involvement. CT or MRI shows demyelination.

▶ Treatment

Treatment is discussed in Chapter 9, Motor Disorders.

ALCOHOLIC CEREBELLAR DEGENERATION

▶ Pathogenesis

A characteristic cerebellar syndrome may develop in chronic alcoholics, probably as a result of nutritional deficiency. Degenerative changes in the cerebellum are largely restricted to the superior vermis (**Figure 8-10**), which is also the site of involvement in Wernicke encephalopathy.

▶ Clinical Features

Alcoholic cerebellar degeneration is most common in men between ages 40 and 60 years. Patients typically have a history of daily or binge drinking lasting 10 or more years with associated dietary inadequacy. Most have experienced other medical complications of alcoholism, such as liver disease, delirium tremens, Wernicke encephalopathy, or polyneuropathy. Cerebellar degeneration usually has an insidious onset and progresses gradually over weeks to months, eventually reaching a plateau of dysfunction. In occasional cases, ataxia appears abruptly.

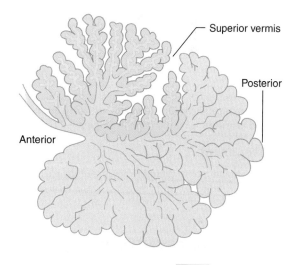

Purkinje cell loss

▲ **Figure 8-10.** Distribution of atrophy in alcoholic cerebellar degeneration. Midsagittal view of the cerebellum showing loss of Purkinje cells, confined largely to the superior vermis.

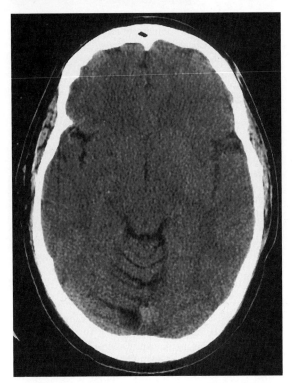

▲ **Figure 8-11.** CT scan in alcoholic cerebellar degeneration, showing marked atrophy of the midline cerebellar vermis with relative sparing of the cerebellar hemispheres. (Used with permission from A. Gean.)

Gait ataxia is universal and almost always the problem that brings the patient to medical attention. The legs are ataxic on heel-knee-shin testing in approximately 80% of patients. Common associated findings include distal sensory deficits in the feet and absent ankle reflexes, which result from polyneuropathy. Ataxia of the arms, nystagmus, dysarthria, hypotonia, and truncal instability are less frequent. CT or MRI may show cerebellar atrophy (**Figure 8-11**).

▶ Treatment

Patients should receive **thiamine** because of the likely role of thiamine deficiency in pathogenesis. Abstinence from alcohol and adequate nutrition may help prevent progression.

TOXIN-INDUCED CEREBELLAR DEGENERATION

Purkinje cells and granule cells of the cerebellum are selectively vulnerable to a variety of toxins. These may cause cerebellar degeneration associated with nystagmus, dysarthria, and ataxia affecting the limbs, trunk, and gait. In addition to alcohol, this syndrome can be produced by phenytoin, lithium, amiodarone, fluorouracil, cytarabine,

toluene, lead, mercury, and thallium. Treatment is discontinuation of the offending agents and, for fluorouracil, administration of thiamine (vitamin B$_1$), but toxin-induced cerebellar syndromes may be irreversible.

HYPOTHYROIDISM

Hypothyroidism can cause a subacute or chronically progressive cerebellar syndrome, which is most common in middle-aged and elderly women. Symptoms evolve over months to years. Systemic symptoms (eg, myxedema) usually precede the cerebellar disorder.

Gait ataxia is universal and is the most prominent finding. Limb ataxia is also common and may be asymmetric. Dysarthria and nystagmus occur less frequently. Other neurologic disorders related to hypothyroidism may coexist with cerebellar involvement, including sensorineural hearing loss, carpal tunnel syndrome, neuropathy, or myopathy.

Diagnosis and treatment are discussed in Chapter 4, Confusional States.

AUTOIMMUNE CEREBELLAR DEGENERATION

▶ Paraneoplastic Cerebellar Degeneration

Autoimmune cerebellar degeneration can occur as a remote (paraneoplastic) effect of systemic cancer. Lung cancer (especially small-cell), ovarian cancer, Hodgkin disease, and breast cancer are the most commonly associated neoplasms.

Paraneoplastic degeneration affects the cerebellar vermis and hemispheres diffusely. The cause appears to be autoimmunity involving **antineural antibodies**, which are directed against either neuronal nuclear antigens or antigens expressed more specifically in the cell membranes or cytoplasm of cerebellar Purkinje cells (**Table 8-10**).

Cerebellar symptoms can appear either before or after the diagnosis of cancer and typically evolve over months. Gait and limb ataxia are prominent, and may be asymmetric. Dysarthria is common but nystagmus is rare. Involvement of additional regions besides the cerebellum may produce dysphagia, dementia, memory disturbance, pyramidal signs, or neuropathy.

Onconeural antibodies can sometimes be detected in the blood, and the CSF may show a mild lymphocytic pleocytosis or elevated protein.

Diagnosis may be difficult when neurologic symptoms precede the discovery of cancer. Dysarthria, dysphagia, and ataxia of the arms help distinguish paraneoplastic cerebellar degeneration from syndromes produced by chronic alcoholism or hypothyroidism. However, Wernicke encephalopathy should always be considered because patients with cancer may suffer from malnutrition.

Treatment is of the underlying tumor, supplemented in some cases by immunotherapy with immunoglobulin G, corticosteroids, cyclophosphamide, tacrolimus, rituximab, mycophenolate, or plasma exchange. The disorder usually

Table 8-10. Autoimmune Cerebellar Degenerations.

Syndrome	Antibody	Associated Neoplasm
Paraneoplastic cerebellar degeneration	Anti-Yo Anti-Hu Anti-Tr Anti-CV2 Anti-Ri Anti-Ma2 Anti-voltage-gated calcium channel (P/Q type)	Breast, uterus, ovary Small cell lung carcinoma Hodgkin disease Small cell lung carcinoma, thymoma Breast Testis, lung Small cell lung carcinoma
Gluten ataxia	Anti-transglutaminase 2, 6	—
Anti-GAD cerebellar ataxia	Anti-glutamic acid decarboxylase	—
Hashimoto encephalopathy	Anti-thyroglobulin, anti-thyroperoxidase, anti-α-enolase	—

Data from Mitoma H et al, Guidelines for treatment of immune-mediated cerebellar ataxias. Cerebellum & Ataxias (2015) 2:14.

progresses steadily, but may stabilize or remit with treatment.

Other Autoimmune Cerebellar Degenerations

Autoimmune cerebellar degeneration also occurs in patients without cancer who produce autoantibodies against transglutaminase, glutamic acid decarboxylase, or thyroid antigens.

Gluten ataxia is manifested by gait ataxia, lower limb ataxia, and nystagmus. It appears to result from autoantibodies against gluten proteins (gliadins) that cross react with transglutaminases in the small intestine (TG2) and brain (TG6). Symptoms of gluten enteropathy (celiac disease) are typically absent, but intestinal biopsy may show immune deposits. MRI may show cerebellar atrophy, and anti-transglutaminase antibodies are commonly present in the blood. The mainstay of treatment is a gluten-free diet.

Anti-glutamic acid decarboxylase (GAD) cerebellar ataxia is associated with autoantibodies against the enzyme (GAD) that synthesizes γ–aminobutyric acid (GABA), the brain's principal inhibitory neurotransmitter. Gait ataxia is the most consistent clinical feature, but limb ataxia, dysarthria, and nystagmus can also occur. Intravenous immunoglobulin and corticosteroids may be beneficial. Anti-GAD antibodies are also implicated in stiff-person syndrome (see Chapter 9, Motor Disorders).

Hashimoto encephalopathy is a steroid-responsive encephalopathy associated with autoimmune thyroiditis. In addition to ataxia, confusional states, seizures, and myoclonus may occur. Patients are typically euthyroid when ataxia is first diagnosed, and MRI shows little or no cerebellar atrophy. Antibodies against thyroid antigens and α-enolase may be detected in the blood. Treatment is with corticosteroids.

AUTOSOMAL DOMINANT SPINOCEREBELLAR ATAXIA

Autosomal dominant spinocerebellar ataxia (**SCA**) encompasses a group of over 40 genetically and clinically heterogeneous disorders (**Table 8-11**).

Genetics

Several types of mutations can produce autosomal dominant SCA, including expansion of **CAG trinucleotide repeats** coding for **polyglutamine (polyQ) tracts**, expansion of tri- or pentanucleotide repeats in noncoding regions, and point mutations. Of these, the polyQ disorders are the most common and best characterized. They affect a wide range of proteins, including ion channels, receptors, enzymes, and cytoskeletal proteins.

A striking feature of polyQ disorders is that the underlying trinucleotide expansion is unstable and tends to enlarge with time. This leads to **anticipation**, in which the age at onset decreases, the disease severity increases, or both, in successive generations.

In addition to SCAs, polyQ disorders include spinal bulbar muscular atrophy (Kennedy disease, see Chapter 9, Motor Disorders) and Huntington disease (see Chapter 11, Movement Disorders).

Pathogenesis

PolyQ expansions confer a **toxic gain of function** on the target protein. The abnormally long polyQ tract predisposes the protein to conformational changes, misfolding, and proteolytic cleavage (**Figure 8-12**). As a consequence, protein fragments are generated that are prone to aggregate and, in some cases, translocate from the cytoplasm to the nucleus. Neuronal dysfunction and death are thought to result from some combination of direct toxicity of abnormal

Table 8-11. Clinical and Genetic Features of Autosomal Dominant Spinocerebellar Ataxias (SCAs).

Syndrome[1]	Clinical Features	Examples[2]	Gene	Protein	Mutation[3]
ADCA I	Cerebellar ataxia + ophthalmoplegia, dementia, extrapyramidal signs, optic atrophy or amyotrophy.	SCA1	ATXN1	Ataxin-1	CAG repeat
		SCA2	ATXN 2	Ataxin-2	CAG repeat
		SCA3/MJD (Machado–Joseph disease)	ATXN3	Ataxin-3	CAG repeat
		SCA8	ATXN8	Ataxin-8	(CTG·CAG) repeat
		SCA28	AFG3L2	ATPase family gene 3-like protein 2	Various missense
ADCA II	Cerebellar ataxia + retinal degeneration	SCA7	ATXN7	Ataxin-7	CAG repeat
ADCA III	Pure cerebellar ataxia	SCA6	CACNA1A	Calcium channel, P/Q-type voltage-gated, α_{1A} subunit	CAG repeat

[1]ADCA, autosomal dominant cerebellar ataxia.
[2]Examples shown are those that constitute ≥3% of SCAs.
[3]CAG repeats code for polyglutamine tracts.

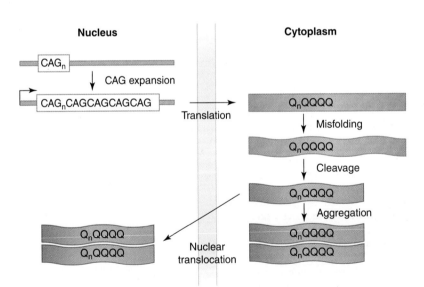

▲ **Figure 8-12.** Proposed mechanisms of polyQ protein processing and toxicity. In polyQ diseases including several autosomal dominant spinocerebellar ataxias, a gene containing a CAG trinucleotide repeat (CAG_n) undergoes mutation by expansion of the repeat. The resulting abnormal protein (Q_nQQQQ) contains an abnormally long polyQ tract, which induces conformational changes that promote misfolding. The misfolded protein is subject to proteolytic cleavage, which generates abnormal and possibly toxic fragments, which may also have an increased tendency to be translocated from the cytoplasm to the nucleus, to aggregate, or both. As a result of these events, neuronal function is impaired, and neurons may eventually die. How neurotoxicity and neuronal death ultimately occur is unknown, but there may be multiple mechanisms, and these may differ across polyQ diseases. Possible contributing factors include direct toxicity of misfolded and cleaved protein monomers or oligomers, or of cytoplasmic or nuclear aggregates (red in figure); impaired proteasomal degradation, axonal transport, or nuclear function; and interactions between polyQ proteins and other cellular proteins.

proteins or their cytoplasmic or nuclear aggregates; impaired proteasomal function, axonal transport, or nuclear function; and protein-protein interactions.

Clinical Findings

The autosomal dominant SCAs show considerable clinical variability, even within a given family. In general, they are associated with an adult-onset, slowly progressive cerebellar syndrome in which gait ataxia is an early and prominent feature. Other manifestations are dysarthria, diplopia, and limb ataxia. Extracerebellar findings are common, including cognitive, pyramidal, extrapyramidal, motor neuron, peripheral nerve, or macular involvement.

The most common SCAs are 1, 2, 3, 6, and 7. SCA1 produces gait ataxia, limb ataxia, and dysarthria, with brainstem involvement but little cognitive abnormality. SCA2 is notable for the association of ataxia and dysarthria with slow saccadic eye movements and polyneuropathy. SCA3 (**Machado–Joseph disease**) is especially common in patients of Portuguese ancestry; ataxia is accompanied by eyelid retraction, reduced blinking, external ophthalmoplegia, dysarthria, dysphagia, and sometimes parkinsonism or peripheral neuropathy. SCA6 is comparatively less severe, progresses more slowly, and is more limited to cerebellar involvement than other SCAs. SCA7 is distinguished by retinal degeneration leading to blindness, in addition to ataxia.

Atrophy of the cerebellum and sometimes also of the brainstem may be apparent on CT or MRI (**Figure 8-13**).

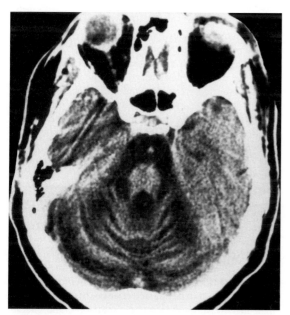

▲ **Figure 8-13.** CT scan in spinocerebellar atrophy, showing an atrophic cerebellum and brainstem. (Used with permission from A. Gean.)

However, definitive diagnosis is by genetic testing. There is no specific treatment, but occupational and physical therapy and devices to assist ambulation may be helpful, and genetic counseling may be indicated.

DENTATORUBRAL-PALLIDOLUYSIAN ATROPHY

Dentatorubral-pallidoluysian atrophy (**DRPLA**) is a dominantly inherited disorder that results from a polyglutamine expansion in the *ATN1* gene coding for the protein atrophin 1. DRPLA causes ataxia, chorea, dementia, seizures, and myoclonus. Because of the prominent extrapyramidal features, this disorder is discussed in Chapter 11, Movement Disorders.

ATAXIA-TELANGIECTASIA

Pathogenesis

Ataxia-telangiectasia (also known as Louis–Bar syndrome) is an inherited autosomal recessive disorder with onset in infancy. It results from loss-of-function mutations in the ataxia-telangiectasia mutated (*ATM*) gene, which codes for a serine/threonine protein kinase related to phosphatidylinositol 3-kinase. Deletions, insertions, and substitutions all have been described. A defect in the repair of DNA double strand breaks is thought to be involved in pathogenesis.

Clinical Findings

Ataxia-telangiectasia is characterized by progressive **cerebellar ataxia**, **oculocutaneous telangiectasia**, **sinopulmonary infections**, and **lymphoid tumors**. Patients typically suffer from progressive pancerebellar degeneration characterized by nystagmus, dysarthria, and gait, limb, and trunk ataxia. Choreoathetosis, loss of vibration and position sense in the legs, areflexia, and disorders of voluntary eye movement are almost universal findings. Mental deficiency is commonly observed in the second decade.

Oculocutaneous telangiectasia usually appears in the teen years. The bulbar conjunctivae are typically affected first, followed by sun-exposed areas of the skin, including the ears, nose, face, and antecubital and popliteal fossae. The vascular lesions, which rarely bleed, spare the central nervous system.

Immunologic impairment usually becomes evident later in childhood, with recurrent sinopulmonary infections in more than 80% of patients. Malignancies occur in approximately one-third of patients and include non-Hodgkin lymphoma, leukemia, and Hodgkin disease.

Other common clinical findings are progeric changes of the skin and hair, hypogonadism, and insulin-resistant diabetes mellitus. The characteristic laboratory abnormalities include decreased circulating levels of IgG2, IgA, and IgE and elevation of α-fetoprotein and carcinoembryonic antigen levels.

Atypical phenotypes may be associated with later (including adult) onset, slower progression, absence of telangiectasia, and movement disorders rather than ataxia as the primary neurologic manifestation.

Because the vascular and immunologic manifestations of ataxia-telangiectasia occur later than the neurologic symptoms, the condition may be confused with Friedreich ataxia, which also manifests in childhood (see later). Ataxia-telangiectasia can be distinguished by its earlier onset (before age 4 years), associated choreoathetosis, and the absence of kyphoscoliosis.

There is no specific treatment for ataxia-telangiectasia, but antibiotics are useful in the management of infections. X-rays should be avoided because of the hypersensitivity to ionizing radiation present in this disorder.

FRAGILE X-ASSOCIATED TREMOR/ATAXIA SYNDROME

Fragile X-associated tremor/ataxia syndrome (FXTAS) is an X-linked disorder caused by gain-of-function mutations (CGG expansions) in the 5′ untranslated region of the fragile X mental retardation 1 (*FMR1*) gene. White matter tracts, including the middle cerebellar peduncles, are prominently involved. FXTAS affects males primarily and presents at an average age of 60 years, with features that include intention tremor and cerebellar ataxia. Diagnosis is by DNA testing.

MULTIPLE SYSTEM ATROPHY

Multiple system atrophy is a neurodegenerative proteinopathy associated with deposition of α-synuclein in affected neurons. It produces autonomic dysfunction and either parkinsonism or ataxia. Multiple system atrophy is discussed in more detail Chapter 11, Movement Disorders.

HEPATOCEREBRAL DEGENERATION

Hepatocerebral degeneration refers to diseases that impair the function of both the liver and brain, including **acquired (non-Wilsonian) hepatocerebral degeneration** (eg, that due to liver cirrhosis with portosystemic shunting) and hereditary disorders. Ataxia may be a feature in both cases. **Wilson disease**, a disorder of copper metabolism characterized by copper deposition in a variety of tissues, is an important cause of hereditary hepatocerebral degeneration. It is an autosomal recessive disorder that results from mutations in the *ATP7B* gene, which codes for the β polypeptide of a copper-transporting ATPase. Because extrapyramidal features are usually the most prominent neurologic manifestations, Wilson disease is discussed in more detail in Chapter 11, Movement Disorders.

PRION DISEASES

Creutzfeldt–Jakob disease (described in Chapter 5, Dementia & Amnesia) and **Gerstmann–Sträussler–Scheinker syndrome** (a rare, autosomal dominant disorder) are prion diseases that can produce ataxia. Cerebellar signs are present in approximately 60% of patients with Creutzfeldt–Jakob disease, and patients present with ataxia in approximately 10% of cases. Cerebellar involvement is diffuse, but the vermis is often most severely affected. In contrast to most other cerebellar disorders, depletion of granule cells is frequently more striking than Purkinje cell loss.

Patients with cerebellar manifestations of Creutzfeldt–Jakob disease typically complain first of gait ataxia. Dementia is usually evident at this time, and cognitive dysfunction always develops eventually. Nystagmus, dysarthria, truncal ataxia, and limb ataxia are all present initially in approximately one-half of patients with the ataxic form of Creutzfeldt–Jakob disease. The course is characterized by progressive dementia, myoclonus, and extrapyramidal and pyramidal dysfunction. Death typically occurs within 1 year after onset.

POSTERIOR FOSSA TUMORS

Tumors of the posterior fossa cause cerebellar symptoms when they arise in the cerebellum or compress it from without. Common posterior fossa tumors in children include **medulloblastoma, cystic astrocytoma, ependymoma**, and **brainstem glioma**, whereas **hemangioblastoma, choroid plexus papilloma, meningioma**, and **metastases** from outside the nervous system (especially the lung and breast) predominate in adults.

▶ Clinical Findings

Patients with cerebellar tumors usually present with headache from increased intracranial pressure or with ataxia. Nausea, vomiting, vertigo, cranial nerve palsies, and hydrocephalus are common. The nature of the clinical findings varies with the location of the tumor. Most metastases are located in the cerebellar hemispheres, causing asymmetric cerebellar signs. Medulloblastomas and ependymomas, on the other hand, tend to arise in the midline, with early involvement of the vermis and hydrocephalus.

Hemangioblastoma may occur as one feature of **von Hippel–Lindau disease**, which results from a dominant mutation in the *VHL* tumor suppressor gene, and may also cause retinal hemangioblastoma, renal or pancreatic cysts, and polycythemia. Ependymomas commonly arise in the fourth ventricle, which predisposes to seeding through the ventricular system and hydrocephalus.

▶ Diagnosis & Treatment

CT scan or MRI is useful for diagnosis, but biopsy may be required for histologic characterization. Methods of treatment include surgical resection, irradiation, and chemotherapy. Corticosteroids are useful in controlling tumor-associated edema. Total resection may be curative for cystic astrocytoma of the cerebellum and meningioma.

Medulloblastoma shows wide variation in prognosis based on molecular subgrouping.

POSTERIOR FOSSA MALFORMATIONS

Congenital anomalies affecting the cerebellum and brainstem include malformations of the hindbrain (cerebellar agenesis, Dandy–Walker malformation, arachnoid cyst) or cranial vault (Arnold–Chiari malformation). Vestibular or cerebellar symptoms presenting in adulthood are most common in type I **Arnold–Chiari malformation**, which consists of downward displacement of the cerebellar tonsils through the foramen magnum. Clinical manifestations are related to cerebellar involvement, obstructive **hydrocephalus**, brainstem compression, and **syringomyelia** (a cyst or syrinx in the spinal cord). Type II Arnold–Chiari malformation is associated with **meningomyelocele** (protrusion of the spinal cord, nerve roots, and meninges through a fusion defect in the vertebral column) and has its onset in childhood. Type III Arnold–Chiari malformation is accompanied by **encephalocele** (herniation of posterior fossa contents through an occipital or cervical bony defect).

Cerebellar ataxia in the type I malformation usually affects the gait and is bilateral; in some cases, it is asymmetric. Hydrocephalus leads to headache and vomiting. Compression of the brainstem by herniated cerebellar tissue may be associated with vertigo, nystagmus, and lower cranial nerve palsies. Syringomyelia typically produces a cape-like distribution of defective pain and temperature sensation.

Arnold–Chiari malformation can be diagnosed by CT or MRI studies that demonstrate cerebellar tonsillar herniation. Patients with headache, neck pain, hydrocephalus, or other symptoms related to compression of the cerebellum or brainstem may benefit from surgical decompression of the foramen magnum. Neuropathic pain may respond to antidepressants or anticonvulsants (see Chapter 12, Seizures & Syncope).

▼ SENSORY ATAXIAS

Sensory ataxia is usually the result of impaired proprioceptive sensation due to lesions of the peripheral sensory nerves (**sensory neuropathy**), dorsal root ganglia (**sensory neuronopathy**), or posterior columns of the spinal cord (**myelopathy**) (**Table 8-12**). Clinical findings include defective joint position and vibration sense in the legs and sometimes the arms, unstable stance with Romberg sign, and a gait of slapping or steppage quality.

SENSORY NEUROPATHY OR NEURONOPATHY

Polyneuropathies that affect **large myelinated sensory fibers** and **sensory neuronopathies** (which target **dorsal root ganglia**) may present with ataxia. Prominent examples

Table 8-12. Causes of Sensory Ataxia.

Sensory neuropathy or neuronopathy[1]
Paraneoplastic (eg, sensory neuronopathy with anti-Hu antibodies)
Other immune-mediated (eg, Sjögren, GALOP, anti-MAG, Miller Fisher, anti-GD1b syndromes)
Infectious (eg, diphtheria delayed radiculoneuropathy, HIV, HTLV-1)
Toxic (eg, pyridoxine, platinum analogs, etoposide, taxol, isoniazid)
Hereditary (eg, Dejerine–Sottas disease/HMSN[2] type III, Refsum disease)
Myelopathy[3]
Acute transverse myelitis
HIV disease (vacuolar myelopathy)
Multiple sclerosis
Tumor or cord compression
Vascular malformations
Combined lesions
Friedreich ataxia
Neurosyphilis (tabes dorsalis)
Nitrous oxide
Vitamin B$_{12}$ deficiency
Vitamin E deficiency (including abetalipoproteinemia)

[1]Involving large, myelinated sensory fibers or dorsal root ganglion neurons.
[2]Hereditary motor and sensory neuropathy.
[3]Involving posterior columns.

include the Hu antibody-positive sensory neuronopathy associated with small-cell lung cancer, sensory neuronopathy from consumption of high doses of pyridoxine, and the Fisher variant of the Guillain–Barré syndrome. These are discussed in more detail in Chapter 10, Sensory Disorders.

MYELOPATHY

Myelopathies that affect the **posterior columns** can also cause ataxia. A common cause of this syndrome is multiple sclerosis, discussed earlier as a cause of cerebellar ataxia and in Chapter 9, Motor Disorders, as a cause of myelopathy.

COMBINED LESIONS

Several diseases can affect both peripheral and central sensory pathways (**Figure 8-14**). Examples include neurosyphilis (tabes dorsalis) and combined systems disease from vitamin B$_{12}$ deficiency, which are discussed elsewhere as causes of dementia (see Chapter 5, Dementia & Amnesia) or sensory disturbance (see Chapter 10, Sensory Disorders). Another example is Friedreich ataxia, discussed next.

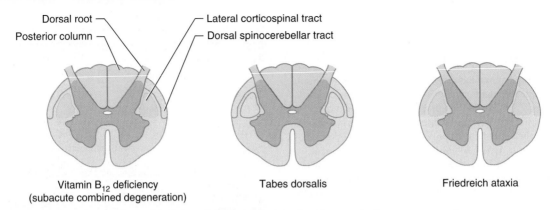

Dorsal root — / Lateral corticospinal tract
Posterior column — / Dorsal spinocerebellar tract

Vitamin B₁₂ deficiency
(subacute combined degeneration) — $Vitamin B_{12}$ deficiency (subacute combined degeneration)

Tabes dorsalis

Friedreich ataxia

▲ **Figure 8-14.** Principal sites of spinal cord disease (blue) in disorders producing sensory ataxia.

FRIEDREICH ATAXIA

Friedreich ataxia, an autosomal recessive disorder with onset usually in childhood, is the most common cause of hereditary ataxia. It results from an expanded GAA trinucleotide repeat in a noncoding region of the *FXN* gene, which causes loss-of-function of a mitochondrial protein, **frataxin**. The key pathologic findings are degeneration of the dorsal root ganglia, large myelinated axons of peripheral sensory nerves, corticospinal tracts, and dentate nuclei of the cerebellum, with secondary involvement of the spinocerebellar tracts, posterior columns, and dorsal nucleus of Clarke.

▶ Clinical Findings

The average age at onset is approximately 13 years, with longer GAA repeats correlating with earlier onset. The initial symptom is usually progressive gait ataxia, followed by limb ataxia, dysarthria, and sensory gait ataxia. Neurologic examination shows knee and ankle areflexia, impaired joint position and vibration sense in the legs, leg (and sometimes arm) weakness, and extensor plantar responses. **Pes cavus** (high-arched feet with clawing of the toes caused by weakness and wasting of the intrinsic foot muscles) is often present, but can also occur in other neurologic disorders (eg, Charcot–Marie–Tooth disease).

Severe progressive **kyphoscoliosis** may lead to chronic restrictive lung disease. **Cardiomyopathy** may result in congestive heart failure, arrhythmia, and death. Other abnormalities include visual impairment from **optic atrophy** and **diabetes mellitus**.

Atypical phenotypes may be seen with smaller GAA expansions and include late (>25 years) or very late (>40 years) onset and preserved reflexes. These syndromes are characterized by slow progression and a paucity of nonneurologic features.

Friedreich ataxia can usually be differentiated from other cerebellar and spinocerebellar degenerations by its early onset and the presence of prominent sensory impairment, areflexia, skeletal abnormalities, and cardiomyopathy. Definitive diagnosis is by genetic testing.

▶ Treatment & Prognosis

There is no current treatment for the neurologic manifestations of Friedreich ataxia. Orthopedic procedures or devices may improve kyphoscoliosis and gait disorder. The average duration of symptomatic illness is approximately 25 years, with death occurring at a mean age of approximately 40 years. Cardiomyopathy and infection are the usual causes of death.

Motor Disorders

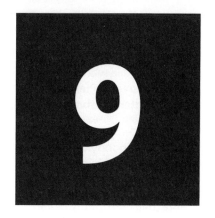

9

(Continued on Next Page)

Normal motor function depends on the transmission of signals from the brain to the brainstem or spinal cord by **upper motor neurons**, and from there to skeletal muscle by **lower motor neurons** (**Figure 9-1**). A lesion that involves this pathway anywhere along its length may impair motor function. Anatomic structures involved in the regulation or execution of motor activity include the pyramidal and extrapyramidal systems, cerebellum, and lower motor neurons in the cranial nerve nuclei of the brainstem and anterior horns of the spinal cord.

The **pyramidal system** (**Figure 9-2**) consists of **upper motor neuron** fibers that descend from the cerebral cortex through the internal capsule, traverse the medullary pyramid, and then mostly decussate, to descend in the lateral corticospinal tract on the opposite side, where they synapse on interneurons and lower motor neurons in the spinal cord.

All other descending influences on lower motor neurons belong to the **extrapyramidal system** and originate primarily in the basal ganglia and cerebellum. Disorders of the basal ganglia (see Chapter 11, Movement Disorders) and cerebellum (see Chapter 8, Disorders of Equilibrium) are considered separately.

The motor fibers in the cranial and peripheral nerves arise from the **lower motor neurons** (**Figure 9-3**). Dysfunction at any point in the peripheral nervous system (anterior horn cell, nerve root, limb plexus, peripheral nerve, or neuromuscular junction) can impair motor function, as can disease of the muscles.

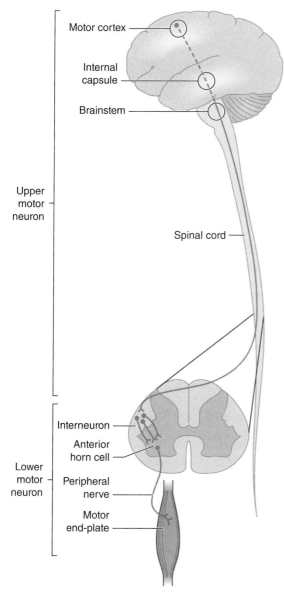

Figure 9-1. Anatomic basis of the upper motor neuron and lower motor neuron concepts.

Labels on figure:
Motor cortex
Internal capsule
Brainstem
Upper motor neuron
Spinal cord
Interneuron
Anterior horn cell
Lower motor neuron
Peripheral nerve
Motor end-plate

Patients with motor deficits generally complain of weakness, heaviness, stiffness, clumsiness, impaired muscular control, or difficulty in executing movements. The term *weakness* is sometimes used in a nonspecific way to denote fatigue or loss of energy, drive, or enthusiasm, and its meaning must therefore always be clarified. The word is properly used to mean loss of muscle *power*, and it is in this sense that it is employed here.

HISTORY OF PRESENT ILLNESS

Mode of Onset

An abrupt onset suggests a vascular disturbance, such as a stroke, or certain toxic or metabolic disturbances, whereas subacute onset over days to weeks is commonly associated with a neoplastic, infective, or inflammatory process (**Table 9-1**). Weakness that evolves slowly over several months or years often has a hereditary, degenerative, endocrinologic, or neoplastic basis.

Course

A progressive increase in the motor deficit from its onset suggests continuing activity of the underlying process. Episodic progression suggests a vascular or inflammatory origin; a steadily progressive course is more suggestive of neoplastic disorder or such degenerative conditions as motor neuron disease. Rapid fluctuation of symptoms over short periods (eg, over the course of the day) is characteristic of myasthenia gravis.

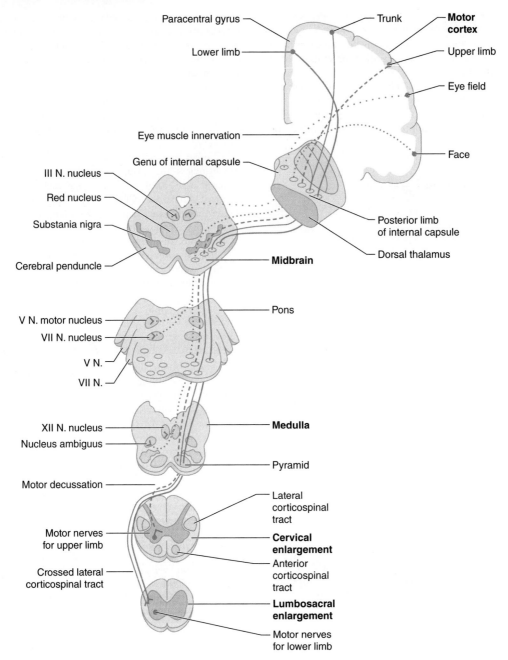

Figure 9-2. Upper motor neuron pathways. Tracts at bottom left are shown outside the cord for clarity only. (Used with permission from McPhee SJ, Hammer GD: *Pathophysiology of Disease: An Introduction to Clinical Medicine*. 6th ed. New York, NY: McGraw-Hill; 2009.)

▶ Distribution of Symptoms

The distribution of weakness and the presence of associated symptoms may indicate the approximate site of the lesion. For example, weakness in the right arm and leg may result from a lesion of the contralateral motor cortex or the corticospinal pathway at any point above the fifth cervical segment of the spinal cord. Associated right facial weakness indicates that the lesion must be above the level of the

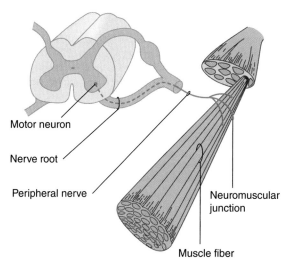

Motor neuron

Nerve root

Peripheral nerve

Neuromuscular
junction

Muscle fiber

▲ **Figure 9-3.** Anatomic components of the motor unit.

Table 9-1. Some Causes of Weakness of Acute or Subacute Onset.

Supraspinal lesions
Stroke
Other structural lesions
Spinal cord lesions
Infective: human immunodeficiency virus (HIV) infection
Inflammatory: transverse myelitis, multiple sclerosis
Compressive: tumor, disk protrusion, abscess
Vascular: infarction, hematomyelia
Anterior horn cell disorders
Poliovirus, coxsackievirus, West Nile virus infection
Peripheral nerve disorders
Guillain–Barré syndrome
Diphtheria
Paralytic shellfish poisoning
Porphyria
Arsenic poisoning
Organophosphate toxicity
Neuromuscular junction disorders
Myasthenia gravis
Botulism
Aminoglycoside toxicity
Muscle disorders
Necrotizing myopathies
Acute hypo- or hyperkalemia
Periodic paralyses

facial (VII) nerve nucleus in the brainstem, and an accompanying aphasia (see Chapter 1, Neurologic History & Examination) or visual field defect (see Chapter 7, Neuro-Ophthalmic Disorders) localizes it to the cerebral hemisphere.

▶ Associated Symptoms

The presence and distribution of any sensory abnormalities also help in localizing the lesion. Sensory abnormalities lateralized to the same side as weakness suggest a hemispheric lesion; a cortical lesion is implied by sensory neglect or inattention, agraphesthesia (inability to identify by touch a number written on the skin), astereognosis (inability to identify by touch an object placed in the hand), abarognosis (inability to judge the weight of an object placed in the hand), or impaired two-point discrimination, when peripheral sensory function is intact. Sensory loss below a particular segmental level on the trunk suggests a spinal cord lesion, whereas distal sensory changes in the limbs favor a peripheral nerve lesion. Diseases of the anterior horn cells, neuromuscular junctions, or muscles are not accompanied by altered sensation.

The character of any associated symptoms may suggest the nature of the lesion. Thus, progressive leg weakness caused by myelopathy is often preceded or accompanied by pain in the back or legs when the myelopathy is due to a compressive lesion—but not when it has a metabolic or hereditary basis.

▶ Severity of Symptoms

The functional severity of a motor deficit is evaluated by determining whether there has been any restriction of daily activities, difficulty in performing previously easy tasks, or reduction in exercise tolerance.

The nature of the functional disturbance depends on the muscles involved. Weakness of proximal muscles in the legs leads to difficulty in climbing or descending stairs or in getting up from a squatting position, whereas proximal weakness in the arms leads to difficulty with such tasks as combing the hair. Distal weakness in the arms may lead to clumsiness, difficulty with such fine motor tasks as doing up buttons or tying shoelaces, and eventually the inability to pick up or grasp objects with the hands, so that even eating becomes difficult or impossible.

Involvement of the muscles supplied by the cranial nerves may lead to diplopia (oculomotor [III], trochlear [IV], or abducens [VI] nerve); difficulty in chewing (trigeminal [V] nerve) or sucking, blowing, or grimacing (facial [VII] nerve); or difficulty in swallowing, with nasal regurgitation and dysarthria (glossopharyngeal [IX], vagus [X], and hypoglossal [XII] nerves).

Weakness of the respiratory muscles leads to tachypnea, the use of accessory muscles of respiration, and anxiety at a stage when arterial blood gases are usually still normal. A vital capacity of less than 1 L in an adult generally calls for ventilatory support, especially if weakness is increasing.

PAST MEDICAL HISTORY

The importance of the past history depends on the patient's present complaint and the nature of any previous illnesses. For example, in a patient with lung cancer, limb weakness may be due to metastasis or to a remote (nonmetastatic) complication of the cancer. Leg weakness in a diabetic may reflect peripheral nerve, plexus, or multiple root involvement, and hand weakness in a myxedematous patient may be associated with carpal tunnel syndrome.

All drugs taken by the patient should be noted. Drugs can cause peripheral neuropathy, impair neuromuscular transmission, or lead to myopathy (**Table 9-2**).

DEVELOPMENTAL HISTORY

When symptoms develop before adult life, it is particularly important to obtain a full developmental history, including details of the delivery, the birth weight, the patient's condition in the neonatal period, and the dates at which motor milestones were attained. Congenital or perinatal cerebral disease accounts for most causes of infantile diplegia (weakness of all four limbs, with the legs more severely affected than the arms).

Table 9-2. Motor Disorders Associated With Drugs.

Drugs that cause motor (or predominantly motor) peripheral neuropathy[1]	
Dapsone	
Imipramine	
Sulfonamides (some)	
Drugs that can impair neuromuscular transmission	
ACTH	Penicillamine
Aminoglycoside antibiotics	Phenothiazines
β-Blockers	Phenytoin
Chloroquine	Polymyxin
Colistin	Procainamide
Corticosteroids	Quinidine, quinine
Lithium	Tetracycline
Magnesium-containing cathartics	
Drugs associated with myopathy	
β-Blockers	ε-Aminocaproic acid
Chloroquine	HMG-CoA reductase
Clofibrate	inhibitors
Corticosteroids	Penicillamine
Drugs causing hypokalemia	Zidovudine
Emetine	

[1]A number of drugs cause mixed sensory and motor neuropathies (see Table 10-2).

FAMILY HISTORY

Hereditary factors may be important, and the patient's family background therefore must be explored. Some types of myopathy, motor neuron disease, and peripheral neuropathy have a genetic basis, as do some spinocerebellar degenerations, hereditary spastic paraparesis, and certain other neurologic disorders. It is sometimes necessary to examine other family members to determine whether the patient's disorder has a hereditary basis.

NEUROLOGIC EXAMINATION

MOTOR SYSTEM

A systematic approach to examining the motor system helps to prevent important abnormalities from being overlooked. A sequential routine for the examination is important.

▶ Muscle Appearance

1. Wasting, or muscle **atrophy,** suggests that weakness is due to a lesion of the lower motor neurons or the muscle itself. The distribution of wasting may help to localize the underlying disorder. Upper motor neuron disorders are not usually accompanied by muscle wasting, though atrophy may occasionally occur with prolonged disuse.
2. **Pseudohypertrophy** of muscles occurs in certain forms of myopathy, but the apparently enlarged muscles are actually weak and flabby.
3. **Fasciculations**—Visible irregular flickerings over the surface of the affected muscle caused by spontaneous contractions of individual motor units—suggest that weakness is due to a lower motor neuron lesion. Fasciculations are most common in anterior horn cell disorders, but may also occur in normal individuals.
4. **Flexor or extensor spasms** of the limbs are sometimes seen in upper motor neuron disorders as a result of impaired supraspinal control of reflex activity.

▶ Muscle Tone

For clinical purposes, tone can be defined as the **resistance of muscle to passive movement of a joint**. Tone depends on the degree of muscle contraction and on the mechanical properties of muscle and connective tissue. The degree of muscle contraction depends, in turn, on the activity of anterior horn cells, which is governed by spinal and supraspinal mechanisms.

Tone is assessed by observing the position of the extremities at rest, by palpating the muscle belly, and particularly by determining the resistance to passive stretch and movement. To assess resistance to passive movement, the patient relaxes while each limb is examined in turn by passively taking the major joints through their full range of movement at different speeds and estimating whether the force required is more or less than normal.

Postural abnormalities may result when disturbances of reflex function increase the activity of certain muscle groups, as exemplified by the typical hemiplegic posture—flexion of the upper limb and extension of the ipsilateral lower limb—of many patients who have had a stroke.

1. **Hypertonia**—Two types of increased tone can be distinguished.
   a. **Spasticity**—consists of an increase in tone that affects different muscle groups to different extents. In the arms, tone is increased more in the flexor and adductor muscles than the extensors and abductors; in the legs, it is greater in the extensor muscles than flexors. The resistance of an affected muscle is not the same throughout the range of movement, but tends to be most marked when passive movement is initiated and then diminishes as the movement continues (the **clasp-knife phenomenon**). The increase in tone is velocity dependent, so that passive movement at high but not low velocities meets increased resistance. Spasticity is caused by an upper motor neuron lesion, such as a stroke that involves the supplementary motor cortex or corticospinal tract. It may not become apparent for several days after onset of an acute lesion.
   b. **Rigidity**—consists of increased resistance to passive movement that is independent of the direction of the movement; that is, it affects agonist and antagonist muscle groups equally (**lead-pipe rigidity**). The term **cogwheel rigidity** is used when there are superimposed ratchet-like interruptions in the passive movement, probably related to underlying tremor. In general, rigidity indicates extrapyramidal dysfunction and is due to a lesion of the basal ganglia (eg, Parkinson disease).
2. **Hypotonia (flaccidity)**—This is characterized by excessive floppiness—a reduced resistance to passive movement—so that the distal portion of the limb is easily waved to and fro when the extremity is passively shaken. In hypotonic limbs, it is often possible to hyper-extend the joints, and the muscle belly may look flattened and feel less firm than usual. Although hypotonia usually relates to pathologic involvement of the lower motor neuron supply to the affected muscles, it can also occur with primary muscle disorders, disruption of the sensory (afferent) limb of the reflex arc, cerebellar disease, and certain extrapyramidal disorders such as Huntington disease, as well as in the acute stage of a pyramidal lesion.
3. **Paratonia**—Some patients seem unable to relax and will move the limb being examined as the physician moves it, despite instructions to the contrary. In more advanced cases, there seems to be rigidity when the examiner moves the limb rapidly but normal tone when the limb is moved slowly. This phenomenon—paratonia—is particularly apt to occur in patients with frontal lobe or diffuse cerebral disease.

▶ Muscle Power

To test muscle power, the patient is asked to resist pressure exerted by the examiner. Based on the history and other findings, muscles particularly likely to be affected are selected for initial evaluation, and other muscles are subsequently examined to determine the distribution of weakness more fully and to shorten the list of diagnostic possibilities. For instance, if an upper motor neuron (pyramidal) lesion is suspected, the extensors and abductors of the upper extremity and flexors of the lower extremity are tested in the most detail, because they will be the most affected. Strength on the two sides is compared so that minor degrees of weakness can be recognized.

1. **Distinction between upper and lower motor neuron lesions**—The distribution of weakness helps to distinguish between dysfunction of the upper or lower motor neurons. Upper motor neuron lesions (eg, stroke) lead to weakness that characteristically involves the extensors and abductors more than the flexors and adductors of the arms—and the flexors more than the extensors of the legs. Lower motor neuron lesions produce weakness of the muscles supplied by the affected neurons; the particular distribution of the weakness may point to lower motor neuron disturbance involving the spinal cord, nerve roots, plexus, or peripheral nerves.
2. **Distinction between myopathic and neuropathic disorders**—Weakness may also result from a primary muscle disorder (myopathy) or from a disorder of lower motor neurons. In patients with a motor deficit in all limbs that is not due to an upper motor neuron lesion, proximal distribution of weakness suggests a myopathic disorder, whereas predominantly distal involvement suggests a neuropathic disturbance.
3. **Neuromuscular junction disorders**—Marked variability in the severity and distribution of weakness over short periods of time (eg, over the course of a day) suggests myasthenia gravis, a disorder of neuromuscular transmission.
4. **Psychogenic disorders**—Apparent weakness that is not organic in nature also shows a characteristic variability; it is often more severe on formal testing than is consistent with the patient's daily activities. Moreover, palpation of antagonist muscles commonly reveals that they contract each time the patient is asked to activate the agonist.

For practical and comparative purposes, power is best graded in the manner shown in **Table 9-3**.

Table 9-3. Grading of Muscle Power According to the System Suggested by the Medical Research Council.

Grade	Muscle Power
5	Normal power
4	Active movement against resistance and gravity
3	Active movement against gravity but not resistance
2	Active movement possible only with gravity eliminated
1	Flicker or trace of contraction
0	No contraction

Used with permission from *Aids to the Investigation of Peripheral Nerve Injuries.* London, UK: H.M. Stationary Office; 1943.

The term **monoplegia** denotes paralysis or severe weakness of the muscles in one limb, and **monoparesis** denotes less severe weakness in one limb, although the two words are often used interchangeably. **Hemiplegia** or **hemiparesis** is weakness in both limbs (and sometimes the face) on one side of the body; **paraplegia** or **paraparesis** is weakness of both legs; and **quadriplegia** or **quadriparesis** (also **tetraplegia, tetraparesis**) is weakness of all four limbs.

COORDINATION

The coordination of motor activity can be impaired by weakness, sensory disturbances, or cerebellar disease and requires careful evaluation.

Voluntary activity is observed with regard to its accuracy, velocity, range, and regularity, and the manner in which individual actions are integrated to produce a smooth complex movement.

In the **finger-nose test**, the patient moves the index finger to touch the tip of his or her nose and then the tip of the examiner's index finger; the examiner can move the target finger about during the test to change its location and should position it so that the patient's arm must extend fully to reach it.

In the **heel-knee-shin test**, the recumbent patient lifts one leg off the bed, flexes it at the knee, places the heel on the other knee, and runs the heel down the shin as smoothly as possible.

Rapid alternating movement is tested by asking the patient to tap repetitively with one hand on the back of the other, to tap alternately with the palm and back of one hand on the back of the other hand or on the knee, to screw an imaginary light bulb into the ceiling with each arm in turn, and to rub the fingers of one hand in a circular polishing movement on the back of the other hand. Other tests of rapid alternating movement include tapping on the ball of the thumb with the tip of the index finger or tapping the floor as rapidly as possible with the sole while keeping

the heel of the foot in place. During all these tests, the examiner looks for irregularities of rate, amplitude, and rhythm and for precision of movements. With pyramidal lesions, fine voluntary movements are performed slowly. With cerebellar lesions, the rate, rhythm, and amplitude of such movements are irregular.

If loss of sensation may be responsible for impaired coordination, the maneuver should be repeated both with eyes closed and with visual attention directed to the limb; with visual feedback, the apparent weakness or incoordination will improve. In patients with cerebellar disease, the main complaint and physical finding are often of incoordination, and examination may reveal little else. Further discussion of cerebellar ataxia and the various terms used to describe aspects of it can be found in Chapter 8, Disorders of Equilibrium.

TENDON REFLEXES

Changes in the tendon (muscle stretch) reflexes may accompany disturbances in motor or sensory function and provide a guide to the cause of any motor deficit. The tendon is tapped with a reflex hammer to produce a sudden brisk stretch of the muscle and its contained spindles. The clinically important stretch reflexes and the nerves, roots, and spinal segments subserving them are indicated in **Table 9-4**. When the reflexes are tested, the limbs on each side should be placed in identical positions and the reflexes elicited in the same manner.

1. **Areflexia**—Apparent loss of the tendon reflexes may merely reflect a lack of clinical expertise by the examiner. Performance of the **Jendrassik maneuver** (an attempt by the patient to pull apart the fingers of the two hands when they are hooked together) or some similar distracting action (such as making a fist with the hand that is not being tested) may allow an

Table 9-4. Tendon (Muscle Stretch) Reflexes.[1]

Reflex	Segmental Innervation	Nerve
Jaw	Pons	Mandibular branch, trigeminal
Biceps	C5, C6	Musculocutaneous
Brachioradialis	C5, C6	Radial
Triceps	C7, C8	Radial
Finger	C8, T1	Median
Knee (patellar)	L3, L4	Femoral
Ankle (Achilles)	S1, S2	Tibial

[1]In the National Institutes of Health system, the reflexes are graded on the following scale: 0, absent; 1, reduced, trace response, or present only with reinforcement; 2 and 3, in lower and upper half of normal range, respectively; 4, increased, with or without clonus.

otherwise unobtainable reflex response to be elicited. A reflex may be lost or depressed by any lesion that interrupts the structural or functional continuity of its reflex arc, as in a radiculopathy or peripheral neuropathy. In addition, reflexes are often depressed during the acute stage of an upper motor neuron lesion, during deep coma, and with cerebellar disease.

2. **Hyperreflexia**—Increased reflexes occur with upper motor neuron lesions, but they may also occur with a symmetric distribution in certain healthy subjects and in patients under emotional stress. The presence of reflex asymmetry is therefore of particular clinical significance. **Clonus** consists of a series of rhythmic reflex contractions of a muscle that is suddenly subjected to sustained stretch; each beat is caused by renewed stretch of the muscle during relaxation from its previous contracted state. **Sustained clonus**—more than three or four beats in response to sudden sustained stretch—is always pathologic and is associated with an abnormally brisk reflex. In hyperreflexic states, the region from which a particular reflex response can be elicited may be enlarged. For example, elicitation of the biceps reflex may be accompanied by reflex finger flexion, or eliciting the finger flexion reflex may cause flexion of the thumb (**Hoffmann sign**).

3. **Reflex asymmetry**—Although the intensity of reflex responses varies considerably among subjects, reflexes should be symmetric in any individual.
   a. **Lateralized asymmetries** of response—reflexes that are brisker on one side of the body than on the other—usually indicate an upper motor neuron disturbance, but sometimes reflect a lower motor neuron lesion on the side with the depressed reflexes.
   b. **Focal reflex deficits** often relate to root, plexus, or peripheral nerve lesions. For example, unilateral depression of the ankle jerk commonly reflects an S1 radiculopathy resulting from a lumbosacral disk lesion.
   c. **Loss of distal tendon reflexes** (especially ankle jerks), with preservation of more proximal ones, is common in polyneuropathies.

SUPERFICIAL REFLEXES

1. **The polysynaptic superficial abdominal reflexes,** which depend on the integrity of the T8-12 spinal cord segments, are elicited by gently stroking each quadrant of the abdominal wall with a blunt object such as a wooden stick. A normal response consists of contraction of the muscle in the quadrant stimulated, with a brief movement of the umbilicus toward the stimulus. Asymmetric loss of the response may be of diagnostic significance. The response may be depressed or lost on one side in patients with an upper motor neuron disturbance affecting that side. Segmental loss of the response may relate to local disease of the abdominal wall or its

innervation, as in a radiculopathy. Bilaterally absent responses are usually of no significance, occurring in the elderly, the obese, multiparous women, and patients who have had abdominal surgery.

2. The **cremasteric reflex,** mediated through the L1 and L2 reflex arcs, consists of retraction of the ipsilateral testis when the inner aspect of the thigh is lightly stroked; it is lost in patients with a lesion involving these nerve roots. It is also lost in patients with contralateral upper motor neuron disturbances.

3. Stimulation of the lateral border of the foot in a normal adult leads to plantar flexion of the toes and dorsiflexion of the ankle. The **Babinski response** consists of dorsiflexion of the big toe and fanning of the other toes in response to stroking firmly the lateral border of the foot, which is part of the S1 dermatome; flexion at the hip and knee may also occur. Such an **extensor plantar response** indicates an upper motor neuron lesion involving the contralateral motor cortex or the corticospinal tract. It can also be found bilaterally in anesthetized or comatose subjects, in patients who have just had a seizure, and in normal infants.

An extensor plantar response can also be elicited, though less reliably, by such maneuvers as pricking the dorsal surface of the big toe with a pin (Bing sign), firmly stroking down the anterior border of the tibia from knee to ankle (Oppenheim maneuver), squeezing the calf muscle (Gordon maneuver) or Achilles tendon (Schafer maneuver), flicking the little toe (Gonda maneuver), or stroking the back of the foot just below the lateral malleolus (Chaddock maneuver). In interpreting responses to these maneuvers, attention must be focused only on the direction in which the big toe first moves.

GAIT

The patient is observed while walking at a comfortable pace. Attention is directed at the stance and posture; the facility with which the patient starts and stops walking and turns to either side; the length of the stride; the rhythm of walking; the presence of normally associated movements, such as swinging of the arms; and any involuntary movements (see Figure 1-25).

Subtle gait disorders become apparent only when the patient is asked to run, walk on the balls of the feet or the heels, hop on either foot, or walk heel-to-toe along a straight line. Gait disorders occur in many neurologic disturbances. A motor or sensory disturbance may lead to an abnormal gait whose nature depends on the site of pathologic involvement.

1. **Apraxic gait**—Apraxic gait occurs in some patients with disturbances, usually bilateral, of frontal lobe function, such as in hydrocephalus or progressive dementing disorders. There is no weakness or incoordination of the limbs, but the patient is unable to stand

unsupported or to walk properly—the feet seem glued to the ground. If walking is possible at all, the gait is unsteady, uncertain, and short-stepped, with marked hesitation ("freezing"), and the legs are moved in a direction inappropriate to the center of gravity.

2. **Corticospinal lesions**—A corticospinal lesion, irrespective of cause, can cause a gait disturbance.

   a. In patients with hemiparesis, the affected leg must be **circumducted** to be advanced. The patient tilts at the waist toward the normal side and swings the affected leg outward as well as forward, thus compensating for any tendency to drag or catch the foot on the ground because of weakness in the hip and knee flexors or ankle dorsiflexors. The arm on the affected side is usually held flexed and adducted. In mild cases, there may be no more than a tendency to drag the affected leg, so that the sole of that shoe tends to be excessively worn.

   b. With severe bilateral spasticity, the legs are brought stiffly forward and adducted, often with compensatory truncal movements (**"scissors-like" gait**). This gait is seen in its most extreme form in children with spastic diplegia from perinatally acquired static encephalopathy. In patients with mild spastic paraparesis, the gait is shuffling, slow, stiff, and awkward, and the feet tend to drag.

3. **Frontal disorders**—Some patients with frontal lobe or white matter lesions have a gait characterized by short, shuffling steps; hesitation in starting ("ignition failure") or turning; unsteadiness; and a wide or narrow base. Sometimes referred to as **marche à petit pas**, this abnormality may be mistaken for a parkinsonian gait, but the wide base, preserved arm swing, absence of other signs of parkinsonism, and accompanying findings of cognitive impairment, frontal release signs, pseudobulbar palsy, pyramidal deficits, and sphincter disturbances should suggest the correct diagnosis. In patients with frontotemporal dementia, however, a parkinsonian gait and other extrapyramidal findings may be present.

4. **Extrapyramidal disorders**.

   a Patients with advanced **parkinsonism** are often stooped, have difficulty in beginning to walk, and may need to lean farther and farther forward while walking in place in order to advance; once in motion, there may be unsteadiness in turning and difficulty in stopping. The gait itself is characterized by small strides, often taken at an increasing rate until the patient is almost running (**festination**), and by loss of the arm swinging that normally accompanies locomotion. At times, as when walking through a doorway, the patient may be unable to advance ("freezing"). Turning may require several small steps. In mild parkinsonism, a mildly slowed or unsteady gait, flexed posture, or reduced arm swinging may be the only abnormality found.

   b. Abnormal posturing of the limbs or trunk is a feature of **dystonia**; it can interfere with locomotion or lead to a distorted and bizarre gait.

   c. **Chorea** can cause an irregular, unpredictable, and unsteady gait, as the patient dips or lurches from side to side. Choreiform movements of the face and extremities are usually evident.

   d. **Tremor** that occurs primarily on standing (orthostatic tremor) may lead to an unsteady, uncertain gait, with hesitancy in commencing to walk.

5. **Cerebellar disorders**—Several gait disorders may occur in cerebellar disorders (see Chapter 8, Disorders of Equilibrium).

   a. **Truncal ataxia** results from involvement of midline cerebellar structures, especially the vermis. The gait is irregular, clumsy, unsteady, uncertain, and broad-based, and the patient walks with feet wide apart for additional support. Turning and heel-to-toe walking are especially difficult. There are often few accompanying signs of a cerebellar disturbance in the limbs. Causes include midline cerebellar tumors and the cerebellar degeneration that can occur with alcoholism or hypothyroidism, as a nonmetastatic complication of cancer, and with certain hereditary disorders.

   b. In extreme cases, with gross involvement of midline cerebellar structures (especially the vermis), the patient cannot stand without falling.

   c. A lesion of one cerebellar hemisphere leads to an unsteady gait in which the patient consistently falls or lurches toward the affected side.

6. **Vestibular disorders**—With unilateral vestibular dysfunction, the patient is unsteady, veering to the affected side. If both sides are affected, the gait becomes especially unsteady in the dark, when visual input is reduced.

7. **Impaired sensation**—Impaired sensation, especially proprioception, also leads to an unsteady gait that is aggravated by walking in the dark or with the eyes closed, as visual input cannot then compensate for the sensory loss. Because of their defective position sense, many patients lift their feet higher than necessary when walking, producing a **steppage gait**. Causes include tabes dorsalis, sensory neuropathies, vitamin B_{12} deficiency, and certain hereditary disorders (see Chapter 10, Sensory Disorders).

8. **Anterior horn cell, peripheral motor nerve, or skeletal muscle disorders**—These disorders lead to gait disturbances if the muscles involved in locomotion are affected. Weakness of the anterior tibial muscles leads to **foot drop**; to avoid catching or scuffing the foot on the ground, the patient must lift the affected leg higher than the other, in a **steppage gait** resembling that of sensory disorders. Weakness of the calf muscles leads to an inability to walk on the balls of

the feet. Weakness of the trunk and girdle muscles, such as occurs in muscular dystrophy, other myopathic disorders, and Kugelberg–Welander syndrome, leads to a **waddling gait** because the pelvis tends to slump toward the non-weight-bearing side.

9. **Unsteady or cautious gait in the elderly**—Many elderly persons complain of unsteadiness when walking and of a fear of falling, but neurologic examination reveals no abnormality. Their gait is cautious, unsteady, and sometimes difficult to initiate. Frontal lobe dysfunction may be responsible, as it may reduce sensory input from several different afferent systems and impair central processing of sensory input; impaired vestibular function may also be important.

10. **Psychogenic gait disorder**—This is suggested by fluctuations of stance and gait, commonly in response to suggestion, frequently accompanied by a sudden buckling at the knees, often without falls. Apart from the bizarre gait, neurologic examination may be normal. Patients apparently unable to stand or walk (**astasia-abasia**) may actually be able to walk on a narrow base, but sway wildly in all directions, often with waving of the arms as if about to fall.

CLINICAL LOCALIZATION OF THE LESION

The findings on examination should indicate whether the motor deficit is due to an upper or lower motor neuron disturbance, impaired neuromuscular transmission, or a primary muscle disorder. With an upper or lower motor neuron disturbance, the clinical findings may also help to localize the lesion to a single level of the nervous system, thereby reducing the number of diagnostic possibilities.

UPPER MOTOR NEURON LESIONS

▶ Signs

The following classic signs of an upper motor neuron lesion occur with involvement of the upper motor neuron at any point; further clinical findings depend on the actual site of the lesion.

1. **Weakness or paralysis**
2. **Spasticity**
3. **Increased tendon reflexes**
4. **Extensor plantar (Babinski) response**
5. **Loss of superficial abdominal reflexes**
6. **Little, if any, muscle atrophy**

▶ Localization of Underlying Lesion

1. A **parasagittal** intracranial lesion produces an upper motor neuron deficit that characteristically affects both legs and may later involve the arms.

2. A discrete lesion of the **cerebral cortex** or its projections may produce a focal motor deficit involving, for example, the contralateral hand. Weakness may be restricted to the contralateral leg in patients with anterior cerebral artery occlusion or to the contralateral face and arm if the middle cerebral artery is involved. A more extensive cortical or subcortical lesion will produce weakness or paralysis of the contralateral face, arm, and leg and may be accompanied by aphasia, a visual field defect, or a sensory disturbance of cortical type.

3. A lesion in the **internal capsule**, where the descending fibers from the cerebral cortex are closely packed, commonly results in a severe hemiparesis involving the contralateral limbs and face.

4. A **brainstem** lesion commonly—but not invariably—leads to bilateral motor deficits, often with accompanying sensory and cranial nerve disturbances, and disequilibrium. A more limited brainstem lesion characteristically leads to an ipsilateral cranial nerve disturbance and contralateral hemiparesis; the cranial nerves affected depend on the level at which the brainstem is involved.

5. A unilateral **spinal cord** lesion above the fifth cervical segment (C5) causes an ipsilateral hemiparesis that spares the face and cranial nerves. Lesions between C5 and the first thoracic segment (T1) affect the ipsilateral arm to a variable extent as well as the ipsilateral leg; a lesion below T1 affects only the ipsilateral leg. If both sides of the spinal cord are involved, quadriparesis or paraparesis usually results. Increased muscle tone (spasticity) may be more prominent than weakness. If there is an extensive but unilateral cord lesion, the motor deficit is accompanied by ipsilateral impairment of vibration and position sense and by contralateral loss of pain and temperature appreciation (**Brown–Séquard syndrome**).

6. With compressive and other focal lesions that involve the **anterior horn cells** in addition to the fiber tracts traversing the cord, the muscles innervated by the affected cord segment weaken and atrophy. Therefore, a focal lower motor neuron deficit exists at the level of the lesion, and an upper motor neuron deficit exists below it—in addition to any associated sensory disturbance.

LOWER MOTOR NEURON LESIONS

▶ Signs

Lower motor neuron lesions produce the following characteristic signs at the affected levels.

1. **Weakness or paralysis**
2. **Wasting and fasciculations** of involved muscles

3. **Hypotonia** (flaccidity)
4. **Loss of tendon reflexes** when neurons subserving them are affected.
5. **Normal abdominal and plantar reflexes**—unless the neurons subserving them are directly involved, in which case reflex responses are lost.

▶ Localization of the Underlying Lesion

In distinguishing weakness from a segmental **spinal cord, anterior horn cell, radicular (nerve root), plexus,** or **peripheral nerve** lesion, the distribution of the motor deficit is important. Only those muscles supplied wholly or partly by the involved structure are weak (**Tables 9-5 and 9-6**). The distribution of any accompanying sensory deficit similarly reflects the location of the underlying lesion (see Chapter 10, Sensory Disorders).

Weakness due to lesions of nerve roots may be difficult to distinguish from weakness caused by spinal cord lesions involving the anterior horn cells. In the latter situation, however, there is more often a bilateral motor deficit at the level of the lesion, a corticospinal or sensory deficit below it, or a disturbance of bladder, bowel, or sexual function.

Disorders affecting the anterior horn cells of the spinal cord commonly cause an extensive lower motor neuron deficit without sensory changes, and this helps to distinguish them from disorders of motor nerves (motor neuropathy).

CEREBELLAR LESIONS

▶ Signs

1. **Hypotonia**
2. **Depressed or pendular tendon reflexes**
3. **Ataxia**—This is a complex movement disorder caused, at least in part, by impaired coordination. It occurs in the limbs on the same side as a lesion affecting the cerebellar hemisphere. With midline lesions, incoordination may not be evident in the limbs, but there is marked truncal ataxia on walking. The term **dysmetria** is used when movements are not adjusted accurately for range, so that, for example, a moving finger overshoots a target at which it is aimed. **Dysdiadochokinesia** denotes rapid alternating movements that are clumsy and irregular in terms of rhythm and amplitude. **Asynergia** or **dyssynergia** denotes the breakdown of complex actions into the individual movements composing them; when asked to touch the tip of the nose with a finger, for example, the patient may first flex the elbow and then bring the hand up to the nose instead of combining the maneuvers into one action. **Intention tremor** occurs during activity and is often most marked as the target is neared. The **rebound phenomenon** is the overshooting of the limb when resistance to a movement or posture is suddenly withdrawn.
4. **Gait disorder**—The gait becomes unsteady in patients with disturbances of either the cerebellar hemispheres or midline structures.

Table 9-5. Innervation of Selected Muscles of the Upper Limbs.

Muscle	Main Root	Peripheral Nerve	Main Action
Supraspinatus	C5	Suprascapular	Abduction of arm
Infraspinatus	C5	Suprascapular	External rotation of arm at shoulder
Deltoid	C5	Axillary	Abduction of arm
Biceps	C5, C6	Musculocutaneous	Elbow flexion
Brachioradialis	C5, C6	Radial	Elbow flexion
Extensor carpi radialis longus	C6, C7	Radial	Wrist extension
Flexor carpi radialis	C6, C7	Median	Wrist flexion
Extensor carpi ulnaris	C7	Radial	Wrist extension
Extensor digitorum	C7	Radial	Finger extension
Triceps	C8	Radial	Extension of elbow
Flexor carpi ulnaris	C8	Ulnar	Wrist flexion
Abductor pollicis brevis	T1	Median	Abduction of thumb
Opponens pollicis	T1	Median	Opposition of thumb
First dorsal interosseous	T1	Ulnar	Abduction of index finger
Abductor digiti minimi	T1	Ulnar	Abduction of little finger

Table 9-6. Innervation of Selected Muscles of the Lower Limbs.

Muscle	Main Root	Peripheral Nerve	Main Action
Iliopsoas	L2, L3	Femoral	Hip flexion
Quadriceps femoris	L3, L4	Femoral	Knee extension
Adductors	L2, L3, L4	Obturator	Adduction of thigh
Gluteus maximus	L5, S1, S2	Inferior gluteal	Hip extension
Gluteus medius and minimus, tensor fasciae latae	L4, L5, S1	Superior gluteal	Hip abduction
Hamstrings	L5, S1	Sciatic	Knee flexion
Tibialis anterior	L4, L5	Fibular (Peroneal)	Dorsiflexion of ankle
Extensor digitorum longus	L5, S1	Fibular (Peroneal)	Dorsiflexion of toes
Extensor digitorum brevis	S1	Fibular (Peroneal)	Dorsiflexion of toes
Peronei	L5, S1	Fibular (Peroneal)	Eversion of foot
Tibialis posterior	L4	Tibial	Inversion of foot
Gastrocnemius	S1, S2	Tibial	Plantar flexion of ankle
Soleus	S1, S2	Tibial	Plantar flexion of ankle

5. **Imbalance of station**
6. **Disturbances of eye movement**—Jerk **nystagmus**, which is commonly seen in patients with a unilateral lesion of the cerebellar hemisphere, is slowest and of greatest amplitude when the eyes are turned to the side of the lesion. Nystagmus is not present in patients with lesions of the anterior cerebellar vermis.
7. **Dysarthria**—Speech becomes dysarthric and takes on an irregular and explosive quality in patients with lesions involving the cerebellar hemispheres. Speech is usually unremarkable when only the midline structures are involved.

▶ Localization of the Underlying Lesion

The relationship of symptoms and signs to lesions of different parts of the cerebellum is considered in Chapter 8, Disorders of Equilibrium.

NEUROMUSCULAR TRANSMISSION DISORDERS

▶ Signs

1. **Normal or reduced muscle tone**
2. **Normal or depressed tendon and superficial reflexes**
3. **No sensory changes**
4. **Weakness**, often patchy in distribution, not conforming to the distribution of any single anatomic structure; frequently involves the cranial muscles and may

fluctuate in severity over short periods, particularly in relation to activity.

▶ Localization of the Underlying Lesion

Pathologic involvement of either the **presynaptic** (eg, botulism) or **postsynaptic** (eg, myasthenia gravis) portion of the neuromuscular junction may impair neuromuscular transmission. Disorders of neuromuscular transmission are discussed later.

MYOPATHIC DISORDERS

▶ Signs

1. **Weakness**, usually most marked **proximally** rather than distally.
2. **No muscle wasting or depression of tendon reflexes**, at least until an advanced stage of the disorder.
3. **Normal abdominal and plantar reflexes.**
4. **No sensory loss or sphincter disturbances.**

▶ Localization of the Underlying Lesion

It is important to determine whether the weakness is congenital or acquired, whether there is a family history of a similar disorder, and whether there is any clinical evidence that a systemic disease may be responsible. The **distribution of affected muscles** is often especially important in distinguishing the various hereditary myopathies (see Myopathic Disorders, later).

INVESTIGATIVE STUDIES

Investigative studies of patients with weakness from focal cerebral deficits are considered in Chapter 2, Investigative Studies. The investigations discussed here may be helpful in evaluating patients with weakness from other causes (**Table 9-7**).

IMAGING

▶ Plain X-Rays of the Spine

Congenital abnormalities and degenerative, inflammatory, neoplastic, or traumatic changes may be revealed by plain X-rays of the spine, but magnetic resonance imaging (MRI) or computed tomography (CT) scan is preferred in patients with suspected cord or root lesions because it provides more detail and visualization of soft tissue structures.

▶ CT Scan or MRI

CT scan of the spine, especially after instilling water-soluble contrast material into the subarachnoid space (**CT myelogram**), may reveal disease involving the spinal cord or nerve roots, but MRI is better in this regard (see Chapter 2, Investigative Studies).

ELECTRODIAGNOSTIC STUDIES

The function of the normal motor unit, which consists of a lower motor neuron and all of the muscle fibers it innervates, may be disturbed at any of several sites in patients with weakness. A lesion may, for example, affect the anterior horn cell or its axon, interfere with neuromuscular transmission, or involve the muscle fibers directly so that they cannot respond normally to neural activation. In each circumstance, characteristic changes in the electrical activity can be recorded from affected muscle by a needle electrode inserted into it and connected to an oscilloscope (**electromyography**, or **EMG**). Depending on the site of pathology, **nerve conduction studies** or the **muscle responses to repetitive nerve stimulation** may also be abnormal (see **Table 9-7** and Chapter 2, Investigative Studies, for further details).

SERUM ENZYMES

Damage to muscle fibers may lead to the release of certain enzymes (creatine kinase [**CK**], aldolase, lactic acid dehydrogenase [**LDH**], and alanine and aspartate transaminases [**ALT** and **AST**]) that can then be detected in increased amounts in serum. Serum CK shows the greatest increase and is the most useful for following the course of

Table 9-7. Investigation of Patients With Weakness of Noncerebral Origin.

Test	Spinal Cord Disorders	Anterior Horn Cell Disorders	Peripheral Nerve or Plexus Disorders	Neuromuscular Junction Disorders	Myopathies
Serum creatine kinase (CK) and other muscle enzymes	Normal	Normal or mildly increased	Normal	Normal	Normal or increased
Electromyography	Reduced number of motor units under voluntary control; with lesions causing axonal degeneration, abnormal spontaneous activity (eg, fasciculations, fibrillations) may be present if sufficient time has elapsed after onset; with reinnervation, motor units may be large, long, and polyphasic			Often normal, but individual motor units may show abnormal variability in size	Small, short, abundant polyphasic motor unit potentials; abnormal spontaneous activity may be conspicuous in myositis
Nerve conduction velocity	Normal	Normal	Slowed, especially in demyelinative neuropathies. May be normal in axonal neuropathies	Normal	Normal
Muscle response to repetitive motor nerve stimulation	Normal	Normal, except in rapidly progressive disease	Normal	Abnormal decrement or increment depending on stimulus frequency and disease	Normal
Muscle biopsy	May be normal in acute stage but subsequently suggestive of denervation			Normal	Changes suggestive of myopathy
Spinal MRI or CT myelography	May be helpful	Helpful in excluding other disorders	Not helpful	Not helpful	Not helpful

muscle disease. It is also present in high concentrations in the heart and brain, however, and damage to these structures can lead to increased serum CK levels. Fractionation of serum CK into isoenzyme forms is useful for determining the tissue of origin. In patients with weakness, elevated serum CK levels are generally indicative of a primary myopathy, especially one that is evolving rapidly. A moderately elevated serum CK may also occur in motor neuron disease, however, and more marked elevations can follow trauma, surgery, intramuscular injections, EMG, or vigorous activity.

MUSCLE BIOPSY

Histopathologic examination of a specimen of weak muscle can help to determine whether the underlying weakness is neurogenic or myopathic. With **neurogenic disorders**, atrophied fibers occur in groups, with adjacent groups of larger, uninvolved fibers. In **myopathies**, atrophy occurs in a random pattern; nuclei of muscle cells may be centrally situated, in contrast to their normal peripheral location; and fibrosis or fatty infiltration may be seen. In addition, the pathologic examination may permit recognition of certain **inflammatory muscle diseases** (eg, polymyositis) for which specific treatment is available and of various congenital or mitochondrial myopathies.

SPINAL CORD DISORDERS (MYELOPATHY)

Spinal cord disorders can lead to motor, sensory, or sphincter disturbances, or to some combination of these deficits. Depending on whether it is unilateral or bilateral, a lesion above C5 may cause an ipsilateral hemiparesis or quadriparesis. With lesions lower in the cervical spinal cord, involvement of the upper limbs is partial, and a lesion below T1 affects only the lower limbs on one or both sides. Disturbances of sensation are considered in detail in Chapter 10, Sensory Disorders, but unilateral involvement of the posterior columns of the cord leads to ipsilateral loss of position and vibration sense. Involvement of the spinothalamic tracts in the anterolateral columns impairs contralateral pain and temperature appreciation below the level of the lesion.

Spasticity is a common accompaniment of upper motor neuron lesions and may be especially troublesome below the level of a myelopathy. When the legs are weak, the increased tone of spasticity may help to support the patient in the upright position. Marked spasticity, however, may lead to deformity, interfere with toilet functions, and cause painful flexor or extensor spasms. Pharmacologic management includes treatment with diazepam, baclofen, dantrolene, or tizanidine, as discussed later under *Traumatic Myelopathy,* but reduction in tone may increase disability from underlying leg weakness.

TRAUMATIC MYELOPATHY

Although spinal cord damage may result from whiplash (recoil) injury, severe injury to the cord usually relates to **fracture-dislocation** in the cervical, lower thoracic, or upper lumbar region, which is commonly associated with local pain. Intervertebral disks may rupture or herniate.

Concomitant cerebral and systemic injuries may complicate evaluation. The most common cause in the United States is motor vehicle accidents, and the group most often affected is young men. The most common site for traumatic spinal cord injury is in the cervical region, particularly at C2 or between C5 and C7; injuries at this level may involve fractures or dislocations.

CLINICAL FINDINGS

▶ Total Spinal Cord Transection

Total transection results in immediate permanent paralysis and loss of sensation below the level of the lesion, including the sacral region. Reflex activity is lost for a variable period, but then increases.

1. In the acute stage ("**spinal shock**"), there is flaccid paralysis with loss of tendon and other reflexes, accompanied by sensory loss and by urinary and fecal retention. Bradycardia and hypotension may also occur.

2. Over the following weeks, as reflex function returns, a **spastic paraplegia or quadriplegia** emerges, with brisk tendon reflexes and extensor plantar responses; however, a flaccid, atrophic (lower motor neuron) paralysis may affect muscles innervated by spinal cord segments at the level of the lesion, where anterior horn cells are damaged. Sensation is reduced at that level and lost below it. The bladder and bowel regain some reflex function, so that urine and feces are expelled at intervals.

3. **Flexor or extensor spasms of the legs** may become increasingly troublesome and are ultimately elicited by even the slightest cutaneous stimulus, especially in the presence of bedsores or a urinary tract infection. Eventually, the patient assumes a posture with the legs in flexion or extension, the former being especially likely with cervical or complete cord lesions.

▶ Less Severe Injury

With lesser injury, the neurologic deficit is less severe, but patients may be left with a mild paraparesis or quadriparesis and/or a distal sensory disturbance that is often less severe than the motor deficit. Sphincter function may also be impaired—urinary urgency and urgency incontinence are especially common. Hyperextension injuries of the neck can lead to focal cord ischemia that causes **bibrachial paresis** (weakness of both arms) with relative sparing of the legs and variable sensory signs.

IMAGING

After trauma, especially to the head, injury to the spinal cord should be assumed until imaging studies prove otherwise. Plain radiographs will reveal misalignments, fractures, and soft tissue swelling, but CT scanning is more sensitive for detecting spinal fractures, especially in the cervical region, and also allows evaluation of the spinal cord. It is therefore preferred in the acute setting. Spinal MRI provides complementary information about the extent and nature of any spinal cord and paraspinal injury and the presence of an epidural hematoma, which is important for treatment and prognosis. It is best performed on stable patients and on those in whom spinal cord injury is suspected despite a normal CT scan. The presence of cardiac pacemakers, metallic foreign bodies, or life support equipment, however, may prohibit MRI.

TREATMENT

Immobilization, Decompression, & Stabilization

Initial treatment consists of immobilization until the nature and extent of the injury are determined. Injury of the spinal cord should be assumed in patients with head injuries until excluded by imaging studies. If there is cord compression, urgent decompressive surgery will be necessary and is best performed within 12 hours of injury. An unstable spine may require surgical fixation, and vertebral dislocation may necessitate spinal traction. Early surgical treatment hastens mobilization, reduces the duration of hospitalization, and lowers complication rates.

General Measures

A clear airway must be ensured and the circulation, blood pressure, and ventilation maintained. Tracheostomy may be required. Respiratory complications such as pneumonia, atelectasis, and pulmonary embolism must be treated vigorously. Respiratory and physical therapy are important. Opiate analgesics will help to relieve pain but may complicate clinical evaluation. Prophylaxis for deep venous thrombosis is with low-molecular-weight heparin. Measures to prevent the occurrence of stress ulcers typically involve the use of proton pump inhibitors. Adequate nutrition should be ensured. Psychologic counselling may be necessary.

Corticosteroids

It is doubtful whether corticosteroids (eg, methylprednisolone 30 mg/kg by intravenous bolus followed by intravenous infusion at 5.4 mg/kg/h for 24 hours), once thought to improve function at 6 months when begun within 8 hours of traumatic spinal cord injury, have any significant beneficial effects. Nevertheless, many physicians administer them routinely, except to patients with penetrating spinal injuries or concomitant severe head injuries.

Treatment of Painful Spasms

Painful flexor or extensor spasms can be treated with drugs that enhance spinal inhibitory mechanisms (baclofen, diazepam) or uncouple muscle excitation from contraction (dantrolene). Baclofen is started with 5 mg orally twice daily, increasing up to 30 mg four times daily; diazepam, 2 mg orally twice daily up to as high as 20 mg three times daily; and dantrolene, 25 mg/d orally to 100 mg four times daily. Tizanidine, a central α_2-adrenergic receptor agonist, may also be helpful by increasing presynaptic inhibition and reducing alpha motoneuron excitability. The daily dose is built up gradually, usually to 8 mg three times daily. Side effects include dryness of the mouth, somnolence, and hypotension, but the drug is usually well tolerated. Patients who fail to benefit from or who cannot tolerate sufficient doses of oral medications may respond to intrathecal infusion of baclofen or to intramuscular administration of botulinum toxin.

All these drugs may increase functional disability by reducing tone. Dantrolene may also increase weakness and should be avoided in patients with severely compromised respiratory function.

Skin Care

Skin care is important; continued pressure on any single area must be avoided.

Bladder & Bowel Disorders

Depending on the severity of injury, catheterization may be necessary initially. Subsequently, the urgency and frequency of the spastic bladder may respond to a parasympatholytic drug such as oxybutynin, 5 mg three times daily. Suppositories and enemas will help maintain regular bowel movements and may prevent or control fecal incontinence.

Experimental Therapeutics

Experimental work has focused recently on enhancing axonal regeneration in the damaged section of the spinal cord through such approaches as neutralization of neurite regrowth inhibitors, use of neurotrophic or growth factors and other neuroprotective agents, implantation of synthetic axonal guidance channels, and cellular therapies. Translational application to patients with spinal cord injuries is possible in the near future.

PROGNOSIS

There is a significant mortality after spinal cord injury, and this is highest in those with cervical injuries, associated head injury, cardiovascular or respiratory inadequacy, and coexisting disorders. The greatest improvement is seen in those with incomplete injury, with most recovery occurring in the first few months.

DEMYELINATING MYELOPATHIES

MULTIPLE SCLEROSIS

▶ Epidemiology

Multiple sclerosis is one of the most common neurologic disorders, affecting approximately 300,000 patients in the United States, and its highest incidence is in young adults. It is defined clinically by the involvement of different parts of the central nervous system at different times—provided that other disorders causing multifocal central dysfunction have been excluded. Initial symptoms generally commence before the age of 55 years, with a peak incidence between ages 20 and 40 years; women are affected nearly twice as often as men.

Epidemiologic studies show that the prevalence of the disease rises with increasing distance from the equator, and no population with a high risk for the disease exists between latitudes 40°N and 40°S. Vitamin D level may also play a role, as may exposure to Epstein–Barr virus. A genetic predisposition is suggested by twin studies, the occasional familial occurrence, and the strong association between the disease and specific HLA alleles. Alleles of *IL2RA* (interleukin-2 receptor α gene) and *IL7RA* (interleukin-7 receptor α gene) have also been proposed as heritable risk factors. Present evidence suggests that the disease has an autoimmune basis.

▶ Pathology

The disorder is characterized pathologically by the development of focal—often perivenular—scattered areas of demyelination, together with reactive gliosis, axonal damage, and neuronal degeneration. These lesions occur in both white and gray matter of the brain and spinal cord and in the optic (II) nerve.

▶ Pathophysiology

The cause of multiple sclerosis is unknown, but tissue damage and neurologic symptoms are thought to be triggered by an immune mechanism directed against myelin antigens. Viral infection or other inciting factors may promote the entry of T cells and antibodies into the central nervous system by disrupting the blood–brain barrier. This leads to increased expression of cell-adhesion molecules, matrix metalloproteinases, and proinflammatory cytokines. These molecules work in concert to attract additional immune cells, break down the extracellular matrix to aid their migration, and activate autoimmune responses against several antigens (eg, myelin basic protein, myelin-associated glycoprotein, myelin oligodendrocyte glycoprotein,

proteolipid protein, α B-crystallin, phosphodiesterases, and S-100). Binding of these target antigens by antigen-presenting cells triggers an autoimmune response that may involve cytokines, macrophages, and complement. Immune attack on myelin denudes axons, which slows nerve conduction. Together with loss of axons and nerve cell bodies, this leads to progressive neurologic symptoms.

▶ Clinical Findings

1. **Initial or presenting symptoms**—Patients can present with any of a variety of symptoms (**Table 9-8**). Common initial complaints are focal weakness, numbness, tingling, or unsteadiness in a limb; sudden loss or blurring of vision in one eye (optic neuritis); diplopia; disequilibrium; or a bladder-function disturbance

Table 9-8. Symptoms and Signs of Multiple Sclerosis.

	Percentage of Patients
Symptoms (at presentation)	
Paresthesia	37
Gait disorder	35
Lower extremity weakness or incoordination	17
Visual loss	15
Upper extremity weakness or incoordination	10
Diplopia	10
Signs	
Absent abdominal reflexes	81
Hyperreflexia	76
Lower extremity ataxia	57
Extensor plantar responses	54
Impaired rapid alternating movements	49
Impaired vibratory sense	47
Optic neuropathy	38
Nystagmus	35
Impaired joint position sense	33
Intention tremor	32
Spasticity	31
Impaired pain or temperature sense	22
Dysarthria	19
Paraparesis	17
Internuclear ophthalmoplegia	11

Adapted with permission from Swanson JW. Multiple sclerosis: update in diagnosis and review of prognostic factors. *Mayo Clin Proc.* 1989;64:577-586. Copyright © Elsevier.

(urinary urgency or hesitancy). Symptoms are often transient, disappearing after a few days or weeks, even though some residual deficit may be found on neurologic examination. Other patients present with an acute or gradually progressive spastic paraparesis and sensory deficit; this should raise concern about the possibility of an underlying structural lesion unless there is evidence on clinical examination of more widespread disease.

2. **Subsequent course**—Months or years may elapse after the initial episode before further symptoms appear. Then, either new symptoms develop or the original ones recur and progress. Relapses may be triggered by infection and, in women, are more likely in the 3 months or so after childbirth (but are reduced during the pregnancy itself). A rise in body temperature can cause transient deterioration in patients with a fixed and stable deficit (Uhthoff phenomenon). With time—and after a number of relapses and usually incomplete remissions—the patient may become increasingly disabled by weakness, stiffness, sensory disturbances, unsteadiness of the limbs, impaired vision, and urinary incontinence.

Based on its course, the disease is divided into a **relapsing-remitting** form (85% of cases), in which progression does not occur between attacks; a **secondary progressive** form (80% of cases after 25 years), characterized by a gradually progressive course after an initial relapsing-remitting pattern; and a **primary progressive** form (10% of cases), marked by gradual progression of disability from clinical onset. A **progressive-relapsing** form, wherein acute relapses occur during a primary progressive course, is rare.

Examination in advanced cases commonly reveals optic atrophy, nystagmus, dysarthria, and upper motor neuron, sensory, or cerebellar deficits in some or all limbs (see Table 9-8). The diagnosis cannot be based on any single symptom or sign but only on a total clinical picture that indicates involvement of different parts of the central nervous system at different times.

▶ Investigative Studies

These may support the clinical diagnosis and exclude other disorders but do not themselves justify a definitive diagnosis of multiple sclerosis.

The cerebrospinal fluid (CSF) is commonly abnormal, with mild lymphocytosis or a slightly increased protein concentration, especially if examined soon after an acute relapse. CSF protein electrophoresis shows the presence of discrete bands in the immunoglobulin G (IgG) region (**oligoclonal bands**) in 90% of patients. The antigens responsible for these antibodies are not known.

If clinical evidence of a lesion exists at only one site in the central nervous system, a diagnosis of multiple sclerosis cannot properly be made unless other regions are affected subclinically. Such subclinical involvement may be detected by the electrocerebral responses evoked by monocular visual stimulation with a checkerboard pattern (**visual evoked potentials**), monaural stimulation with repetitive clicks (**brainstem auditory evoked potentials**), or electrical stimulation of a peripheral nerve (**somatosensory evoked potentials**).

MRI may also detect subclinical lesions and has become nearly indispensable in confirming the diagnosis (**Figure 9-4**). T1-weighted images may reveal hypointense "black holes" that probably represent areas of permanent axonal damage; hyperintense lesions are also found. Gadolinium-enhanced T1-weighted images may highlight areas of inflammation with breakdown of the blood–brain barrier. T2-weighted images provide information about **disease burden** or **lesion load** (ie, total number of lesions); lesions typically appear as areas of high signal intensity. Other MRI techniques, including measures of cerebral atrophy, magnetization transfer imaging, magnetic resonance spectroscopy, and diffusion tensor imaging, provide yet more relevant information. The MRI of healthy subjects sometimes shows "unidentified bright objects" that resemble the lesions of multiple sclerosis but are without clinical correlates or significance; the imaging findings must therefore be interpreted in the clinical context in which they were obtained.

Spinal MRI or CT myelography may be necessary to exclude a single congenital or acquired surgically treatable lesion in patients with spinal involvement and no evidence of disseminated disease. The region of the foramen magnum must be visualized to exclude the possibility of a lesion such as Arnold–Chiari malformation, in which part of the cerebellum and the lower brainstem are displaced into the cervical canal, producing mixed pyramidal and cerebellar deficits in the limbs.

▶ Diagnosis

The diagnosis of multiple sclerosis requires evidence that at least two different regions of the central white matter have been affected at different times. Multiple sclerosis can be diagnosed straightaway in patients with at least two typical attacks and two MRI lesions. Typical attacks are characterized clinically by symptoms or signs typical of an acute inflammatory demyelinating event in the CNS, lasting at least 24 hours and occurring in the absence of fever or infection. If imaging has been performed in patients with typical attacks but shows no abnormality, the diagnosis of multiple sclerosis should be made only when other possibilities have been excluded.

If only one clinical attack has occurred, the MRI findings may be used to provide evidence of dissemination. To fulfill the criterion of **dissemination in space**, MRI should demonstrate at least one T2 lesion in at least two of four characteristic locations (juxtacortical, periventricular, infratentorial, and spinal cord); in patients with brainstem or spinal cord syndromes, lesions within the symptomatic region are excluded. To show **dissemination in time** in a patient with only one attack, the simultaneous presence on

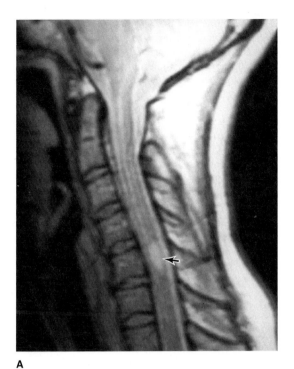

A

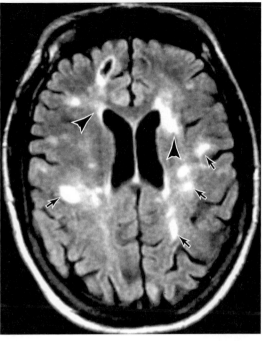

B

▲ **Figure 9-4.** (**A**) A mid-sagittal T2-weighted MRI of the cervical spinal cord in a young woman with multiple sclerosis. An abnormal region of high signal intensity (**arrow**) is seen. (Used with permission from RA Heyman.) (**B**) Axial T2-weighted MR brain image of a patient with multiple sclerosis showing multiple, primarily punctate, white matter plaques (**arrows**); note the typical location in the periventricular region (**arrowheads**). (Used with permission from RA. Heyman.)

MRI of asymptomatic gadolinium-enhancing and non-enhancing lesions at any time is sufficient; alternatively, it is necessary to await development of a new T2 or gadolinium-enhancing lesion on follow-up MRI or a second clinical attack. Diagnosis of primary progressive disease requires at least one year of progressive disease plus two of the following: (1) at least one typical T2 brain lesion, (2) at least two spinal T2 lesions, and (3) positive CSF oligoclonal bands, increased IgG index, or both.

In patients with only a single clinical event and who do not satisfy criteria for multiple sclerosis, a **clinically isolated syndrome (CIS)** is diagnosed. These patients are at increased risk for developing multiple sclerosis and are sometimes offered treatment as if they had the disease in the hope of delaying progression to clinically definite disease. Follow-up MRI should be considered 6 to 12 months later to determine whether any new lesions have occurred.

▶ Treatment

The treatment approach is summarized in **Table 9-9**.

1. **Relapsing-remitting disease—Corticosteroids** may hasten recovery from acute relapses, but the extent of the recovery itself is unchanged. Treatment is therefore generally reserved for attacks that lead to acute change in functional ability, such as by causing visual or gait dysfunction. Long-term corticosteroid administration does not prevent relapses and should not be used because of unacceptable side effects. There is no standard schedule of treatment with corticosteroids, but the regimen most commonly used is intravenous methylprednisolone (1 g daily) for 5 days, followed by an oral prednisone taper (1 mg/kg/d for 1 week, with rapid reduction over the ensuing 1-2 weeks). **Plasmapheresis** is sometimes helpful when patients have severe relapses that are unresponsive to corticosteroids.

   Treatment on an indefinite basis with **interferon** β-**1a** (30 μg intramuscularly once weekly, or 44 μg subcutaneously three times per week) or **interferon** β-**1b** (0.25 mg subcutaneously every other day) reduces the relapse rate. **Glatiramer acetate** (a mixture of random polymers simulating the amino acid composition of myelin basic protein) given by subcutaneous injection (20 mg daily) appears to be equally effective. In addition to their effect on relapses, interferon β-1a and glatiramer acetate may also delay the onset of significant disability in patients with relapsing disease.

Table 9-9. Treatment of Multiple Sclerosis or Clinically Isolated Demyelinating Events Suggestive of Multiple Sclerosis. Selection of treatment is individualized depending on convenience (oral agents), safety (interferons), or efficacy (intravenously administered agents).

Acute episode, including relapse[1]
• Methylprednisolone, 1 g IV daily × 3-5 days
• Prednisone, 1,000 mg PO daily × 3-5 days
• Dexamethasone, 160 mg PO daily × 3-5 days
Relapse prevention, first-line treatment[2]
• Interferon
β-1a (Rebif), 44 µg SC 3 times per week
β-1a (Avonex), 30 µg IM once per week
β-1b (Betaseron, Extavia), 0.25 mg SC on alternate days
• Glatiramer acetate (Copaxone), 20 mg SC daily
• Fingolimod (Gilenya), 0.5 mg PO daily[3]
• Teriflunomide (Aubagio), 14 mg PO daily[4]
• Dimethyl fumarate (Tecfidera), 240 mg PO twice daily
• Ocrelizumab (Ocrevus), 300 mg IV on day 1 and day 15; then 600 mg IV every 6 months
• Natalizumab (Tysabri), 300 mg IV monthly[5]
• Alemtuzumab, 12 mg IV per day for 5 days; subsequently (after 1 year) 12 mg IV per day for 3 days; may or may not require further dosing
Relapse prevention for disease activity despite use of first-line treatment
• Fingolimod, 0.5 mg PO daily
• Teriflunomide (Aubagio), 14 mg PO daily[4]
• Dimethyl fumarate (Tecfidera), 240 mg PO twice daily
• Mitoxantrone, 12 mg/m² IV every 3 months; maximum lifetime dose, 140 mg/m²
• Natalizumab (Tysabri), 300 mg IV monthly[5]
• Rituximab, 1000 mg IV on day 1 and day 15; subsequently (after 24 weeks) 1000 mg IV every 24 weeks
• Ocrelizumab (Ocrevus), 300 mg IV on day 1 and day 15; then 600 mg IV every 6 months
• Alemtuzumab, 12 mg IV per day for 5 days; subsequently (after 1 year) 12 mg IV per day for 3 days; may or may not require further dosing
High disease activity (typically with multiple gadolinium-enhancing lesions on MRI)
• Natalizumab (Tysabri), 300 mg IV monthly
• Rituximab, 1000 mg IV on day 1 and day 15; subsequently (after 24 weeks) 1000 mg IV every 24 weeks
• Ocrelizumab (Ocrevus), 300 mg IV on day 1 and day 15; then 600 mg IV every 6 months
• Alemtuzumab, 12 mg IV per day for 5 days; subsequently (after 1 year) 12 mg IV per day for 3 days; may or may not require further dosing

[1]For corticosteroid-refractory relapses, plasmapheresis or IVIG may be used.
[2]High-dose high-frequency interferons, fingolimod, and glatiramer acetate are more efficacious than once weekly interferon.
[3]Heart rate should be monitored for 6 hours after the first dose of fingolimod or if restarted after an interval of ≥2 weeks.
[4]Pregnancy category X; if patient becomes pregnant, need to wash out drug.
[5]Need to monitor JC antibody status every 6 months.

Interferons may cause a flu-like syndrome and (in the case of interferon β-1b) injection site reactions. Glatiramer acetate is generally tolerated well but may produce erythema at injection sites, and approximately 15% of patients experience transient episodes of flushing, dyspnea, chest tightness, palpitations, and anxiety after injections. All three of these agents are approved for use in relapsing-remitting multiple sclerosis. They are expensive, but their cost must be balanced against the reduced need for medical care and reduced time lost from work that follows their use.

Natalizumab, an α4 integrin antibody, reduces the relapse rate when given intravenously once each month. It is given without other immune-modulating therapies to patients with relapsing-remitting disease poorly responsive to other therapies or with an aggressive initial course. It has rarely been associated with progressive multifocal leukoencephalopathy, but if JC virus antibody testing is negative, the risk is low. **Alemtuzumab**, a monoclonal antibody directed at CD52 (a protein on the surface of immune cells), is given by intravenous infusion for 5 consecutive days and then for 3 consecutive days one year later. It markedly reduces the relapse rate but may have serious side effects such as autoimmune disorders (eg, thrombocytopenia) and anti-glomerular basement membrane disease; life-threatening infusion reactions may also occur, and there is an increased risk of malignancies (including thyroid cancer, melanoma, and blood cancers).

Oral therapies are now available and are preferred by some, although their long-term safety profile is less clear. There are no trials comparing the efficacy of these newer agents. **Fingolimod** (0.5 mg daily) reduces relapses and disease progression; it also reduces MRI lesion activity and loss of brain volume in relapsing-remitting disease. Its mechanism of action is unknown but probably involves prevention of lymphocyte migration into the central nervous system. It is generally safe and well tolerated, but is contraindicated after recent myocardial infarction or with certain other cardiac disturbances. Adverse effects include headache, fatigue, back pain, diarrhea, respiratory tract infections, elevation of liver enzymes, blood pressure effects, macular edema, and—on initiation of therapy—transient bradycardia and slowed atrioventricular conduction. Therefore, heart rate should be monitored for 6 hours after the first dose, or if fingolimod is restarted after interruption of use for 2 weeks or more. Skin and certain other cancers have also been reported. At least until further experience has accumulated, use of fingolimod is probably best restricted to patients with active relapsing-remitting disease who are intolerant of β interferons and glatiramer acetate; it is also prescribed for newly diagnosed patients with active relapsing disease who prefer treatment with oral rather than parenteral medications, provided they understand the associated risks. Another oral agent, **dimethyl fumarate** (120 mg twice daily for 1 week, then 240 mg twice daily), also reduces relapse rate. Side effects include flushing, gastrointestinal complaints (eg, diarrhea, nausea, abdominal pain), and a reduced peripheral lymphocyte count. Relapse rate and disease progression are reduced by **teriflunomide**, an immunomodulatory drug (taken orally in a daily dose of 7 or 14 mg). It has risks of hepatotoxicity and teratogenicity; side effects include alopecia, nausea, diarrhea, paresthesias, flu-like symptoms, elevated serum transaminases, and peripheral neuropathy.

Ocrelizumab, which targets B cells, is particularly effective in reducing the relapse rate and lessening progression of disability in relapsing-remitting disease. It was approved for use by the U.S. Food and Drug Administration while this book was in production. It is given by intravenous infusion. The most common complications are infusion reactions and respiratory tract infections.

2. **Primary or secondary progressive multiple sclerosis—** Optimal treatment in these forms of the disease is less clear. Until recently, there was no established treatment for primary progressive multiple sclerosis, but **ocrelizumab** has now been shown to slow disease progression both clinically and by imaging studies in that disorder. It is given by intravenous infusion; infusion reactions and respiratory tract infections may occur.

Interferon β-1b (and probably interferon β-1a) are effective in reducing the progression rate as determined clinically and by MRI in secondary progressive disease, but there is only limited experience with glatiramer acetate in this setting. Mitoxantrone probably reduces the clinical attack rate and may help to reduce disease progression in patients whose clinical condition is worsening. Treatment with cyclophosphamide, azathioprine, or methotrexate may help to arrest the course of secondary progressive disease, but studies are inconclusive. Pulse therapy with high-dose intravenous methylprednisolone (1 g/d once a month) is also sometimes effective and may carry a lower risk of long-term complications than the cytotoxic drugs.

3. **General health and symptomatic treatment—** Exercise and physical therapy are important, but excessive exertion must be avoided, particularly during periods of acute relapse. Fatigue is a serious problem for many patients and sometimes responds to amantadine or one of the selective serotonin reuptake inhibitor antidepressants. Treatment for spasticity (discussed earlier) is often needed, as is aggressive bladder and bowel management. Treatment for other aspects of advanced multiple sclerosis such as cognitive deficits, pain, tremor, and ataxia is generally less successful.

▶ **Prognosis**

At least partial recovery from an acute episode can be anticipated, but it is impossible to predict when the next relapse will occur. Features that tend to imply a more favorable prognosis include female sex, onset before 40 years of age, and presentation with visual or somatosensory, rather than pyramidal or cerebellar, dysfunction. Although some degree of disability is likely to result eventually, approximately one-half of patients are only mildly or moderately disabled 10 years after the onset of symptoms.

NEUROMYELITIS OPTICA

This relapsing disorder (formerly known as Devic disease and once considered a variant of multiple sclerosis) is associated with a specific antibody marker, NMO-IgG, that targets the water channel aquaporin-4. The disorder is characterized by optic neuritis and acute myelitis associated with MRI changes that extend over at least three segments of the spinal cord. Some patients with isolated myelitis or optic neuritis are also antibody positive. Seropositivity suggests a poor visual outcome. Unlike multiple sclerosis, the MRI typically does not show widespread white matter involvement, although such changes do not exclude the diagnosis.

Acute attacks are treated with intravenous methylprednisolone (1 g daily) for 5 days, followed by an oral prednisone taper (1 mg/kg/d for 1 week, with rapid reduction over the ensuing 1-2 weeks). If the response is poor, plasmapheresis is undertaken. Treatment with intravenous immunoglobulins is generally unhelpful. Treatment is otherwise with long-term immunosuppressive therapy, which may reduce the frequency of attacks and stabilize the disorder, but their use is empiric and off-label. Rituximab (1 g by intravenous infusion, given twice separated by 2 weeks, with re-treatment typically every 6 months) may be effective. Alternatively, mycophenolate mofetil (usually 1000 mg orally twice daily) can be given. Finally, azathioprine (~2 mg/kg orally) can be used; a typical daily dose is 150 mg. Azathioprine is usually titrated until the total peripheral white cell count declines to approximately 3000/μL while the absolute neutrophil count is maintained above 1000/μL. Treatment is usually continued indefinitely as recurrence of disease activity typically follows treatment discontinuation. There is no evidence favoring one therapy over another.

ACUTE DISSEMINATED ENCEPHALOMYELITIS

▶ **Pathogenesis**

Neurologic symptoms and signs develop over a few days in association with a nonspecific viral infection, after immunization, or without obvious antecedents, when it then may represent the initial manifestation of multiple sclerosis. Pathologically, perivascular areas of demyelination are scattered throughout the brain and spinal cord, with an associated inflammatory reaction. Lesions are all of similar age, and the brain appears swollen.

Clinical Findings

The disorder has its highest incidence in childhood. It is usually monophasic but relapses occur in rare instances. Initial symptoms often consist of headache, fever, and confusion; examination reveals meningeal irritation. Multifocal neurologic deficits are common. The patient is commonly encephalopathic: disturbances of consciousness range from somnolence to coma; seizures may occur. Flaccid weakness and sensory disturbance of the legs, extensor plantar responses, and urinary retention are common manifestations of spinal cord involvement. Other neurologic signs may indicate involvement of the optic nerves or cranial nerves, cerebral hemispheres, brainstem, or cerebellum; cerebellar ataxia is often conspicuous (especially when associated with varicella), but optic neuritis, hemiparesis and other long-tract signs, aphasia, and even movement disorders may also occur.

The neurologic deficit resolves spontaneously, at least in part, over a few weeks or months. Many patients make a virtually complete recovery, but some are left with severe residual deficits. Measles-associated disease is often especially severe.

Investigative Studies

The CSF is occasionally normal but in many cases shows an increased mononuclear cell count; protein concentration may be increased, but glucose concentration is normal. Oligoclonal bands, a nonspecific finding, are sometimes present. CT scans are often normal but MRI is helpful: T2-weighted images and FLAIR sequences show asymmetric high-signal lesions particularly in the hemispheric white matter, optic nerves, basal ganglia, thalamus, cerebellum, brainstem, or spinal cord. There may be mass effect and edema. On T1-weighted images, low-signal lesions are found in the white matter and—depending on their age—may enhance uniformly with gadolinium (**Figure 9-5**). Gadolinium enhancement is variable, however, and enhancing and non-enhancing lesions may occur in the same scan. Gray matter abnormalities may also be present.

Differential Diagnosis

The diagnosis is based on the clinical and neuroimaging features. Infective meningitis, encephalitis, and other inflammatory disorders (eg, multiple sclerosis) must be excluded. Long-term follow-up helps to confirm the diagnosis; relapses suggest alternative possibilities, such as multiple sclerosis.

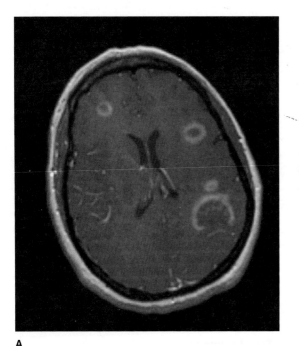
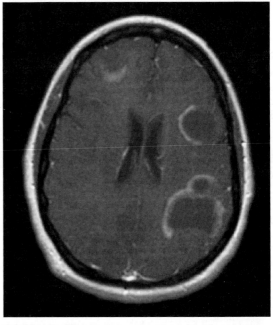

A   B

▲ **Figure 9-5.** Gadolinium-enhanced T1 axial MRI in a patient with acute disseminated encephalomyelitis, showing evolution of the lesions. The MRI in B was obtained 7 days after that in A. (Used with permission from A. DiBernardo.)

Treatment

Broad-spectrum antibiotics and acyclovir are often administered until bacterial infections and herpes simplex virus encephalitis are excluded by diagnostic studies. High-dose intravenous methylprednisolone (30 mg/kg/d, up to a maximum dose of 1 g daily, for 5 days) is then usually given. Treatment with intravenous immunoglobulins or plasmapheresis is sometimes helpful in patients with an inadequate response to methylprednisolone. Treatment is otherwise symptomatic.

OTHER INFECTIVE OR INFLAMMATORY MYELOPATHIES

SPINAL EPIDURAL ABSCESS

Pathogenesis

Epidural abscess—that is, located within the spinal canal but outside the dura mater—may occur as a sequel to skin infection, septicemia, vertebral osteomyelitis, intravenous drug abuse, spinal trauma or surgery, epidural anesthesia, or lumbar puncture. Predisposing factors include diabetes, alcoholism, acquired immunodeficiency syndrome (AIDS), and iatrogenic immunosuppression.

The most common causative organisms are *Staphylococcus aureus,* streptococci, gram-negative bacilli, and anaerobes. Neurologic complications result from compression of the spinal cord or its blood supply, obstructed venous drainage, inflammatory reactions, and vasculitis.

Clinical Findings

Fever, backache and tenderness, pain in the distribution of a spinal nerve root, headache, and malaise are early symptoms, followed by rapidly progressive paraparesis, sensory disturbances in the legs, and urinary and fecal retention. Spinal epidural abscess is a neurologic emergency that requires prompt diagnosis and treatment.

Investigations

MRI with gadolinium enhancement is the imaging study of choice and should be sufficient to determine the extent of the abscess. The entire spine is best imaged because patients may have more than one lesion, and lesions are not necessarily contiguous. CT myelography may reveal a block. Laboratory investigations reveal a peripheral leukocytosis and increased erythrocyte sedimentation rate. Spinal tap should not be performed at the site of a suspected abscess, as it may disseminate the infection from the epidural to subarachnoid space. The CSF typically shows a mild pleocytosis with increased protein but normal glucose concentration. Blood cultures and cultures of the excised abscess or its aspirate help to identify the causal organism.

Treatment

Treatment involves surgery and antibiotics. Early surgical decompression and drainage improve the long-term outlook and should be considered when MRI shows evidence of cord compression or when any neurologic deficit is progressing. With the advent of MRI, however, spinal epidural abscess is diagnosed increasingly before it has compressed the spinal cord and at a time when treatment with intravenous antibiotics alone is successful. Nafcillin or vancomycin is administered to cover staphylococcal or streptococcal infection, and a third- or fourth-generation cephalosporin such as ceftazidime or cefepime, respectively, to cover gram-negative infections; other agents are added or substituted based on the clinical context and results of Gram stain of excised material. The results of culture of the necrotic material that makes up the abscess may subsequently alter the antibiotic regimen. The antibiotic dosages are those used to treat bacterial meningitis, as given in Chapter 4, Confusional States. Intravenous antibiotics are usually continued for 4 to 6 weeks, but treatment for 6 to 8 weeks is required in the presence of vertebral osteomyelitis or when the response to treatment has been slow.

Follow-up MRI is obtained after about 4 weeks when the patient is improving but at any time if deterioration is occurring.

Prognosis

Uncontrolled sepsis may result in a fatal outcome. Delayed diagnosis or treatment and suboptimal management may lead to irreversible paraparesis or paraplegia, which occurs in up to 20% of cases, depending on the series. The most important prognostic indicator is the patient's clinical status before decompressive surgery; the more severe the preoperative deficit, the less recovery is to be expected. Delayed diagnosis is usually reflected by a more severe deficit and thus a poorer prognosis.

ACUTE TRANSVERSE MYELITIS

This syndrome results from a variety of infectious (bacterial, viral, fungal, parasitic) and noninfectious inflammatory disorders (multiple sclerosis, neuromyelitis optica, acute disseminated encephalomyelitis, systemic autoimmune diseases, idiopathic) that produce anatomic and functional disruption of the spinal cord. Children and young adults are affected most often. Clinical findings include bilateral sensory, motor, and autonomic deficits in the limbs and trunk; a discrete sensory level corresponding to the site of inflammation in the spinal cord; a course of hours to days; an inflammatory CSF profile (pleocytosis and/or an increased IgG index; an accompanying low CSF glucose suggests an infective cause); and an MRI showing an intrinsic spinal cord lesion that usually enhances with gadolinium administration. Compressive lesions of the spinal cord, such as spinal epidural abscess, must be excluded, usually by MRI, as they require specific treatment.

Treatment is with corticosteroids, typically methylprednisolone (1 g intravenously daily for 3-5 days), although their benefit has not been rigorously established. Plasma exchange, intravenous immunoglobulins, or cyclophosphamide may be useful in steroid-unresponsive patients, but their utility remains to be established. Patients tend to improve over several months, but may have residual deficits, and mortality rates in excess of 30% have been reported. Recurrences may occur, depending on the underlying cause.

SYPHILIS

Syphilis can produce meningovasculitis resulting in spinal cord infarction. Vascular myelopathies are discussed later in this chapter.

TUBERCULOSIS

Tuberculosis may lead to vertebral disease (**Pott disease**) with secondary compression of the spinal cord, meningitis with secondary arteritis and cord infarction, or cord compression by a tuberculoma. Such complications assume great importance in certain parts of the world, especially Asia and Africa, and among such groups as the homeless and intravenous drug users, who are at increased risk for contracting tuberculosis. Tuberculous meningitis is considered in more detail in Chapter 4, Confusional States.

AIDS

A disorder of the spinal cord, **vacuolar myelopathy,** is found at autopsy in about 30-40% of patients with AIDS; in most, it was asymptomatic. Vacuolation of white matter in the spinal cord is most pronounced in the thoracic lateral and posterior columns. Although attributed to direct involvement by human immunodeficiency virus-1 (HIV-1), the correlation between the presence and extent of HIV-1 infection and spinal pathology is poor. A metabolic basis therefore has been suggested. Myelopathy in patients with AIDS also may be caused by lymphoma, cryptococcal infection, or herpesviruses.

Most patients with vacuolar myelopathy have coexisting HIV-associated dementia. The myelopathy usually presents clinically in the late stages of AIDS. Symptoms progress over weeks to months and include leg weakness, ataxia, incontinence, erectile dysfunction, and paresthesias. There is typically no back pain. Examination shows paraparesis, lower extremity monoparesis, or quadriparesis; spasticity; increased or decreased tendon reflexes; Babinski signs; and diminished vibration and position sense. Sensation over the trunk is usually normal, and a sensory level is difficult to define. MRI of the spinal cord is usually normal. Treatment is with combination antiretroviral therapy (cART), but whether this helps to arrest the myelopathy is not clear. Spasticity and incontinence require symptomatic measures.

OTHER VIRAL INFECTIONS

▶ Tropical Spastic Paraparesis

A retrovirus, human T-lymphotropic virus type I (HTLV-I), appears to be the cause of **tropical spastic paraparesis,** a disorder found especially in the Caribbean, off the Pacific coast of Colombia, and in the Seychelles, southern Japan, Melanesia, the Middle East, and parts of Africa. Transmission of the virus occurs in breast milk, during sexual intercourse, and by exposure to contaminated blood products. The spinal cord in the thoracic region is affected particularly, and MRI may show an atrophic cord in this region. Clinical features include spastic paraparesis, impaired vibration and joint position sense, and bowel and bladder dysfunction. A clinically similar myelopathy may also follow infection with human T-lymphotropic virus type II (HTLV-II). The precise pathogenesis is uncertain, specific therapy is lacking, and treatment is symptomatic (primarily for spasticity and a spastic bladder). Preventive therapy is also important; patients should avoid sharing needles or syringes and breast-feeding, use condoms to prevent sexual transmission, and not donate blood, sperm, or other tissues.

▶ Herpesvirus

Herpesviruses can also produce myelopathy, which commonly affects spinal nerve roots as well as the cord (**radiculomyelopathy**), especially in immunocompromised patients, such as those with AIDS. **Cytomegalovirus** causes a myelopathy characterized by demyelination of the posterior columns of the spinal cord and by cytomegalic cells that contain Cowdry type A inclusion bodies. MRI may show increased T2 signal with enhancement. The CSF usually contains a lymphocytosis and increased protein concentration, but is sometimes normal. Viral identification may be possible by polymerase chain reaction in CSF and by antibody studies. Treatment is with antiviral drugs such as ganciclovir and foscarnet. Herpes zoster and herpes simplex types 1 and 2 may respond to treatment with acyclovir (see Chapter 4, Confusional States).

TETANUS

▶ Pathogenesis

Tetanus is a disorder of neurotransmission associated with infection by *Clostridium tetani*. The organism typically becomes established in a wound, where it elaborates a toxin that is transported retrogradely along motor nerves into the spinal cord or, with wounds to the face or head, the brainstem. The toxin is also disseminated through the bloodstream to skeletal muscle, where it gains access to additional motor nerves. In the spinal cord and brainstem, tetanus toxin interferes with release of the inhibitory neurotransmitters glycine and GABA, resulting in motor nerve hyperactivity. Autonomic nerves are also disinhibited.

Clinical Findings

After an incubation period of up to 3 weeks, tetanus usually presents with **trismus** (lockjaw), difficulty in swallowing, or spasm of the facial muscles that resembles a contorted smile (**risus sardonicus**). Painful muscle spasms and rigidity progress to involve both axial and limb musculature and may cause apneic episodes and hyperextended posturing (**opisthotonos**). Laryngospasm and autonomic instability are potential life-threatening complications.

Investigations

Although the diagnosis is usually made clinically, the presence of continuous motor unit activity or absence of the normal silent period in the masseter muscle after elicitation of the jaw-jerk reflex is a helpful electromyographic finding. The serum CK may be elevated, and myoglobinuria may occur. The organisms can be cultured from a wound in only a minority of cases.

Prevention

1. **Immunization**—Tetanus is preventable through immunization with tetanus toxoid. Tetanus toxoid is usually administered routinely to infants and children in the United States, in combination with pertussis vaccine and diphtheria toxoids. In children under age 7 years, three doses of tetanus toxoid are administered at intervals of at least 1 month, followed by a booster dose 1 year later. For older children and adults, the third dose is delayed for at least 6 months after the second, and no fourth dose is required. Immunization lasts for 5 to 10 years.

2. **Wound care**—Debridement of wounds is important to remove necrotic tissue and spores. Patients with open wounds should receive an additional dose of tetanus toxoid if they have not received a booster dose within 10 years—or if the last booster dose was more than 5 years ago and the risk of infection with *C. tetani* is moderate or high. A moderate likelihood of infection is associated with wounds that penetrate muscle, those sustained on wood or pavement, human bites, and non-abdominal bullet wounds. High-risk wounds include those acquired in barnyards or near sewers or other sources of waste material, and abdominal bullet wounds. To neutralize unbound toxin, patients with moderate- or high-risk wounds should also be given

tetanus immune globulin (3,000-6,000 units intramuscularly at a site other than that injected with tetanus toxoid, with part of the dose injected around the wound).

Treatment

The treatment of tetanus includes hospitalization in an intensive care unit to monitor respiratory and circulatory function, tetanus immune globulin to neutralize the toxin, and metronidazole (500 mg intravenously every 6 hours) for 7 to 10 days for the infection itself. Penicillin G can also be used but is an antagonist of GABA. Diazepam, 10 to 30 mg intravenously or intramuscularly every 4 to 6 hours, is useful for treating painful spasms and rigidity, as is intravenous infusion of propofol. Intrathecal baclofen has also been used. Neuromuscular blockade with vecuronium or pancuronium, with mechanical ventilation, may be required when these measures fail.

Autonomic hyperactivity can be treated with intravenous administration of the mixed α- and β-adrenergic receptor antagonist labetalol (up to 1 mg/min) or with morphine sulfate (0.5-1 mg/kg/h). Magnesium sulfate, which also blocks neurotransmitter release at the neuromuscular junction, can also be used and helps to control muscle spasms as well.

Prognosis

Fatality rates of 10% to 60% are reported. Lower fatality rates are most likely to be achieved by early diagnosis, prompt institution of appropriate treatment before the onset of spasms, and possibly by using intrathecal—in addition to intramuscular—tetanus immune globulin. Among patients who recover, approximately 95% do so without long-term sequelae.

CHRONIC ADHESIVE ARACHNOIDITIS

This inflammatory disorder is usually idiopathic but can follow subarachnoid hemorrhage; meningitis; intrathecal administration of penicillin, radiologic contrast materials, and certain forms of spinal anesthetic; trauma; and surgery. It can occur at any level, but now occurs most commonly in the lumbosacral region.

The usual initial complaint is of constant radicular pain, but in other cases paresthesias or lower motor neuron weakness occur. Eventually, depending on the level of involvement, a spastic ataxic paraparesis develops, with sphincter involvement and sexual dysfunction.

CSF protein is elevated, and the cell count may be increased, but these changes are not reliable indicators of the disease. MRI shows thickened and clumped nerve roots. Treatment with corticosteroids or nonsteroidal anti-inflammatory analgesics may be helpful. Surgery may be indicated in cases with localized spinal cord involvement.

VASCULAR MYELOPATHIES

SPINAL CORD INFARCTION

▶ Pathogenesis

This rare event most commonly involves the **anterior spinal artery (Figure 9-6)**. This artery, which supplies the anterior two-thirds of the cord, is itself supplied by only a limited number of feeding vessels, whereas the **paired posterior spinal arteries** receive numerous feeders at many different levels. Thus, anterior spinal artery syndrome usually results from interrupted flow in a single feeder. Other patterns of involvement include central and posterior spinal artery syndromes and a transverse syndrome. Causes include trauma, dissecting aortic aneurysm, aortography, polyarteritis nodosa, and hypotensive crisis. Because the anterior spinal artery is particularly well supplied in the cervical region, infarcts almost always occur more caudally.

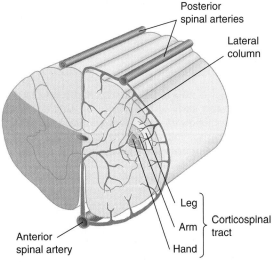

▲ **Figure 9-6.** Blood supply to the cervical spinal cord (shown in transverse section). **Left:** Major territories supplied by the anterior spinal artery (dark shading) and the posterior spinal artery (light shading). **Right:** Pattern of supply by intramedullary arteries. From the pial vessels (around the circumference of the cord), radially oriented branches supply much of the white matter and the posterior horns of the gray matter. The remaining gray matter and the innermost portion of the white matter are supplied by the central artery (located in the anterior median fissure), which arises from the anterior spinal artery. The descending corticospinal tract is supplied by both the anterior and posterior spinal arteries.

▶ Clinical Findings

The acute onset of a flaccid, areflexic paraparesis is followed, as spinal shock wears off after a few days or weeks, by a spastic paraparesis with brisk tendon reflexes and extensor plantar responses in patients with an **anterior spinal artery syndrome**. In addition, there is dissociated sensory impairment—pain and temperature appreciation are lost below the level of the lesion, but vibration and position sense are spared because the posterior columns are supplied by the posterior spinal arteries. Bladder, bowel, and sexual dysfunction may occur. Hypotension, a recognized cause of spinal cord ischemia, may also follow infarction. Neurologic deficits are typically bilateral, but unilateral involvement sometimes occurs depending on the integrity of the collateral blood supply and on whether the occlusion involves a branch of the anterior spinal artery going to one side of the cord. Treatment is symptomatic. Mortality relates to the underlying cause. Survivors may show some improvement; most remain chair-bound, however, and only a minority regain the ability to walk unaided.

Posterior spinal artery infarction leads to unilateral loss of vibration and joint position sense below the level of the lesion, sometimes accompanied by mild, transient weakness. It is rare.

▶ Investigations

Spinal MRI is important in excluding other causes for symptoms. In patients with spinal cord ischemia, it may show T2 signal abnormalities in a vascular territory, but the findings are sometimes normal soon after symptom onset. Diffusion-weighted MRI, however, reveals restricted diffusion.

Depending on the clinical context, additional studies are performed to exclude other diagnostic possibilities.

▶ Differential Diagnosis

A subacute, asymmetric myelopathy sometimes develops as a consequence of a vasculitic process; the cerebrospinal fluid shows a pleocytosis, and clinical benefit may follow corticosteroid therapy. An even more insidious, asymmetric ischemic myelopathy may result from compression of the anterior spinal artery or its major feeder, as by degenerative disease of the spine. The resulting disorder may simulate amyotrophic lateral sclerosis when there is a combined upper and lower motor neuron deficit, without sensory changes.

Compressive myelopathies can be excluded by imaging studies, which should be undertaken urgently. An inflammatory transverse myelitis is suggested by progression of symptoms over several hours; clinical and MRI involvement that exceeds a vascular territory; and the CSF findings (pleocytosis or elevated IgG levels).

HEMATOMYELIA

Hemorrhage into the spinal cord is rare; it is caused by trauma, a vascular anomaly, a bleeding disorder, or anticoagulant therapy. A severe cord syndrome develops acutely and is usually associated with blood in the CSF. The prognosis depends on the extent of the hemorrhage and the rapidity with which it occurs.

SPINAL EPIDURAL OR SUBDURAL HEMORRHAGE

Spinal epidural or subdural hemorrhage may occur spontaneously or in relation to trauma or tumor and as a complication of anticoagulation, aspirin therapy, thrombocytopenia, coagulopathy, epidural catheters, or lumbar puncture. Hemorrhage after lumbar puncture—usually epidural in location—is more likely when a disorder of coagulation is present. Therefore, the platelet count, prothrombin time, and partial thromboplastin time should be determined before lumbar puncture, and if anticoagulant therapy is to be instituted, it should be delayed for at least 1 hour after the procedure. Patients with fewer than 20,000 platelets/µL or those with rapidly falling counts to less than 50,000/µL should undergo platelet transfusion before lumbar puncture.

Spinal epidural hemorrhage usually presents with back pain that may radiate in the distribution of one or more spinal nerve roots; it is occasionally painless. Paraparesis or quadriparesis, sensory disturbances in the lower limbs, and bowel and bladder dysfunction may develop rapidly, necessitating urgent CT scan or MRI and surgical evacuation of the hematoma.

ARTERIOVENOUS MALFORMATION (AVM) OR FISTULA

This may present with spinal subarachnoid hemorrhage or with myelopathy. Most of these lesions involve the lower spinal cord. Symptoms include motor and sensory disturbances in the legs and disorders of sphincter function. Leg or back pain is often conspicuous.

On examination, there may be an upper or lower motor neuron deficit or a mixed motor deficit in the legs. Sensory deficits are usually extensive but occasionally radicular. The signs indicate an extensive lesion in the longitudinal axis of the cord. In patients with cervical lesions, symptoms and signs may also be present in the arms. A bruit is sometimes audible over the spine, and there may be a segmentally-related cutaneous angioma.

Spinal MRI shows multiple flow voids (**Figure 9-7**), but can rarely be normal; myelography reveals serpiginous filling defects caused by enlarged vessels. The diagnosis is confirmed by selective spinal arteriography. Most lesions are extramedullary (dural), posterior to the spinal cord, and can be treated by embolization or by ligation of feeding

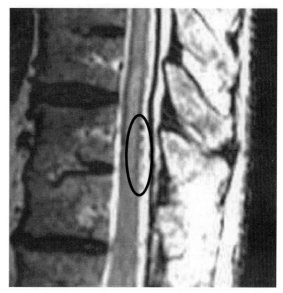

Figure 9-7. Spinal MRI, sagittal view, T2-weighted image, demonstrating multiple flow voids (within circle) in the posterior subarachnoid space in a patient with an arteriovenous fistula. (Used with permission from A. DiBernardo.)

vessels and excision of the anomalous arteriovenous nidus of the malformation. Left untreated, the patient is likely to become increasingly disabled until chair-bound or bed-bound.

NUTRITIONAL MYELOPATHIES

Subacute combined degeneration of the cord as a result of **vitamin B$_{12}$ deficiency** is characterized by an upper motor neuron deficit in the limbs that is usually preceded by sensory symptoms and signs caused by posterior column involvement (see Chapter 10, Sensory Disorders). In addition to the myelopathy, there may be optic atrophy, mental changes, or peripheral neuropathy. **Nitrous oxide toxicity** can produce a similar syndrome, as can **copper deficiency.**

CERVICAL SPONDYLOSIS

Cervical spondylosis is characterized by any or all of the following:

1. Pain and stiffness in the neck
2. Pain in the arms, with or without a segmental motor or sensory deficit
3. Upper motor neuron deficit in the legs

PATHOGENESIS

Cervical spondylosis results from chronic cervical disk degeneration, with herniation of disk material, secondary calcification, and associated osteophytic outgrowths. It can lead to impingement on one or more nerve roots on either or both sides and to myelopathy related to compression, vascular insufficiency, or recurrent minor trauma to the cord. Cervical spondylosis is the most common cause of myelopathy in patients over the age of 50 years,

CLINICAL FEATURES

Symptoms usually develop insidiously, although acute presentation may follow a seemingly minor neck injury, as from a motor vehicle accident. Patients often present with neck pain and limitation of head movement or with occipital headache. Presentation with a gait disturbance is also common. In some cases, radicular pain and other sensory disturbances occur in the arms, and there is weakness of the arms or legs. Dysfunction of bladder function (urgency, frequency, retention, incontinence) may be troublesome, as also may bowel and sexual disturbances. The quality of life often is impaired significantly.

Examination commonly reveals restricted lateral flexion and rotation of the neck, sometimes with crepitus. There may be a segmental pattern of weakness or dermatomal sensory loss in one or both arms, along with depression of those tendon reflexes mediated by the affected root(s). Cervical spondylosis tends to affect particularly the C5 and C6 nerve roots, so there is commonly weakness of muscles (eg, deltoid, supra- and infraspinatus, biceps, brachioradialis) supplied from these segments, pain or sensory loss about the shoulder and outer border of the arm and forearm, and depressed biceps and brachioradialis reflexes. If there is an associated myelopathy, upper motor neuron weakness develops in one or both legs, with concomitant changes in tone and reflexes. There may also be posterior column or spinothalamic sensory deficits.

INVESTIGATIVE STUDIES

Plain X-rays show osteophyte formation, narrowing of disk spaces, and encroachment on the intervertebral foramina. However, such findings are common in asymptomatic middle-aged or elderly subjects, and the extent of radiologic abnormality correlates poorly with the presence or severity of pain. Spinal MRI, CT scanning, or CT myelography confirms the diagnosis, provides a measure of central canal narrowing, and excludes other structural causes of myelopathy. The CSF obtained at the time of myelography is usually normal, but the protein concentration may be increased, especially if there is a block in the subarachnoid space. Needle electromyography is helpful in identifying a radiculopathy and determining whether degenerative anatomic abnormalities of the cervical spine are clinically significant.

DIFFERENTIAL DIAGNOSIS

Spondylotic myelopathy may resemble myelopathy caused by such disorders as multiple sclerosis, motor neuron disease, subacute combined degeneration, spinal cord tumor, syringomyelia, hereditary spastic paraplegia, or other disorders affecting the cervical spinal cord. Moreover, degenerative changes in the spine are common in the middle-aged and elderly and may coincide with one of these other disorders. The combination of bladder and gait disturbances may lead to a mistaken diagnosis of normal-pressure hydrocephalus, but the clinical context and imaging findings should help to distinguish these disorders.

TREATMENT

A cervical collar to restrict neck movements may relieve severe pain. Pain may also respond to simple analgesics, nonsteroidal anti-inflammatory drugs, muscle relaxants, tricyclic antidepressants (taken at night), or anticonvulsants. Provocative activities must be avoided. Physical therapy may help once pain is less severe and increasing mobilization is desirable. Patients with cervical radiculopathy and severe pain are sometimes helped by epidural steroid injections, but complications include spinal cord or cerebral infarction.

Operative treatment may prevent progression of neurologic deficits; it may also be required if radicular pain is severe, persistent, and unresponsive to conservative measures and if imaging reveals root compression. Operative treatment is indicated for acute or progressive spinal cord compression, and should be undertaken early if there is sphincter disturbance.

CONGENITAL SPINAL ANOMALIES

A combination of corticospinal and cerebellar signs may occur in the limbs of patients with congenital skeletal abnormalities such as **platybasia** (flattening of the base of the skull) or **basilar invagination** (an upward bulging of the margins of the foramen magnum). **Syringomyelia** (cavitation of the cord), which can be congenital or acquired, may lead to a lower motor neuron deficit, a dissociated sensory loss in the arms, and upper motor neuron signs in the legs. Because the sensory findings are so characteristic, this disorder, which is frequently associated with Arnold–Chiari malformation, is discussed in detail in Chapter 10, Sensory Disorders.

SPINAL CORD TUMORS

ETIOLOGY

Tumors can be divided into two groups: **intramedullary** (10%) and extramedullary (90%). **Ependymomas** are the most common type of intramedullary tumor; the various types of **gliomas** make up the remainder. Extramedullary tumors can be either extradural or intradural in location.

Among the primary extramedullary tumors, **neurofibromas** and **meningiomas** are relatively common and are benign; they can be intra- or extradural. Carcinomatous metastases (especially from bronchus, breast, or prostate), lymphomatous or leukemic deposits, and myeloma are usually extradural.

PATHOGENESIS OF MYELOPATHY

Myelopathy may occur in patients with malignant neoplasms because of spinal cord compression or direct involvement by the primary tumor or by metastases, ischemic or hemorrhagic complications of the neoplasm or its treatment, complications of radiation or chemotherapy, secondary infection (especially in immunocompromised patients), or a paraneoplastic disorder.

▶ Opportunistic Infection

Immunocompromised patients are at particular risk of infection, often with unusual agents that may cause a myelopathy, such as varicella-zoster virus, cytomegalovirus, Epstein–Barr virus, or herpes simplex virus. Treatment of infective myelopathies was discussed earlier in this chapter.

▶ Paraneoplastic Disorders

In **paraneoplastic necrotizing myelopathy**, the most common antibody is anti-Hu; other antibodies may also be found, but sometimes no antibody can be identified. The underlying tumor is commonly a cancer of the lung or breast, lymphoma, or leukemia. Patients present with a rapidly ascending flaccid paraplegia. The myelopathy is often accompanied by an encephalopathy and neuropathy (**paraneoplastic encephalomyelitis**). The MRI findings are usually nonspecific or normal, but may show swelling of the spinal cord. The CSF may contain inflammatory cells. Treatment is of the underlying malignancy, but improvement of the myelopathy is uncommon. Immunosuppressive therapies are often prescribed, with limited benefit.

▶ Spinal Cord Compression

Common causes of cord compression are disk protrusion, trauma, and tumors; in certain parts of the world, tuberculous disease of the spine is also a frequent cause. Rare but important causes of cord compression include epidural abscess and hematoma. The present section will be restricted to a consideration of tumors, as other causes are considered elsewhere in this chapter.

CLINICAL FINDINGS

Irrespective of its nature, a spinal tumor can lead to cord dysfunction and a neurologic deficit by direct compression, ischemia secondary to arterial or venous obstruction, or, in the case of intramedullary lesions, by invasive infiltration.

Table 9-10. Clinical Features of Spinal Cord Compression by Extradural Metastasis.

Sign or Symptom	Initial Feature (%)	Present at Diagnosis (%)
Pain	96	96
Weakness	2	76
Sensory disturbance	0	51
Sphincter dysfunction	0	57

Data from Gilbert RW, Kim JH, Posner JB. Epidural spinal compression from metastatic tumor: diagnosis and treatment. *Ann Neurol.* 1978;3:40-51.

▶ Symptoms

Symptoms may develop insidiously and progress gradually or—as with spinal cord compression from metastatic carcinoma—exhibit a rapid course.

Pain is conspicuous—and usually the initial abnormality—in many patients with extradural lesions; it can be radicular, localized to the back, or experienced diffusely in an extremity and is characteristically aggravated by coughing or straining (**Table 9-10**).

Motor symptoms (heaviness, weakness, stiffness, or focal wasting of one or more limbs) may develop, or there may be paresthesias or numbness, especially in the legs. When sphincter disturbances occur, they usually are particularly disabling.

▶ Signs

Localized **spinal tenderness** to percussion is sometimes present. Involvement of anterior roots leads to an appropriate lower motor neuron deficit, and of posterior roots leads to dermatomal sensory changes at the level of the lesion. Dysfunction of pathways traversing the cord may cause an upper motor neuron deficit below the level of the lesion and a sensory deficit with an upper level on the trunk. The distribution of signs varies with lesion level and may take the form of Brown-Séquard or central cord syndrome (see Figures 10-5 and 10-7).

INVESTIGATIVE STUDIES

The CSF is often xanthochromic, due to a greatly increased protein concentration rather than hemorrhage, with normal or elevated white blood cell count and normal or depressed glucose concentration. MRI or CT myelography delineates and localizes the lesion.

TREATMENT

Extradural metastases must be treated urgently. Depending on the primary neoplasm, they are best managed by analgesics, corticosteroids, radiotherapy, and hormonal treatment; decompressive laminectomy is often unnecessary. Intradural (but extramedullary) lesions are best removed if possible. Intramedullary tumors are treated by decompression and surgical excision when feasible and by radiotherapy.

PROGNOSIS

The prognosis depends on the cause and severity of the cord compression before it is relieved. Cord compression by extradural metastasis is usually manifested first by pain and may progress rapidly to impair motor, sensory, and sphincter function. Therefore, any patient with cancer and spinal or radicular pain must be investigated immediately. Reliance on motor, sensory, or sphincter disturbances to make the diagnosis will delay treatment and worsen the outcome.

ANTERIOR HORN CELL DISORDERS

Disorders that predominantly affect the anterior horn cells are characterized clinically by wasting and weakness of the affected muscles without accompanying sensory changes. Electromyography shows changes that are characteristic of chronic partial denervation: abnormal spontaneous activity in resting muscle and a reduction in the number of motor units under voluntary control; signs of reinnervation may also be present. Motor conduction velocity is usually normal but may be slightly reduced, and sensory conduction studies are normal. Muscle biopsy shows the histologic changes of denervation. Serum CK may be mildly elevated, but it never reaches the extremely high values seen in some muscular dystrophies.

IDIOPATHIC DISORDERS

The clinical features and outlook depend in part on the patient's age at onset. The cause of these disorders is unknown, but some have a genetic basis.

MOTOR NEURON DISEASE IN CHILDREN

Three forms of spinal muscular atrophy (SMA-I, II, and III) occur in infants and children, and mutations in the survival of motor neuron 1 (*SMN1*) gene have been identified in 95% of patients. A nearby gene, coding for neuronal apoptosis inhibitory protein (NAIP), is also affected in 45% of patients with SMA-I and 18% of those with SMA-II and SMA-III. NAIP may modify disease severity. The survival of motor neuron 2 (*SMN2*) gene, a homolog of *SMN1*, is also a disease modifier of spinal muscular atrophy; it improves survival. In SMA, production of survival motor neuron (SMN) protein, critical for the maintenance of motor neurons, is diminished.

A new disease-modifying therapy has recently been approved for use in the United States and elsewhere.

Intrathecally administered nusinersen (Spinraza), an antisense oligonucleotide (ie, a synthetic string of nucleotides that binds to target RNA and regulates gene expression), alters the splicing of SMN2 pre-mRNA to increase production of full-length, fully functional SMN protein. Its use slowed or halted disease progression; improved motor performance and development, allowing motor milestones to be achieved or maintained when this would otherwise not be expected; and reduced mortality. Its most common side effects are upper or lower respiratory infections, constipation, headache, and back pain; thrombocytopenia and renal toxicity may also occur.

▶ Infantile Spinal Muscular Atrophy (Werdnig–Hoffmann Disease or SMA-I)

This autosomal recessive disorder usually manifests within the first 3 months of life. The infant is floppy and may have difficulty with sucking, swallowing, or ventilation. Examination reveals impaired swallowing or sucking, atrophy and fasciculation of the tongue, and muscle wasting in the limbs that is sometimes obscured by subcutaneous fat. The tendon reflexes are normal or depressed, and the plantar responses may be absent. There is no sensory deficit. The disorder is rapidly progressive, generally leading to death from respiratory complications by approximately 3 years of age unless treated with nusinersen.

▶ Intermediate Spinal Muscular Atrophy (Chronic Werdnig–Hoffmann Disease or SMA-II)

This autosomal recessive disorder usually begins clinically in the latter half of the first year of life. The extremities become wasted and weak; bulbar weakness is less common. Progression occurs slowly, ultimately leading to severe disability with kyphoscoliosis and contractures, but the course is more benign than in the infantile variety, and many patients survive into adulthood. Treatment is with nusinersen and also is supportive, directed particularly at the prevention of scoliosis and other deformities.

▶ Juvenile Spinal Muscular Atrophy (Kugelberg–Welander Disease or SMA-III)

This disorder develops in childhood or early adolescence, on a sporadic or hereditary (usually autosomal recessive) basis. It particularly affects the proximal limb muscles, with generally little involvement of the bulbar musculature. It follows a gradually progressive course, leading to disability in early adult life. The proximal weakness may lead to a mistaken diagnosis of muscular dystrophy, but serum CK determination, electromyography, and muscle biopsy will differentiate the disorders. Treatment is with nusinersen. Noninvasive ventilatory support has extended survival.

MOTOR NEURON DISEASE IN ADULTS

These disorders are characterized by degeneration of anterior horn cells in the spinal cord, motor nuclei of the lower cranial nerves in the brainstem, and corticospinal and corticobulbar pathways.

▶ Epidemiology

Motor neuron disease in adults generally begins between the ages of 30 and 60 years and has an annual incidence of approximately 2 per 100,000, with a male predominance, except in familial cases. Occasional familial cases have a juvenile onset. The disorder usually occurs sporadically but may be familial in 5% to 10% of cases.

▶ Pathogenesis

Genetics Approximately 90% to 95% of cases are sporadic and of unknown cause; no robust environmental risk factors have emerged. Approximately 20% of familial cases show autosomal dominant inheritance of motor neuron disease (with upper and lower motor neuron signs) related to mutations in the copper/zinc superoxide dismutase (*SOD1*) gene. Other autosomal dominant forms are associated with mutations in senataxin (*SETX*), fused in sarcoma (*FUS*), vesicle-associated membrane protein-associated protein B (*VAPB*), angiogenin (*ANG*), TAR DNA-binding protein (*TARDP*), homolog of *S. cerevisiae* FIG4 (*FIG4*), ataxin 2 (*ATXN2*), profilin 1 (*PFN1*), or valosin-containing protein (*VCP*). Autosomal recessive motor neuron disease is linked in some cases to alsin (*ALSN*), and both dominant and recessive inheritance have been seen with mutations in optineurin (*OPTN*). An X-linked mutation occurs in ubiquilin 2 (*UBQLN2*).

Vascular endothelial growth factor (*VEGF*) gene polymorphisms may increase the risk of motor neuron disease. Other susceptibility genes include heavy neurofilament subunit (*NEFH*), peripherin (*PRPH*), and dynactin (*DCTN1*).

A GGGGCC hexanucleotide repeat is present within the noncoding region of the *C9ORF72* gene on chromosome 9q21, and accounts for many familial and some sporadic cases, discussed later. C9ORF72 is an RNA-binding protein and provides a new target for therapy.

Mechanisms The pathophysiologic basis of motor neuron disease is uncertain, but several mechanisms have been proposed, based largely on studies in animal models with *SOD1* mutations. Because these are gain-of-function mutations, the mechanisms inferred generally involve a toxic effect of the mutated protein.

CELLULAR MECHANISMS Although motor neurons are the primary cellular target, studies in which mutant *SOD1* is expressed selectively in different cell types indicate that non-neuronal cells also contribute to the pathogenesis of motor neuron disease. Involvement of **neurons** appears to determine the age at onset and early course of disease, whereas **microglia** and **astrocytes** influence the subsequent rate of progression.

MOLECULAR MECHANISMS Several explanations have been offered for the toxicity of mutant *SOD1*—and, perhaps, of factors involved in sporadic motor neuron disease. These are not mutually exclusive, as multiple mechanisms might operate in concert, or different mechanisms might underlie different forms of the disease. With *SOD1* mutations, an early pathogenic step is **abnormal folding** and **aggregation** of the mutant protein, as in other neurodegenerative proteinopathies (see Chapter 5, Dementia & Amnestic Disorders). How this leads to disease is disputed.

Excitotoxicity The principal excitatory neurotransmitter, glutamate, is toxic to neurons when present in excessive amounts. In motor neuron disease, spinal cord astrocytes express reduced levels of the EAAT2 excitatory amino acid (glutamate) transporter, which is the major site through which extracellular glutamate is cleared. This could expose motor neurons to toxic concentrations of glutamate.

Endoplasmic Reticulum Stress Mutant *SOD1* accumulates in the endoplasmic reticulum, where it may interfere with the degradation of misfolded proteins or the synthesis of normal proteins.

Proteasome Inhibition The proteasome is a large protein complex involved in proteolytic degradation and elimination of abnormal cellular proteins. The production of large amounts of mutant *SOD1* may overwhelm the ability of the proteasome to perform its normal function.

Mitochondrial Damage Mutant *SOD1* associates with the outer mitochondrial membrane, which might inhibit the production of ATP or the ability of mitochondria to regulate intracellular calcium levels.

Secretion of Mutant SOD1 *SOD1* released into the extracellular space may activate microglia, resulting in immune-mediated injury of motor neurons.

Increased Production of Superoxide Mutant *SOD1* may stimulate increased production of toxic superoxide radicals by glial cell NADPH oxidase.

Impaired Axonal Transport Anterograde and retrograde axonal transport may be disrupted by the accumulation of misfolded *SOD1* or other proteins.

Microvascular Dysfunction Loss of tight junctions between capillary endothelial cells could cause microhemorrhages that allow toxins such as iron to escape into the extravascular compartment and damage motor neurons.

▶ Classification

Five varieties of adult-onset motor neuron disease can be distinguished clinically by their predominant distribution (**limb** or **bulbar** musculature) and whether deficits

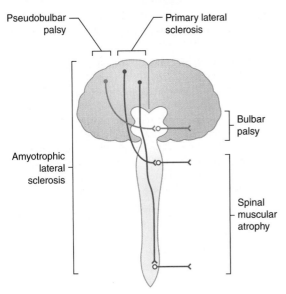

Pseudobulbar palsy — Primary lateral sclerosis

Bulbar palsy

Amyotrophic lateral sclerosis

Spinal muscular atrophy

▲ **Figure 9-8.** Adult-onset motor neuron disease syndromes. Upper motor neurons are shown with filled circles and lower motor neurons with open circles for cell bodies. Cerebral cortex is indicated with dark, brainstem white, and spinal cord light shading.

are from **upper** or **lower** motor neuron involvement (**Figure 9-8**).

1. **Progressive bulbar palsy**—Predominant bulbar (brainstem) involvement from lesions affecting the motor nuclei of cranial nerves (ie, lower motor neurons) in the brainstem.

2. **Pseudobulbar palsy**—Predominant bulbar involvement due primarily to upper motor neuron disease (ie, to bilateral involvement of corticobulbar pathways). A pseudobulbar palsy can occur in any disorder that causes bilateral corticobulbar disease (eg, vascular dementia or progressive supranuclear palsy), however, and not just in motor neuron disease.

3. **Progressive spinal muscular atrophy**—There is primarily a lower motor neuron deficit in the limbs, caused by anterior horn cell degeneration in the spinal cord. Familial forms have been recognized.

4. **Primary lateral sclerosis**—A purely upper motor neuron (corticospinal) deficit is found in the limbs.

5. **Amyotrophic lateral sclerosis**—A mixed upper and lower motor neuron deficit is present in the limbs. Bulbar involvement of the upper or lower motor neuron type may also occur. Both primary lateral sclerosis and progressive spinal muscular atrophy are considered to be variants of amyotrophic lateral sclerosis because, at autopsy, abnormalities of both upper and lower motor neurons are likely. Cognitive and behavioral changes also occur in some patients.

▶ Clinical Findings

1. **Bulbar muscles**—In approximately 20% of patients with amyotrophic lateral sclerosis, the initial symptoms are related to weakness of bulbar muscles. Bulbar involvement is somewhat more common in familial cases and is generally characterized by difficulty in swallowing, chewing, coughing, breathing, and speaking (dysarthria). In progressive bulbar palsy, examination may reveal drooping of the palate, a depressed gag reflex, a pool of saliva in the pharynx, a weak cough, and a wasted and fasciculating tongue. The tongue is contracted and spastic in pseudobulbar palsy and cannot be moved rapidly from side to side. The extraocular muscles are not involved.

2. **Limb muscles**—Patients may first present with weakness of the upper (approximately 40% of patients) or lower extremity (40%) muscles. Limb involvement is characterized by easy fatigability, weakness, stiffness, twitching, wasting, and muscle cramps, and there may be vague sensory complaints and weight loss.

3. **Other systems**—Amyotrophic lateral sclerosis and frontotemporal dementia (see Chapter 5, Dementia & Amnestic Disorders) overlap clinically, pathologically, and genetically. The GGGGCC hexanucleotide repeat in the non-coding region of the *C9orf72* gene on chromosome 9q21 occurs in at least 40% of familial cases of amyotrophic lateral sclerosis cases, 25% of familial cases of frontotemporal dementia, and 5% to 10% of apparently sporadic cases of these disorders. Cognitive and behavioral alterations are common in patients with amyotrophic lateral sclerosis, including personality change, irritability, lack of insight, and deficits in executive function. In other instances, parkinsonian or dysautonomic features may be present. Sensory and sphincteric functions are characteristically spared. The CSF is normal.

▶ Diagnosis

Diagnostic criteria for amyotrophic lateral sclerosis have been established by the World Federation of Neurology. Criteria vary depending on the level of certainty of the diagnosis, as shown in **Table 9-11**. Definitive diagnosis requires the presence of upper and lower motor neuron signs in the bulbar region and at least two other spinal regions (cervical, thoracic, or lumbosacral), or in three spinal regions. Alternative causes of signs and symptoms must be excluded.

▶ Differential Diagnosis

Other noninfective disorders of anterior horn cells (discussed later) must be excluded: They have different prognostic and therapeutic implications. Multifocal motor neuropathy is also an important consideration; its clinical features and treatment are discussed later in this chapter.

Table 9-11. Clinical Diagnosis of Amyotrophic Lateral Sclerosis: Revised El Escorial Criteria of the World Federation of Neurology.

Diagnostic Certainty	Clinical and Other Features[1]
Clinically definite	Upper and lower motor neuron signs in the bulbar and two spinal regions or in three spinal regions (cervical, thoracic, lumbosacral)
Clinically probable	Upper and lower motor neuron signs in two or more regions; the regions may differ, but some upper motor neuron signs must be rostral to the lower motor neuron deficit
Clinically probable, laboratory supported	Upper and lower motor neuron signs in one region, or upper motor neuron signs in one region, but lower motor neuron signs are found by EMG criteria in at least two limbs, and neuroimaging and electrodiagnostic studies exclude other causes
Clinically possible	Upper and lower motor neuron signs in only one region or upper motor neuron signs alone in two or more regions or lower motor neuron signs rostral to upper motor neuron signs. Other diagnostic possibilities must be excluded.
Suspected	Lower (but not upper) motor neuron signs in at least two regions

[1]The body is divided into a cranial region and three spinal regions (cervical, thoracic, and lumbosacral).

Cervical spondylosis can mimic amyotrophic lateral sclerosis when it produces lower motor neuron signs in the arms and upper motor neuron signs in the legs, but can be distinguished by the absence of clinical and electromyographic evidence of lower motor neuron involvement in the legs.

▶ Treatment

1. **Edaravone (Radicava)**, a free-radical scavenger, is a new FDA-approved treatment for amyotrophic lateral sclerosis based on a clinical trial in Japan showing slowed clinical progression in early-stage disease. It is administered intravenously (60 mg infused over 1 hour) on 10 days per month after an initial loading dose over 14 days. It is contraindicated in patients with a sulfite allergy. Adverse effects include contusion, gait disturbance, and headache.

2. **Riluzole** (50 mg orally twice daily) may reduce the mortality rate and slow progression of amyotrophic lateral sclerosis, possibly because it blocks NMDA receptor-mediated glutamatergic transmission. However, it probably prolongs survival by only about 2 or 3 months.

Adverse effects include fatigue, dizziness, gastrointestinal symptoms, reduced pulmonary function, and an increase in liver enzymes.

3. **Symptomatic measures** may include muscarinic anti-cholinergic drugs (eg, glycopyrrolate, trihexyphenidyl, amitriptyline, transdermal hyoscine, or atropine) if drooling of saliva is troublesome. Refractory drooling may respond to injection of botulinum toxin into the parotid and other salivary glands. Braces or a walker may improve mobility, and physical therapy may prevent contractures. Occupational therapy may facilitate daily activities in those with physical limitations.

4. **Diet**—A semiliquid diet or feeding via nasogastric tube may be required for severe dysphagia. Percutaneous endoscopic gastrostomy (PEG) is indicated for dysphagia with accelerated weight loss due to insufficient caloric intake, dehydration, or choking on food. For optimal safety, it should be offered when the patient's vital capacity is more than 50% of predicted.

5. **Ventilation**—Noninvasive or invasive ventilation may be necessary as hypoventilation develops. With respiratory therapy, patients are more likely to try non-invasive ventilation and to use it for longer. Palliative care to relieve distress without prolonging life then becomes an important consideration and requires detailed discussion with the patient and family. Such discussions are best initiated early in the course of the disease, with continuing discussion as the disease advances.

6. **Other**—Treatment with celecoxib, coenzyme Q-10, creatine, gabapentin, insulin growth factor-1, lamotrigine, lithium, minocycline, topiramate, valproic acid, verapamil, and vitamin E has been studied experimentally in the hope of slowing disease progression, but no benefit was found. Stem cell-based treatments are under investigation.

▶ Prognosis

Motor neuron disease is progressive and usually has a fatal outcome within 3 to 5 years, most commonly from respiratory failure. Some familial cases progress more slowly. In general, patients with bulbar involvement have a poorer prognosis than those in whom dysfunction is limited to the extremities. Patients with primarily upper motor neuron involvement (primary lateral sclerosis) often survive longer despite severe quadriparesis and spasticity. Survival and quality of life improve when patients are followed in a specialized multidisciplinary clinic.

OTHER NONINFECTIVE ANTERIOR HORN CELL DISORDERS

Bulbospinal neuronopathy (Kennedy disease) is a sex-linked recessive disorder associated with an expanded CAG trinucleotide repeat sequence in the androgen receptor (*AR*) gene. There is gradual but progressive degeneration of lower motor neurons in the brainstem nuclei and spinal cord; endocrine disturbances also occur and include late-onset gynecomastia and testicular atrophy. The disorder has a more benign prognosis than the other motor neuron diseases. Its clinical characteristics include tremor (resembling essential tremor), cramps, fasciculations, bulbar and both proximal and distal limb weakness, and twitching movements of the chin that are precipitated by pursing of the lips. Severity of weakness and earlier disease onset correlate with CAG repeat length. There is no effective treatment.

Juvenile (and adult-onset) spinal muscular atrophy can occur in patients with **hexosaminidase deficiency**, an autosomal recessive disorder involving the *HEXA* gene. The clinical findings are varied and may include spasticity, dystonia, and ataxia. Rectal biopsy may be abnormal, and reduced hexosaminidase A is found in serum and leukocytes.

Patients with **monoclonal gammopathy** may present with pure motor syndromes. Plasmapheresis and immunosuppressive drug treatment (with dexamethasone and cyclophosphamide) may be beneficial in such cases.

Anterior horn cell disease may occur as a rare paraneoplastic complication of **lymphoma.** Both men and women are affected, and the symptoms typically have their onset after the diagnosis of lymphoma has been established. The principal manifestation is weakness, which primarily affects the legs, may be patchy in its distribution, and spares bulbar and respiratory muscles. The reflexes are depressed, and sensory abnormalities are minor or absent. Neurologic deficits usually progress over months, followed by spontaneous improvement and, in some cases, resolution.

INFECTIVE ANTERIOR HORN CELL DISORDERS

POLIO VIRUS INFECTION

Poliomyelitis due to infection with polio virus became rare in developed countries with the introduction of immunization programs. The usual route of infection is fecal-oral, and the incubation period varies between 5 and 35 days.

Neurologic involvement follows a prodromal phase of fever, myalgia, malaise, and upper respiratory or gastrointestinal symptoms in a small number of cases. This involvement may consist merely of aseptic meningitis but in some instances leads to weakness or paralysis due to involvement of lower motor neurons in the spinal cord and brainstem. Weakness develops over the course of one or a few days, sometimes in association with recrudescence of fever, and is accompanied by myalgia and signs of meningeal irritation. The weakness is asymmetric in distribution and can be focal or unilateral; the bulbar and respiratory muscles may be affected either alone or in association with limb muscles. Tone is reduced in the affected muscles, and tendon reflexes may be lost. There is no sensory deficit.

CSF pressure is often mildly increased, and spinal fluid analysis characteristically shows a polymorphonuclear or lymphocytic pleocytosis, slightly elevated protein concentration, and normal glucose level. Diagnosis may be confirmed by virus isolation from the stool or nasopharyngeal secretions—and less commonly from the CSF. A rise in viral antibody titer in convalescent-phase serum, compared with serum obtained during the acute phase of the illness, is also diagnostically helpful. A clinically similar disorder is produced by coxsackie virus infection.

There is no specific treatment. Management is purely supportive, with attention directed particularly to respiratory function. With time, there is often useful recovery of strength even in severely weakened muscles.

POSTPOLIO SYNDROME

The **postpolio syndrome** is characterized by the occurrence some years after the original illness of increasing weakness in previously involved or seemingly uninvolved muscles. Muscle pain and ease of fatigue are common. Slow progression occurs and may lead to increasing restriction of daily activities. The postpolio syndrome probably relates to loss of anterior horn cells with aging from a pool that was depleted by the original infection. There is no specific treatment.

WEST NILE VIRUS INFECTION

West Nile virus infection is acquired from infected mosquitos. Its most common manifestation is meningoencephalitis. Acute paralytic poliomyelitis is another manifestation and is characterized by acute, focal or generalized, asymmetric weakness or by a rapidly ascending quadriplegia that may be mistaken for the Guillain–Barré syndrome. Electrodiagnostic studies may be helpful in showing the nature and extent of involvement, distinguishing the disorder from a neuropathy, and guiding prognosis. Examination of the CSF is also helpful; there is a pleocytosis, often with a predominance of neutrophils, and viral-specific IgM antibodies are also found. Treatment is supportive, as in paralytic polio virus infection.

NERVE ROOT AND PLEXUS LESIONS

ACUTE INTERVERTEBRAL DISK PROLAPSE

LUMBAR DISK PROLAPSE

Acute prolapse of a lumbar disk (**Figure 9-9**) generally leads to back and radicular pain (L5 or S1) in the leg, often accompanied by numbness and paresthesias (**Table 9-12**). Weakness may also occur, depending on the root affected. An L5 radiculopathy causes weakness of dorsiflexion of the foot and toes, whereas S1 root involvement produces weakness of plantar flexion of the foot and a depressed ankle jerk. Movement of the spine is restricted, and there is local back tenderness and palpable spasm of the

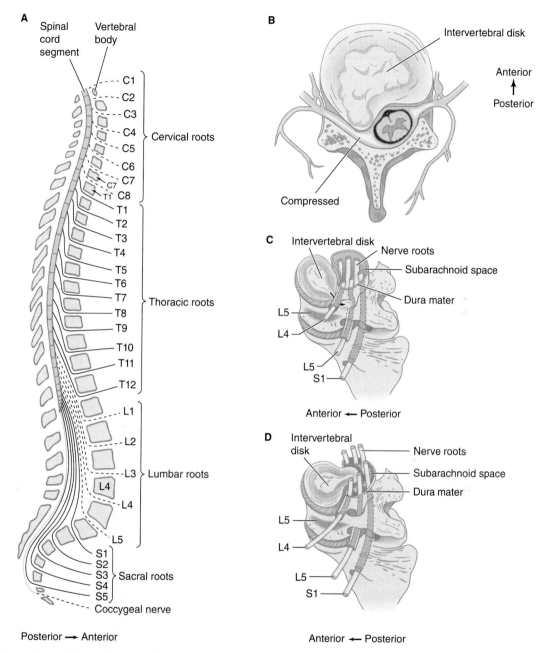

Figure 9-9. (**A**) Lateral view of the vertebral column, showing the levels at which the various nerve roots exit; nerves exit above their numbered vertebral body in the cervical spine but below in the lumbar spine. (**B**) Lateral disk prolapse in cervical spine, causing compression of exiting nerve root and compressing cervical cord. (**C**) Lateral disk prolapse in lumbar spine, causing compression of the root exiting at the next lower vertebral level (eg, L4 disk compresses the L5 nerve root). (**D**) Central disk prolapse in lumbar spine, causing bilateral root compression.

Table 9-12. The Most Common Patterns of Weakness, Sensory Symptoms, and Reflex Changes in Patients with Nerve Root Lesions.[1]

	C5	C6	C7	C8	L4	L5	S1
Weak muscle(s)	Deltoids > biceps	Biceps	Triceps, finger extensors	Finger extensors plus abductors of index and fifth fingers	Quadriceps	Great toe extensor	Plantar flexors (tested standing: "get up on toes")
Pattern of sensory changes	Lateral upper arm	Thumb	Middle finger(s)	Little finger	Medial shin	Medial foot, great toe	Lateral foot, small toe
Depressed reflex		Biceps	Triceps		Knee		Ankle

[1]Overlap and individual variation occur. In some cases, single nerve lesions may produce a similar syndrome (eg, L5 vs. common fibular [peroneal] nerve). If a peripheral nerve lesion is suspected, see Tables 9-5 and 9-6.

paraspinous muscles. Straight-leg raising in the supine position is restricted, often to approximately 20 or 30 degrees of hip flexion, from a normal value of approximately 80 or 90 degrees, because of reflex spasm of the hamstring muscles (**Lasègue sign**). A centrally prolapsed disk may cause bilateral symptoms and signs and sphincter involvement. The symptoms and signs of a prolapsed lumbar intervertebral disk may begin suddenly or insidiously and may follow trauma. Pelvic and rectal examination and imaging of the spine help to exclude causes such as tumors.

Bed rest on a firm mattress for 2 or 3 days followed by gradual mobilization often permits symptoms to settle, but persisting pain, an increasing neurologic deficit, or any evidence of sphincter dysfunction should lead to CT, MRI, or CT myelography, followed by surgical treatment. Drug treatment for pain includes aspirin or acetaminophen with 30 mg of codeine, two doses three or four times daily, or other nonsteroidal analgesics such as ibuprofen or naproxen. Muscle spasm may respond to cyclobenzaprine 10 mg orally three times daily or as needed and tolerated, or diazepam 5 to 10 mg orally three times daily or as tolerated.

CERVICAL DISK PROLAPSE

Acute protrusion of a cervical disk can occur at any age, often with no preceding trauma, and leads to neck and radicular arm pain, exacerbated by head movement. With lateral herniation of the disk, a motor, sensory, or reflex deficit may occur in a radicular (usually C6 or C7) distribution on the affected side (see Table 9-12); with more centrally directed herniations, the spinal cord may also be involved (see Figure 9-9), leading to a spastic paraparesis and sensory disturbance in the legs, sometimes accompanied by impaired sphincter function. The diagnosis is confirmed by CT scanning, MRI, or CT myelography. Surgical treatment may be needed.

CERVICAL SPONDYLOSIS

This disorder was described earlier as a cause of myelopathy.

TRAUMATIC AVULSION OF NERVE ROOTS

ERB-DUCHENNE PARALYSIS

Traumatic avulsion of the C5 and C6 roots can occur at birth from traction on the head during delivery of the shoulder. It can also result from injuries causing excessive separation of the head and shoulder. It leads to loss of shoulder abduction and elbow flexion. In consequence, the affected arm is held internally rotated at the shoulder, with a pronated forearm and extended elbow. The biceps and brachioradialis reflexes are lost, but sensory impairment is usually inconspicuous and confined to a small area overlying the deltoid muscle.

KLUMPKE PARALYSIS

Involvement of the C8 and T1 roots causes paralysis and wasting of the small muscles of the hand and of the long finger flexors and extensors. Horner syndrome is sometimes an associated finding. Such lower plexus paralysis often follows a fall that has been arrested by grasping a fixed object with one hand or may result from traction on the abducted arm.

BRACHIAL PLEXOPATHY

NEURALGIC AMYOTROPHY (IDIOPATHIC BRACHIAL PLEXOPATHY)

This disorder, also referred to as **Parsonage–Turner syndrome**, typically begins with severe pain about the shoulder followed within a few days by weakness, reflex changes, and sensory disturbances in the arm, often involving the C5 and C6 segments especially. Symptoms and signs are unilateral in approximately 70% of patients. The motor deficit sometimes corresponds to the territory of an individual nerve, especially the axillary, suprascapular, or radial nerve, but in other instances appears to arise in the brachial plexus (**Figure 9-10**). Wasting of the affected

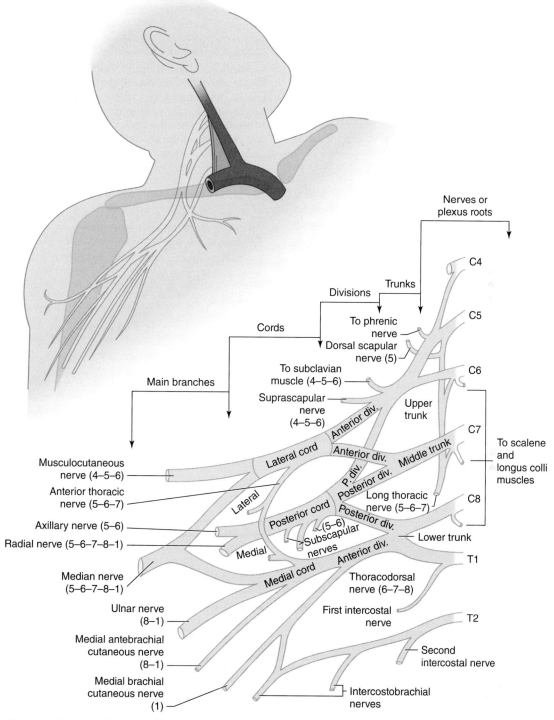

▲ **Figure 9-10.** Brachial plexus. The numbers in parentheses refer to the segmental origin of the nerves depicted.
(Used with permission from Waxman SG. *Clinical Neuroanatomy.* 26th ed. New York, NY: McGraw-Hill; 2010.)

muscles is often profound. Recurrences occur in approximately 25% of patients.

The cause is unknown, but may be autoimmune in nature. Neuralgic amyotrophy sometimes follows minor injury, injections, inoculations, or mild systemic infections, but whether these are of etiologic relevance is unclear. Hereditary neuralgic amyotrophy occurs occasionally as an autosomal dominant disorder characterized by recurrent symptoms beginning in the second or third decade of life. In some cases, it results from mutations in the gene (*SEPT9*) coding for septin 9, a cytoskeleton-interacting GTPase.

Treatment is symptomatic. The combination of a non-steroidal anti-inflammatory drug and an opiate is often effective treatment for pain in the acute phase, whereas persisting pain may respond to an anticonvulsant or tricyclic antidepressant. Recovery occurs over the ensuing weeks and months but may be incomplete.

CERVICAL RIB SYNDROME

The C8 and T1 roots or the lower trunk of the brachial plexus may be compressed by a cervical rib or band arising from the seventh cervical vertebra. This leads to weakness and wasting of intrinsic hand muscles, especially those in the thenar eminence, accompanied by pain and numbness in the appropriate dermatomal distribution (often like that of an ulnar nerve lesion but extending up the medial border of the forearm). The subclavian artery may also be compressed; this forms the basis of **Adson test** for diagnosing the disorder. The radial pulse decreases in amplitude when the seated patient turns the head to the affected side and inhales deeply. A positive Adson test, however, also can be seen in normal subjects; a supraclavicular bruit during the maneuver supports the diagnosis of subclavian artery compromise.

X-rays of the neck or chest often show the cervical rib or a long transverse process of the seventh cervical vertebra. A band may only be visualized by CT scan or MRI. Electromyography reveals chronic partial denervation in hand muscles beyond the territory of individual peripheral nerves. Nerve conduction studies show no evidence of peripheral nerve disease, but there is a small or absent ulnar sensory nerve action potential on stimulation of the little finger. Treatment is by surgical excision of the rib or band.

OTHER CAUSES OF BRACHIAL PLEXOPATHY

Brachial plexopathy may result from neoplastic infiltration (especially by breast or lung cancer) or follow radiation therapy, median sternotomy, or trauma. Electrophysiologic studies are important in defining the extent of involvement and localizing the lesion, as well as in distinguishing radiation from other causes of plexopathy. The absence of electrodiagnostic abnormalities despite an adequate examination suggests an incorrect diagnosis and raises the possibility of conversion reactions, malingering, or so-called nonneurogenic thoracic outlet syndrome (a controversial and disputed entity).

LUMBOSACRAL PLEXOPATHY

A disorder similar to idiopathic brachial plexopathy occasionally affects the lumbosacral plexus. Treatment is symptomatic. Lumbosacral plexopathy can also be caused by neoplasms (colorectal or gynecologic cancers, sarcomas, or lymphomas) or radiation. Intrapartum maternal lumbosacral plexopathy is an uncommon but important cause of acute foot drop developing during labor. It occurs mostly in short women and relates to compression of the lumbosacral trunk by the fetal head at the pelvic brim. Most patients recover completely within 6 months.

▼ DISORDERS OF PERIPHERAL NERVE

The term **peripheral neuropathy** designates a disturbance in function of one or more peripheral nerves. Several types of peripheral neuropathy are distinguishable by the extent of involvement.

Depending on the underlying cause, there may be selective involvement of motor, sensory, or autonomic fibers or more diffuse involvement of all fibers in the nerve.

The clinical deficit is usually a mixed one, and sensory symptoms and signs are often the initial—and most conspicuous—feature. Further discussion of these disorders and their treatment is therefore deferred to Chapter 10, Sensory Disorders, except where presentation is typically with acute motor deficits. For convenience, however, the root and peripheral nerve supply of the major limb muscles is set forth in Tables 9-5 and 9-6 to facilitate evaluation of patients presenting with focal weakness of lower motor neuron type.

POLYNEUROPATHY

In polyneuropathy, because there is symmetric and simultaneous involvement of several nerves, the deficits resulting from individual nerves cannot be recognized clinically. Polyneuropathies are discussed in Chapter 10, Sensory Disorders, but brief mention is made here of those neuropathies in which patients present with acute weakness.

ACUTE INFLAMMATORY POLYRADICULONEUROPATHY (GUILLAIN–BARRÉ SYNDROME)

This disorder commonly presents with weakness that is often symmetric and most often begins in the legs. The speed and extent of progression vary, but in severe cases there is marked weakness of all limbs and bilateral facial weakness. There may also be subjective sensory complaints, although objective sensory disturbances are usually far less conspicuous than motor deficits. Autonomic involvement is common and may lead to a fatal outcome, as may aspiration pneumonia or impaired respiration from weakness. Further details about this disorder are given in the following chapter.

CRITICAL ILLNESS POLYNEUROPATHY

A polyneuropathy may develop in patients with sepsis and multiorgan failure and often is first manifest by unexpected difficulty in weaning them from a mechanical ventilator. In more advanced cases, wasting and weakness of the extremities occur and the tendon reflexes are lost. Sensory abnormalities are overshadowed by the motor deficit.

Electrophysiologic studies reveal an axonal neuropathy, unlike classic Guillain–Barré syndrome. The underlying pathogenesis is obscure. The polyneuropathy is associated with the use of neuromuscular blocking agents or corticosteroids. Treatment is supportive. The long-term outlook is good in patients who recover from the underlying critical illness.

DIPHTHERITIC POLYNEURITIS

Infection with *Corynebacterium diphtheriae* can occur either in the upper respiratory tract or by infection of a skin wound, and neuropathy results from a neurotoxin that is released by the organism. **Diphtheria toxin** kills cells by inactivating eukaryotic elongation factor-2 and thereby blocking protein synthesis.

Palatal weakness may develop 2 to 3 weeks after infection of the throat, and cutaneous diphtheria may be followed by focal weakness of neighboring muscles after a similar interval. Impaired pupillary responses to accommodation may occur approximately 4 to 5 weeks after infection and a generalized sensorimotor polyneuropathy after 1 to 3 months. The polyneuropathy may follow a biphasic course, with further deterioration occurring 5 to 6 weeks after onset. The weakness may be asymmetric and is often more marked proximally than distally. The tendon reflexes may be depressed or absent. Respiratory paralysis occurs in severe cases. Recovery usually occurs over 2 to 3 months but takes longer in severe cases.

In patients with diphtheritic polyneuritis, the CSF protein content is increased and a mild pleocytosis is sometimes found. Electrophysiologic studies show a slowing of nerve conduction velocity, but this may not be manifest until the patient has begun to improve clinically. Treatment consists of early administration of equine diphtheria antitoxin without awaiting the results of bacterial culture, provided the patient is not hypersensitive to horse serum. A 2-week course of penicillin or erythromycin usually eradicates the infection but does not alter the incidence of serious complications. In patients with marked weakness, supportive measures, including ventilatory assistance, are necessary.

PARALYTIC SHELLFISH POISONING

Bivalve molluscan shellfish, especially mussels and clams found on the East and West Coasts of the United States, may be dangerous to eat, especially in the summer months. They feed on poisonous varieties of plankton and come to contain **saxitoxin** and other toxins, which block sodium channels—and therefore action potentials—in motor and sensory nerves and in muscle. The toxins are not destroyed by heating or freezing.

Headaches, tingling of the lips and tongue, and a rapidly progressive acute peripheral neuropathy, with sensory symptoms and a rapidly ascending paralysis, begin within 30 minutes after eating affected shellfish and may lead to respiratory paralysis and death. There is no available antitoxin, but with proper supportive care (including mechanical ventilation if necessary) the patient recovers completely. A cathartic or enema may help remove unabsorbed toxin.

PORPHYRIA

Acute polyneuropathy may occur with the hereditary hepatic porphyrias. Attacks can be precipitated by drugs (eg, barbiturates, estrogens, sulfonamides, griseofulvin, phenytoin, and succinimides) that can induce the enzyme δ-aminolevulinic acid synthetase, or by infection, a period of fasting, or, occasionally, menses or pregnancy. They usually last for 1 to 2 weeks but can be life-threatening.

Colicky abdominal pain—sometimes also felt in the back or thighs—frequently precedes neurologic involvement, and there may also be anxiety, agitation, acute confusion or delirium, and convulsions. Weakness, the major neurologic manifestation, results from a predominantly motor polyneuropathy that causes a symmetric disturbance that is sometimes more marked proximally than distally. It may begin in the upper limbs and progress to involve the lower limbs or trunk. Progression is variable in rate and extent and can lead to complete flaccid quadriparesis with respiratory paralysis over a few days. Sensory loss is less conspicuous and extensive; muscle pain is sometimes prominent. The tendon reflexes may be depressed or absent. Fever, excessive sweating, persistent tachycardia, hypertension, hyponatremia (attributed to inappropriate secretion of antidiuretic hormone), and peripheral leukocytosis may accompany acute attacks, and patients may become dehydrated.

The CSF may show a slight increase in protein concentration and a slight pleocytosis. The diagnosis is confirmed by demonstrating increased levels of porphobilinogen and δ-aminolevulinic acid in the urine or deficiency of porphobilinogen deaminase in red blood cells (**acute intermittent porphyria**) or of coproporphyrinogen oxidase in lymphocytes (**hereditary coproporphyria**).

Treatment with hemin (4 mg/kg by intravenous infusion over 15 minutes once daily for 3 to 14 days depending on response) is effective in improving the clinical state. Alternatively, or as a temporary measure, intravenous dextrose is given to suppress the heme biosynthetic pathway. Propranolol helps to control tachycardia and hypertension. The best index of progress is the heart rate. The abdominal and mental symptoms (but not the neuropathy) may be helped by chlorpromazine or another phenothiazine; benzodiazepines may relieve anxiety. Pain relief may require opiates. Patients with impaired respiratory function, depressed level of consciousness, or convulsions should be followed in an intensive care unit. Respiratory failure may necessitate tracheostomy and mechanical ventilation. Recovery from paralysis is gradual and may not be complete.

Any precipitant should be removed: Precipitating medications should be discontinued, infections should be treated, and inadequate diets corrected. Preventing future acute attacks by avoiding known precipitants is important. Cigarette smoking and consumption of alcohol should be stopped. Identification of the responsible genetic mutation in an affected patient allows for genetic screening of other family members to prevent acute attacks in those with occult disease. Different genes have been implicated in different porphyrias: many different mutations of the porphobilinogen deaminase (*PBGD*) gene lead to acute intermittent porphyria.

ACUTE ARSENIC OR THALLIUM POISONING

Acute arsenic or thallium poisoning can produce a rapidly evolving sensorimotor polyneuropathy, often with an accompanying or preceding gastrointestinal disturbance and crampy abdominal pain. Arsenic may also cause a skin rash, with increased skin pigmentation and marked exfoliation, together with the presence of Mees lines (transverse white lines) on the nails in long-standing cases. Thallium can produce a scaly rash and hair loss. Sensory symptoms, often painful, are usually an early manifestation of polyneuropathy; this is followed by symmetric motor impairment, which is usually more marked distally than proximally and occurs in the legs rather than the arms.

The CSF protein may be increased, with little or no change in cell content, and the electrophysiologic findings sometimes resemble those of Guillain–Barré syndrome, especially in the acute phase of the disorder. The diagnosis of arsenic toxicity is best established by measuring the arsenic content of hair protected from external contamination (eg, pubic hair). Urine also contains arsenic in the acute phase. The diagnosis of thallium poisoning is made by finding thallium in body tissues or fluids, especially in urine. The degree of neurologic recovery depends on the severity of intoxication. Chelating agents are of uncertain value.

ORGANOPHOSPHATE POLYNEUROPATHY

Organophosphate compounds are widely used as insecticides and are also the active principles in the nerve gas of chemical warfare. They have a variety of **acute toxic effects**, particularly manifestations of cholinergic crisis caused by inhibition of acetylcholinesterase. In the 1 to 4 days after acute exposure, some patients develop an **intermediate syndrome** characterized by weakness of respiratory, neck, and proximal limb muscles. Its pathogenesis is unclear, and treatment is supportive. Some organophosphates also induce a **delayed polyneuropathy** that generally begins approximately 1 to 3 weeks after acute exposure.

Cramping muscle pain in the legs is usually the initial symptom of neuropathy, sometimes followed by distal numbness and paresthesias. Progressive leg weakness then occurs, along with depression of the tendon reflexes. Similar deficits may develop in the upper limbs after several days. Sensory disturbances occur in some instances, initially in the legs and then the arms, but are often mild or inconspicuous.

Examination shows a distal, symmetric, predominantly motor polyneuropathy, with wasting and flaccid weakness of distal leg muscles. In some patients, involvement may be severe enough to cause quadriplegia, whereas in others the weakness is much milder. Mild pyramidal signs also may be present. Objective evidence of sensory loss is usually slight.

The acute effects of organophosphate poisoning may be prevented by the use of protective masks and clothing. Treatment after exposure includes decontamination of the skin with bleach or soap and water and intravenous administration of atropine to block muscarinic cholinergic receptors (2 to 6 mg every 5 minutes for adults, until bronchoconstriction is relieved and secretions can be cleared). Once the effects of atropine become apparent, pralidoxime is administered (1 g every hour for up to 3 hours in adults) intramuscularly or slowly (over 30 minutes) intravenously to reactivate acetylcholinesterase. There is no treatment for the neuropathy other than supportive care. Recovery of peripheral nerve function may occur with time, but central deficits are usually permanent and may govern the extent of functional recovery.

MONONEUROPATHY MULTIPLEX

This term signifies that there is involvement of several nerves but in an asymmetric manner and at different times, so that the individual nerves involved can usually be identified until the disorder reaches an advanced stage. Comment here is restricted to two disorders characterized by motor involvement in the absence of sensory symptoms and signs.

LEAD TOXICITY

Lead toxicity is common among persons in certain occupations and may also occur in those using lead-containing paints or who ingest contaminated alcohol. Inorganic lead can produce dysfunction of both the central and peripheral nervous systems. In children, who can develop toxicity by ingesting lead-containing paints that flake off old buildings or furniture, acute encephalopathy is the major neurologic feature.

The peripheral neuropathy is predominantly motor, and in adults it is more severe in the arms than legs. It typically affects the radial nerves, although other nerves may also be affected, leading to an asymmetric progressive motor disturbance. Sensory loss is usually inconspicuous or absent. There may be loss or depression of tendon reflexes. Systemic manifestations of lead toxicity include anemia, constipation, colicky abdominal pain, gum discoloration, and nephropathy. The extent to which exposed workers develop minor degrees of peripheral nerve damage as a result of lead toxicity is not clear. Similarly, there is no agreement about the lowest concentration of blood lead that is associated with damage to the peripheral nerves.

The optimal approach to treatment is not known, but intravenous or intramuscular edetate calcium disodium (EDTA) and oral penicillamine have been used, as has dimercaprol (BAL).

MULTIFOCAL MOTOR NEUROPATHY

This disorder is characterized by progressive asymmetric wasting and weakness, by electrophysiologic evidence of multifocal motor demyelination with partial motor conduction block but normal sensory responses, and by the presence of antiglycolipid (usually anti-GM1 IgM) antibodies in the serum of many patients. Arm and hand weakness is typical. Cramps and fasciculations sometimes occur. There is no sensory loss or upper motor neuron involvement. The disorder typically has an insidious onset and chronic course, but variants occur with a more acute onset. For the diagnosis to be established, electrophysiologic studies should demonstrate a motor deficit in the distribution of two or more named nerves and related to conduction block outside of common entrapment sites. A variant with involvement of only a single nerve has been described (monofocal motor neuropathy). The conduction block results from demyelination, but axonal excitability changes also contribute to conduction failure. Treatment with prednisone and plasmapheresis has been disappointing, but patients may improve after treatment with human immunoglobulin 2 g/kg intravenously given over 3 to 5 days every 4 to 6 weeks. If this fails, cyclophosphamide 1 g/m² intravenously once per month for 6 months is sometimes worthwhile. Improvement is sometimes associated with a decrease in anti-GM1 antibody levels.

MONONEUROPATHY SIMPLEX

In mononeuropathy simplex only a single peripheral nerve is involved. Most of the common mononeuropathies entail both motor and sensory involvement (as discussed in Chapter 10, Sensory Disorders). Accordingly, only Bell palsy, which leads primarily to a motor deficit, is discussed here.

BELL PALSY

Facial weakness of lower motor neuron type caused by idiopathic facial (VII) nerve involvement outside the central nervous system, without evidence of more widespread neurologic disease, has been designated Bell palsy. Its cause is unclear, but it occurs more commonly in pregnant women and diabetics. Reactivation of herpes simplex virus type 1 or varicella-zoster virus infection in the geniculate ganglion may injure the facial nerve and cause Bell palsy in at least some patients.

Facial weakness is often preceded or accompanied by pain about the ear. Weakness generally comes on abruptly but may progress over several hours or even a day or so. Depending on the site of the lesion, there may be impairment of taste, lacrimation, or hyperacusis. There may be paralysis of all muscles supplied by the affected nerve (**complete palsy**) or variable weakness in different muscles (**incomplete palsy**). Clinical examination reveals no abnormalities beyond the territory of the facial nerve.

Most patients recover completely without treatment, over several days or months. A poor prognosis for complete recovery is suggested by severe pain at onset and complete palsy when the patient is first seen. Nevertheless, permanent disfigurement or some other complication affects only about 10% of patients.

Treatment with acyclovir or other antiviral agents confers no benefit. Treatment with corticosteroids (prednisone 60 or 80 mg/d orally for 3 days, tapering over the next 7 days), beginning within 5 days after the onset of palsy, increases the proportion of patients who recover completely over time. Surgical procedures to decompress the facial nerve are generally of no benefit. If eye closure is not possible, the eye should be protected with lubricating drops and a patch.

Other conditions that can produce facial palsy include tumors, herpes zoster infection of the geniculate ganglion (Ramsay Hunt syndrome), Lyme disease, AIDS, sarcoidosis, or any inflammatory process involving the subarachnoid space, such as infective or neoplastic meningitis. Facial palsies that are bilateral or are associated with another cranial neuropathy merit lumbar puncture and brain MRI to search for an underlying cause.

DISORDERS OF NEUROMUSCULAR TRANSMISSION

MYASTHENIA GRAVIS

PATHOGENESIS

Myasthenia gravis is caused by variable block of neuromuscular transmission related to an immune-mediated decrease in the number of functioning nicotinic acetylcholine receptors (**Figure 9-11**). In approximately 80% of

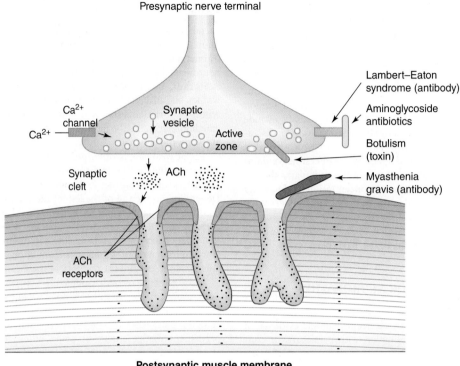

Presynaptic nerve terminal

Lambert–Eaton syndrome (antibody)

Aminoglycoside antibiotics

Botulism (toxin)

Myasthenia gravis (antibody)

Ca²⁺ channel

Ca^{2+}

Synaptic vesicle

Active zone

Synaptic cleft

ACh

ACh receptors

Postsynaptic muscle membrane

▲ **Figure 9-11.** Sites of involvement in disorders of neuromuscular transmission. At left, normal transmission involves depolarization-induced influx of calcium (Ca) through voltage-gated channels. This stimulates release of acetylcholine (ACh) from synaptic vesicles at the active zone and into the synaptic cleft. ACh binds to ACh receptors and depolarizes the postsynaptic muscle membrane. At right, disorders of neuromuscular transmission result from blockage of Ca channels (Lambert–Eaton syndrome or aminoglycoside antibiotics), impairment of Ca-mediated ACh release (botulinum toxin), or antibody-induced internalization and degradation of ACh receptors (myasthenia gravis).

cases, **antibodies to the skeletal muscle nicotinic acetylcholine receptor** are present and lead to loss of receptor function. Some patients seronegative for these antibodies have antibodies against the **muscle-specific receptor tyrosine kinase** (MuSK), which is involved in the clustering of acetylcholine receptors during development and is also expressed in mature neuromuscular junctions. A similar disorder can occur in patients receiving penicillamine for rheumatoid arthritis; it frequently remits when the drug is discontinued.

CLINICAL FINDINGS

Myasthenia gravis can occur at any age and is sometimes associated with thymic tumor, thyrotoxicosis, rheumatoid arthritis, or disseminated lupus erythematosus. More common in females than males, it is characterized by **fluctuating weakness** and **easy fatigability** of voluntary muscles; muscle activity cannot be maintained, and initially powerful movements weaken readily. There is a predilection for the external ocular muscles and certain other cranial

muscles, including the masticatory, facial, pharyngeal, and laryngeal muscles. Respiratory and limb muscles may also be affected.

▶ History

Onset is usually insidious, but the disorder is sometimes unmasked by a concurrent infection, which exacerbates symptoms. Exacerbations may also occur in pregnancy or before the menstrual periods. Symptoms may be worsened by quinine, quinidine, procainamide, propranolol, phenytoin, lithium, tetracycline, calcium channel blockers, penicillamine, and aminoglycoside antibiotics, which should be avoided or used with caution.

Myasthenia follows a slowly progressive course. Patients present with ptosis, diplopia, difficulty in chewing or swallowing, nasal speech, respiratory difficulties, or weakness of the limbs (**Table 9-13**). Symptoms often fluctuate in intensity during the day, and this diurnal variation is superimposed on longer-term spontaneous relapses and remissions that may last for weeks.

Table 9-13. Presenting Symptoms in Myasthenia Gravis.

Symptom	Percentage of Patients
Diplopia	41
Ptosis	25
Dysarthria	16
Lower-extremity weakness	13
Generalized weakness	11
Dysphagia	10
Upper-extremity weakness	7
Masticatory weakness	7

Data from Herrmann C Jr. Myasthenia gravis—current concepts. *West J Med.* 1985;142:797-809.

▶ Examination

Clinical examination confirms the weakness and fatigability of affected muscles. The weakness does not conform to the distribution of any single nerve, root, or level of the central nervous system. In more than 90% of cases the **extraocular muscles** are involved, leading to often asymmetric ocular palsies and ptosis, and in 15% of all cases the symptoms and signs are restricted to these muscles. Pupillary responses are not affected. Sustained activity of affected muscles leads to temporarily increased weakness. Thus, sustained upgaze for 2 minutes can lead to increased ptosis, with power in the affected muscles improving after a brief rest. In advanced cases, affected muscles may show mild atrophy. Sensation is normal, and there are usually no reflex changes.

DIAGNOSIS

The diagnosis can generally be confirmed by antibody and electrophysiologic studies (see later) and by the benefit that follows administration of anticholinesterase drugs; the power of affected muscles is influenced at a dose that has no effect on normal muscles and slight, if any, effect on muscles weakened by other causes.

The most commonly used pharmacologic test for patients with obvious ptosis or ophthalmoparesis is the edrophonium (**Tensilon**) **test.** Edrophonium is given intravenously in a dose of 10 mg (1 mL), of which 2 mg is given initially as a test dose and the remaining 8 mg approximately 30 seconds later if the test dose is well tolerated. In myasthenic patients, there is an obvious improvement in the strength of weak muscles that lasts for approximately 5 minutes. Alternatively, 1.5 mg of neostigmine can be given intramuscularly, with a response that lasts for about 2 hours. Atropine sulfate (0.6 mg intravenously) should be available to counteract the muscarinic cholinergic side effects of increased salivation, diarrhea, and nausea. Atropine does not affect nicotinic cholinergic function at the neuromuscular junction.

INVESTIGATIVE STUDIES

MRI and CT scans of the chest, with and without contrast, may reveal a thymoma; normal studies do not exclude this possibility. Blood studies should include thyroid function tests. Impaired neuromuscular transmission can be detected electrophysiologically by a **decremental response** of muscle to repetitive supramaximal stimulation (at 2 or 3 Hz) of its motor nerve, but normal findings do not exclude the diagnosis. Single-fiber electromyography shows increased variability in the interval between two muscle fiber action potentials from the same motor unit in clinically weak muscles. Measuring serum acetylcholine receptor and anti-MuSK antibody levels is very helpful, because increased values are found in 80% to 90% of patients with generalized myasthenia gravis. MuSK antibodies are present in 5% to 10% cases and are associated with more severe disease. Patients with titin or ryanodine antibodies as well as acetylcholine receptor antibodies generally have a thymoma and severe, late-onset myasthenia. Lipoprotein receptor-related protein (LRP4) antibodies are present in about 3% of myasthenic patients, usually those with mild disease. Neither MuSK nor LRP4 antibodies are associated with thymic disease. Other antibodies have also been detected in some patients with myasthenia.

TREATMENT

Medications (referred to earlier) that impair neuromuscular transmission should be avoided. The following approaches to treatment are recommended.

▶ Anticholinesterase Drugs

Treatment with these drugs provides symptomatic benefit without influencing the course of the underlying disease. The mainstay of treatment is pyridostigmine, at doses individually determined but usually between 30 and 120 mg (average, 60 mg) about every 4 hours. A long-acting preparation (Mestinon TS, 180 mg) can be used at bedtime in patients with persistent, severe weakness upon awakening. Glycopyrrolate (1 mg), propantheline (15 mg), or hyoscyamine sulfate (0.125 mg) taken three times daily may ameliorate side effects such as bowel hypermotility or hypersalivation. Overmedication can lead to increased weakness, which, unlike myasthenic weakness, is unaffected or enhanced by intravenous edrophonium. Such a **cholinergic crisis** may be accompanied by pallor, sweating, nausea, vomiting, salivation, colicky abdominal pain, and miosis.

▶ Thymectomy

Thymectomy should be performed in all patients with thymoma. It should also be performed in patients without a thymoma who are younger than 60 to 65 years of age, and considered in those older, with weakness that is not restricted to the extraocular muscles. Thymectomy leads to symptomatic benefit or remission by an uncertain mechanism in many patients, but its beneficial effect may not be evident immediately.

Thymectomy is not recommended for those with MuSK or LRP4 antibodies; its benefit is unclear in those with purely ocular myasthenia. It is often withheld in those with generalized disease who are antibody negative, but it may be considered when there is a poor response to immunosuppressive drugs.

Corticosteroids

Corticosteroids are indicated for patients who have responded poorly to anticholinesterase drugs and have already undergone thymectomy, but may initially exacerbate weakness. For this reason, high-dose prednisone or prednisolone is often started while patients are hospitalized for plasmapheresis or intravenous immune globulin (IVIG) therapy. Alternatively, steroids are started in the outpatient setting at a low dose that is increased gradually (up to 60 to 80 mg on alternate days) to avoid an initial deterioration. An initial high dose of prednisone can be tapered gradually to a relatively low-maintenance level (5-15 mg/d) as improvement occurs. Alternate-day treatment is helpful in reducing the incidence of side effects, which are described (as clinical findings) in the section on hyperadrenalism (Cushing syndrome) in Chapter 4, Confusional States.

Azathioprine

This drug can be used in patients with severe or progressive disease despite thymectomy and treatment with anticholinesterases. It is often given in combination with corticosteroids, which can then be given in reduced dose or withdrawn. When steroids are contraindicated or refused, azathioprine can be given alone. If possible, patients should first be screened for mutations in the thiopurine methyltransferase (*TPMT*) gene that cause TPMT deficiency, or the level of enzyme activity should be measured. Patients homozygous for a mutant allele (3 per 1000 subjects) have absent enzyme levels and should not receive azathioprine—they cannot metabolize it and consequently may develop severe toxicity. Patients heterozygous for the mutant allele generally have low enzyme activity, but can tolerate azathioprine in low doses. The usual dose of azathioprine is 2 to 3 mg/kg/d, increased from a lower initial dose. Benefit may take a year to manifest.

Plasmapheresis

Plasmapheresis may be used to achieve temporary improvement in patients deteriorating rapidly or in myasthenic crisis and in certain special circumstances, such as before surgery that is likely to produce postoperative respiratory compromise. Clinical improvement begins within a few days and relates to removal of acetylcholine receptor antibodies from the circulation.

Intravenous Immunoglobulins

Intravenous immunoglobulins also have been used to provide temporary benefit, usually after 7 to 10 days, in circumstances similar to those in which plasmapheresis is used.

Mycophenolate Mofetil

This agent selectively inhibits proliferation of T and B lymphocytes and has been used as an immunosuppressant with only modest side effects, including diarrhea, nausea, abdominal pain, fever, leukopenia, and edema. Several studies indicate that many patients with mild to moderate myasthenia gravis improve or are able to lower their corticosteroid intake in response to this medication (unlabeled use; 1 g twice daily by mouth), but usually after a delay of 6 to 12 months.

Other Immunomodulating Agents

Methotrexate, cyclosporine, tacrolimus, and rituximab are other second-line immunomodulating agents that have been used in refractory myasthenia gravis, based on anecdotal reports of benefit.

PROGNOSIS

Most patients can be managed successfully with drug treatment. The disease may have a fatal outcome because of respiratory complications, such as aspiration pneumonia, related to weakness of the intercostal muscles or diaphragm.

MYASTHENIC AND CHOLINERGIC CRISIS

Patients with increasing weakness of the respiratory muscles that necessitates intubation or assisted ventilation are said to be in myasthenic crisis. They require admission to the intensive care unit and treatment with intravenous immunoglobulins or by plasma exchange; these modalities are equally effective, and selection depends on the available facilities, physician preference, and clinical context. Long-term immunomodulating therapy is also commenced if not already initiated. Myasthenic crisis may be precipitated by infection or other factors such as exposure to certain medications (eg, aminoglycoside agents, beta blockers, or neuromuscular blockers), or may occur without apparent cause. Any precipitating causes should be identified and treated vigorously.

Myasthenic crisis must be distinguished from cholinergic crisis, in which weakness is exacerbated by excessive anticholinesterase medication; in this latter circumstance, ventilatory support via endotracheal intubation is required until the crisis resolves on its own. The edrophonium (Tensilon) test demonstrates worsening of the weakness caused by cholinergic crisis, but improvement of that due to myasthenia gravis.

MYASTHENIC SYNDROME (LAMBERT–EATON SYNDROME)

This is characterized by variable weakness due to defective release of acetylcholine at the neuromuscular junctions.

PATHOGENESIS

The disorder is often associated with an underlying neoplasm and sometimes with such autoimmune diseases as pernicious anemia; occasionally no cause is found. In the paraneoplastic disorder, antibodies directed against tumor antigens cross-react with voltage-gated calcium channels involved in acetylcholine release, leading to a **presynaptic** disturbance of neuromuscular transmission (see Figure 9-11).

CLINICAL FINDINGS

Weakness occurs, especially of the proximal muscles of the limbs. Unlike myasthenia gravis, the extraocular muscles are spared, and power steadily increases if a contraction is maintained. Autonomic disturbances, such as dry mouth, constipation, and impotence, may occur.

DIAGNOSIS

The diagnosis is confirmed electrophysiologically by the **incremental response** to repetitive nerve stimulation. The size of the muscle response increases remarkably to stimulation of its motor nerve at high rates—even in muscles not clinically weak. The presence of **autoantibodies to the P/Q subtype of voltage-gated calcium channels**, found on the presynaptic membrane of the neuromuscular junction, is highly sensitive and specific to the Lambert–Eaton syndrome of any etiology.

TREATMENT

An underlying neoplasm must be sought, and screening repeated after 3 to 6 months if initially negative. Treatment of the underlying condition, often a small-cell lung cancer, improves myasthenic syndrome.

Plasmapheresis or intravenous immunoglobulin therapy may lead to short-term symptomatic benefit, but treatment must be repeated to sustain it. Immunosuppressive drug therapy (corticosteroids, mycophenolate, and azathioprine as described for myasthenia gravis) may lead to improved muscle strength. Benefit has been shown in small series of cases rather than documented in randomized controlled trials.

Guanidine hydrochloride (25 mg/kg/d in three or four divided doses to a maximum of 1,000 mg/d) is sometimes helpful by enhancing the release of acetylcholine in seriously disabled patients, but adverse effects include bone marrow suppression and renal failure.

The response to treatment with an anticholinesterase drug such as pyridostigmine, alone or in combination with guanidine, is variable but usually disappointing.

3,4-Diaminopyridine, a potassium channel antagonist that enhances the release of acetylcholine at the neuromuscular junction, used in doses up to 25 mg orally four times daily, may improve weakness and autonomic dysfunction, but its use for this purpose is not approved in the United States. Paresthesias are a common side effect, and seizures may occur.

BOTULISM

PATHOGENESIS

The toxin of *Clostridium botulinum* can cause neuromuscular paralysis by preventing the release of acetylcholine at neuromuscular junctions and autonomic synapses (see Figure 9-11). Botulism occurs most commonly after ingestion of home-canned food contaminated with the toxin; it occurs rarely from infected wounds. The shorter the latent period between ingestion of toxin and onset of symptoms, the greater the dose of toxin and the risk for further involvement of the nervous system.

CLINICAL FINDINGS

Fulminating weakness begins 12 to 72 hours after ingestion of the toxin and characteristically is manifested by diplopia, ptosis, facial weakness, dysphagia, nasal speech, and then difficulty with respiration; weakness usually occurs last in the limbs. In addition to weakness, blurring of vision is characteristic, the pupils being dilated and unreactive, and there may be dryness of the mouth, paralytic ileus, and postural hypotension. There is no sensory deficit, and the tendon reflexes are usually unchanged unless the involved muscles are quite weak. Symptoms can progress for several days after their onset.

In infants, enteric infection with local production of the toxin leads to a different clinical picture with hypotonia, constipation, progressive weakness, and a poor suck. This is now the most common form of botulism in the United States.

INVESTIGATIVE STUDIES

When the diagnosis is suspected, the local health authority should be notified and samples of the patient's serum and the contaminated food (if available) sent to be assayed for toxin. The most common types of toxin encountered clinically are A, B, and E. Electrophysiologic studies may help confirm the diagnosis, as the evoked muscle response tends to increase in size progressively with repetitive stimulation of motor nerves at fast rates.

TREATMENT

Patients should be hospitalized, because respiratory insufficiency can develop rapidly and necessitates ventilatory assistance. Treatment with **trivalent antitoxin (ABE)** is commenced once it is established that the patient is not allergic to horse serum, but the effect on the course of the disease is unclear.

In wound botulism, antibiotic therapy is often prescribed but is of unclear benefit; either penicillin G (3 million units IV every 4 hours in adults) or metronidazole (500 mg IV every 8 hours in patients allergic to penicillin) is typically administered, but the regimen may need to be altered depending on the results of wound culture.

Guanidine hydrochloride (25-30 mg/kg/d in divided doses), a drug that facilitates release of acetylcholine from nerve endings, is sometimes helpful in improving muscle strength; anticholinesterase drugs are generally of no value.

In infants, **human-derived botulinum immune globulin** should be given intravenously as soon as possible. Nursing and supportive care are important.

AMINOGLYCOSIDE ANTIBIOTICS

Large doses of antibiotics such as kanamycin and gentamicin can produce a clinical syndrome rather like botulism, because the release of acetylcholine from nerve endings is prevented. This effect may be related to calcium channel blockade (see Figure 9-11). Symptoms resolve rapidly as the responsible drug is eliminated from the body. Note that these antibiotics are particularly dangerous and best avoided in patients with preexisting disturbances of neuromuscular transmission such as myasthenia gravis.

▼ MYOPATHIC DISORDERS

MUSCULAR DYSTROPHIES

The muscular dystrophies are a group of inherited myopathic disorders characterized by progressive muscle weakness and wasting. They are subdivided clinically by their mode of inheritance, age at onset, distribution of involved muscles, rate of progression, and long-term outlook (**Table 9-14**). Various genes have been associated with the different muscular dystrophies. These skeletal muscle genes encode sarcolemmal (eg, sarcoglycans), cytoskeletal (eg, dystrophin), cytosolic, extracellular matrix, and nuclear membrane proteins. Abnormalities of these proteins may lead to a greater susceptibility to necrosis of muscle fibers, but the molecular mechanisms

involved are not yet clear. Genetic heterogeneity for the same phenotype has led to subdivision of the main clinical disorders, but the basis for the different clinical phenotypes is unknown.

There is no specific treatment for the muscular dystrophies. Patients should lead as normal a life as possible. Deformities and contractures often can be prevented or ameliorated by physical therapy and orthopedic procedures. Prolonged bed rest must be avoided, as inactivity often leads to worsening of disability.

DUCHENNE DYSTROPHY

The most common form of muscular dystrophy, Duchenne dystrophy is an X-linked disorder that predominantly affects males. The responsible genetic defect has been identified and forms the basis of a diagnostic test. The gene, located on the short arm of the X chromosome, codes for the protein **dystrophin,** which is absent or profoundly reduced in muscle from patients with the disorder. The absence of dystrophin from synaptic regions of cerebral cortical neurons may contribute to the cognitive impairment associated with the disorder.

Symptoms begin by age 5 years, and patients are typically severely disabled by adolescence, with death occurring in the third or fourth decade. Toe walking, waddling gait, and an inability to run are early symptoms. Weakness is most pronounced in the proximal lower extremities but also affects the proximal upper extremities. In attempting to rise from a supine to standing position, patients characteristically must use their arms to climb up their bodies (**Gowers sign**). **Pseudohypertrophy** of the calves caused by fatty infiltration of muscle is common. The heart is involved late in the course, and cognitive impairment is a frequent accompaniment. Death is usually from respiratory insufficiency or cardiac arrhythmias. Serum CK levels are exceptionally high.

Management should involve monitoring of cardiac and respiratory function; and of weight, nutritional status, and bone status for patients on long-term corticosteroids (serum calcium, phosphate, alkaline phosphatase, and vitamin D levels, and measurement of bone mineral density). Orthopedic procedures may be needed.

No definitive treatment is available, but prednisone 0.75 mg/kg/d orally may improve muscle strength for up to 3 years. Side effects include weight gain, cushingoid appearance, and hirsutism; the long-term effects of prednisone in this disorder are uncertain. Deflazacort (0.9 mg/kg/d), an analogue of prednisone, is probably as effective as prednisone but with fewer side effects.

Treatment with eteplirsen increases muscle dystrophin in the 10% to 15% of patients with Duchenne dystrophy who have a mutation of the dystrophin gene amenable to exon 51 skipping. In the United States, the Food and Drug Administration has approved the drug for treatment of

Table 9-14. The Muscular Dystrophies.

Disorder	Inheritance	Onset Age (Years)	Distribution	Prognosis	Serum CK	Notes
Duchenne dystrophy	X-linked recessive	1–5	Pelvic, then shoulder girdle; later, limb and respiratory muscles	Rapid progression; die within about 15 years after onset	Marked increase	Pseudohypertrophy of muscles may occur at some stage; cardiac involvement, skeletal deformities, and muscle contractures occur; cognitive impairment is common
Becker dystrophy	X-linked recessive	5–25	Pelvic, then shoulder girdle	Slow progression; may have normal life span	Increase	Usually no cardiac involvement, skeletal deformities, or contractures
Limb-girdle (Erb) dystrophy	Autosomal recessive or dominant, or sporadic	10–30	Pelvic or shoulder girdle initially, with later spread to other muscles	Variable severity and rate of progression; may cause severe disability in middle life	Mild increase	Variable clinical expression; hypertrophy of calves may occur; normal intellectual function; cardiac involvement is rare; many subtypes have been described
Facioscapulohumeral dystrophy	Autosomal dominant	Any age	Face and shoulder girdle initially; later, pelvic girdle and legs	Slow progression; minor disability; usually normal life span	Often normal	Aborted or mild cases are common; muscle hypertrophy, contractures, and deformities are rare
Emery–Dreifuss dystrophy	X-linked recessive or autosomal dominant or recessive	5–10	Humeroperoneal or scapuloperoneal	Variable	Increase	Variable expression; contractures, skeletal deformities, cardiomyopathy, cardiac conduction defects are common; no pseudohypertrophy
Distal myopathy	Autosomal dominant or recessive	40–60	Onset distally in extremities; proximal involvement later	Slow progression	Often normal	
Ocular dystrophy	Autosomal dominant (may be recessive or sporadic)	Any age (usually 5–30)	Extraocular muscles. Mild weakness of face, neck, and arms may occur	Not known	Often normal	
Oculopharyngeal dystrophy	Autosomal dominant	Any age	As in the ocular form, but with dysphagia	Not known	Often normal	
Paraspinal dystrophy	Unknown	≥40	Paraspinal muscles	Variable progression	Mild increase	Leads to back pain and marked kyphosis
Congenital myopathy	Autosomal recessive or dominant	Infancy or childhood	Proximal limb muscles; extraocular muscles in some forms	Slow progression	Normal	Includes nemaline, central core, myotubular, centronuclear, and mitochondrial myopathies; may be diagnosed by muscle biopsy
Myotonic dystrophy	Autosomal dominant	Any age (usually 20–40)	Facial and sternomastoid muscles and distal muscles in the extremities	Variable severity and progression	Normal or mild increase	Associated features include myotonia, cataracts, gonadal atrophy, endocrinopathies, cardiac abnormalities, intellectual changes; asymptomatic carriers of the gene may sometimes be detected by clinical examination, slit lamp examination for lenticular abnormalities, or electromyography

such patients, but it is unclear whether treatment confers any clinical benefit; the issue is under further study.

BECKER DYSTROPHY

This is also X-linked and is associated with a pattern of weakness similar to that in Duchenne dystrophy. Its average onset (11 years) and age at death (45 years) are later, however. Cardiac and cognitive impairment do not occur, and serum CK levels are less strikingly elevated than in Duchenne dystrophy. Dystrophin levels in muscle are normal, but the protein is qualitatively altered. It is not clear whether corticosteroids have any role in treatment of this dystrophinopathy.

LIMB-GIRDLE DYSTROPHY

Previously a catchall designation that probably subsumed a variety of disorders, including undiagnosed cases of other dystrophies, it is (in classic form) inherited in autosomal recessive fashion, although autosomal dominant and sporadic forms also exist. Patients with different genetic mutations may be clinically indistinguishable, and patients with the same mutation may show marked phenotypic variation, even within the same family. The disorder begins clinically between late childhood and early adulthood. In contrast to Duchenne and Becker dystrophies, the shoulder and pelvic girdle muscles are affected to a more nearly equal extent. Pseudohypertrophy is not seen, and serum CK levels are less elevated.

FACIOSCAPULOHUMERAL DYSTROPHY

This is an autosomal dominant disorder that usually has its onset in adolescence and is compatible with a normal life span. The genetic defect involves contraction of repeated DNA sequences on chromosome 4, together with single-nucleotide polymorphisms that create a polyadenylation site for a homeobox gene, *DUX4*. Contraction produces a more open chromatin structure, promoting transcription of *DUX4*, whereas polyadenylation enhances stability of the *DUX4* transcript. As a result, levels of the transcript are increased, consistent with a toxic gain of protein function. The clinical severity of this condition is highly variable. Weakness is typically confined to the face, neck, and shoulder girdle, but foot drop can occur. Winged scapulae are common. The heart is not involved, and serum CK levels are normal or only slightly elevated.

EMERY–DREIFUSS MUSCULAR DYSTROPHY

This disorder occurs in X-linked recessive, autosomal dominant, and autosomal recessive forms. A variety of different genes are involved. Clinical onset in childhood is followed by slow progression, with development of contractures, weakness and wasting (particularly of triceps and biceps in the arms, and of peronei and tibialis anterior in the legs, with later spread to the girdle muscles), cardiac conduction abnormalities, and cardiomyopathy. The serum CK is usually mildly increased. Cardiac function should be monitored and a pacemaker inserted if necessary. Physical therapy is important to maintain mobility.

DISTAL MYOPATHY

The autosomal dominant variety typically presents after age 40 years, although onset may be earlier and symptoms more severe in homozygotes. Small muscles of the hands and feet, wrist extensors, and the dorsiflexors of the foot are affected. The precise pattern of involvement varies in the different subtypes of the disorder. The course is slowly progressive. Distal myopathies with autosomal recessive inheritance or occurring sporadically present with progressive leg weakness in adolescents or young adults. Late-onset variants also occur; in one, there is selective involvement of the posterior calves.

OCULAR DYSTROPHY

This is typically an autosomal dominant disorder, although recessive and sporadic cases also occur. Some cases are associated with deletions in mitochondrial DNA. Onset is usually before age 30 years. Ptosis is the earliest manifestation, but progressive external ophthalmoplegia subsequently develops; facial weakness is also common, and subclinical involvement of limb muscles may occur. The course is slowly progressive. The extent to which ocular dystrophy is distinct from oculopharyngeal dystrophy is unclear in many cases.

OCULOPHARYNGEAL DYSTROPHY

An autosomal dominant disorder related to mutations in the *PABPN1* gene, this is found with increased frequency in certain geographic areas, including Quebec and the southwestern United States. It most often begins in the third to fifth decade. Findings include ptosis, total external ophthalmoplegia, dysphagia, facial weakness, and often proximal limb weakness. Serum CK is normal or mildly elevated. Dysphagia is particularly incapacitating and may require nasogastric feeding or gastrostomy.

PARASPINAL DYSTROPHY

Progressive paraspinal weakness may develop after the age of 40 years in patients of either sex, some of whom may have a family history of the disorder. Back pain and a marked kyphosis (**bent spine syndrome** or **camptocormia**) are characteristic. The serum CK is mildly elevated. CT scans show fatty replacement of paraspinal muscles.

CONGENITAL MYOPATHIES

The congenital myopathies are a heterogeneous group of rare and relatively nonprogressive disorders that usually begin in infancy or childhood but may not become clinically apparent until adulthood. Most are characterized by predominantly proximal muscle weakness, hypotonia, hyporeflexia, and normal serum CK; many are inherited.

Congenital myopathies are classified according to ultrastructural histopathologic features and are diagnosed by muscle biopsy. They include **nemaline** myopathy, characterized by rod-shaped bodies in muscle fibers, which are also seen in some patients with AIDS-related myopathy (see later); **central core** disease, which may be associated with malignant hyperthermia as a complication of general anesthesia; **myotubular** or **centronuclear** myopathy; and **mitochondrial** myopathies, such as Kearns–Sayre–Daroff syndrome, a cause of progressive external ophthalmoplegia (see Chapter 7, Neuro-Ophthalmic Disorders). No treatment is available for any of these disorders.

MITOCHONDRIAL MYOPATHIES

The mitochondrial myopathies are a clinically heterogeneous group of disorders caused by defective oxidative phosphorylation and accompanied by structural mitochondrial abnormalities on skeletal muscle biopsy. Their morphologic signature is the "**ragged red fiber**" seen with the modified Gomori stain, containing accumulations of abnormal mitochondria (**Figure 9-12**). Since the first reported pathogenic mutation of human mitochondrial DNA in the 1980s, many other mutations have been described, including point mutations and large-scale deletions.

Patients may present with **Kearns–Sayre–Daroff syndrome** (progressive external ophthalmoplegia, pigmentary degeneration of the retina, and cardiomyopathy) or with limb weakness that is exacerbated or induced by

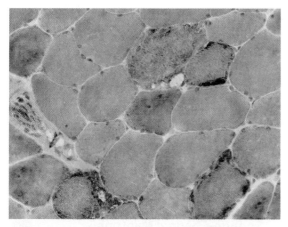

▲ **Figure 9-12.** Ragged-red muscle fibers seen on trichrome stain of muscle biopsy obtained in a 65-year-old woman with a mitochondrial myopathy. (Used with permission from A. Hiniker.)

activity. In other patients, the symptoms and signs are of central neurologic dysfunction and may include myoclonic epilepsy (myoclonic epilepsy, ragged red fiber syndrome [**MERRF**]) or the combination of mitochondrial myopathy, encephalopathy, lactic acidosis, and strokelike episodes (**MELAS**). These various syndromes are caused by separate abnormalities of mitochondrial DNA. Investigations may include muscle biopsy, measurement of serum and CSF lactate, and imaging studies. Genetic testing on peripheral leukocytes is important when the mitochondrial DNA mutation is expressed in hematopoietic cells, such as in MELAS. Treatment is generally supportive.

Mitochondrial DNA depends for its proper function on various factors encoded by nuclear DNA. Mutations in nuclear genes may thus affect mitochondrial function. This is exemplified by mutations in the gene for thymidine phosphorylate, which lead to an autosomal recessive disorder called mitochondrial neurogastrointestinal encephalomyopathy (**MNGIE**), manifest by gastrointestinal dysmotility and skeletal muscle abnormalities.

MYOTONIC DISORDERS

In **myotonia**, an abnormality of the muscle fiber membrane (sarcolemma) causes marked delay before the affected muscles can relax after a contraction; this leads to apparent muscle stiffness. On examination, it is frequently possible to demonstrate myotonia by difficulty in relaxing the hand after sustained grip or by persistent contraction after percussion of the belly of a muscle such as in the thenar eminence. Electromyography of affected muscles may reveal characteristic high-frequency discharges of potentials that wax and wane in amplitude and frequency, producing over the EMG loudspeaker a sound like that of a dive bomber or chain saw.

MYOTONIC DYSTROPHIES

▶ **Myotonic Dystrophy Type 1**

Myotonic dystrophy type 1 (DM1) is a dominantly inherited disorder that usually is manifests in the third or fourth decade, although it may appear in infancy or early childhood. The gene defect is an expanded trinucleotide (CTG) repeat in an untranslated region of the gene coding for dystrophia myotonica protein kinase (*DMPK*) on chromosome 19. This expanded trinucleotide repeat forms the basis of a diagnostic test; repeat lengths greater than 34 repeats are abnormal, but the disease does not become symptomatic until repeat length is greater than 50. Prenatal testing during at-risk pregnancies can be performed. Myotonia accompanies weakness and wasting of the facial, sternomastoid, and distal limb muscles (**Figure 9-13**). There may also be cataracts, frontal baldness, testicular atrophy, diabetes mellitus, cardiac abnormalities, respiratory disturbances,

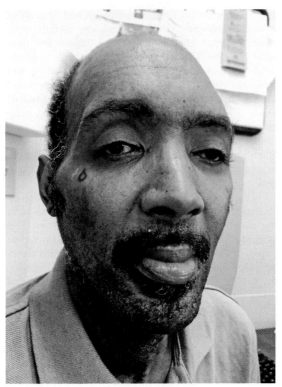

▲ **Figure 9-13.** A 48-year-old man with myotonic dystrophy, cataracts, frontal baldness, and wasting of the temporalis, facial, and sternocleidomastoid muscles.

sleep apnea/hypopnea, intellectual and behavioral changes, hypogammaglobulinemia, and sudden death. A severe electrocardiographic abnormality and the presence of atrial tachyarrhythmia predict sudden death.

A congenital form also occurs in the infants of affected mothers and is characterized by floppiness, facial weakness, poor suck, and respiratory failure that may lead to death in the neonatal period. Before birth, polyhydramnios and reduced fetal movement may be noted.

Myotonic Dystrophy Type 2

Patients with **myotonic dystrophy type 2** (DM2), sometimes designated **proximal myotonic myopathy,** have myotonia, cataracts, primarily proximal weakness (neck and finger flexors, followed by hip flexors and extensors, and elbow extensors), and a less severe course than those with DM1. The disorder is dominantly inherited and results from an expanded CCTG repeat in a noncoding (intronic) region of the gene for zinc finger protein-9 (*ZNF9*) on chromosome 3. Onset is commonly in young adults. A congenital form does not occur. A variant with more severe muscle involvement and hearing loss has been described.

Diagnosis

Diagnosis is generally based on clinical suspicion and confirmed by genetic testing. EMG shows myopathic changes and myotonic discharges. Serum levels of muscle enzymes may be elevated. Muscle biopsy is usually unnecessary. ECG permits cardiac conduction defects to be identified and monitored.

Treatment

Management includes the use of assistive devices as needed for weakness and the management of complications such as cataracts or cardiac arrhythmias. If necessary, myotonia can be treated with phenytoin (100 mg three times daily). Other drugs that may help myotonia, such as procainamide 0.5 to 1 g four times daily or mexiletine 150 to 200 mg three times daily, may have undesirable effects on cardiac conduction. There is no treatment for the weakness that occurs, and pharmacologic maneuvers do not influence the natural history.

NONDYSTROPHIC MYOTONIAS

The nondystrophic myotonias are caused by dysfunction of certain skeletal muscle ion channels. They include myotonia congenita, paramyotonia congenita, and the sodium-channel myotonias. These disorders are manifest primarily by muscle stiffness resulting from myotonia but—depending on the disorder—pain, weakness, and fatigue may also be conspicuous.

Myotonia Congenita

Myotonia congenita is usually inherited as a dominant disorder (**Thomsen disease**) that relates to a mutation in the *CLCN1* skeletal muscle chloride channel gene. Many different mutations have been identified. Generalized myotonia without weakness is usually present from birth, but symptoms may not develop until early childhood. Muscle stiffness is enhanced by cold and inactivity and relieved by exercise. Muscle hypertrophy, sometimes pronounced, is also a feature. A recessive form with later onset (**Becker disease**, not to be confused with Becker muscular dystrophy) is associated with slight weakness—especially on initiating a movement—and with atrophy of distal muscles. It is also due to a *CLCN1* mutation. Drugs acting specifically on the CLCN1 channel are not available, but treatment with mexiletine or phenytoin may help the myotonia.

Paramyotonia Congenita and Sodium-Channel Myotonias

These are allelic, autosomal dominant disorders caused by point mutations in the skeletal muscle voltage-gated sodium channel gene, *SCN4A*.

Paramyotonia is characterized by episodic muscle cramps and weakness that is exacerbated markedly by cold and exercise and becomes symptomatic in childhood. The facial, tongue, and hand muscles are most affected, and the lower limbs much less so. The myotonia can last up to several minutes, but weakness may persist for hours and even days. Muscle hypertrophy is sometimes present.

Patients with **sodium-channel myotonias** are typically not sensitive to cold (although this occurs in some cases), but their myotonia is worsened with potassium ingestion. Weakness does not occur. The myotonia tends to occur about 10 or more minutes after the onset of exercise and is improved with acetazolamide treatment. In some cases, myotonia is severe and may impair respiration.

▶ Diagnosis

Various electrophysiologic test protocols can aid diagnosis. Sarcolemmal excitability is measured indirectly by changes in size of the compound muscle action potential after varying periods of exercise, and the effect of muscle cooling is noted. Distinct patterns have been recognized and have been used to direct genetic testing.

▶ Treatment

There is insufficient evidence to make treatment recommendations for these disorders, but sodium-channel blockers to reduce the excitability of cell membranes may be of some benefit. Mexiletine is often favored, but it may cause cardiac arrhythmias or gastrointestinal disturbances, and is sometimes ineffective.

INFLAMMATORY MYOPATHIES

Muscle biopsy is important in confirming the diagnosis of an inflammatory myopathy and facilitating recognition of unusual varieties such as eosinophilic, granulomatous, and parasitic myositis.

TRICHINOSIS, TOXOPLASMOSIS, & SARCOIDOSIS

These disorders may lead to an inflammatory disorder of muscle, but this is uncommon. Treatment is of the underlying cause.

POLYMYOSITIS & DERMATOMYOSITIS

▶ Pathogenesis

Polymyositis and dermatomyositis are immune-mediated inflammatory myopathies characterized by destruction of muscle fibers and inflammatory infiltration of muscles (**Table 9-15**). There are immunologic and histopathologic differences between the two disorders. Dermatomyositis is a microangiopathy affecting skin and muscle: lysis of endomysial capillaries is caused by activation and deposition of complement, leading to muscle ischemia. Inflammatory infiltrates occur especially in the perimysial region and include CD4+ cells. In polymyositis, muscle fibers expressing major histocompatibility complex (MHC) class I antigens are invaded by clonally expanded CD8+ cytotoxic T cells, leading to necrosis. Infiltrates are predominantly intrafascicular.

Table 9-15. The Inflammatory Myopathies.

	Polymyositis	Dermatomyositis	Inclusion Body Myositis
Sex	Females > males	Females > males	Males > females
Age	Usually adults	Any age	Usually after age 50 years
Onset	Acute or insidious	Acute or insidious	Insidious
Distribution of weakness	Proximal > distal	Proximal > distal	Selective (see text)
Course	Often rapid	Often rapid	Gradual
Serum creatine kinase	Often very high	Often very high	Normal or mild increase (<12-fold)
EMG	Myopathic ± neurogenic	Myopathic ± neurogenic	Myopathic ± neurogenic
Response to treatment	Good	Good	Poor
Skin changes	No	Yes	No
Increased incidence of cancer	No	Yes	No
Biopsy	Intrafascicular inflammatory infiltrates with CD8+ T cells	Perifascicular and often perivascular inflammatory infiltrates, composed of B cells and CD4+ T cells	Endomysial inflammation with infiltrates of CD8+ T cells; intracellular inclusions, rimmed vacuoles

Clinical Findings

Polymyositis can occur at any age; it progresses at a variable rate and leads to symmetric weakness, wasting, and myalgia, especially of the proximal limb and girdle muscles.

Dermatomyositis is also characterized by muscle weakness but is distinguished clinically by the presence of an erythematous rash over the eyelids, about the eyes (**heliotrope rash**), or on the extensor surfaces of the joints (**Gottron sign** or **papules; Figure 9-14**). Other cutaneous manifestations also occur, including periungual lesions, calcinosis, photodistributed poikiloderma, and scalp lesions resembling psoriasis. The skin lesions may precede or accompany muscle involvement.

Polymyositis/dermatomyositis may be manifest also by interstitial pulmonary disease, dysphagia, Raynaud phenomenon, arthralgia, malaise, weight loss, and a low-grade fever. It has been reported in association with various autoimmune disorders, including scleroderma, lupus erythematosus, rheumatoid arthritis, and Sjögren syndrome. In addition, approximately 25% of patients with adult-onset dermatomyositis have an associated malignancy (most often ovarian, lung, gastrointestinal, or nasopharyngeal carcinoma). The association with malignancy is less in polymyositis.

Diagnosis

The serum CK is generally elevated in patients with polymyositis or dermatomyositis, sometimes to very high levels, but normal values do not exclude the diagnosis. Levels of other muscle enzymes, such as lactic dehydrogenase, aldolase, and aspartate and alanine aminotransferase, are commonly also increased. Antibodies to aminoacyl-transfer ribonucleic acid (tRNA) synthetase enzymes are present in about 30% of patients with polymyositis or

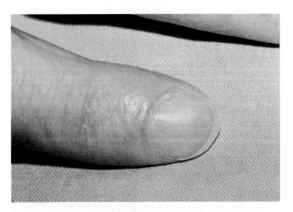

▲ **Figure 9-14.** Gottron papules over the extensor aspect of the finger joints in a patient with dermatomyositis and colon cancer.

dermatomyositis. The most common of these is the anti-Jo-1 antibody, the presence of which is associated with an incomplete response to treatment. Antibodies to signal recognition particle (SRP) occur in some patients with severe polymyositis, who usually respond poorly to treatment; antibodies to Mi-2, a nuclear helicase, are found in occasional patients with dermatomyositis and are associated with a good treatment response. The frequency with which these antibodies are present varies in different studies, with the type of inflammatory muscle disease, and with the patient population.

Electromyography reveals a myopathic process (in about 90% cases) but not its cause. An abundance of short, low-amplitude, polyphasic motor unit potentials is found, as in any myopathic process, but abnormal spontaneous activity is often conspicuous as well.

Muscle biopsy usually shows muscle fiber necrosis and infiltration with inflammatory cells and is important for accurate diagnosis. Additional studies are performed to exclude malignancy depending on the individual circumstances.

Treatment

Response to treatment can be predicted in part by the results of antibody studies. A prolonged interval before diagnosis (more than 18 months) or initiation of treatment (6 to 12 months) is associated with a worse outcome. Treatment is with anti-inflammatory drugs. Prednisone is commonly used in an initial dose of 60 or 80 mg/d, along with potassium supplements and frequent antacids if necessary. As improvement occurs and serum CK values decline, the prednisone dose is gradually tapered to maintenance levels that usually range between 10 and 20 mg/d. Patients may need to continue this regimen for 2 to 3 years, however; too rapid a reduction in dose may lead to relapse. Improvements in strength indicate clinical response more reliably than serum muscle enzyme levels.

Corticosteroid-sparing agents may be introduced at the start of treatment or later. Methotrexate (15 mg/wk, increased after 3 months to 25 mg/wk, if necessary) and azathioprine (50 mg/d, increasing gradually to up to 2.5 mg/kg daily depending on response and tolerance) have been used, either alone or in combination with corticosteroids; they are particularly useful in corticosteroid-resistant patients. As remission occurs, glucocorticoids are usually stopped before azathioprine or methotrexate are withdrawn gradually over about 6 months.

Newer immunosuppressants, such as mycophenolate mofetil, have been used in refractory cases, but experience is limited. Intravenous immunoglobulin therapy can also be used in refractory cases of dermatomyositis, but its utility in polymyositis is less clear.

Physical therapy may help to prevent contractures, and, as the patient responds to anti-inflammatory drugs, active exercise may hasten recovery.

INCLUSION-BODY MYOSITIS

Epidemiology

This disorder is more common in men than women and has an insidious onset, usually after 50 years of age. Its incidence is unclear, but it is being recognized with increasing frequency.

Etiology

The etiology of the myositis is unknown, but accumulating evidence suggests a T-cell-mediated myocytotoxicity and probably a multifactorial genetic susceptibility to the disease. Associated disorders include various autoimmune disturbances, diabetes mellitus, and diffuse peripheral neuropathy.

Clinical Findings

Inclusion-body myositis produces weakness of the lower and then the upper extremities. Weakness and atrophy of the quadriceps and of the forearm flexor and extensor muscles are characteristic. The disease is progressive and is associated with early depression of the knee reflexes. Muscle pain occurs in some patients. Distal weakness also develops, but is usually less severe than proximal weakness. Dysphagia from involvement of the cricopharyngeal muscles is common.

Diagnosis

Serum CK levels may be normal or mildly increased. The EMG reveals nonspecific findings suggestive of an inflammatory myopathy. The diagnosis is confirmed by histologic examination of biopsied muscle, showing endomysial inflammation, vacuolated muscle fibers, muscle fiber inclusions of beta-amyloid, and intranuclear and intracytoplasmic filaments by electron microscopy or with immunohistologic staining.

Differential Diagnosis

A familial disorder with onset in young adults, characterized by slowly progressive weakness, especially of distal muscles, and with histologic features resembling inclusion-body myositis (vacuolar myopathy with inclusions) has been described. The family history helps to distinguish this **hereditary inclusion-body myopathy** from the sporadic disorder, as does the lack of inflammatory changes on histologic examination. Table 9-15 summarizes the differences between inclusion-body myositis, polymyositis, and dermatomyositis.

Treatment

Immunosuppressive or immunomodulatory therapies should be tried, but usually provide little or no benefit. Conflicting reports on the utility of intravenous globulin therapy make its role unclear. Physical therapy is important in maintaining and improving strength. Assistive appliances such as walkers should be provided as needed. Patients may eventually become chair-bound and require help with the activities of daily life.

AIDS

Several forms of myopathy can occur in patients with either symptomatic or otherwise asymptomatic HIV-1 infection (**Table 9-16**). These disorders can be distinguished by muscle biopsy.

Polymyositis

This most common AIDS-related myopathy may be caused by autoimmune mechanisms triggered by HIV-1 infection. It resembles polymyositis in patients without HIV-1 infection (see earlier) and may respond to treatment with corticosteroids.

Inclusion-Body Myositis-Like Syndrome

Patients with AIDS may also develop a myopathy resembling inclusion-body myositis, apparently because the virus triggers an immune response similar to that occurring in sporadic inclusion-body myositis; there does not seem to be direct infection of the muscle.

Muscle-Wasting Syndrome

This sometimes relates to **type II muscle fiber atrophy;** malnutrition, cachexia, immobility, or remote effects of AIDS-related tumors may have a pathogenic role. Proximal muscle weakness is the major finding, and serum CK is normal.

Rod-Body (Nemaline) Myopathy

Rod-body myopathy is a noninflammatory disorder characterized by rod-shaped bodies and selective loss of thick filaments. Clinical features include proximal muscle weakness and moderate elevation of serum CK. Treatment with corticosteroids or plasmapheresis may be helpful.

Table 9-16. Myopathies Related to HIV-1 Infection or Its Treatment.

Polymyositis
Inclusion-body myositis
Muscle-wasting syndrome/type II muscle fiber atrophy
Rod-body (nemaline) myopathy
Vasculitic processes
Opportunistic infections of muscle
Zidovudine-induced mitochondrial myopathy
Fat accumulation (in HIV-associated lipodystrophies)
Myositis (in immune restoration inflammatory syndrome)
Acute rhabdomyolysis

Vasculitic Myopathy

Vasculitic processes may involve the muscles (and nerves); treatment in AIDS patients usually involves antiretroviral and immunomodulatory agents including intravenous immunoglobulins and corticosteroids.

Infective Myopathy

Opportunistic infections of muscle are well recognized and may present as pyomyositis; muscle toxoplasmosis may lead to a subacute painful myopathy. Treatment is directed against the offending organisms.

Mitochondrial Myopathy

A myopathy in which muscle biopsy specimens show the **ragged red fibers** indicative of damaged mitochondria can occur in patients receiving zidovudine for treatment of AIDS and may coexist with polymyositis. The disorder is characterized clinically by proximal muscle weakness, myalgia, and moderate to marked elevation of serum CK; it is thought to result from a toxic effect of zidovudine on muscle. Mild symptoms may be controlled with nonsteroidal anti-inflammatory drugs or corticosteroids, and more severe involvement may respond to discontinuing zidovudine. If there is no response, a muscle biopsy should be performed to look for other causes of myopathy.

Treatment-Related Myopathies

Patients with HIV-1 infection treated with **combination antiretroviral therapy (cART)** may develop a **lipodystrophy**; muscle biopsy (performed for unrelated reasons) then shows fatty accumulation in muscle. In the **immune reconstitution inflammatory syndrome (IRIS)**, HIV-1-infected patients receiving cART develop inflammatory responses that may lead to a myositis resembling polymyositis.

Acute Rhabdomyolysis

This sometimes occurs in patients with HIV-1 infection and causes myalgia, muscle weakness, and an elevated serum CK; it may also relate to medication or opportunistic infection.

POLYMYALGIA RHEUMATICA

Polymyalgia rheumatica, which is more common in women than in men, generally occurs in patients older than 50 years and is best regarded as a variant of **giant cell arteritis**. It is characterized by muscle pain and stiffness, particularly about the neck and girdle muscles, that is sometimes so severe that it interferes with the simple activities of daily life such as turning over in bed. Headache, anorexia, weight loss, and low-grade fever may be conjoined, and the erythrocyte sedimentation rate is

increased. Serum enzymes, electromyography, and muscle biopsy are normal.

There is usually a dramatic response to treatment with corticosteroids in low dosage (eg, prednisone 15-20 mg/d orally). Treatment is monitored by clinical parameters and sedimentation rate and may need to be continued for 2 years or more if serious complications are to be avoided, as noted for giant cell arteritis (see Chapter 6, Headache & Facial Pain). Relapses may occur when the daily dose of prednisone is reduced to about 5 mg or less. Methotrexate is the most commonly used corticosteroid-sparing agent.

METABOLIC MYOPATHIES

HYPOKALEMIA

Proximal myopathic weakness may result from **chronic hypokalemia,** and once the metabolic disturbance has been corrected, power usually returns to normal within a few weeks. **Acute hypo- or hyperkalemia** may also lead to muscle weakness that is rapidly reversed by correcting the metabolic disturbance.

PERIODIC PARALYSES

The **periodic paralysis syndromes,** which may be familial (dominant inheritance), are characterized by episodes of flaccid weakness or paralysis with preserved ventilation that may be associated with abnormalities of the serum potassium level. Strength is normal between attacks. Electromyography during attacks shows reduced or absent motor unit recruitment. These disorders are **channelopathies** in which there is abnormal, often potassium-sensitive, muscle-membrane excitability. Mutations in genes encoding three ion channels—*CACNA1S, SCN4A,* and *KCNJ2*—are responsible for most cases.

Hypokalemic Periodic Paralysis

In the **hypokalemic form,** attacks tend to occur on awakening, after exercise, or after a heavy meal, and may last for several days. A progressive myopathy may develop late in the disease course. The disorder is commonly due to a mutation in the gene encoding the α_{1S} subunit of the L-type (dihydropyridine-sensitive) skeletal muscle calcium channel (*CACNA1S*). The clinical disorder is genetically heterogeneous and may also be caused by mutations in the α subunit of the type IV voltage-gated sodium channel (*SCN4A*), which is more typically associated with hyperkalemic periodic paralysis (see later). In some families, no genetic cause has been identified.

The disorder should be distinguished from hyperkalemic periodic paralysis by measurement of the serum potassium level during an attack, from thyrotoxic periodic paralysis by tests of thyroid function, and from cardiodysrhythmic periodic paralysis (discussed later) by the electrocardiographic findings.

Acetazolamide (250-750 mg daily), dichlorphenamide (50-100 mg daily), or oral potassium supplements may prevent attacks, as also may a low salt and low carbohydrate diet. Ongoing attacks may be arrested by potassium chloride given orally or even intravenously if the ECG can be monitored and kidney function is satisfactory. Excessive exertion should be avoided.

Thyrotoxic (Hypokalemic) Periodic Paralysis

Hypokalemic periodic paralysis may be associated with hyperthyroidism, particularly in young Asian men. The clinical features of the disorder are as described earlier. Treatment of the thyroid disorder may prevent recurrences. All patients with suspected hypokalemic periodic paralysis should therefore be screened for thyroid disease.

Hyperkalemic Periodic Paralysis

This disorder usually manifests in the first decade of life. Attacks associated with **hyperkalemia** tend to come on after exercise but are usually much briefer than those of hypokalemic periodic paralysis, typically lasting for less than 1 hour. They may also occur with cold exposure or when fasting. Several attacks may occur during the course of a day. The serum potassium during an attack is increased. A progressive myopathy may develop in later years.

The disorder is inherited in an autosomal dominant manner. Many affected families have mutations in the gene encoding the α subunit of the type IV voltage-gated sodium channel (SCN4A); several allelic mutations have been recognized and account for some phenotypic variation, such as the presence of myotonia or paramyotonia.

Attacks often require no treatment, as they are short lived. Severe attacks may be terminated by intravenous calcium gluconate (1-2 g), intravenous diuretics (furosemide 20-40 mg), or glucose, and daily acetazolamide or chlorothiazide may help prevent further episodes. Attacks may be prevented or reduced in frequency by avoiding potassium-rich foods and avoiding excessive carbohydrate intake. Acetazolamide (250-750 mg daily) or dichlorphenamide (50-100 mg daily) may also be helpful. Special precautions may need to be taken for patients requiring general anesthesia.

Cardiodysrhythmic Periodic Paralysis

This disorder, also referred to as Andersen–Tawil syndrome, results from mutations in the gene for an inwardly rectifying potassium channel (KCNJ2). The disorder is inherited in autosomal dominant fashion, generally manifests before the age of 20 years, and is characterized by periodic paralysis, ventricular arrhythmias, and facial or skeletal deformities. The QT or QU interval is prolonged

on the electrocardiogram. Serum potassium levels may be increased, decreased, or normal at the time of paralytic attacks, which may be triggered by rest following exertion.

Paramyotonia Congenita

This is a dominantly inherited disorder, related to mutation of the SCN4A gene, discussed earlier; attacks of hyperkalemic periodic paralysis may also occur.

Normokalemic Periodic Paralysis

This disorder is similar clinically to the hyperkalemic variety, but the plasma potassium level is normal in attacks; treatment is with acetazolamide. It is sometimes unresponsive to treatment; in severe attacks, it may be impossible to move the limbs, but respiration and swallowing are rarely affected.

OSTEOMALACIA

Proximal muscle weakness may also occur in osteomalacia, often with associated bone pain and tenderness, mild hypocalcemia, and elevated serum alkaline phosphatase. Strength improves after treatment with vitamin D.

ENDOCRINE MYOPATHIES

Myopathy may occur in association with hyper- or hypothyroidism, hyper- or hypoparathyroidism, hyper- or hypoadrenalism, hypopituitarism, and acromegaly. Treatment is that of the underlying endocrine disorder.

ALCOHOLIC MYOPATHIES

ACUTE NECROTIZING ALCOHOLIC MYOPATHY

Heavy binge drinking may result in an acute necrotizing myopathy that develops over 1 or 2 days. Presenting symptoms include muscle pain, weakness, and sometimes dysphagia. On examination, the affected muscles are swollen, tender, and weak. Weakness is proximal in distribution and may be asymmetric or focal. Serum CK is moderately to severely elevated, and myoglobinuria may occur. As hypokalemia and hypophosphatemia can produce a similar syndrome in alcoholic patients, serum potassium and phosphorus concentrations should be determined. With abstinence from alcohol and a nutritionally adequate diet, recovery can be expected over a period of weeks to months.

CHRONIC ALCOHOLIC MYOPATHY

Chronic myopathy characterized by proximal weakness of the lower limbs may develop insidiously over weeks to months in alcoholic patients. Muscle pain is not a prominent feature. Cessation of drinking and an improved diet are associated with clinical improvement over several months in most cases.

DRUG-INDUCED MYOPATHIES

Myopathy can occur with administration of medications such as corticosteroids, chloroquine, clofibrate, emetine, ε-aminocaproic acid, certain β-blockers, bretylium tosylate, colchicine, statins (HMG-CoA reductase inhibitors), zidovudine, and drugs that cause potassium depletion. Common variants in the gene for a solute carrier organic anion transporter (*SLCO1B1*) are strongly associated with an increased risk of statin-induced myopathy. Symptoms of drug-induced myopathy vary from an asymptomatic increase in serum CK levels to acute rhabdomyolysis, depending on the causal agent and the individual patient. Necrotizing myopathies are due mainly to lipid-lowering drugs, and mitochondrial myopathies to antiretroviral nucleoside analogues. Corticosteroid myopathy is particularly common. Drug-induced myopathies are usually reversible if the causal agent is discontinued.

CRITICAL ILLNESS MYOPATHY

Patients in the intensive care unit may develop weakness both proximally and distally in the limbs from primary muscle involvement. Histopathologic examination reveals a diffuse non-necrotizing cachectic myopathy, a selective loss of thick (myosin) filaments, or an acute necrotizing myopathy. The myopathy may coexist with a neuropathy. Its cause is uncertain, but it is associated with the use of nondepolarizing neuromuscular blockers and corticosteroids. Serum CK is sometimes increased, especially if muscle necrosis has occurred. Electrophysiologic findings may be suggestive of muscle involvement and help to distinguish myopathy from neuropathy or disorders of the neuromuscular junction. Muscle biopsy may be definitive but is not always revealing. Prognosis is good except when muscle necrosis is conspicuous. Treatment is supportive. Sepsis must be treated aggressively.

MYOGLOBINURIA

This can result from muscle injury or ischemia (irrespective of its cause) and leads to a urine that is dark red. The following causes are important:

1. Excessive unaccustomed **exercise**, leading to muscle necrosis (rhabdomyolysis) and thus to myoglobinuria, sometimes on a familial basis
2. **Crush injuries**
3. **Muscle infarction**
4. Prolonged **tonic-clonic convulsions**
5. **Polymyositis**
6. Chronic **potassium depletion**
7. An acute **alcoholic binge**
8. Certain **viral infections** associated with muscle weakness and pain
9. **Hyperthermia**
10. **Metabolic myopathies** (eg, muscle glycogen phosphorylase deficiency [McArdle disease])

Serum CK levels are elevated, often greatly. Myoglobin can be detected in the urine by the dipstick test for heme pigment; a positive test indicates the presence of myoglobin in the urine unless red blood cells are present. In severe cases, myoglobinuria may lead to renal failure, and peritoneal dialysis or hemodialysis may then be necessary. Otherwise, treatment consists of increasing the urine volume by hydration. The serum potassium level must be monitored, as it may rise rapidly.

MOTOR-UNIT HYPERACTIVITY STATES

Disorders affecting the central or peripheral nervous system at a variety of sites can produce abnormal, increased activity in the motor unit (**Table 9-17**).

CENTRAL NERVOUS SYSTEM DISORDERS

STIFF-PERSON SYNDROME

This is a rare, usually sporadic, and slowly progressive disorder manifested by tightness, stiffness, and rigidity of axial and proximal limb muscles with superimposed painful spasms.

▶ Pathogenesis

An immune-mediated defect in central **GABAergic transmission** has been proposed as the cause of the disorder. In approximately 60% of patients, the blood and cerebrospinal fluid contain autoantibodies against **glutamic acid decarboxylase (GAD)**, which is involved in synthesis of the neurotransmitter γ-aminobutyric acid (GABA), and is concentrated in pancreatic β-cells and GABAergic neurons of the central nervous system. Another 10% of patients have an associated neoplasm and circulating autoantibodies against the synaptic vesicle-associated protein, **amphiphysin**. In these patients, symptoms may improve after removal of the tumor. Antibodies against postsynaptic markers at GABAergic synapses—GABA$_A$ receptor-associated protein and gephyrin—have also been identified in some patients. No clinical difference has been found between patients with and without autoantibodies.

▶ Clinical Findings

Stiff-person syndrome sometimes has an autoimmune basis, and it may be associated with other autoimmune

Table 9-17. Motor-Unit Hyperactivity States.

Site of Pathology	Syndrome	Clinical Features	Treatment
Central nervous system	Stiff-person syndrome	Rigidity, spasms	Diazepam, baclofen, sodium valproate, vigabatrin, gabapentin, immunosuppression
	Tetanus	Rigidity, spasms	Diazepam
	Hyperekplexia	Exaggerated startle, falls, stiffness	Clonazepam
Peripheral nerve	Cramps	Painful contraction of single muscle relieved by passive stretch	Phenytoin, carbamazepine, oxcarbazepine, baclofen; quinine if other treatments fail
	Neuromyotonia	Stiffness, myokymia, delayed relaxation	Phenytoin, carbamazepine
	Tetany	Chvostek sign Trousseau sign Carpopedal spasm	Calcium, magnesium, correction of alkalosis
	Hemifacial spasm	Involuntary hemifacial contraction	Carbamazepine, botulinum toxin, decompressive surgery
Muscle	Myotonia	Delayed relaxation, percussion myotonia	Mexiletine, phenytoin, carbamazepine, procainamide
	Malignant hyperthermia	Rigidity, fever	Dantrolene

disorders such as thyroiditis, myasthenia gravis, and pernicious anemia. Many patients have type 1 diabetes mellitus.

Patients with stiff person syndrome have muscle rigidity caused by sustained, involuntary contraction of agonist and antagonist muscles. Axial and proximal limb muscles are affected in particular, resulting in abnormal posture and gait and frequent falls. Rigidity typically disappears during sleep. Examination may show tight muscles, a slow or cautious gait, and hyperreflexia. In some patients, symptoms have a restricted distribution, for example, to one limb.

Painful spasms are often provoked by sudden movement, startle, or emotional upset and may be accompanied by hyperhidrosis and increased blood pressure. Paroxysmal dysautonomia may be manifest also by tachypnea and even respiratory arrest—perhaps due to stiffness of the respiratory muscles—and sometimes leads to sudden death. Some patients also have focal or generalized seizures.

Diagnosis

Electromyography reveals continuous motor-unit activity in the paraspinal or leg muscles that varies with the clinical state.

Differential Diagnosis

Stiff-person syndrome can be distinguished from tetanus (discussed later) by its more gradual onset, the absence of trismus (lockjaw), and its rapid response to diazepam.

Treatment

The paraneoplastic disorder may remit following treatment of the underlying malignancy. Symptomatic treatment is with drugs that enhance GABAergic transmission, such as diazepam 5 to 30 mg or clonazepam 1 to 6 mg orally four times daily. Baclofen, vigabatrin, sodium valproate, and gabapentin also may be helpful for relieving symptoms in some patients. Treatment with corticosteroids is helpful in refractory or severe cases, and intravenous immunoglobulin therapy or plasmapheresis is sometimes effective in patients who are otherwise unresponsive to treatment. There are also anecdotal reports of benefit with rituximab. The abrupt withdrawal of symptomatic measures may be life-threatening.

TETANUS

Tetanus, a disorder of central inhibitory neurotransmission caused by a toxin produced by *Clostridium tetani*, is discussed earlier in this chapter.

STARTLE SYNDROMES

In **hyperekplexia**, startle reflexes to an unexpected stimulus are excessive; startle-induced falls may occur and relate to a transient generalized stiffness that follows the startle reflex for a few seconds. In such patients, continuous stiffness is present in the neonatal period, resolving with time. The disorder may occur on a sporadic or familial (autosomal dominant or recessive) basis, associated usually with mutations in the α1 subunit of the glycine receptor gene (*GLRA1*).

Autosomal recessive forms may also relate to mutations in a glycine transporter (*SLC6A5*) or the gene encoding the beta-subunit of the glycine receptor (*GLRB*), whereas mutations in the postsynaptic anchoring protein gephyrin (*GPHN*) or a Rho-like GTPase (*ARHGEF9*) have been observed in sporadic cases. The abnormal startle reflex seems to originate in the brainstem, but a cortical basis has sometimes been suggested. In some patients with a minor form of the disorder, excessive startle reflexes are the only abnormality; the genetic and pathophysiologic bases of this form are unknown. Patients with hereditary or sporadic hyperekplexia often respond favorably to clonazepam, which potentiates effects of the inhibitory transmitter GABA. In occasional patients, hyperekplexia is symptomatic and relates to diffuse acquired cerebral or brainstem pathology.

Neuropsychiatric startle syndromes (eg, Jumping Frenchman of Maine, latah, miryachit) are also described and, in some instances, involve mimicking behaviors and cultural or familial factors.

PERIPHERAL NERVE DISORDERS

CRAMPS

These involuntary and typically painful contractions of a muscle or portion of a muscle are thought to arise distally in the motor neuron. Palpable knot-like hardening of the muscle may occur. Cramps are characteristically relieved by passive stretching of the affected muscle. They usually represent a benign condition and are common at night or during or after exercise.

However, cramps may also be a manifestation of peripheral vascular disease, motor neuron disease or polyneuropathy, metabolic disturbances (pregnancy, uremia, hypothyroidism, adrenal insufficiency), or fluid or electrolyte disorders (dehydration, hemodialysis). They may also be an adverse effect of radiation therapy or various medications. If a reversible underlying cause cannot be found, daytime cramps may respond to treatment with vitamin B supplementation, diphenhydramine (up to 50 mg each night), certain calcium-channel blockers, and certain anti-seizure drugs (phenytoin 300 to 400 mg/d orally or carbamazepine 200 to 400 mg orally three times a day; other drugs sometimes used are baclofen and oxcarbazepine). For none of these medications is there convincing evidence of efficacy. Open-label studies suggest that levetiracetam and gabapentin are occasionally helpful.

Nocturnal cramps may respond to locally applied heat or cold, or to a single oral bedtime dose of quinine sulfate (325 mg), phenytoin (100-300 mg), carbamazepine (200-400 mg), or diazepam (5-10 mg). However, because it may uncommonly cause serious hematologic abnormalities such as hemolytic uremic syndrome–thrombotic thrombocytopenia purpura, disseminated intravascular coagulation, and a bleeding diathesis, quinine should not be prescribed routinely unless the cramps are disabling and fail to respond to other approaches. Occasional patients respond to vitamin B complex or calcium-channel blockers, such as diltiazem or verapamil, but evidence for efficacy is limited or anecdotal.

NEUROMYOTONIA

Neuromyotonia (**Isaacs syndrome**) is a rare, sporadic disorder that produces continuous muscle stiffness, rippling muscle movements (**myokymia**), and delayed relaxation after muscle contraction. Some cases have an autosomal dominant mode of inheritance; in others, the neuromyotonia occurs as a paraneoplastic disorder, or in association with other autoimmune diseases or with hereditary motor and sensory neuropathies. It may also follow irradiation of the nervous system. In acquired neuromyotonia, antibodies against voltage-gated potassium channels are often found in the serum and CSF. Symptoms may be controlled with phenytoin 300 to 400 mg/d orally or carbamazepine 200 to 400 mg orally three times a day.

TETANY

Tetany—not to be confused with tetanus (see earlier)—is a hyperexcitable state of peripheral nerves usually associated with hypocalcemia, hypomagnesemia, or alkalosis. Signs of tetany (Chvostek sign, Trousseau sign, carpopedal spasm) are described in the section on hypocalcemia in Chapter 4, Confusional States. Treatment is by correction of the underlying electrolyte disorder.

HEMIFACIAL SPASM

Hemifacial spasm is characterized by repetitive, involuntary contractions of some or all of the muscles supplied by one facial (VII) nerve. Symptoms often commence in the orbicularis oculi and then spread to the cheek and levator anguli oris muscles. The contractions initially are brief but become more sustained as the disorder progresses; they may be provoked by blinking or voluntary activity. Slight facial weakness may also be found on examination. The disorder commonly relates to the presence of an anomalous blood vessel compressing the intracranial facial nerve, but MRI should be performed to exclude other structural lesions. The involuntary movements have been attributed to ephaptic transmission and ectopic excitation of demyelinated fibers in the compressed segment, to altered excitability of the facial nerve nucleus in the brainstem, or to both mechanisms. Treatment with carbamazepine or phenytoin is occasionally helpful. Injection of botulinum toxin A into the affected muscles suppresses the contractions temporarily but must be repeated every 3 or 4 months for sustained benefit. Microvascular decompressive procedures are often curative.

Table 9-18. Distinction Between Neuroleptic Malignant Syndrome, Malignant Hyperthermia, and Heat Stroke.

	Neuroleptic Malignant Syndrome	Malignant Hyperthermia	Heat Stroke
Hyperthermia	+	+	+
Muscle rigidity	+	+	Rare
Sweating	+	+	Rare
Genetic predisposition	−	+[1]	−
Precipitant	Neuroleptics	Halothane, succinylcholine	Heat exposure, exercise
Onset	Hours–days	Minutes–hours	Minutes–hours
Treatment	Dantrolene, dopamine agonists	Dantrolene	Rapid external cooling

[1]MHS1 mutation associated with the *RYR1* gene, chromosome 19, is most common.
Tachycardia, coagulopathy, acidosis, myoglobinuria, and altered mental status may occur in all three conditions and therefore are not reliable distinguishing features.
Data from Lazarus A, Mann SC, Caroff SN. *The Neuroleptic Malignant Syndrome and Related Conditions.* Washington, DC: American Psychiatric Association; 1989.

MUSCLE DISORDERS

MYOTONIA

Disorders that produce myotonia are discussed earlier.

MALIGNANT HYPERTHERMIA

Susceptibility to this disorder, which is often inherited in autosomal dominant fashion, may result from a mutation in the ryanodine receptor gene (*RYR1*) or less commonly in the α_{1S} subunit of the L-type (dihydropyridine-sensitive) skeletal muscle calcium channel (*CACNA1S*) or unidentified genes at other sites. The clinical abnormality is thought to result from abnormal excitation-contraction coupling in skeletal muscle. Symptoms are usually precipitated by administration of neuromuscular blocking agents (eg, succinylcholine) or inhalational anesthetics. Clinical features include **rigidity**, **hyperthermia**, **metabolic acidosis**, and **myoglobinuria**. Mortality rates as high as 70% have been reported. The disorder must be distinguished from neuroleptic malignant syndrome (**Table 9-18** and Chapter 11, Movement Disorders), which is manifested by rigidity, fever, altered mental status, and autonomic dysfunction.

Treatment includes prompt cessation of anesthesia, administration of the excitation-contraction uncoupler dantrolene (1-2 mg/kg intravenously every 5-10 minutes as needed, to a maximum dose of 10 mg/kg), reduction of body temperature, and correction of acidosis with intravenous bicarbonate. Patients who require surgery and are known or suspected to have malignant hyperthermia should be pretreated with dantrolene (four 1-mg/kg oral doses) on the day before surgery. Preoperative administration of atropine (which can also cause hyperthermia) should be avoided, and the anesthetics used should be restricted to those known to be safe in this condition (nitrous oxide, opiates, barbiturates, droperidol).

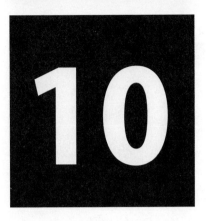

10

Sensory Disorders

(Continued on Next Page)

APPROACH TO DIAGNOSIS

In order to interpret the history and clinical signs of patients with disorders of **somatic sensation,** the functional anatomy of the sensory components of the nervous system must be understood. As used here, somatic sensation refers to the sensations of touch or pressure, vibration, joint position, pain, and temperature, and to more complex functions that rely on these primary sensory modalities (eg, two-point discrimination, stereognosis, graphesthesia); it excludes **special senses** such as smell, vision, taste, and hearing.

FUNCTIONAL ANATOMY OF THE SOMATIC SENSORY PATHWAYS

The sensory pathway between peripheral tissues (eg, skin or joints) and the cerebral cortex involves three neurons and two central synapses (**Figure 10-1**).

First-order sensory neurons from the limbs and trunk have cell bodies in the **dorsal root ganglia.** Each of these neurons sends a peripheral process that terminates in a free nerve ending or encapsulated sensory receptor and a central process that enters the spinal cord. **Sensory receptors** are relatively specialized for particular sensations and, in addition to free nerve endings (pain, itch), include Meissner corpuscles, Merkel corpuscles, and hair cells (touch); Krause end-bulbs (cold); and Ruffini corpuscles (heat). First-order sensory neurons synapse centrally at a site that depends on the type of sensation. Fibers mediating touch, pressure, or postural sensation in the limbs and trunk ascend in the **posterior columns** of the spinal cord to the medulla, where they synapse in the **gracile** and **cuneate nuclei.** Other fibers that mediate touch and those subserving pain, temperature, and itch appreciation in the limbs and trunk synapse on neurons in the **posterior horns** of the spinal cord, particularly in the **substantia gelatinosa.** First-order sensory neurons from the face, which have cell bodies in the trigeminal (gasserian) ganglion, travel in the trigeminal (V) nerve and enter the pons. Fibers mediating facial touch and pressure synapse in the **main trigeminal (V) nerve sensory nucleus**, whereas those conveying facial pain and temperature synapse in the **spinal trigeminal (V) nerve nucleus**.

Second-order sensory neurons with cell bodies in the gracile and cuneate nuclei cross the midline and ascend in the **medial lemniscus.** Second-order sensory neurons that arise in the posterior horns of the spinal cord cross the midline and

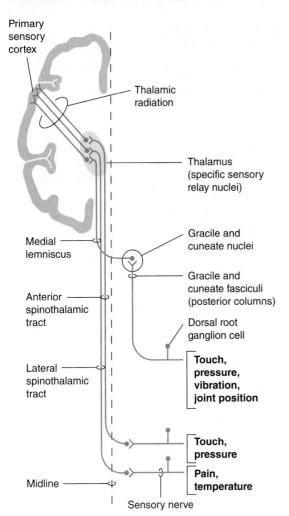

Primary sensory cortex

Thalamic radiation

Thalamus (specific sensory relay nuclei)

Medial lemniscus

Gracile and cuneate nuclei

Gracile and cuneate fasciculi (posterior columns)

Anterior spinothalamic tract

Dorsal root ganglion cell

Touch, pressure, vibration, joint position

Lateral spinothalamic tract

Touch, pressure

Pain, temperature

Midline

Sensory nerve

▲ **Figure 10-1.** Sensory pathways conveying touch, pressure, vibration, joint position, pain, and temperature sensation. (Used with permission from Barrett KE, Barman SM, Boitano S, Brooks H. *Ganong's Review of Medical Physiology*. 23rd ed. New York, NY: McGraw-Hill; 2010.)

ascend in the anterolateral part of the cord: fibers mediating touch pass upward in the **anterior spinothalamic tract**, whereas pain, itch, and temperature fibers generally travel in the **lateral spinothalamic tract**. Second-order sensory neurons from the limbs and trunk are joined in the brainstem by fibers from the face: those that mediate facial touch and pressure sensation project from the main trigeminal (V) nerve sensory nucleus via the **trigeminal lemniscus**, and those that convey facial pain, itch, and temperature project from the spinal trigeminal (V) nerve nucleus via the **trigeminotha-lamic tract**, to the ipsilateral **thalamus**. In the thalamus, medial lemniscal and spinothalamic fibers synapse in the

ventral posterolateral (VPL) nucleus; spinothalamic fibers also synapse in the **ventral posteroinferior (VPI) nucleus** and **intralaminar (ILa) nuclei**; and fibers in the trigeminal lemniscus and trigeminothalamic tract synapse in the **ventral posteromedial (VPM) nucleus**. In addition, some second-order spinothalamic sensory neurons send collaterals to the reticular formation.

Third-order sensory neurons project from the thalamus to the ipsilateral cerebral cortex. Fibers from VPL, VPI, and VPM travel primarily to the **primary somatosensory cortex** in the postcentral gyrus; fibers from ILa also project to the striatum, cingulate gyrus, and prefrontal cortex.

HISTORY

Sensory disturbances may consist of loss of sensation, abnormal sensations, or pain. The term **paresthesia** denotes abnormal spontaneous sensations, such as burning, tingling, or pins and needles, whereas **dysesthesia** denotes any unpleasant sensation produced by a stimulus that is normally painless. The term **numbness** is often used by patients to describe a sense of heaviness, weakness, or deadness in part of the body—and sometimes to signify any sensory impairment; the meaning must be clarified whenever this word is used.

It is important to determine the location of sensory symptoms; their mode of onset and progression; whether they are constant or episodic in nature; whether any factors specifically produce, enhance, or relieve them; and whether there are any accompanying symptoms.

The **location** of symptoms may reflect their origin. For example, sensory disturbances involving all the limbs suggest peripheral neuropathy, a cervical cord or brainstem lesion, or a metabolic disturbance such as hyperventilation syndrome. Involvement of one entire limb, or of one side of the body, suggests a central (brain or spinal cord) lesion. A hemispheric or brainstem lesion may cause lateralized sensory symptoms, but the face is also commonly affected. In addition, there may be other symptoms and signs, such as aphasia, apraxia, and visual field defects with hemispheric disease, or dysarthria, weakness, vertigo, diplopia, disequilibrium, and ataxia with brainstem disorders. Involvement of part of a limb or a discrete region of the trunk raises the possibility of a nerve or root lesion, depending on the precise distribution. With a root lesion, symptoms may show some relationship to neck or back movements, and pain is often conspicuous.

The **course** of sensory complaints provides a guide to their cause. Intermittent or repetitive transient symptoms may represent sensory seizures, ischemic phenomena, or metabolic disturbances such as those accompanying hyperventilation. Intermittent localized symptoms that occur at a consistent time may suggest the diagnosis or an exogenous precipitating factor. For example, the pain and paresthesias of carpal tunnel syndrome (median nerve compression at the wrist) characteristically occur at night and awaken the patient from sleep.

SENSORY EXAMINATION

Various sensory modalities are tested in turn, and the distribution of any abnormality is plotted with particular reference to the normal root and peripheral nerve territories. Complete loss of touch appreciation is **anesthesia**, partial loss is **hypesthesia**, and increased sensitivity is **hyperesthesia**. The corresponding terms for pain appreciation are **analgesia**, **hypalgesia**, and **hyperalgesia** or **hyperpathia**; **allodynia** refers to the misperception of a trivial tactile sensation as pain.

PRIMARY SENSORY MODALITIES

▶ Light Touch

The appreciation of light touch is evaluated with a wisp of cotton wool that is brought down carefully on a small region of skin. The patient lies with eyes closed, and indicates each time the stimulus is felt. The appreciation of light touch depends on fibers that traverse the posterior column of the spinal cord in the gracile (leg) and cuneate (arm) fasciculi ipsilaterally (Figures 10-1 and **10-2**), passing to the medial lemniscus of the brainstem (**Figure 10-3**), and on fibers in the contralateral anterior spinothalamic tract.

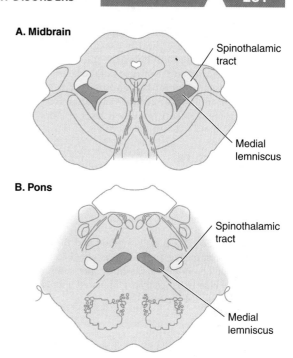

A. Midbrain
Spinothalamic tract

Medial lemniscus

B. Pons
Spinothalamic tract

Medial lemniscus

C. Medulla
Spinothalamic tract

Medial lemniscus

▲ **Figure 10-3.** Sensory pathways in the brainstem. In the medulla, spinothalamic fibers conveying pain and temperature sensation are widely separated from medial lemniscal fibers mediating touch and pressure; these pathways converge as they ascend in the pons and midbrain.

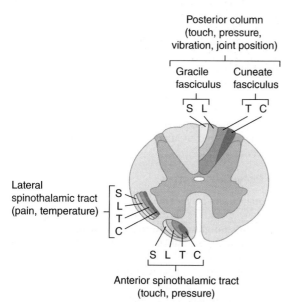

Posterior column (touch, pressure, vibration, joint position)

Gracile fasciculus | Cuneate fasciculus
S L | T C

Lateral spinothalamic tract (pain, temperature)
S
L
T
C

S L T C

Anterior spinothalamic tract (touch, pressure)

▲ **Figure 10-2.** Location and lamination of sensory pathways in the spinal cord. C (cervical), T (thoracic), L (lumbar), and S (sacral) indicate the level of origin of fibers within each tract.

▶ Pinprick & Temperature

Pinprick appreciation is tested by asking the patient to indicate whether the point of a pin (not a hypodermic needle, which may puncture the skin and draw blood) feels sharp or blunt. Appreciation of sharpness must be distinguished from appreciation of pressure or touch. The pin—a potential source of infection—should be handled with care and discarded after use. **Temperature** appreciation is evaluated by applying containers of hot or cold water to the skin. For convenience, cold can be tested by

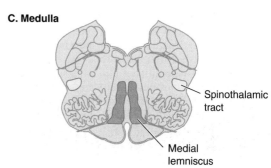

application of the side of a metal tuning fork to different bodily regions; testing of heat is usually omitted from the routine examination. Pinprick and temperature appreciation depend on the integrity of the lateral spinothalamic tracts (see Figures 10-1 and 10-2). The afferent fibers cross in front of the central canal after ascending for two or three segments from their level of entry into the cord.

Deep Pressure

Deep pressure sensibility is evaluated by pressure on the tendons, such as the Achilles tendon at the ankle.

Vibration

A tuning fork (128 Hz) is set in motion and then placed over a bony prominence; the patient is asked to indicate whether vibration, rather than simple pressure, is felt. Many healthy elderly patients have impaired appreciation of vibration below the knees.

Joint Position

The patient is asked to indicate the direction of small passive movements of the terminal interphalangeal joints of the fingers and toes. Patients with severe impairment of joint position sense may exhibit slow, continuous movement of the fingers (**pseudoathetoid movement**) when attempting to hold the hands outstretched with eyes closed. For clinical purposes, both joint position sense and the ability to appreciate vibration are considered to depend on fibers carried in the posterior columns of the spinal cord, although this is not strictly true for vibration.

COMPLEX SENSORY FUNCTIONS

Romberg Test

The patient assumes a steady stance with feet together, arms outstretched, and eyes closed and is observed for any tendency to sway or fall. The test is positive (abnormal) if unsteadiness is markedly increased by eye closure—as occurs, for example, in tabes dorsalis. A positive test is indicative of grossly impaired joint position sense in the legs.

Two-Point Discrimination

The ability to distinguish simultaneous touch at two neighboring points depends on the integrity of the central and peripheral nervous system, the degree of separation of the two points, and the part of the body that is stimulated. The patient indicates whether he or she is touched by one or two compass points, while the distance between the points is varied in order to determine the shortest distance at which they are recognized as different points. The threshold for two-point discrimination approximates 4 mm at the fingertips and may be several centimeters on the back. When peripheral sensory function is intact, impaired two-point discrimination suggests a disorder affecting the sensory cortex.

Graphesthesia, Stereognosis, & Barognosis

Agraphesthesia, the inability to identify a number traced on the skin of the palm of the hand despite normal cutaneous sensation, implies a lesion involving the contralateral parietal lobe. The same is true of inability to distinguish between various shapes or textures by touch (**astereognosis**) or impaired ability to distinguish between different weights (**abarognosis**).

Bilateral Sensory Discrimination

In some patients with apparently normal sensation, simultaneous stimulation of the two sides of the body reveals an apparent neglect of (or inattention to) sensation from one side, usually because of an underlying contralateral cerebral lesion.

SENSORY CHANGES & THEIR SIGNIFICANCE

The nature and distribution of any sensory change must be determined. Failure to find clinical evidence of sensory loss in patients with sensory symptoms should not imply that the symptoms necessarily have a psychogenic basis. Sensory symptoms often develop well before the onset of sensory signs.

PERIPHERAL NERVE LESIONS

Mononeuropathy

In patients with a lesion of a single peripheral nerve, sensory loss is usually less than predicted on anatomic grounds because of overlap from adjacent nerves. Moreover, depending on the type of lesion, the fibers in a sensory nerve may be affected differently. Compressive lesions, for example, tend to affect preferentially the large fibers subserving touch.

Polyneuropathy

In patients with polyneuropathies, sensory loss is generally symmetric and is greater distally than proximally (**stocking-and-glove sensory loss** or **length-dependent neuropathy**). The loss generally will have progressed almost to the knees before the hands are affected. Sensory loss may then be accompanied by a motor deficit and reflex changes. Diabetes mellitus, amyloidosis, and certain other metabolic disorders (eg, Tangier disease, a recessive trait characterized by the near absence of high-density lipoproteins) preferentially involve small nerve fibers subserving pain and temperature appreciation; in a pure small-fiber sensory neuropathy, the tendon reflexes are unaffected and no motor deficit occurs.

ROOT LESIONS

Nerve root involvement produces impaired cutaneous sensation in a segmental pattern (**Figure 10-4**), but because of overlap there is generally no sensory loss unless two or more adjacent roots are affected. Pain is often a conspicuous feature with compressive root lesions. Depending on the level affected, there may be loss of tendon reflexes (C5-C6, biceps and brachioradialis; C7-C8, triceps; L3-L4, knee; S1, ankle), and if the anterior roots are also involved, weakness and muscle atrophy may occur.

SPINAL CORD LESIONS

In patients with spinal cord lesions, there may be a transverse sensory level. Physiologic areas of increased sensitivity do occur, however, at the costal margin, over the breasts, and in the groin, and these must not be taken as abnormal. Therefore, the level of a sensory deficit affecting the trunk is best determined by careful sensory testing over the back rather than the chest and abdomen.

▶ Central Cord Lesion

With a central cord lesion, such as occurs in syringomyelia, after trauma, and with certain tumors, there is characteristically a loss of pain and temperature appreciation with sparing of other modalities. This loss is due to the interruption of fibers conveying pain and temperature that cross from one side of the cord to the spinothalamic tract on the other. Such a loss is usually bilateral, may be asymmetric, and involves only the fibers of the involved segments. It may be accompanied by lower motor neuron weakness in the muscles supplied by the affected segments and sometimes by a pyramidal and posterior column deficit below the lesion (**Figure 10-5**).

▶ Anterolateral Spinal Cord Lesion

Lesions involving the anterolateral portion of the spinal cord (lateral spinothalamic tract) can cause contralateral impairment of pain and temperature appreciation in segments below the level of the lesion. The spinothalamic tract is laminated, with fibers from the sacral segments the outermost. Intrinsic cord (intramedullary) lesions often spare the sacral fibers, whereas extramedullary lesions, which compress the cord, tend to involve these fibers as well as those arising from more rostral levels.

▶ Anterior Spinal Cord Lesion

With destructive lesions involving predominantly the anterior portion of the spinal cord, pain and temperature appreciation are impaired below the level of the lesion from lateral spinothalamic tract involvement. In addition, weakness or paralysis of muscles supplied by the involved segments of the cord results from damage to anterior horn cells. With more extensive disease, involvement of the corticospinal tracts in the lateral funiculi may cause a pyramidal deficit below the lesion. There is relative preservation of posterior column function (**Figure 10-6**). Ischemic myelopathies caused by occlusion of the anterior spinal artery take the form of anterior spinal cord lesions.

▶ Posterior Column Lesion

A patient with a posterior column lesion may complain of a tight or bandlike sensation in the regions corresponding to the level of spinal involvement and sometimes also of paresthesias (like electric shocks) radiating down the extremities on neck flexion (**Lhermitte sign**). There is loss of vibration and joint position sense below the level of the lesion, with preservation of other sensory modalities. The deficit may resemble that resulting from involvement of large fibers in the posterior roots.

▶ Spinal Cord Hemisection

Lateral hemisection of the spinal cord leads to **Brown–Séquard syndrome.** Below the lesion, there is an ipsilateral pyramidal deficit and disturbed appreciation of vibration and joint position sense; contralateral loss of pain and temperature appreciation begins two or three segments below the lesion (**Figure 10-7**). Hyperalgesia and spontaneous pain are sometimes prominent ipsilaterally.

BRAINSTEM LESIONS

With brainstem lesions, sensory disturbances may be accompanied by a motor deficit, cerebellar signs, and cranial nerve palsies.

With lesions involving the spinothalamic tract in the dorsolateral medulla and pons, pain and temperature appreciation are lost in the limbs and trunk on the opposite side of the body. When such a lesion is medullary, it also typically involves the spinal trigeminal nucleus, impairing pain and temperature sensation on the same side of the face as the lesion. The result is a **crossed sensory deficit** that affects the ipsilateral face and contralateral limbs. In contrast, spinothalamic lesions above the spinal trigeminal nucleus affect the face, limbs, and trunk contralateral to the lesion. With lesions affecting the medial lemniscus, there is loss of touch and proprioception on the opposite side of the body. In the upper brainstem, the spinothalamic tract and medial lemniscus run together so that a single lesion may cause loss of all superficial and deep sensation over the contralateral side of the body (see Figure 10-3).

THALAMIC LESIONS

Thalamic lesions may lead to loss or impairment of all forms of sensation on the contralateral side of the body, and this may have a distribution that differs from the area of symptomatic involvement. Spontaneous pain, sometimes with a particularly unpleasant quality, may occur on the affected side. Patients may describe it as burning,

Peripheral nerve   **Nerve root**

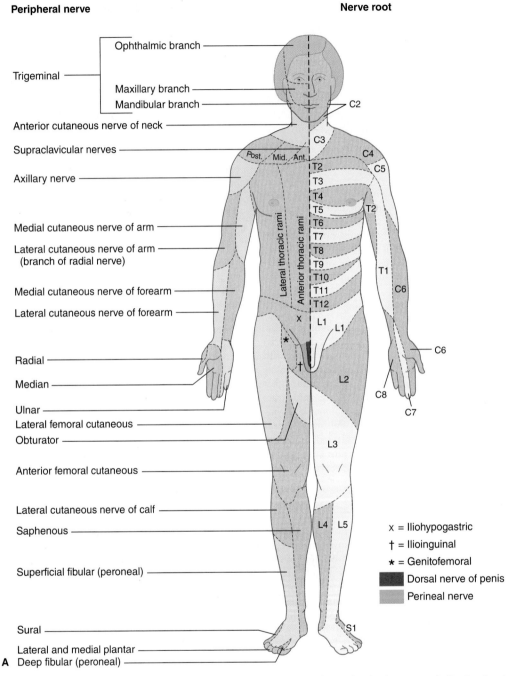

Ophthalmic branch

Trigeminal

Maxillary branch

Mandibular branch

C2

Anterior cutaneous nerve of neck

C3

Supraclavicular nerves

Post. Mid. Ant.

C4

Axillary nerve

C5

T2

T3

T4

T5

T6

Medial cutaneous nerve of arm

T7

Lateral cutaneous nerve of arm
(branch of radial nerve)

T8

T9

T10

T1

Medial cutaneous nerve of forearm

T11

C6

Lateral cutaneous nerve of forearm

T12

X

L1

L1

★

C6

Radial

Median

L2

Ulnar

C8

Lateral femoral cutaneous

C7

Obturator

Anterior femoral cutaneous

L3

Lateral cutaneous nerve of calf

Saphenous

L4 L5

x = Iliohypogastric

† = Ilioinguinal

Superficial fibular (peroneal)

★ = Genitofemoral

Dorsal nerve of penis

Perineal nerve

Sural

S1

Lateral and medial plantar

A   Deep fibular (peroneal)

Lateral thoracic rami

Anterior thoracic rami

▲ **Figure 10-4.** (**A**) Cutaneous innervation (anterior view). The segmental or radicular (nerve root) distribution is shown on the left side of the body, and the peripheral nerve distribution on the right side of the body. (**B**) Cutaneous innervation (posterior view). The segmental or radicular (nerve root) distribution is shown on the left side of the body, and the peripheral nerve distribution on the right side of the body. Segmental maps show differences depending on how they were constructed (single root stimulation or section; local anesthetic injection into single dorsal root ganglia). For details of radial, median, ulnar, fibular (peroneal), and femoral nerves, see Appendix.

Nerve root

Peripheral nerve

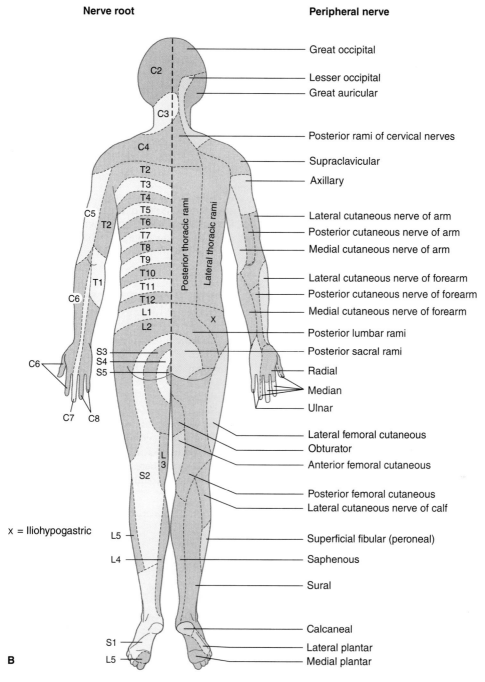

- Great occipital
- Lesser occipital
- Great auricular
- Posterior rami of cervical nerves
- Supraclavicular
- Axillary
- Lateral cutaneous nerve of arm
- Posterior cutaneous nerve of arm
- Medial cutaneous nerve of arm
- Lateral cutaneous nerve of forearm
- Posterior cutaneous nerve of forearm
- Medial cutaneous nerve of forearm
- Posterior lumbar rami
- Posterior sacral rami
- Radial
- Median
- Ulnar
- Lateral femoral cutaneous
- Obturator
- Anterior femoral cutaneous
- Posterior femoral cutaneous
- Lateral cutaneous nerve of calf
- Superficial fibular (peroneal)
- Saphenous
- Sural
- Calcaneal
- Lateral plantar
- Medial plantar

x = Iliohypogastric

B

▲ **Figure 10-4.** (*Continued*)

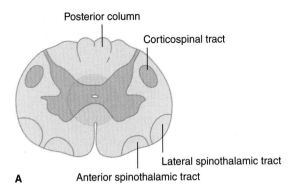

A

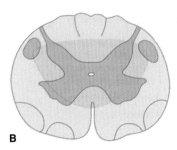

B

▲ **Figure 10-5.** Central cord lesions (blue) of moderate (**A**) or marked (**B**) extent. Less extensive lesions impair pain and temperature appreciation by interrupting incoming sensory fibers as they cross to the contralateral spinothalamic tract; involvement of anterior horn cells causes lower motor neuron weakness. These deficits are restricted to dermatomes and muscles innervated by the involved spinal cord segments. More extensive lesions also produce disturbances of touch, pressure, vibration, and joint position sense because of involvement of the posterior columns and cause pyramidal signs because of corticospinal tract involvement, especially affecting the arms (see lamination of corticospinal tract in Figure 9-6). These deficits occur below the level of the lesion.

tearing, knifelike, or stabbing, but often have difficulty characterizing it. Any form of cutaneous stimulation can lead to painful or unpleasant sensations. Such a thalamic syndrome (**Dejerine–Roussy syndrome**) can also occasionally result from lesions of the white matter of the parietal lobe or from spinal cord lesions, as discussed later.

LESIONS OF THE SENSORY CORTEX

Disease limited to the sensory cortex impairs discriminative sensory function on the opposite side of the body. Patients may be unable to localize stimuli on the affected side or to recognize the position of different parts of the body. They may not be able to recognize objects by touch or to estimate their size, weight, consistency, or texture. Cortical sensory disturbances are usually more conspicuous in the hands than in the trunk or proximal portions of the limbs.

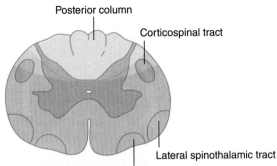

▲ **Figure 10-6.** Anterior spinal cord lesion (blue) associated with occlusion of the anterior spinal artery. Clinical features are similar to those seen with severe central cord lesions (see Figure 10-5B), except that posterior column sensory functions are spared and the defect in pain and temperature sensation extends to sacral levels.

DISTINCTION BETWEEN ORGANIC & PSYCHOGENIC SENSORY DISTURBANCES

Psychogenic disturbances of sensation may be associated with such psychiatric disturbances as conversion disorder. They may take any form but most often are restricted to **loss of cutaneous sensation.** There may be several characteristic features.

Nonorganic sensory loss does not conform in its distribution to any specific **neuroanatomic pattern.** It may surround a bony landmark or involve an area defined by surface landmarks rather than innervation. Indeed, it is not uncommon for there to be an apparent loss of sensation in one or more extremities, with circumferential margins in

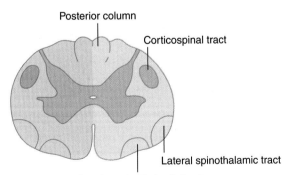

▲ **Figure 10-7.** Spinal cord lesion (blue) in Brown–Séquard syndrome. Lateral hemisection of the spinal cord causes ipsilateral pyramidal dysfunction and impairment of posterior column sensory function below the level of the lesion, and contralateral impairment of pain and temperature sensation with an upper limit slightly below the level of the lesion.

the axilla or groin; organic sensory loss with such a margin is unusual. Organic peripheral sensory loss over the trunk or face does not usually extend to the midline but stops 3 to 5 cm before it, because of overlap in the innervation on the two sides; with nonorganic disturbances, apparent sensory loss commonly stops precisely at the midline.

There is often a **sudden transition** between areas of nonorganic sensory loss and areas with normal sensation. By contrast, with organic disturbances, there is usually an area of altered sensation between insensitive areas and adjacent areas with normal sensibility.

In nonorganic disturbances, there may be a **dissociated loss** that is difficult to interpret on an anatomic basis. For example, there may be a total loss of pinprick appreciation but preserved temperature sensation. Moreover, despite the apparent loss of posterior column function, the patient may be able to walk normally or maintain the arms outstretched without difficulty or pseudoathetoid movements.

In nonorganic sensory disturbances, appreciation of **vibration** may be impaired on one side but not the other side of a bony midline structure, such as the skull or sternum. The vibrations are in fact conducted to both sides by the bone, so that even if there is a hemisensory disturbance, the vibrations are appreciated on either side in patients with organic sensory disorders.

Finally, it should be noted that sensory disturbances are often **suggested** to the patient by the examiner's own expectations. Such findings can be particularly misleading because they may be neuroanatomically correct. One helpful approach is to have the patient outline on the body the extent of any perceived sensory disturbance before formal sensory testing is undertaken.

PERIPHERAL NERVE LESIONS

Sensory symptoms are usually a conspicuous feature in patients with peripheral nerve lesions (**Table 10-1**). Sensory impairment may be in a distal stocking-and-glove pattern in patients with polyneuropathies or may follow

Table 10-1. Causes of Peripheral Neuropathy.

Idiopathic inflammatory neuropathies	Drug-induced and toxic neuropathies
Acute idiopathic polyneuropathy (Guillain–Barré syndrome)	Alcohol
Chronic inflammatory demyelinating polyneuropathy	Therapeutic drugs (see Table 10-2)
Metabolic and nutritional neuropathies	Toxins
Diabetes	Organic compounds
Other endocrinopathies	Hexacarbons
Hypothyroidism	Organophosphates
Acromegaly	Heavy metals
Uremia	Arsenic
Liver disease	Lead
Vitamin B$_{12}$ deficiency	Thallium
Infective and granulomatous neuropathies	Gold
AIDS	Platinum
Leprosy	Tryptophan (contaminant)
Diphtheria	**Hereditary neuropathies**
Sarcoidosis	Idiopathic
Sepsis and multiorgan failure	Hereditary motor and sensory neuropathies
Vasculitic neuropathies	Hereditary sensory and autonomic neuropathies
Systemic necrotizing vasculitis	Familial amyloidosis
Granulomatosis with polyangiitis (Wegener granulomatosis)	Friedreich ataxia
Giant cell arteritis	Hereditary neuropathy with liability to pressure palsies
Rheumatoid arthritis	Metabolic
Systemic lupus erythematosus	Porphyria
Sjögren syndrome	Metachromatic leukodystrophy
Scleroderma	Krabbe disease
Mixed connective tissue disease	Abetalipoproteinemia
Neoplastic and paraproteinemic neuropathies	Tangier disease
Compression and infiltration by tumor	Refsum disease
Paraneoplastic syndromes	Fabry disease
Paraproteinemias	**Entrapment neuropathies**
Amyloidosis	

the pattern of individual peripheral nerves in patients with mononeuropathies (see Figure 10-4).

CLASSIFICATION

MONONEUROPATHY SIMPLEX

This term signifies involvement of a single peripheral nerve.

MONONEUROPATHY MULTIPLEX

In this disorder, several individual nerves are affected, usually at random and noncontiguously. Clinical examination reveals a clinical deficit attributable to involvement of one or more isolated peripheral nerves, except when mononeuropathy multiplex is extensive and the resulting deficits become confluent.

POLYNEUROPATHY

The term *polyneuropathy* denotes a disorder in which the function of several peripheral nerves is affected at the same time. This leads to a predominantly distal and symmetric deficit, with loss of tendon reflexes except when small fibers are selectively involved. Polyneuropathies are sometimes subclassified according to the primary site at which the nerve is affected.

In **distal axonopathies (axonal neuropathies)**, the axon is the principal pathologic target; most polyneuropathies fall into this category.

Myelinopathies (demyelinating neuropathies) are conditions that involve the myelin sheath surrounding the axon. These disorders include acute idiopathic polyneuropathy (Guillain–Barré syndrome), chronic inflammatory demyelinating neuropathy, diphtheria, certain paraneoplastic and paraproteinemic states, and various hereditary conditions including metachromatic leukodystrophy, Krabbe disease, and types 1 and 3 Charcot–Marie–Tooth hereditary motor and sensory neuropathy (CMT-1 and 3).

Finally, certain disorders, termed **neuronopathies,** principally affect nerve cell bodies in the anterior horn of the spinal cord or dorsal root ganglion. Examples are type 2 CMT hereditary motor and sensory neuropathy, pyridoxine-induced neuropathy, and some paraneoplastic syndromes.

CLINICAL FINDINGS

SENSORY DISTURBANCES

Involvement of sensory fibers can lead to numbness and impaired sensation; abnormal spontaneous sensations, such as pain and paresthesias; and perverted sensations such as hyperpathia (amplified response to a normally painful stimulus).

▶ Pain

Pain is a conspicuous feature of certain neuropathies, especially if **small fibers** within the nerves are affected. The precise mechanism of its genesis is unclear. Polyneuropathies associated with prominent pain include those related to diabetes, alcoholism, porphyria, Fabry disease, amyloidosis, rheumatoid arthritis, and acquired immunodeficiency syndrome (AIDS), as well as dominantly inherited sensory neuropathy and paraneoplastic sensory neuronopathy. Pain is also a feature of many entrapment neuropathies and of idiopathic brachial plexopathy.

▶ Dissociated Sensory Loss

Dissociated sensory loss is impairment of some sensory modalities, such as pain and temperature, with preservation of others, such as light touch, vibration, and joint position sense. Although the presence of a dissociated sensory loss often indicates a spinal cord lesion, it also occurs in peripheral neuropathies when there is selective involvement of peripheral nerve fibers of a certain size, such as occurs in amyloid neuropathy, leprous neuritis, or hereditary sensory neuropathy. **Small fiber** disease is commonly associated with disproportionate impairment of pain and temperature appreciation, spontaneous pain, and autonomic dysfunction. **Large fiber** disease, by contrast, results in defective touch, vibration, and joint position sense, early loss of tendon reflexes, and prominent motor symptoms.

MOTOR DEFICITS

Peripheral nerve lesions may cause weakness of muscles innervated by the nerve, accompanied in severe cases by wasting and fasciculation. There may be difficulty in the performance of fine tasks; this is compounded by any accompanying sensory loss. The clinical findings reflect a lower motor neuron deficit, and it is the distribution of these signs and the presence of accompanying sensory and reflex changes that suggest they may be due to peripheral nerve involvement.

TENDON REFLEXES

These are impaired or lost if reflex arcs are interrupted on either the afferent or efferent side (C5-C6, biceps and brachioradialis; C7-C8, triceps; L3-L4, knee; S1, ankle). The ankle reflexes are usually the first to be lost in patients with polyneuropathies, but may also be absent in healthy elderly subjects.

AUTONOMIC DISTURBANCES

Autonomic disturbances are particularly conspicuous in some peripheral neuropathies—especially Guillain–Barré syndrome and neuropathies related to diabetes, renal failure, porphyria, certain paraneoplastic disorders, and amyloidosis. Symptoms include postural hypotension, tachycardia, cold extremities, impaired thermoregulatory sweating, bladder and bowel dysfunction, and impotence.

ENLARGED NERVES

Palpably enlarged peripheral nerves raise the possibility of leprosy, amyloidosis, hereditary motor and sensory neuropathies, Refsum disease, acromegaly, or chronic inflammatory demyelinating polyneuropathy.

EVALUATION OF PATIENTS

TIME COURSE

Polyneuropathy that develops acutely over a few days usually relates to an inflammatory process, as in the Guillain–Barré syndrome. It may also relate to an underlying neoplasm, to infections such as diphtheria, to metabolic disorders such as acute intermittent porphyria, or to exposure to such toxic substances as thallium or triorthocresyl phosphate. A chronic course with a gradual evolution over several years is typical of many hereditary or metabolic polyneuropathies but also characterizes chronic inflammatory demyelinating polyneuropathy.

Mononeuropathy of acute onset is likely to be traumatic or ischemic in origin, whereas one evolving gradually is more likely to relate to entrapment (ie, compression by neighboring anatomic structures) or to recurrent minor trauma.

AGE AT ONSET

Polyneuropathy that develops during childhood or early adult life often has a hereditary basis, but may also relate to an underlying inflammatory disorder. Polyneuropathy developing later is more likely to result from a metabolic, toxic, or inflammatory disorder, or from an underlying neoplasm.

Mononeuropathy presenting in the neonatal period is likely to be developmental in origin or related to birth injury; one presenting in later life may relate to entrapment or injury that is often occupationally determined.

OCCUPATIONAL HISTORY

Various **industrial toxins** can lead to peripheral neuropathy, including carbon disulfide, *n*-hexane, ethylene oxide, methyl bromide, acrylamide, triorthocresyl phosphate and certain other organophosphates, DDT, arsenic, lead, and thallium. A mononeuropathy is sometimes the first clinical manifestation of an occupationally related polyneuropathy, but it may also develop in response to entrapment or recurrent minor occupational trauma. For example, **carpal tunnel syndrome** is more common in persons who do heavy manual labor or develop repetitive motion injury as a result of computer terminal use, and a lesion of the deep palmar branch of the ulnar nerve may relate to repeated pressure on the palm of the hand by, for example, punching down heavily on a stapler or using heavy equipment such as a pneumatic road drill.

MEDICAL HISTORY

▶ Metabolic Disorders

Peripheral neuropathy may relate to metabolic disorders such as diabetes mellitus, uremia, liver disease, myxedema, acromegaly, metachromatic leukodystrophy, or Fabry disease. That caused by diabetes is especially important and may take the form of an entrapment mononeuropathy, acute ischemic mononeuropathy, distal sensorimotor polyneuropathy, subacute proximal motor polyradiculoplexopathy (diabetic amyotrophy), thoracoabdominal radiculopathy, or autonomic neuropathy.

▶ Neoplasm

The peripheral nerves, spinal nerves, and limb plexuses may be compressed or infiltrated by extension of primary tumors or metastatic lymph nodes. Neoplastic disease can also lead to a nonmetastatic (**paraneoplastic**) sensory or sensorimotor polyneuropathy or to Lambert–Eaton syndrome, a disorder of neuromuscular transmission discussed in Chapter 9, Motor Disorders.

▶ Connective Tissue Disorders

Polyarteritis nodosa, rheumatoid arthritis, Churg–Strauss syndrome, and granulomatosis with polyangiitis (formerly Wegener granulomatosis) may be associated with mononeuropathy multiplex or, less commonly, polyneuropathy or cranial neuropathy. Polyneuropathy is more common in systemic lupus erythematosus. Rheumatoid arthritis may cause focal entrapment or compressive mononeuropathies in the vicinity of affected joints.

▶ Infection With Human Immunodeficiency Virus

Acquired immune deficiency syndrome (AIDS) is commonly associated with a distal, symmetric, primarily sensory polyneuropathy. Less frequently, AIDS is associated with an acute or chronic inflammatory demyelinating polyneuropathy, polyradiculopathy, mononeuropathy multiplex, or autonomic neuropathy. Neuropathies are also seen with asymptomatic human immunodeficiency virus-1 (HIV-1) infection and HIV-1 seroconversion.

DRUG & ALCOHOL HISTORY

Some of the drugs that cause peripheral neuropathy are listed in **Table 10-2**; motor or sensory fibers are involved selectively with certain drugs.

Table 10-2. Selected Drugs Inducing Peripheral Neuropathy.

Sensory neuropathy
Chloramphenicol
Cisplatin
Docetaxel
Pyridoxine
Taxol
Predominantly sensory neuropathy
Ethambutol
Hydralazine
Metronidazole
Misonidazole
Motor neuropathy
Dapsone
Imipramine
Sulfonamides (some)
Mixed sensory and motor neuropathy
Amiodarone
Chloroquine
Disulfiram
Gold
Indomethacin
Isoniazid
Nitrofurantoin
Penicillamine
Perhexiline
Phenytoin
Thalidomide
Tryptophan (contaminant)
Vincristine

FAMILY HISTORY

Polyneuropathies may have a hereditary basis, as is discussed later in this chapter in the section on hereditary neuropathies.

DIFFERENTIAL DIAGNOSIS

Peripheral neuropathies can lead to a motor or sensory deficit or both. The preservation of sensation and tendon reflexes distinguishes the motor deficit of pure pyramidal lesions, spinal muscular atrophies, myopathies, or disorders of neuromuscular transmission from that caused by peripheral nerve involvement. Other distinguishing features are discussed in Chapter 9, Motor Disorders.

Myelopathies are characterized by a pyramidal deficit below the level of the lesion as well as by distal sensory loss. In tabes dorsalis, there is often a history of syphilitic infection, and examination reveals other stigmas of syphilis. In addition, tactile sensation is preserved.

Radiculopathies are distinguished from peripheral neuropathies by the distribution of motor or sensory deficits (see Figure 10-4). The presence of neck or back pain that radiates to the extremities in a radicular distribution also suggests a root lesion.

INVESTIGATIVE STUDIES

Laboratory studies in patients with peripheral neuropathy are directed at confirming the diagnosis and revealing any underlying cause.

Electromyography may reveal evidence of denervation in the affected muscles and can be used to determine whether any motor units remain under voluntary control. **Nerve conduction studies** permit conduction velocity to be measured in motor and sensory fibers (see Chapter 2, Investigative Studies). On the basis of electrodiagnostic or histopathologic studies, peripheral neuropathies can be divided into demyelinating or axonal neuropathies. In **demyelinating neuropathies,** electromyography typically reveals little or no evidence of denervation, but there is conduction block or marked slowing of maximal conduction velocity in affected nerves. In **axonal neuropathies**, electromyography shows that denervation has occurred, especially distally in the extremities, but maximal nerve conduction velocity is normal or slowed only slightly.

Determination of a complete blood count, erythrocyte sedimentation rate, serum urea nitrogen and creatinine, fasting blood glucose, serum vitamin B_{12}, serum protein, protein electrophoresis and immunoelectrophoresis, liver and thyroid function blood tests, and serologic test for syphilis (FTA or MHA-TP), rheumatoid factor, and antinuclear antibody may help to identify the cause of a peripheral nerve disorder, as also may chest x-ray. Depending on the clinical circumstances, serologic tests for Lyme disease, hepatitis, infection with HIV, or paraneoplastic antibodies may be required. Genetic studies may also be necessary after appropriate genetic counseling.

If toxic causes are suspected, a 24-hour urine collection followed by analysis for heavy metals may be helpful, and hair and fingernail clippings can be analyzed for arsenic. Examination of a fresh specimen of urine for porphobilinogen and δ-aminolevulinic acid is necessary when porphyria is suspected.

TREATMENT

DISEASE-SPECIFIC TREATMENT

Treatment of the underlying cause may limit the progression of or even reverse the neuropathy. Disease-specific treatments are discussed later under individual disorders.

VENTILATORY ASSISTANCE

Respiratory function must be monitored—particularly in acute idiopathic polyneuropathy (Guillain–Barré syndrome), chronic inflammatory demyelinating polyneuropathy, and diphtheritic neuropathy—and preparations made to assist ventilation if the forced vital capacity reaches 15 mL/kg, the mean inspiratory force reaches −40 mm Hg, dyspnea becomes evident, or the oxygen saturation of arterial blood declines.

TRAUMA PREVENTION

Nursing care is important in patients with severe motor or sensory deficits to prevent **decubitus ulcers, joint contractures,** and additional **compressive peripheral nerve damage**. In patients with severe **dysesthesia,** a cradle (metal bar frame) can be used to keep the bedclothes from touching sensitive areas of the skin.

Extremities with **sensory loss** must be protected from repeated minor trauma, such as thermal injury, that can destroy tissues. The temperature of hot surfaces should be checked with a part of the body in which sensation is preserved, and the setting of water heaters must be reduced to prevent scalding. The skin and nails must be cared for meticulously.

PAIN RELIEF

Patients with sensory disorders may suffer from especially severe pain, which can impair quality of life. Treatment of this pain is important.

Duloxetine (60 mg once daily) or **venlafaxine** (titrated up to 75 mg two to three times daily in standard formulation or as the equivalent dose once daily in the extended release formulation) is often helpful; both are selective serotonin and norepinephrine reuptake inhibitors.

Pregabalin (150 mg increasing after 1 week to 300 mg daily in divided doses; maximum, 600 mg daily) also relieves neuropathic pain.

Phenytoin 300 mg/d, **carbamazepine** up to 1200 mg/d, or **mexiletine** 600 to 900 mg/d can sometimes relieve the lancinating pain of certain neuropathies. If the pain is constant, burning, or dysesthetic, **amitriptyline** 25 to 100 mg at bedtime is often helpful, as are other tricyclic agents.

Gabapentin (300 mg three times daily, with subsequent increments depending on response and tolerance) is effective in treating various neuropathic pain disorders; pain relief may similarly occur with **lamotrigine, topiramate,** or **sodium valproate**, but this has been documented less well. Lamotrigine requires slow dose titration to avoid skin rashes and other complications. Combined gabapentin and nortriptyline may be more effective than either drug given alone for neuropathic pain (diabetic neuropathy or postherpetic neuralgia). This drug combination is therefore recommended in patients who show a partial response to either drug given alone and require additional pain relief.

Topical **capsaicin** is also helpful in neuropathic pain syndromes.

AUTONOMIC DISTURBANCES

Dysautonomic symptoms may be troublesome in some polyneuropathies, especially diabetic polyneuropathy. Waist-high elastic hosiery, dietary salt supplementation, and treatment with fludrocortisone 0.1 to 0.5 mg/d orally may relieve **postural hypotension,** but the patient must be monitored to prevent recumbent hypertension. Other medications that may be helpful include clonidine, midodrine, dihydroergotamine, octreotide, or β-blockers. The utility of droxidopa in peripheral dysautonomias is unclear. Instructing the patients to sleep in a semierect rather than recumbent position is helpful because dysautonomic patients are often unable to conserve salt and water when recumbent.

POLYNEUROPATHIES

IDIOPATHIC INFLAMMATORY NEUROPATHIES

ACUTE IDIOPATHIC POLYNEUROPATHY (GUILLAIN–BARRÉ SYNDROME)

Guillain–Barré syndrome is an acute or subacute polyneuropathy that can follow minor infective illnesses, inoculations, or surgical procedures or may occur without obvious precipitants. Clinical and epidemiologic evidence suggests an association with preceding *Campylobacter jejuni* infection. It may also occur in association with Zika virus infection. Its precise cause is unclear, but an immunologic basis is likely. Both demyelinating and axonal forms occur, with distinctive clinical and electrophysiologic features. The **demyelinative** form is more common in the United States, but an axonal variant is encountered occasionally (**acute motor sensory axonal neuropathy**). In northern China, a related axonal form occurs frequently (**acute motor axonal neuropathy** or **AMAN**). The axonal variants are caused by antibodies to gangliosides on the axon membrane, including anti-GM1, anti-GM1b, anti-GD1a, anti-GD1b, and (in AMAN) anti-GalNAC-GD1a antibodies. The **Miller Fisher syndrome**, another subtype, is characterized by ophthalmoplegia, ataxia, and areflexia, and is associated with anti-GQ1b antibodies (see Chapter 8, Disorders of Equilibrium); it is sometimes associated with a brainstem encephalitis (**Bickerstaff encephalitis**).

Clinical Features

Diagnostic features are summarized in **Table 10-3**. Patients commonly present with **ascending weakness** that is symmetric, usually begins in the legs, is often more marked

Table 10-3. Diagnostic Criteria for Guillain–Barré Syndrome.

Required for diagnosis
Progressive weakness of more than one limb
Distal areflexia with proximal areflexia or hyporeflexia
Supportive of diagnosis
Progression for up to 4 weeks
Relatively symmetric deficits
Mild sensory involvement
Cranial nerve (especially VII) involvement
Recovery beginning within 4 weeks after progression stops
Autonomic dysfunction
No fever at onset
Increased CSF protein after 1 week
CSF white blood cell count ≤10/μL
Nerve conduction slowing or block by several weeks
Against diagnosis
Markedly asymmetric weakness
Bowel or bladder dysfunction (at onset or persistent)
CSF white blood cell count >50 or PMN count >0/μL
Well-demarcated sensory level
Excluding diagnosis
Isolated sensory involvement
Another polyneuropathy that explains clinical picture

Data from Asbury AK, Cornblath DR. Assessment of current diagnostic criteria for Guillain-Barré syndrome. *Ann Neurol.* 1990; 27(suppl):S21-S24.

proximally than distally, and may be life-threatening, especially if the muscles of respiration or swallowing are involved. Some patients present instead with weakness about the bulbar, neck, and shoulder muscles, or with an acute pandysautonomia. Muscle wasting develops if axonal degeneration has occurred. Sensory complaints, although usually less marked than motor symptoms, are also frequent. The deep tendon reflexes are typically absent. There may be marked autonomic dysfunction, with tachycardia, cardiac irregularities, labile blood pressure, disturbed sweating, impaired pulmonary function, sphincter disturbances, paralytic ileus, and other abnormalities.

Investigative Studies

The cerebrospinal fluid (CSF) often shows an increased protein concentration but normal cell count (**cytoalbuminologic dissociation**), but abnormalities may not occur in the first week. Electrophysiologic studies may reveal marked slowing of motor and sensory conduction velocity or evidence of denervation and axonal loss. The time course of the electrophysiologic changes does not necessarily parallel any clinical developments. When HIV-1 infection is suspected because of the clinical context in which

the neuropathy has developed, the presence of high-risk factors, or a CSF pleocytosis, appropriate serologic studies should be performed.

Treatment

Plasmapheresis reduces the time required for recovery and may decrease the likelihood of residual neurologic deficits. It is best instituted early, and it is indicated especially in patients with a severe or rapidly progressive deficit or respiratory compromise. **Intravenous immunoglobulin** (400 mg/kg/d for 5 days) is equally effective and should be used in preference to plasmapheresis in adults with cardiovascular instability and in children; the two therapies are not additive.

Therapy is otherwise symptomatic, the aim being to prevent such complications as respiratory failure or vascular collapse. For this reason, patients who are severely affected are best managed in intensive care units, where facilities are available for monitoring and assisted respiration if necessary (eg, if the forced vital capacity reaches 15 mL/kg, the mean inspiratory force reaches –40 mm Hg, the patient is short of breath, or the blood oxygen saturation declines). Paroxysmal hypertension may necessitate treatment with labetalol or nitroprusside. Volume replacement or treatment with pressor agents is sometimes required to counter hypotension, and low-dose heparin may help to prevent pulmonary embolism. Cardiac arrhythmias are common and—depending on their nature—may require treatment. Corticosteroids may affect the outcome adversely or delay recovery, and are not indicated. Physical therapy and rehabilitation are important aspects of treatment.

Prognosis

Symptoms and signs cease to progress by approximately 4 weeks into the illness. The disorder is self-limiting, and improvement occurs over the weeks or months after onset. Approximately 70% of patients recover completely, 25% are left with mild neurologic deficits, and 5% die, usually as a result of respiratory failure. The prognosis is poorer when there is evidence of preceding *Campylobacter jejuni* infection, and a more protracted course and less complete recovery are also likely when axonal degeneration is the primary pathology. Advanced age, the need for ventilatory support, or more rapid onset of symptoms may also predict a poorer prognosis.

CHRONIC INFLAMMATORY DEMYELINATING POLYNEUROPATHY

Chronic inflammatory demyelinating polyneuropathy is clinically similar to Guillain–Barré syndrome except that it follows a chronic progressive course, or a course characterized by relapses, and no improvement is apparent within the 6 months after onset. Its cause is not known. Its clinical

Table 10-4. Clinical Features of Chronic Inflammatory Demyelinating Polyneuropathy.

Clinical Features	Percentage of Patients
Weakness, hyporeflexia, or areflexia	94
Distal upper extremity	85
Distal lower extremity	85
Proximal upper extremity	74
Proximal lower extremity	68
Respiratory muscles	11
Neck	4
Face	2
Sensory deficit on examination	
Distal lower extremity	83
Distal upper extremity	68
Paresthesia	
Upper extremity	79
Lower extremity	72
Face	6
Pain	
Lower extremity	17
Upper extremity	15
Dysarthria	9
Dysphagia	9
Impotence	4
Incontinence	2

Adapted with permission from Dyck PJ, Lais AC, Ohta M, et al. Chronic inflammatory polyradiculopathy. *Mayo Clin Proc.* 1975;50:621-637. Copyright © Elsevier.

features are summarized in **Table 10-4**. It must be distinguished from certain hereditary demyelinating neuropathies, discussed later in this chapter.

Examination of the CSF reveals findings resembling those in Guillain–Barré syndrome: the protein is elevated while the white-cell count is normal. The electrophysiologic findings indicate a demyelinative neuropathy with superimposed axonal degeneration. Laboratory studies may help to identify disorders causing neuropathy, such as diabetes.

The disorder is often responsive to treatment with **corticosteroids** (prednisone 60-100 mg/d for 2-4 weeks, then gradually tapered to 5-20 mg every other day), which may be required on a long-term basis. Treatment with **intravenous immunoglobulin** (1 g/kg daily for 2 days with a single additional infusion at 3 weeks, or 400 mg/kg/d for 5

consecutive days for a total of 2 g, with subsequent courses as needed to maintain benefit) is also effective as initial or later therapy. When used as initial therapy, it has the advantage of fewer side effects (but greater expense) than prednisone. Its precise mode of action is unknown. Plasma exchange is another effective immunomodulator therapy, but is more difficult to administer. In nonresponsive patients, treatment with methotrexate, azathioprine, or cyclophosphamide may be helpful, but claims of benefit from these agents or from cyclosporine, interferon-β, or interferon-α require confirmation by randomized trials.

METABOLIC & NUTRITIONAL NEUROPATHIES

DIABETES MELLITUS

Peripheral nerve involvement in diabetes is common and may take several forms (**Table 10-5**), which can occur in isolation or in any combination. The incidence of peripheral nerve involvement may be influenced by the adequacy of diabetes control, which should, in any event, be optimized.

▶ Clinical Features

Distal **polyneuropathy** is the most common manifestation and may be mixed (sensory, motor, and autonomic; 70% of cases) or predominantly sensory (30%). Symptoms are

Table 10-5. Neuropathies Associated With Diabetes.

Type	Distribution
Polyneuropathy	
Mixed sensory, motor, and autonomic	Symmetric, distal, lower > upper limbs
Primarily sensory	
Mononeuropathy multiplex	Variable
Polyradiculopathy/plexopathy	
Diabetic amyotrophy	Asymmetric, proximal (pelvic girdle and thighs)
Thoracoabdominal radiculopathy	Chest, abdomen
Mononeuropathy simplex	
Peripheral	Ulnar, median, radial, lateral femoral cutaneous, sciatic, fibular (peroneal), other nerves
Cranial	Oculomotor (III) > abducens (VI) > trochlear (IV) nerve
	Facial (VII) nerve

generally more common in the legs than arms and consist of numbness, pain, or paresthesias. It may be diagnosed presymptomatically by the presence of depressed tendon reflexes and impaired appreciation of vibration in the legs. In severe cases, there is distal sensory loss in all limbs and some accompanying motor disturbance.

Diabetic **dysautonomia** leads to many symptoms, including postural hypotension, disturbances of cardiac rhythm, impaired thermoregulatory sweating, and disturbances of bladder, bowel, gastric, and sexual function.

Diabetic **mononeuropathy multiplex** is usually characterized by pain and weakness and often has a vascular basis. The clinical deficit depends on the nerves that are affected.

Diabetic **amyotrophy** is due to radiculoplexopathy, polyradiculopathy, or polyradiculoneuropathy. Pain, weakness, and atrophy of pelvic girdle and thigh muscles are typical, with absent quadriceps reflexes and little sensory loss.

Diabetic **mononeuropathy simplex** is typically abrupt in onset and often painful.

CSF protein concentration is typically increased in diabetic polyneuropathy and mononeuropathy multiplex.

▶ Treatment & Prognosis

No specific treatment exists for the peripheral nerve complications of diabetes except when the patient has an entrapment neuropathy and may benefit from a decompressive procedure. The treatment of pain or autonomic disturbances was outlined earlier. Diabetic amyotrophy usually improves spontaneously. It is important that the control of diabetes is optimized.

OTHER ENDOCRINOPATHIES

▶ Hypothyroidism

Hypothyroidism is associated with entrapment neuropathy, especially carpal tunnel syndrome (median nerve entrapment; see later), but rarely causes a polyneuropathy. Polyneuropathy may be mistakenly diagnosed in patients with proximal limb weakness caused by hypothyroid myopathy or in patients with delayed relaxation of tendon reflexes, a classic manifestation of hypothyroidism that is independent of neuropathy. Other neurologic manifestations of hypothyroidism include an acute confusional state (see Chapter 4, Confusional States), dementia (see Chapter 5, Dementia & Amnestic Disorders), and cerebellar ataxia (see Chapter 8, Disorders of Equilibrium).

▶ Acromegaly

This also frequently produces carpal tunnel syndrome and, less often, polyneuropathy. Because many acromegalic patients are also diabetic, it may be difficult to determine which disorder is primarily responsible for polyneuropathy in a given patient.

UREMIA

A symmetric sensorimotor polyneuropathy, predominantly axonal in type, may occur in uremia. It affects the legs more than the arms, is more marked distally than proximally, and relates to the severity of impaired renal function. Restless legs, muscle cramps, and burning feet may be associated. The neuropathy may improve markedly with renal transplantation. Carpal tunnel syndrome (see later) may also occur with renal disease and may develop distal to the arteriovenous fistulas placed in the forearm for access during hemodialysis. In patients on chronic hemodialysis, it often relates to amyloidosis and the accumulation of β_2-microglobulin.

LIVER DISEASE

Primary biliary cirrhosis may lead to a sensory neuropathy that is probably of the axonal type. A predominantly demyelinative polyneuropathy can occur with chronic liver disease. There does not appear to be any correlation between the neurologic findings and the severity of the hepatic dysfunction.

VITAMIN B$_{12}$ DEFICIENCY

Vitamin B$_{12}$ deficiency is associated with symmetric distal sensory and mild motor impairment and loss of tendon reflexes. Because controversy exists about the relative importance of polyneuropathy and myelopathy in producing this syndrome, vitamin B$_{12}$ deficiency is considered in more detail later, in the section on myelopathies. Polyradiculoneuropathy, polyneuropathy, and myelopathy may follow bariatric surgery and relate to nutritional deficiencies, including but not limited to vitamin B$_{12}$.

INFECTIVE & GRANULOMATOUS NEUROPATHIES

HIV INFECTION

Neuropathy is a common complication of HIV-1 infection (**Table 10-6**); involvement of peripheral nerves is seen at autopsy in approximately 40% of patients with AIDS. It may be a consequence of HIV infection or of secondary infection with other organisms (eg, cytomegalovirus, varicellazoster virus, *Treponema pallidum*), have an immunologic basis, or relate to nutritional deficiency or medication.

Distal symmetric **sensorimotor** or **predominantly sensory polyneuropathy** is the most common neuropathy associated with HIV-1 infection. Axons, rather than myelin, are primarily affected. The cause is unknown, but in some patients, vitamin B$_{12}$ deficiency or exposure to neurotoxic drugs (which should be discontinued if possible) may be responsible in part. Other causes of neuropathy should be excluded. HIV-1 is rarely identified in the affected nerves. Sensory symptoms predominate and

Table 10-6. Neuropathies Associated With AIDS.

Type	Stage of HIV-1 Infection	Immune Status	Distribution
Sensorimotor polyneuropathy	Early or late	Competent or suppressed	Symmetric, distal, lower > upper limbs
Inflammatory demyelinating polyneuropathy	Early	Competent	Proximal > distal limbs
Lumbosacral polyradiculopathy	Late	Suppressed	Proximal lower limbs, sphincters
Mononeuropathy multiplex	Early or late	Competent or suppressed	Cranial (eg, facial nerve), peripheral (eg, fibular nerve)
Mononeuropathy simplex	Early	Competent	Cranial (eg, facial nerve), peripheral (eg, fibular nerve)
Autonomic neuropathy	Early or late	Competent or suppressed	Diffuse

include pain and paresthesias affecting especially the feet. Weakness is a minor or late feature. Ankle and sometimes knee reflexes are absent. The course is typically progressive. Combination antiretroviral therapy (cART) may help in improving sensory function. Pain may be controlled pharmacologically, as described earlier. Plasmapheresis is of no benefit.

Inflammatory demyelinating polyneuropathy may occur early in HIV-1 infection and follow an acute course (symptoms reaching their nadir within 4 weeks) or, in patients with severe infection, a chronic course (progression for longer than 4 weeks). The neuropathy may be immune mediated, but sometimes results from direct, secondary viral infection, as from cytomegalovirus. It is characterized by proximal, and sometimes distal, weakness with less pronounced sensory disturbances, and areflexia or hyporeflexia. The CSF is abnormal, with an elevated protein concentration and often a lymphocytic pleocytosis (unlike the findings in Guillain–Barré syndrome or chronic inflammatory demyelinating polyneuropathy in patients without HIV-1 infection). Some patients improve spontaneously or stabilize, and others may respond to corticosteroids, plasmapheresis, or intravenous immunoglobulin.

Lumbosacral polyradiculopathy occurs late in the course of HIV-1 infection, usually in patients with prior opportunistic infections. Cytomegalovirus infection is the cause, at least in some instances. Clinical features usually develop over several weeks and include diffuse, progressive leg weakness, back pain, painful paresthesias of the feet and perineum, lower extremity areflexia, and early urinary retention. The course may be fulminant, with ascending paralysis leading to respiratory failure, but is sometimes more benign, especially when the etiology is unclear. CSF findings include mononuclear or polymorphonuclear pleocytosis, elevated protein concentration, and decreased glucose level; a positive test for cytomegalovirus by polymerase chain reaction provides further support. It is always important to exclude

meningeal lymphomatosis, cord compression, or syphilis as the underlying cause, as these require specific treatment and affect the prognosis. Patients with cytomegalovirus infection may respond to ganciclovir 2.5 mg/kg intravenously every 8 hours for 10 days, then 7.5 mg/kg/d 5 d/wk. An alternative approach is with foscarnet; in severe cases, both drugs are given. Some worsening in the first 2 weeks of ganciclovir therapy does not indicate treatment failure. The CSF should be re-examined after 3 weeks to determine whether the polymorphonuclear cell count has declined; if it has not, foscarnet should replace ganciclovir.

Mononeuropathy multiplex affects multiple cranial and peripheral nerves, resulting in focal weakness and sensory loss. This may have an autoimmune basis or neoplastic or infectious causes (eg, cytomegalovirus infection), or result from vasculopathy. In early HIV-1 infection, mononeuropathy multiplex may be a self-limited disorder restricted to a single limb, with spontaneous stabilization or improvement. Late in AIDS, several limbs may be affected in a progressive fashion.

Mononeuropathy simplex tends to occur acutely in early HIV-1 infection and improve spontaneously. It may present as unilateral or bilateral facial palsy. A vascular cause is probable.

Autonomic neuropathy tends to occur late in HIV-1 infections and may lead to syncopal episodes, orthostatic hypotension, disturbances of sphincter or sexual function, impaired thermoregulatory sweating, and diarrhea. The dysautonomia may relate to central or peripheral pathology. Treatment is symptomatic (as discussed in an earlier section).

Medication-related neuropathy may result from treatment with the antiretroviral drugs zalcitabine (ddC), didanosine (ddI), and stavudine (d4T), after approximately 4 months unless other coexisting conditions make the patient more susceptible. It is an axonal sensory neuropathy, characterized by distal tingling, numbness, and pain. Other drugs that may be associated with a neuropathy in

AIDS patients include isoniazid, ethambutol, vincristine, vinblastine, Taxol, thalidomide, and the statins.

LEPROSY

Leprosy is one of the most frequent causes of peripheral neuropathy worldwide. In turn, neuropathy is the most disabling manifestation of leprosy. *Mycobacterium leprae* affects the skin and peripheral nerves because its growth is facilitated by the cooler temperatures present at the body surface.

In **tuberculoid leprosy**, the immune response is adequate to confine the infection to one or more small patches of skin and their associated cutaneous and subcutaneous nerves. This produces a hypopigmented macule or papule over which sensation is impaired; pain and temperature appreciation are most affected. Anhidrosis occurs with involvement of autonomic fibers. Sensory deficits occur most often in the distribution of the digital, sural, radial, and posterior auricular nerves, whereas motor findings usually relate to involvement of the ulnar or fibular (peroneal) nerve. Involved nerves are often enlarged.

Lepromatous leprosy is a more widespread disorder that results in a symmetric, primarily sensory polyneuropathy that disproportionately affects pain and temperature sense. Its distribution is distinctive in that exposed areas of the body—especially the ears; nose; cheeks; dorsal surfaces of the hands, forearms, and feet; and lateral aspects of the legs—are preferentially involved. Unlike most polyneuropathies, that caused by leprosy tends to spare the tendon reflexes. Associated findings include resorption of the digits, trophic ulcers, and cyanosis and anhidrosis of the hands and feet.

Treatment depends on the type of leprosy, but typically involves dapsone, rifampicin, and clofazimine. The most recent guidelines of the World Health Organization (http://www.who.int/lep/mdt/regimens/en/index.html) should be followed. In the United States, further information can be obtained from the National Hansen's Disease Program of the US Department of Health and Human Services (http://www.hrsa.gov/hansensdisease/).

DIPHTHERIA

Corynebacterium diphtheriae infects tissues of the upper respiratory tract and produces a toxin that causes demyelination of peripheral nerves. Within approximately 1 month after infection, patients may develop a cranial motor neuropathy with prominent impairment of ocular accommodation. Blurred vision is the usual presenting complaint. Extraocular muscles and the face, palate, pharynx, and diaphragm may also be affected, but the pupillary light reflex is preserved. Recovery typically occurs after several weeks. A more delayed syndrome that commonly has its onset 2 to 3 months after the primary infection takes the form of a symmetric distal sensorimotor polyneuropathy. Most patients recover completely. Diphtheritic neuropathy is discussed in more detail in Chapter 9, Motor Disorders.

SARCOIDOSIS

Sarcoidosis can produce mononeuropathy or, rarely, polyneuropathy. The mononeuropathy commonly involves cranial nerves, especially the **facial nerve**. In some instances, a small-fiber neuropathy leads to pain, dysesthesias, and autonomic involvement. Clinical evaluation for extraneural disease, x-rays of the lungs and bones, examination of the CSF, and determination of serum levels of angiotensin-converting enzyme are helpful in establishing the diagnosis of sarcoidosis. Treatment with prednisone, 60 mg/d orally followed by tapering doses, may speed recovery.

SEPSIS & MULTIORGAN FAILURE

Patients with sepsis and multiorgan failure may develop a **critical illness polyneuropathy**. This manifests primarily by weakness and is therefore discussed in Chapter 9, Motor Disorders.

NEUROPATHIES IN VASCULITIS & COLLAGEN VASCULAR DISEASE

Systemic vasculitides and collagen vascular diseases can produce polyneuropathy, mononeuropathy simplex, mononeuropathy multiplex, or entrapment neuropathy (**Table 10-7**).

SYSTEMIC NECROTIZING VASCULITIS

This includes **polyarteritis nodosa** and allergic angiitis and granulomatosis (**Churg–Strauss syndrome**). Neuropathy occurs in approximately 50% of patients, most often as mononeuropathy multiplex, which may manifest with pain of acute onset in one or more cranial or peripheral nerves. Distal symmetric sensorimotor polyneuropathy is less common. Treatment should begin as soon as the diagnosis is made; it includes prednisone 60 to 100 mg/d orally and cyclophosphamide 2 to 3 mg/d orally.

GRANULOMATOSIS WITH POLYANGIITIS (WEGENER GRANULOMATOSIS)

Mononeuropathy multiplex or polyneuropathy occurs in up to 30% of cases. Treatment is the same as for systemic necrotizing vasculitis.

GIANT CELL ARTERITIS

This disorder is considered in detail in Chapter 6, Headache & Facial Pain. Mononeuropathy affecting cranial nerves innervating the extraocular muscles can occur.

Table 10-7. Neuropathies Associated With Vasculitis and Collagen Vascular Disease.

Disease	Polyneuropathy	Mononeuropathy Simplex or Multiplex[1]	Entrapment Neuropathy[1]
Vasculitis			
Systemic necrotizing vasculitis[2]	+	+	–
Granulomatosis with polyangiitis	+	+	–
Giant cell arteritis	–	+ (III, VI, IV)	–
Collagen vascular disease			
Rheumatoid arthritis	+	+	+ (M, U, R)
Systemic lupus erythematosus	+	+	–
Sjögren syndrome	+	+ (V, III, VI)	+ (M)
Progressive systemic sclerosis	–	+ (V)	–
Mixed connective-tissue disease	+	+ (V)	–

+, present; –, absent.
[1]Commonly affected nerves: III, oculomotor; IV, trochlear; V, trigeminal; VI, abducens; M, median; R, radial; U, ulnar.
[2]Includes polyarteritis nodosa and Churg–Strauss syndrome.

RHEUMATOID ARTHRITIS

Rheumatoid arthritis produces entrapment neuropathy (most commonly involving the median nerve) in approximately 45% of patients and distal symmetric sensorimotor polyneuropathy in about 30%. Mononeuropathy multiplex is a frequent feature in cases complicated by necrotizing vasculitis.

SYSTEMIC LUPUS ERYTHEMATOSUS

This is discussed in Chapter 4, Confusional States, as a cause of acute confusional states. Neuropathy occurs in up to 20% of patients. The most common pattern is a distal, symmetric sensorimotor polyneuropathy. An ascending, predominantly motor polyneuropathy (Guillain–Barré syndrome, see earlier) can also occur, as may mononeuropathy simplex or multiplex, which often affects the ulnar, radial, sciatic, or fibular (peroneal) nerve.

SJÖGREN SYNDROME

Sjögren syndrome involves the peripheral nerves in approximately 20% of cases. Distal symmetric sensorimotor polyneuropathy is most common, entrapment neuropathy (affecting especially the median nerve) is also frequent, and mononeuropathy multiplex can occur.

SCLERODERMA & MIXED CONNECTIVE-TISSUE DISEASE

Progressive systemic sclerosis (scleroderma) and mixed connective-tissue disease may produce cranial mononeuropathy, which most often involves the trigeminal (V) nerve.

NEOPLASTIC & PARAPROTEINEMIC NEUROPATHIES

COMPRESSION & INFILTRATION BY TUMOR

Nerve compression is a common complication of multiple myeloma, lymphoma, and carcinoma. Tumorous invasion of the epineurium may occur with leukemia, lymphoma, and various cancers, particularly carcinoma of the breast or pancreas.

PARANEOPLASTIC SYNDROMES

Carcinoma (especially small-cell cancer of the lung) and lymphoma may be associated with neuropathies that are thought to be immunologically mediated, based on the detection of autoantibodies to neuronal antigens in several cases.

▶ Sensory or Sensorimotor Polyneuropathy

This occurs with both carcinoma and lymphoma. It can be either an acute or chronic disorder, is sometimes asymmetric, and may be accompanied by prominent pain. The CSF is typically acellular but protein concentration may be mildly elevated. Among patients with a chronic sensorimotor polyneuropathy of uncertain cause, approximately 10% have a monoclonal gammopathy; many such patients eventually develop a hematologic malignancy, as discussed later. Treatment of the malignancy may improve the neuropathy.

▶ Sensory Neuronopathy

Carcinoma can also cause sensory neuronopathy, which primarily affects the cell bodies of sensory neurons in the dorsal root ganglion and is associated with the presence of anti-Hu (or ANNA-1) antibodies (see Chapter 8, Disorders of Equilibrium). This rare condition may be the presenting manifestation of cancer. Initial symptoms of pain and numbness usually begin distally but sometimes begin proximally or in the face. The disorders often progress over days or several weeks, leading to marked sensory ataxia and impairment of all sensory modalities. Motor involvement is late, and autonomic dysfunction is uncommon. The CSF may have an inflammatory formula. Treatment of the underlying tumor is usually unrewarding.

▶ Motor Neuronopathy, Guillain–Barré Syndrome, & Other Motor Disorders

Lymphoma may be complicated by motor neuronopathy, a disorder of anterior horn cells. Hodgkin disease and angio-immunoblastic lymphadenopathy are sometimes associated with Guillain–Barré syndrome, which responds to treatment as in patients without malignancy. These and other paraneoplastic motor disorders (including the Lambert–Eaton myasthenic syndrome, neuromyotonia, and stiff-person syndrome) are discussed in Chapter 9, Motor Disorders.

▶ Autonomic Neuropathy

An autonomic neuropathy may occur as a paraneoplastic disorder, especially in patients with small-cell lung cancer. It relates most often to anti-Hu antibodies but may also occur with an antibody against ganglionic acetylcholine receptors (anti-nAChR). It is underdiagnosed, often develops in the setting of other paraneoplastic syndromes, and has a poor prognosis. Symptoms may include hypotension, orthostatic hypotension, hypoventilation, abnormal thermoregulatory sweating, sleep apnea, gastroparesis, intestinal pseudo-obstruction, and cardiac arrhythmias, sometimes leading to sudden death. Affected patients do not improve with immunotherapy even after treatment of the underlying tumor.

PARAPROTEINEMIAS

Patients with paraproteinemic demyelinating neuropathy, especially a chronic distal sensory neuropathy, may have a malignant plasma cell dyscrasia. The paraprotein is likely to underlie the neuropathy when it is an immunoglobulin (Ig)M. When it is IgG or IgA, the neuropathy may be clinically and electrophysiologically indistinguishable from chronic inflammatory demyelinating polyradiculoneuropathy and similar in its response to treatment.

Polyneuropathy is a common complication of **multiple myeloma.** Patients affected by lytic myeloma are usually men. The clinical picture is of a distal symmetric sensorimotor polyneuropathy. All sensory modalities are affected, pain is a frequent feature, and the reflexes are depressed. The disorder is usually progressive and leads to death within 2 years.

Sclerotic myeloma may be accompanied by a chronic demyelinating polyneuropathy. Motor involvement predominates, but vibration and position sense may also be impaired, and the reflexes are depressed. Pain is less common than in the neuropathy of lytic myeloma, and symptoms may improve with treatment of the underlying cancer or by plasmapheresis.

The **POEMS syndrome** (polyneuropathy, organomegaly, endocrinopathy, M protein, and skin changes) may complicate plasma cell dyscrasias, especially osteosclerotic myeloma. The sensorimotor polyneuropathy may show certain distinctive electrophysiologic features, such as conduction slowing that is more marked in intermediate than distal nerve segments, and often responds to treatment. Local irradiation or resection of an isolated plasmacytoma should be considered, as should melphalan with or without corticosteroids.

A sensorimotor polyneuropathy similar to that observed with lytic myeloma may also occur in **Waldenström macroglobulinemia** or **benign monoclonal gammopathy**. Treatment with immunosuppressant drugs and plasmapheresis is sometimes helpful.

AMYLOIDOSIS

Nonhereditary amyloidosis occurs as an isolated disorder (primary generalized amyloidosis) or in patients with multiple myeloma and may be associated with polyneuropathy. Polyneuropathy is also a feature of hereditary amyloidosis. Amyloid neuropathies are considered later in the section on hereditary neuropathies.

DRUG-INDUCED & TOXIC NEUROPATHIES

ALCOHOLISM

Polyneuropathy is one of the most common neurologic complications of chronic alcoholism; it can occur alone or in combination with other alcohol-related neurologic disorders, such as Wernicke encephalopathy (see Chapter 4, Confusional States) or the Korsakoff amnestic syndrome (see Chapter 5, Dementia & Amnestic Disorders). Controversy exists concerning the relative contributions of direct neurotoxicity of alcohol and associated nutritional (especially **thiamine**) deficiency in producing polyneuropathy.

Alcoholic polyneuropathy is typically a symmetric distal sensorimotor neuropathy. The legs are most affected, resulting in defective perception of vibration and touch and depressed or absent ankle reflexes. In some cases, distal weakness is pronounced, and autonomic dysfunction may occur. When pain occurs, it may respond to the treatment described earlier for painful neuropathy.

Abstinence from alcohol and thiamine repletion can halt the progression of symptoms.

OTHER DRUGS

As indicated in Table 10-2, a large number of drugs may cause neuropathies and most merit no additional comment here. With regard to **isoniazid,** a widely used antituberculous agent that interferes with pyridoxine metabolism, the polyneuropathy principally affects the sensory neurons. High doses, hereditary variations in drug metabolism, and malnutrition predispose to this complication. Spontaneous improvement occurs when administration of the drug is halted. Isoniazid-induced neuropathy can be prevented by concurrent administration of pyridoxine 100 mg/d orally.

Pyridoxine (vitamin B_6) toxicity may cause a sensory neuronopathy that disproportionately impairs vibration and position sense. This disorder usually occurs in patients taking at least 200 mg of pyridoxine daily—approximately 100 times the minimum daily requirement. Sensory ataxia, Romberg sign, Lhermitte sign, and ankle areflexia are common findings. Pain is less common, and motor involvement is unusual. Symptoms are usually reversible over months to years if the abuse ceases, but an irreversible syndrome has also been reported after intravenous administration of high doses of pyridoxine.

TOXINS

Organic compounds implicated as causes of polyneuropathy include **hexacarbons** present in solvents and glues (eg, *n*-hexane, methyl *n*-butyl ketone) and **organophosphates** used as plasticizers or insecticides (eg, triorthocresyl phosphate). Sensory involvement is most striking in *n*-hexane neuropathy, whereas neuropathy caused by triorthocresyl phosphate primarily affects motor nerves. Organophosphate neuropathy is discussed in more detail in Chapter 9, Motor Disorders.

Heavy metals may also be responsible for polyneuropathy. Neuropathy caused by lead, arsenic, and thallium is discussed in Chapter 9, Motor Disorders. Gold, which is used to treat rheumatoid arthritis, may cause a symmetric polyneuropathy, and cisplatin (a platinum analogue with anticancer activity) may produce a sensory neuropathy.

HEREDITARY NEUROPATHIES

HEREDITARY MOTOR & SENSORY NEUROPATHIES

These are designated **Charcot–Marie–Tooth (CMT) hereditary neuropathies**. They constitute a genetically heterogeneous group of disorders having a similar clinical phenotype. There is weakness and wasting of distal muscles in the limbs, with or without sensory loss; pes cavus and reduced or absent tendon reflexes also occur. They are divided into **demyelinating (CMT-1)** and **neuronal (CMT-2)** types, the latter sparing sensory neurons and resembling progressive spinal muscular atrophy (see Chapter 9, Motor Disorders). Both types have an autosomal dominant pattern of inheritance, although apparently sporadic cases occur.

CMT-1 has its onset in the first decade, follows a slowly progressive course, and is of variable severity. The nerves are often palpably thickened. Nerve conduction velocities are markedly reduced. CMT-1 is subdivided on the basis of the genetic findings, but the most common forms result from duplication of or mutations in the gene for peripheral myelin protein-22 (*PMP22*) in CMT1A or for myelin protein zero (*MPZ*) in CMT1B.

CMT-2 is generally less severe than CMT-1, is associated with normal or near-normal nerve conduction velocities, and does not cause nerve enlargement. The most common mutations are in the gene for mitofusin 2 (*MFN2*), but mutations in various other genes, including *MPZ*, have also been reported. X-linked dominant (CMT-X) and autosomal recessive (CMT-4) variants have been described.

Dejerine–Sottas disease (HMSN3; CMT-3) has its onset by 2 years of age with delayed motor milestones, is characterized by a severe sensorimotor neuropathy that frequently extends to the proximal muscles, and is associated with skeletal abnormalities such as scoliosis. There is severe demyelination of the nerves. It has autosomal recessive or dominant inheritance, and the responsible mutations involve the same genes associated with CMT-1.

HEREDITARY SENSORY & AUTONOMIC NEUROPATHIES

These neuropathies also take a variety of forms. In hereditary sensory and autonomic neuropathy (HSAN) type I, there is dominant inheritance, a gradually progressive course from onset in early adulthood, and symmetric loss of distal pain and temperature perception, with relative preservation of light touch. Perforating ulcers over pressure points and painless infections of the extremities are common. The tendon reflexes are depressed, but there is little, if any, motor disturbance. This phenotype is associated with mutations in the genes coding for serine palmitoyltransferase long-chain subunits (*SPTLC1* and *SPTLC2*), the GTPase atlastin family (*ATL1* and *ATL3*), or DNA methyltransferase 1 (*DNMT1*).

In **HSAN type II,** inheritance is recessive, onset is in infancy or early childhood, progression is slow, all sensory modalities are affected, autonomic involvement is variable, and tendon reflexes are lost. Four subtypes are recognized. The affected genes are lysine-deficient protein kinase 1 (*WNK1*); family with sequence similarity 134, member B (*FAM134B*); kinesin family member 1A (*KIF1A*); and voltage-gated sodium channel type IX, alpha subunit (*SCN9A*).

HSAN type III (Riley–Day syndrome, familial dysautonomia) is a progressive recessive disorder that commences in infancy. It is characterized by conspicuous autonomic dysfunction (absent tearing, and labile temperature and blood pressure), absent taste sensation, impaired pain and temperature sensation, and areflexia. The disorder, which has an increased prevalence in persons of Ashkenazi Jewish origin, is linked to mutations in the gene for inhibitor of kappa light polypeptide gene enhancer in B cells, kinase complex-associated protein (*IKBKAP*).

HSAN type IV is associated with congenital insensitivity to pain and absent sweating and has been related to recessive mutations in the gene encoding a receptor tyrosine kinase for nerve growth factor (*NTRK1*). Many of these patients have cognitive dysfunction. Death from hyperpyrexia may occur.

HSAN type V resembles type IV, but cognitive abnormalities do not occur. The mutation is in the nerve growth factor β-subunit gene (*NGFB*).

Other, less common forms have also been described.

AMYLOIDOSIS

Polyneuropathy can occur in both hereditary and nonhereditary forms of amyloidosis. Because small-diameter sensory and autonomic nerve fibers are especially likely to be involved, **pain** and **temperature** sensation and **autonomic functions** are prominently affected. Clinical presentation is commonly with distal paresthesias, dysesthesias, and numbness; postural hypotension; impaired thermoregulatory sweating; and disturbances of bladder, bowel, or sexual function. Distal weakness and wasting eventually occur. The tendon reflexes are often preserved until a relatively late stage. Entrapment neuropathy, especially **carpal tunnel syndrome,** may develop as a consequence of amyloid deposits.

In primary amyloidosis, the diagnosis is made by identifying amyloid deposits in the tissues; examination of abdominal fat aspirate is usually the initial step. Treatment has included alkylating agents or autologous peripheral blood stem-cell transplantation. In hereditary (familial) amyloidosis, genetic testing for transthyretin (*TTR*) mutations is more useful for establishing the diagnosis than analysis of tissues for amyloid deposition. Treatment by orthotopic liver transplantation is effective.

FRIEDREICH ATAXIA

Friedreich ataxia usually has an autosomal recessive mode of inheritance but occasionally occurs with dominant inheritance. It is usually caused by an expanded GAA trinucleotide repeat in a noncoding region of the gene for **frataxin** (*FXN*), a mitochondrial protein. An ataxic gait develops, followed by clumsiness of the hands and other signs of cerebellar dysfunction. Involvement of peripheral sensory fibers leads to sensory deficits of the limbs, with depressed or absent tendon reflexes. There may also be leg weakness and extensor plantar responses from central

motor involvement. This condition is considered in detail in Chapter 8, Disorders of Equilibrium.

HEREDITARY NEUROPATHY WITH LIABILITY TO PRESSURE PALSIES

This is a genetically heterogeneous disorder that relates most commonly to deletion in the peripheral myelin protein 22 (*PMP22*) gene. Inheritance is as an autosomal dominant trait with variable expression. Patients present with simple or multiple mononeuropathies that occur after mild pressure or stretch of nerves, and electrophysiologic studies reveal that abnormalities are more widespread than is evident clinically. Patients should be advised to avoid prolonged sitting with legs crossed or leaning on the elbows, and not to engage in activities involving repetitive movements of the wrist. Protective pads worn at the elbows or knees are sometimes worthwhile.

METABOLIC DISORDERS

In **acute intermittent porphyria,** which is transmitted by recessive inheritance, the initial neurologic manifestation is often a polyneuropathy that usually involves motor more than sensory fibers. Sensory symptoms and signs may be predominantly proximal or distal. The peripheral nerves may also be affected in **variegate porphyria.** Neuropathy caused by porphyria is considered further in Chapter 9, Motor Disorders.

Two autosomal recessive lipidoses are associated with polyneuropathy with a typical onset in infancy or childhood. These are **metachromatic leukodystrophy,** which results from deficiency of the enzyme arylsulfatase A, and **Krabbe disease,** due to galactocerebroside β-galactosidase deficiency.

Lipoprotein deficiencies that cause polyneuropathy include **abetalipoproteinemia,** which is associated with acanthocytosis, malabsorption, retinitis pigmentosa, and cerebellar ataxia, and **Tangier disease,** which produces cataract, orange discoloration of the tonsils, and hepatosplenomegaly. These are autosomal recessive conditions.

Refsum disease (previously HMSN IV) is an autosomal recessive disorder related to impaired metabolism of phytanic acid, resulting from mutations in the *PHYH* gene (encoding phytanoyl-CoA hydroxylase) in 90% of cases and from mutations in the *PEX7* gene (encoding the PTS2 receptor) in 10% or less of cases. The disorder is characterized by polyneuropathy, cerebellar ataxia, retinitis pigmentosa, and ichthyosis. Sensorineural deafness, anosmia, and cardiac arrhythmias may also occur. Treatment is by restricting dietary intake of phytol. Plasmapheresis to reduce body stores of phytanic acid may also help at the initiation of treatment, especially if there is acute weakness or a cardiac arrhythmia.

Fabry disease is an X-linked recessive disease caused by deficiency of the enzyme α-galactosidase-A, which leads to the accumulation of α-D-galactosyl moieties in different cells and tissues. This results in a painful sensory and autonomic (ie, a small-fiber) neuropathy, angiokeratomas, renal and cardiac disease, and an increased incidence of stroke. White matter lesions may be present on brain MRI. Multiple mutations of the α-galactosidase-A (*GLA*) gene have been found. The diagnosis can be confirmed in males by a low α-galactosidase-A activity in leukocytes or plasma. Mutation analysis is required for the diagnosis of female carriers.

Pharmacologic measures (discussed earlier) may be helpful in treating pain, especially treatment with gabapentin or amitriptyline. Enzyme replacement therapy with agalsidase β or α, a recombinant human α-galactosidase A enzyme, also merits consideration. It should probably be given to all hemizygous males with low or undetectable levels of α-galactosidase-A, regardless of whether clinical features of the disease are present, but there is no agreement about this. Enzyme replacement therapy is important in reducing pain and, once started, should be continued indefinitely; it may help to stabilize or improve cardiac and renal function, although this remains unclear. Antiplatelet agents help to prevent ischemic stroke, as discussed in Chapter 13, Stroke.

ENTRAPMENT NEUROPATHIES

Certain peripheral nerves are particularly susceptible to mechanical injury at vulnerable sites. The term **entrapment neuropathy** is used when the nerve is compressed, stretched, or angulated by adjacent anatomic structures to such an extent that dysfunction occurs. There are numerous entrapment neuropathies, and in many the initial or most conspicuous clinical complaints are of sensory symptoms or pain. Some of the more common syndromes are described next.

UPPER LIMB ENTRAPMENT SYNDROMES

MEDIAN NERVE COMPRESSION

Compression of the median nerve is common in the carpal tunnel at the wrist. **Carpal tunnel syndrome** may occur during pregnancy and as a complication of trauma, degenerative arthritis, tenosynovitis, diabetes mellitus, myxedema, and acromegaly. Early symptoms are pain and paresthesias confined to a median nerve distribution in the hand, that is, involving primarily the thumb, index, and middle fingers and the lateral half of the ring finger (see Appendix). There may be pain in the forearm and, in occasional patients, more proximally. Symptoms are often particularly troublesome at night and may awaken the patient from sleep. As the neuropathy advances, weakness and atrophy may eventually develop in the thenar muscles.

Examination reveals impaired cutaneous sensation in the median nerve distribution in the hand and, with motor involvement, weakness and wasting of the abductor pollicis brevis and opponens pollicis muscles (see Appendix). There may be a positive **Tinel sign** (percussion of the nerve at the wrist causes paresthesias in its distribution) or a positive response to the **Phalen maneuver** (flexion of the wrist for 1 minute exacerbates or reproduces symptoms).

The diagnosis can generally be confirmed by electrophysiologic studies. If the symptoms fail to respond to local corticosteroid injections or simple maneuvers such as wearing a nocturnal wrist splint, surgical decompression of the carpal tunnel may be necessary.

INTERDIGITAL NEUROPATHY

Interdigital neuropathy may lead to pain in one or two fingers, and examination reveals hyperpathia or impaired cutaneous sensation in the appropriate distribution of the affected nerve or nerves. Such a neuropathy may result from entrapment in the intermetacarpal tunnel of the hand, direct trauma, tenosynovitis, or arthritis.

Treatment by local infiltration with corticosteroids is sometimes helpful, but in severe cases neurolysis may be necessary.

ULNAR NEUROPATHY

Ulnar nerve dysfunction at the **elbow** leads to paresthesias, hypesthesia, and nocturnal pain in the little finger and ulnar border of the hand. Pain may also occur about the elbow. Symptoms are often intensified by elbow flexion or use of the arm.

Examination may reveal sensory loss on the ulnar aspect of the hand and weakness of the adductor pollicis, the deep flexor muscles of the fourth and fifth digits, and the intrinsic hand muscles (see Appendix). The lesion may result from external pressure, from entrapment within the cubital tunnel, or from cubitus valgus deformity causing chronic stretch injury of the nerve. Electrodiagnostic studies may localize the lesion.

Avoiding pressure on or repetitive flexion and extension of the elbow, combined in some instances with splinting the elbow in extension, is sometimes sufficient to arrest progression and alleviate symptoms. Surgical decompression or ulnar nerve transposition to the flexor surface of the arm may also be helpful, depending on the cause and severity of the lesion and duration of symptoms.

An ulnar nerve lesion may also develop in the **wrist** or **palm** of the hand in association with repetitive trauma, arthritis, or compression from ganglia or benign tumors. Involvement of the deep terminal branch in the palm leads to a motor deficit in ulnar-innervated hand muscles other than the hypothenar group, whereas a more proximal palmar lesion affects the latter muscles as well; there is no sensory deficit. With lesions at the wrist involving either the ulnar nerve itself or its deep and superficial branches, both sensory and motor changes occur in the hand. Sensation over the dorsal surface of the hand is unaffected, however, because the cutaneous branch to this region arises proximal to the wrist. Surgical treatment is helpful in relieving compression from a ganglion or benign tumor.

RADIAL NEUROPATHY

The radial nerve may be compressed in the axilla by pressure from crutches or other causes; this is frequently seen in alcoholics and drug addicts who have fallen asleep with an arm draped over some hard surface (so-called "Saturday night palsy"). The resulting deficit is primarily motor, with weakness or paralysis occurring in the muscles supplied by the nerve, but sensory changes may also occur, especially in a small region on the back of the hand between the thumb and index finger (see Appendix).

Treatment involves preventing further compression of the nerve. Recovery usually occurs spontaneously and completely, except when a very severe injury has resulted in axonal degeneration. Physical therapy and a wrist splint may be helpful until recovery occurs.

THORACIC OUTLET SYNDROME

A cervical rib or band or other anatomic structure may compress the lower part of the brachial plexus. Symptoms include pain, paresthesias, and numbness in a C8 and T1 distribution (see Figure 10-4). There may be diffuse weakness of the intrinsic hand muscles, often particularly involving the muscles in the thenar eminence and thereby simulating carpal tunnel syndrome. The section on cervical rib syndrome in Chapter 9, Motor Disorders, contains further details.

LOWER LIMB ENTRAPMENT SYNDROMES

FIBULAR (PERONEAL) NEUROPATHY

Fibular (peroneal) nerve lesions can follow trauma or pressure about the knee at the fibular head. The resulting weakness or paralysis of foot and toe extension—and foot eversion—is accompanied by impaired sensation over the dorsum of the foot and the lower anterior aspect of the leg (see Appendix). The ankle reflex is preserved, as is foot inversion.

Treatment is purely supportive. The nerve must be protected from further injury or compression. Patients with foot drop may require a brace until recovery occurs. Recovery occurs spontaneously with time and is usually complete unless the injury was severe enough to cause marked axonal degeneration.

TIBIAL NEUROPATHY

The **posterior tibial nerve** or its branches can be compressed between the floor and the ligamentous roof of the **tarsal tunnel**, which is located at the ankle immediately below and behind the medial malleolus. The usual complaint is of burning in the foot, especially at night, sometimes accompanied by weakness of the intrinsic foot muscles. The diagnosis can usually be confirmed electrophysiologically. If treatment with local injection of corticosteroids is not helpful, surgical decompression may be necessary.

FEMORAL NEUROPATHY

Isolated femoral neuropathy may occur in association with diabetes mellitus, vascular disease, bleeding diatheses (eg, hemophilia or treatment with anticoagulant drugs), or retroperitoneal neoplasms. Weakness of the quadriceps muscle is accompanied by a reduced or absent knee reflex, and sensory disturbances may also occur in the anterior and medial aspects of the thigh and medial part of the lower leg. Treatment is of the underlying cause.

SAPHENOUS NEUROPATHY

The saphenous nerve is the terminal sensory branch of the femoral nerve and supplies cutaneous sensation to the medial aspect of the leg about and below the knee (see Figure 10-4). Mechanical injury to the nerve can occur at several points along its course; patients complain of pain or impaired sensation in the distribution of the nerve. Weakness in quadriceps function (ie, extension at the knee; see Appendix) indicates femoral, rather than saphenous, nerve involvement. There is no specific treatment, but the nerve should be protected from further injury.

LATERAL FEMORAL CUTANEOUS NEUROPATHY

The lateral femoral cutaneous nerve supplies sensation to the outer border of the thigh (see Appendix). Its function can be impaired by excessive angulation or compression by neighboring anatomic structures, especially in pregnancy or other conditions that cause exaggerated lumbar lordosis. This leads to pain and paresthesias in the lateral thigh, where examination reveals impaired sensation. This syndrome, known as **meralgia paresthetica**, is best treated with symptomatic measures such as simple analgesics taken orally. Its course is often self-limited, but in occasional cases it progresses to a patch of permanent, painless numbness.

OBTURATOR NEUROPATHY

Trauma to the obturator nerve—for example, by pelvic fracture or a surgical procedure—can lead to pain radiating from the groin down the inner aspect of the thigh. An obturator hernia or osteitis pubis may cause a similar disorder; there is accompanying weakness of the adductor thigh muscles (see Appendix).

ROOT & PLEXUS LESIONS

COMPRESSIVE & TRAUMATIC LESIONS

The clinical disturbances resulting from acute intervertebral disk prolapse, cervical spondylosis, traumatic plexopathy, cervical rib syndrome, and neuralgic amyotrophy are discussed in Chapter 9, Motor Disorders. In addition to these conditions, patients with metastatic cancer may develop root or plexus lesions from compression by tumor or as a result of trauma induced by radiation therapy.

Root lesions are typically compressive in nature and usually occur in the setting of neoplastic meningitis, which is discussed in Chapter 4, Confusional States.

Brachial plexopathy can result from **tumor infiltration**, especially by lung or breast cancer, causing severe arm pain and sometimes dysesthesia. Because involvement of the lower trunk of the plexus is most common, symptoms usually occur within the C8 and T1 dermatomes, and Horner syndrome (see Chapter 7, Neuro-Ophthalmic Disorders) is present in approximately 50% of cases. **Radiation injury**, rather than direct invasion by tumor, should be suspected when the upper trunk of the brachial plexus (C5 and C6 nerve roots) is involved, weakness is a prominent presenting symptom, arm swelling occurs, or symptoms develop within 1 year after completion of radiation therapy with a total dose of more than 60 Gy. MRI findings of thickening and diffuse enhancement of the brachial plexus without a focal mass lesion support a radiation-induced plexopathy, as does the finding of myokymic discharges on electromyography.

Lumbosacral plexopathy is usually seen in patients with colorectal, cervical, uterine, or ovarian carcinoma or sarcoma. Clinical features that suggest **tumor invasion** include early and severe pain, unilateral involvement, leg swelling, and a palpable rectal mass. **Radiation injury** is more commonly associated with early prominent leg weakness and bilateral symptoms.

TABES DORSALIS

This type of **neurosyphilis**, now rare, is characterized mainly by sensory symptoms and signs that indicate marked involvement of the posterior roots, especially in the lumbosacral region, with resulting degeneration in the posterior columns of the spinal cord. Common complaints are of unsteadiness, sudden lancinating somatic pains, and urinary incontinence. Visceral crises characterized by excruciating abdominal pain also occur.

Examination reveals marked impairment of vibration and joint position sense in the legs, together with an ataxic gait and Romberg sign. Deep pain sensation is impaired, but superficial sensation is generally preserved. The bladder is often palpably enlarged; because it is flaccid and insensitive, there is overflow incontinence. Tendon reflexes

are lost, and the limbs are hypotonic. Sensory loss and hypotonicity may lead to the occurrence of **hypertrophic (Charcot) joints**. In many patients, there are other signs of neurosyphilis, including Argyll Robertson pupils, optic atrophy, ptosis, a variable ophthalmoplegia, and, in some cases, pyramidal and mental changes from cerebral involvement (taboparesis), as discussed in Chapter 5, Dementia & Amnestic Disorders. Treatment is of the underlying infection.

LYME DISEASE

Lyme disease, like syphilis, is a spirochetal infection that produces both central and peripheral nervous system disease. Central nervous system involvement is manifested by meningitis or meningoencephalitis (see Chapter 4, Confusional States). Lyme disease is also associated with inflammatory mono- or polyradiculopathy, brachial plexopathy, mononeuropathy (including facial palsy), and mononeuropathy multiplex. The radiculopathy results in pain, sensory loss, or dysesthesia in affected dermatomes; it also causes focal weakness. One or more cervical, thoracic, or lumbar nerve roots may be involved. Electromyography can confirm the presence of radiculopathy, and serologic testing establishes Lyme disease as the cause. Treatment is described in Chapter 4.

MYELOPATHIES

Myelopathies may present with pain or various sensory complaints and with motor disturbances. The clinical findings should suggest the level of the lesion, but further investigation is necessary to delineate it more fully and determine its nature. Compressive, ischemic, inflammatory, demyelinative, and traumatic myelopathies are discussed in Chapter 9, Motor Disorders.

SYRINGOMYELIA

Syringomyelia is cavitation of the spinal cord. **Communicating syringomyelia**, with communication between the central canal of the cord and the cavity, is a hydrodynamic disorder of the CSF pathways. In **noncommunicating syringomyelia**, there is cystic dilation of the cord, which is not in communication with the CSF pathways.

Syringomyelia may be asymptomatic, being discovered incidentally on imaging studies. When symptomatic, the clinical disturbance depends on the site of cavitation. Typically, there is a **dissociated sensory loss** at the level of the lesion; pinprick and temperature appreciation are impaired, but light touch sensation is preserved (see Figure 10-5). The sensory loss may be reflected by the presence of painless skin ulcers, scars, edema, hyperhidrosis, neuropathic joints, resorption of the terminal phalanges, and other disturbances. Weakness and wasting of muscles occur at the level of the lesion because of the involvement of the anterior horns of the spinal cord (see Figure 10-5).

A pyramidal deficit and sphincter disturbances sometimes occur below the level of the lesion because of gliosis or compression of the descending corticospinal pathways. The tendon reflexes may be depressed at the level of the lesion—because of interruption of their afferent, central, or efferent pathways—and increased below it. **Scoliosis** is a common accompaniment of cord cavitation.

Cavitation commonly occurs in the cervical region, causing a **capelike** distribution of sensory loss over one or both shoulders, diffuse pain in the neck, and radicular pain in the arms; involvement of the T1 segment frequently leads to ipsilateral Horner syndrome. If the cavitation involves the lower brainstem (**syringobulbia**), there may also be ipsilateral tongue wasting, palatal weakness, vocal cord paralysis, dissociated trigeminal sensory loss, and other evidence of brainstem involvement.

Communicating syringomyelia is often associated with developmental anomalies of the brainstem and foramen magnum region (such as **Arnold–Chiari malformation**; see Chapter 8, Disorders of Equilibrium) or with chronic arachnoiditis of the basal cisterns. Arnold–Chiari malformation can lead to hydrocephalus, cerebellar ataxia, pyramidal and sensory deficits in the limbs, and abnormalities of the lower cranial nerves, alone or in any combination. CT scans reveal a small posterior fossa and enlarged foramen magnum; other skeletal abnormalities may be present at the base of the skull and upper cervical spine. MRI reveals the syrinx and the Arnold–Chiari malformation, with caudal displacement of the fourth ventricle and herniation of the cerebellar tonsils through the foramen magnum.

Noncommunicating syringomyelia is often due to trauma, intramedullary tumors (such as ependymomas or hemangioblastomas), or spinal arachnoiditis (**Figure 10-8**). Posttraumatic syringomyelia generally occurs in patients with preexisting, severe neurologic deficits from spinal trauma after an interval of several years, although rarely it develops after only a few months. Presentation is with increase in a previously stable deficit; weakness, impaired sensation, and spasticity are often conspicuous, and pain, often radicular, may be distressing. Focal cord enlargement is found on MRI in patients with cavitation related to previous injury or to intramedullary neoplasms. The presence of arachnoiditis, cord compression, or spinal stenosis implies a worse prognosis than otherwise.

Treatment depends on the underlying cause. Decompression of a distended syrinx may provide transient benefit. In the case of communicating syringomyelia associated with Arnold–Chiari malformation, removal of the posterior rim of the foramen magnum and amputation of the cerebellar tonsils are sometimes helpful. The cord cavity should be drained, and, if necessary, an outlet should be made for the fourth ventricle; the use of syrinx shunts is more controversial. Posttraumatic syringomyelia is treated

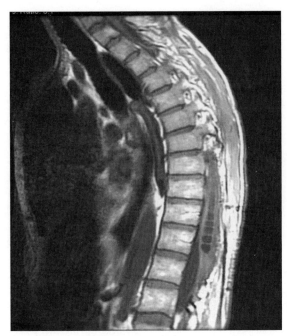

▲ **Figure 10-8.** Sagittal T1-weighted spinal MRI demonstrating a large septated syrinx in the lumbar cord of a patient with disseminated tuberculosis. (Used with permission from A. DiBernardo.)

by surgery if it is causing a progressive neurologic deficit or intolerable pain. A variety of surgical approaches have been used, including various draining procedures from the cord cavity, myelotomy, and formation of surgical meningocele. Radicular pain and sensory disturbances are usually helped, whereas spasticity and motor deficits respond less satisfactorily.

SUBACUTE COMBINED DEGENERATION

Vitamin B$_{12}$ deficiency (Figure 10-9) may result from impaired absorption by the gastrointestinal tract such as occurs in **pernicious anemia** or because of gastrointestinal surgery, sprue, or infection with fish tapeworm; it can also be caused by a strictly vegetarian diet. Vitamin B$_{12}$ deficiency can lead to subacute combined degeneration of the posterior and lateral columns of the spinal cord.

Clinical onset is with distal paresthesias and weakness in the extremities (involvement of the hands occurs relatively early), followed by the development of spastic paraparesis, with ataxia from impaired postural sensation in the legs. Lhermitte sign may be present, and examination reveals a combined posterior column (vibration and joint position sense) and pyramidal deficit in the legs. Plantar responses are extensor, but tendon reflexes may be increased or depressed, depending on the site and

Treatment is with vitamin B_{12} given by intramuscular injection daily (1,000 µg) for 2 weeks, then weekly (100 µg) for 2 months, and monthly (100 µg) thereafter. Note that folic acid supplements do not help the neurologic disorder; in addition, they may mask associated anemia.

A similar disorder may result from **nitrous oxide abuse,** which leads to inactivation of vitamin B_{12}. Management is focused on the prevention of further exposure to nitrous oxide.

Copper deficiency can also lead to subacute combined degeneration. The copper deficiency may follow total parenteral hyperalimentation, copper insufficiency with enteral feeding, malabsorption, gastric surgery, or excessive zinc ingestion, which inhibits the intestinal absorption of copper. Low serum copper and ceruloplasmin levels and urinary copper excretion confirm the diagnosis. Treatment involves copper supplementation and modification of any risk factors, which leads to stabilization of the neurologic deficit.

CEREBRAL DISORDERS

Sensory symptoms may relate to diverse diseases involving the brainstem or cerebral hemispheres (eg, stroke). The clinical features of the sensory deficit have been described earlier in this chapter and, together with the nature and extent of any accompanying neurologic signs, should suggest the probable site of the lesion.

PAIN SYNDROMES

Pain from infective, inflammatory, or neoplastic processes is a feature of many visceral diseases and may be a conspicuous component of certain neurologic or psychiatric diseases. It can also occur with no obvious cause.

In evaluating patients with pain, it is important to determine the level of the nervous system at which the pain arises and whether it has a primary neurologic basis. In the history, attention is focused on the mode of onset, duration, nature, severity, and location of the pain; on any associated symptoms; and on factors that precipitate or relieve the pain.

Treatment depends on the underlying cause and clinical context of the pain and is discussed later. A brief comment is necessary, however, about **stimulation-produced analgesia** and, in particular, about spinal cord stimulation ("dorsal column stimulation") and peripheral nerve stimulation. These approaches were based on principles encapsulated by the **gate control theory,** in which activation of large myelinated fibers was held to interrupt nociceptive transmission in the spinal cord, but their precise mechanism of action is uncertain. Spinal cord stimulation is known to affect certain neurotransmitter systems, particularly substance P and γ-aminobutyric acid (GABAergic) systems.

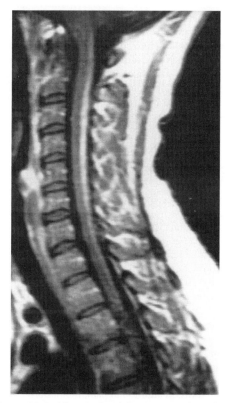

▲ **Figure 10-9.** Vitamin B_{12} deficiency myelopathy in a 30-year-old woman, wheelchair-bound with an 18-month history of progressive myelopathy. Vitamin B_{12} level: 60 pg/mL. Gadolinium-enhanced, T1-weighted cervical and upper thoracic MRI image shows marked enhancement of the posterior cord. (Used with permission from R. Laureno.)

severity of the involvement. Signs of cord involvement can be accompanied by centrocecal scotoma or optic atrophy from optic (II) nerve involvement, by behavioral or psychiatric changes, or by peripheral neuropathy. The neurologic manifestations are often accompanied by **macrocytic megaloblastic anemia,** but this is not invariably present.

The serum vitamin B_{12} level is low in untreated cases, and serum **homocysteine** and methylmalonic acid levels are elevated. In pernicious anemia, gastric achlorhydria is usual, and anti-intrinsic factor and gastric parietal cell antibodies confirm the diagnosis. Hematologic findings may be normal, however, especially if folic acid supplements have been given. Electrophysiologic studies may confirm peripheral nerve involvement, and median- or tibial-derived somatosensory evoked potentials may show abnormalities indicative of posterior column dysfunction. Spinal MRI sometimes shows abnormalities in the posterior columns.

PERIPHERAL NERVE PAIN

Pain arising from peripheral nerve lesions is usually localized to the site of nerve injury or confined to the territory of the affected nerve. It may have a burning quality, and when mixed (motor and sensory) nerves are involved, there may be an accompanying motor deficit. **Painful peripheral neuropathies** include those caused by diabetes, polyarteritis, alcoholic-nutritional deficiency states, and the various entrapment neuropathies. Treatment of pain associated with peripheral neuropathies was discussed earlier.

Reflex sympathetic dystrophy is a general term that denotes sympathetically mediated pain syndromes precipitated by a wide variety of tissue injuries, including soft tissue trauma, bone fractures, and myocardial infarction. The designation **complex regional pain syndrome (CRPS), type 1**, is now used (in preference to reflex sympathetic dystrophy) for pain that follows injury but spreads beyond the site of trauma in a distribution that does not conform to that of an individual peripheral nerve, is greater than would be expected from the injury, and may progress with time (sometimes to the opposite limb). It has been attributed to a post-traumatic neuralgia associated with distal degeneration of small-diameter peripheral axons. **CRPS type 2**, or **causalgia**, designates the severe persistent pain, often burning in quality, that results from **nerve trauma.** Such pain is associated with exquisite tenderness. Onset of pain may be at any time within the first 6 weeks or so after nerve injury. The cause is uncertain, but it has been attributed to ephaptic transmission between efferent sympathetic and afferent somatic fibers at the site of injury. Other proposed mechanisms involve inflammatory reactions and changes in the central mechanisms subserving pain.

In both types of CRPS, pain may be accompanied by swelling, increased sweating, and vasoconstriction of the affected extremity, which is commonly kept covered up and still by the patient; allodynia, hyperalgesia, muscle atrophy, and osteoporosis may also occur. No other cause for the symptoms and signs is apparent.

Treatment is largely empirical; studies to support specific therapeutic regimens are lacking. Medical approaches to treatment include physical and occupational therapy, with emphasis on increasing activity of the involved limb. Relaxation therapy or biofeedback may help, as also may topical lidocaine or capsaicin cream. Various pharmacologic approaches have been tried singly or in combination, with doses tailored to the individual. These include tricyclic antidepressants, serotonin-norepinephrine reuptake inhibitors (eg, duloxetine or venlafaxine), nonsteroidal anti-inflammatory drugs, gabapentin, pregabalin, lamotrigine, and opioids. If these measures do not provide satisfactory relief, a therapeutic trial of prednisone (starting with 1 mg/kg daily for 3 days) is sometimes undertaken. Addition of calcitonin or a bisphosphonate may be useful.

Sympathetic blockade by injection of local anesthetics into the sympathetic chain or by regional infusion of reserpine or guanethidine provides temporary benefit to some patients. One such procedure sometimes produces permanent cessation of pain; in other instances, repeated sympathetic blocks may be required. Surgical sympathectomy is beneficial in up to 75% of cases. Spinal cord stimulation has been effective in some instances for the treatment of either type of CRPS when other measures, including opiates, have been unhelpful.

RADICULAR PAIN

Radicular pain is caused most commonly by mechanical root compression from disk protrusion, spinal stenosis, or congenital anomalies, but infective, inflammatory, and neoplastic causes require exclusion. Herpes zoster infection is considered separately. The pain is localized to the distribution of one or more nerve roots and is often exacerbated by coughing, sneezing, and other maneuvers that cause **increased intraspinal pressure**. It is also exacerbated by maneuvers that **stretch** the affected roots. Passive straight-leg raising leads to stretching of the sacral and lower lumbar roots, as does passive flexion of the neck. Spinal movements that narrow the intervertebral foramina can aggravate root pain. **Extension and lateral flexion** of the head to the affected side may thus exacerbate cervical root symptoms. In addition to pain, root lesions can cause paresthesias and numbness in a dermatomal distribution (see Figure 10-4); they can also cause segmental weakness and reflex changes, depending on the level affected (see Chapter 9, Motor Disorders, Table 9-12). Useful modes of treatment for mechanical causes include immobilization, nonsteroidal anti-inflammatory drugs or other analgesics, and surgical decompression.

THALAMIC PAIN

Depending on their extent and precise location, thalamic lesions may lead to a burning, unpleasant pain in all or part of the contralateral half of the body. It is aggravated by emotional stress and tends to develop during partial recovery from a sensory deficit caused by the underlying thalamic lesion. Mild cutaneous stimulation may produce very unpleasant and painful sensations. This combination of sensory loss, spontaneous pain, and perverted cutaneous sensation is called **Dejerine–Roussy** syndrome. Similar pain can be produced by a lesion of the parietal lobe or the sensory pathways at any point in the cord (posterior columns or spinothalamic tract) or brainstem. Treatment with analgesics, anticonvulsants (carbamazepine, phenytoin, gabapentin, pregabalin, and lamotrigine), or tricyclic antidepressants, serotonin-norepinephrine reuptake inhibitors, mexiletine, baclofen, and phenothiazines, either alone or in combination, is occasionally helpful, according to anecdotal observations. Opioids are sometimes used but carry the risk of dependency and addiction.

BACK & NECK PAIN

Spinal disease occurs most commonly in the neck or low back and can cause local or root pain, or both, and pain referred to other parts of the involved dermatomes. Pain from the lower lumbar spine, for example, is often referred to the buttocks. Conversely, pain may be referred to the back from the viscera, especially the pelvic organs. Local pain may lead to protective reflex muscle spasm, which in turn causes further pain and may result in abnormal posture, limitation of movement, and local spinal tenderness.

The history may suggest the underlying cause, and physical examination will define any neurologic involvement. Investigative studies may include complete blood count and erythrocyte sedimentation rate (especially if infective or inflammatory disorders or myeloma is suspected); determination of serum protein and protein electrophoresis; and measurement of serum calcium, phosphorus, alkaline and acid phosphatase, and uric acid. Electromyography may indicate the extent and severity of root involvement and provides a guide to prognosis. A CT scan, MRI of the spine, or CT myelogram may be necessary, especially if neoplasm is suspected, neurologic deficits are progressive, pain persists despite conservative treatment measures, or there is evidence of cord involvement. At myelography, CSF can be obtained for laboratory examination.

LOW BACK PAIN

Low back pain is a common cause of time lost from work. It has many causes. Routine immediate imaging of patients with acute or subacute low back pain who have no clinical features suggestive of serious underlying disorder does not improve the clinical outcome and is therefore unnecessary.

▶ Trauma

Unaccustomed exertion or activity—or lifting heavy objects without adequate bracing of the spine—can cause musculoskeletal pain that improves with rest. Clinical examination commonly reveals spasm of the lumbar muscles and restricted spinal movement. Management includes local heat, bed rest on a firm mattress, nonsteroidal anti-inflammatory drugs or other analgesics, and muscle-relaxant drugs (eg, diazepam 2 mg three times daily, increased gradually until symptoms are relieved or to the highest dose tolerated). Vertebral fractures that follow more severe injury and lead to local pain and tenderness can be visualized at radiography. If spinal cord involvement is suspected—for example, because of leg weakness after injury—the patient must be immobilized until imaged

to determine whether fracture dislocation of the vertebral column has occurred.

▶ Prolapsed Lumbar Intervertebral Disk

This most commonly affects the **L5-S1** or the **L4-L5** disk. The prolapse may relate to injury, but commonly follows minor strain or normal activity. Protruded disk material may press on one or more nerve roots and thus produce radicular pain, a segmental motor or sensory deficit, or a sphincter disturbance in addition to a painful stiff back. The pain may be reproduced by percussion over the spine or sciatic nerve, by passive straight leg raising, or by extension of the knee while the hip is flexed. Bilateral symptoms and signs suggest that disk material has protruded centrally, and this is more likely to cause sphincter involvement than is lateral protrusion.

An L5 radiculopathy causes weak dorsiflexion of the foot and toes, whereas an S1 root lesion leads to a depressed ankle reflex and weakness of plantar flexion of the foot (see Chapter 9, Motor Disorders, Table 9-12). In either case, spinal movements are restricted, there is local tenderness, and Lasègue sign (reproduction of the patient's pain on stretching the sciatic nerve by straight leg raising) is positive. The L4 root is occasionally affected, but involvement of a higher lumbar root should arouse suspicion of other causes of root compression.

Pelvic and rectal examination and spinal MRI or CT and CT myelography help to exclude other diseases, such as local tumors or metastatic neoplastic deposits.

Symptoms often resolve with simple analgesics, diazepam, and bed rest on a firm mattress for 2 to 3 days, followed by gradual mobilization. Bed rest for longer than 2 to 3 days provides no additional benefit. Nonsteroidal anti-inflammatory drugs may be helpful for acute back pain but are often ineffective or provide only minor or transient benefits in patients with root compression. Epidural steroid injection is of uncertain benefit and associated with potentially serious adverse effects.

Persisting pain, an increasing neurologic deficit, or any evidence of sphincter dysfunction should lead to MRI, CT scanning, or CT myelography, and surgical treatment if indicated by the results of these procedures. The presence of structural abnormalities does not mandate surgical treatment unless the clinical circumstances are appropriate—degenerative abnormalities are common in asymptomatic subjects, especially with advancing age, and may therefore be of no clinical relevance.

Continuing pain despite surgery may result from inadequate decompression, recurrent herniation of disk material, root compression or damage relating to the operative procedure, surgery at the wrong level, infective or inflammatory complications of surgery, or spinal instability. Often, however, no specific cause can be identified, and most patients do not require further surgery. Chronic pain in this setting may, however, respond to spinal cord stimulation. There is a high risk that patients will not return to work.

Lumbar Osteoarthropathy

This tends to occur in later life and may cause low back pain that is increased by activity. MRI is the preferred mode of imaging; abnormalities vary in severity, and their clinical relevance is not always clear. Many asymptomatic elderly subjects have degenerative changes of the lumbar spine. In patients with mild symptoms, a surgical corset is helpful, whereas in more severe cases operative treatment may be necessary.

Even minor changes may cause root or cord dysfunction in patients with a congenitally narrowed spinal canal (**spinal stenosis**), leading to the syndrome of **intermittent claudication of the spinal cord or cauda equina**. Similar symptoms may result from ossification of the ligamentum flavum, epidural lipomatosis, Pott disease, osteomyelitis, rheumatoid arthritis, or post-traumatic stenosis of the spinal canal. They may also occur with dural arteriovenous fistulas. The syndrome is characterized by pain, sometimes accompanied by weakness or radicular sensory disturbances in the legs, that occurs with activity or with certain postures and is relieved by rest.

Patients with mild to moderate symptoms related to spinal stenosis should be treated conservatively with pain medication, nonsteroidal anti-inflammatory agents, and physical therapy to reduce the lumbar lordosis. Muscle relaxants and antidepressant drugs are often prescribed also. Studies to examine the relative merits and cost-effectiveness of these approaches are lacking. Bed rest is to be avoided. If symptoms are severe, decompressive surgery is indicated when conservative treatment for 3 to 6 months has been unhelpful or there is a significant motor deficit or symptoms of **cauda equina syndrome** (compression of lumbosacral nerve roots in the spinal canal, below the end of the spinal cord [conus medullaris]). Such surgery leads to pain relief, but the rapidity and extent of recovery is variable. Complications include epidural hematomas, inadequate decompression with residual stenosis, instability, and reossification with renewed nerve compression. Up to 25% of patients undergoing surgical decompression will require reoperation in the following 10 years.

Ankylosing Spondylitis

Backache and stiffness, followed by progressive limitation of movement, characterize this disorder, which occurs predominantly in young men. Characteristic early radiologic findings consist of sclerosis and narrowing of the sacroiliac joints. Treatment is with nonsteroidal anti-inflammatory agents, especially indomethacin or aspirin. Physical therapy, including postural exercises, is also important.

Neoplastic Disease

Extradural malignant tumors are an important cause of back pain and should be suspected if there is persistent pain that worsens despite bed rest. They may eventually lead to spinal cord compression or a cauda equina syndrome, depending on the level of involvement. The diagnosis is confirmed by spinal MRI or CT and CT myelography. CSF cytology may be diagnostic with leptomeningeal involvement, but is sometimes negative initially. Benign osteogenic tumors also produce back pain; treatment is by excision.

Infections

Tuberculous and pyogenic infections of the vertebrae or intervertebral disks can cause progressive low back pain and local tenderness. Although there are sometimes no systemic signs of infection, the peripheral white cell count and erythrocyte sedimentation rate are elevated. Spinal imaging may show disk space narrowing and a soft tissue mass, but is sometimes normal initially.

Bone infection (osteomyelitis) requires long-term antimicrobial therapy; surgical debridement and drainage may also be needed. Spinal epidural abscess (see Chapter 9, Motor Disorders) similarly presents with localized pain and tenderness, sometimes associated with osteomyelitis. Cord compression may occur with the onset of a rapidly progressive flaccid paraplegia. MRI, CT scanning, or CT myelography, followed by operative treatment, are undertaken urgently if there is cord compression. In early cases without neurologic involvement, treatment with antibiotics alone may be sufficient.

Osteoporosis

Low back pain is a common complaint in patients with osteoporosis, and vertebral fractures may occur spontaneously or after trivial trauma. Pain may be helped by a brace to support the back. It is important that patients keep active, stop tobacco smoking, and take a diet containing adequate amounts of calories, calcium, vitamin D, and protein. Estrogen therapy may be helpful in postmenopausal women, but is less widely used than previously. The bisphosphonates alendronate and risedronate may be helpful and have reduced the incidence of fractures in randomized trials. Other antiresorptives include raloxifene, a selective estrogen receptor modulator, and the bisphosphonate zoledronic acid. In special circumstances, parathyroid hormone, calcitonin, or strontium is helpful.

Paget Disease of the Spine

Paget disease, which is characterized by excessive bone destruction and repair, is of unknown cause but may have a familial basis. Pain is commonly the first symptom. Vertebral involvement may also lead to evidence of cord or root compression. The serum calcium and phosphorus levels are normal, but the alkaline phosphatase is markedly increased. Urinary hydroxyproline and calcium are increased when the disease is active. X-rays show expansion and increased density of the involved bones, and fissure fractures may be evident in the long bones.

In active, progressive disease, treatment with calcitonin or bisphosphonates reduces osteoclastic activity. Decompressive surgery is sometimes necessary for neurologic complications.

Congenital Anomalies

Minor spinal anomalies can cause pain because of altered mechanics or alignment or because reduction in the size of the spinal canal renders the cord or roots more liable to compression by degenerative or other changes. Children or young adults with congenital defects in spinal fusion (**spinal dysraphism**) occasionally present with pain, a neurologic deficit in one or both legs, or sphincter disturbances. Treatment is of the underlying disorder.

Congenital **spinal stenosis** may lead to the syndrome of neurogenic claudication, but symptoms usually develop only in later life when minor degenerative changes have come to be superimposed on the congenital anomaly, as discussed earlier.

Arachnoiditis

Severe pain in the back and legs can result from inflammation and fibrosis of the arachnoid layer of the spinal meninges (arachnoiditis), which may be idiopathic or causally related to previous surgery, infection, myelography, or long-standing disk disease. There is no adequate treatment, but operation may be possible if the arachnoiditis is localized. Spinal cord stimulation may provide symptomatic relief. This condition is considered in more detail in Chapter 9, Motor Disorders.

Referred Pain

Disease of the hip joints may cause pain in the back and thighs that is enhanced by activity; examination reveals limitation of movement at the joint with a positive **Patrick sign** (hip pain on external rotation of the hip), and radiographs show degenerative changes. Aortic aneurysms, cardiac ischemia, visceral and genitourinary disease (especially pelvic disorders in women), and retroperitoneal masses can also cause back pain. There are often other symptoms and signs that suggest the underlying disorder. Moreover, there is no localized spinal tenderness or restriction of motility. Treatment is of the underlying cause.

Nonspecific Chronic Back Pain

In many patients with chronic back pain, there are no objective clinical signs or obvious causes of pain despite detailed investigations. In some cases, the pain may have a postural basis; in others, it may be a somatic manifestation of a psychiatric disorder. Pain that initially had an organic basis is often enhanced or perpetuated by nonorganic factors and leads to disability out of proportion to the symptoms.

Nonsteroidal anti-inflammatory drugs may provide short-term symptomatic relief. There is some controversy about the chronic use of narcotic analgesics in patients with persisting low back pain, but such agents are generally best avoided. Treatment with tricyclic antidepressant drugs is sometimes helpful, and psychiatric evaluation may be worthwhile. Bedrest is not recommended and provides no greater benefit than symptom-limited activity. Unnecessary surgical procedures must be avoided.

NECK PAIN

Neck pain is a common problem in the general population; surveys indicate that approximately one-third of the adult population has experienced it over the previous year, and in some instances, it lasts for more than 6 months.

Congenital abnormalities of the cervical spine, such as hemivertebrae or fused vertebrae, basilar impression, and instability of the atlantoaxial joint, can cause neck pain. The traumatic, infective, and neoplastic disorders mentioned previously as causes of low back pain can also affect the cervical spine, producing pain in the neck. Rheumatoid arthritis may involve the spine, especially in the cervical region, leading to pain, stiffness, and reduced mobility; spinal cord compression may result from displacement of vertebrae or atlantoaxial subluxation and can be life-threatening if not treated by fixation.

Cervical injuries are an important cause of neck pain. **Whiplash** flexion-extension injuries commonly result from automobile accidents. Other occult cervical injuries such as disk clefts and fissures may be responsible for symptoms in some instances, but are difficult to recognize. Management of persistent symptoms after whiplash injuries is controversial. Conservative therapeutic measures are appropriate. Other approaches sometimes advocated include block of cervical facet joints with bupivacaine and injection into the joints of depot corticosteroids, but the response is variable and often short-lived. Subluxed cervical facet joints are another well-recognized complication of automobile accidents. Even minor trauma may lead to cervical fractures in an apparently ankylosed region in patients with diffuse idiopathic skeletal hyperostosis, but major neurologic deficits are common in such circumstances.

Acute Cervical Disk Protrusion

Patients commonly present with neck and radicular arm pain that is exacerbated by head movement, accompanied by muscle spasm. The pathophysiology of the pain is unclear; pressure on nerve roots is unlikely to be the sole cause because pain may resolve with time and conservative measures despite persisting compression. With lateral herniation of the disk, there may also be segmental motor, sensory, or reflex changes, usually at the C6 or C7 level, on the affected side (see Figure 9-9 and Table 9-12). With more centrally directed herniations, spastic paraparesis and a sensory disturbance in the legs, sometimes accompanied by impaired sphincter function, can occur as a result of spinal cord involvement. The diagnosis is confirmed by CT scan, MRI, or CT myelography. However, these imaging studies often show abnormalities in asymptomatic subjects in middle or later life, so that any disk protrusion may be incidental and unrelated to patients' symptoms. Electromyography may help to establish that anatomic abnormalities are of functional relevance.

Treatment recommendations have limited objective evidence and are based on anecdotal experience. In mild cases, postural modification, the temporary nocturnal use of a soft collar, and immobilization of the neck in a collar for brief periods during the day often helps. Activities that provoke pain should be avoided. Acetaminophen or nonsteroidal anti-inflammatory drugs may relieve pain, and—when pain persists and disturbs sleep—a tricyclic antidepressant and muscle relaxants are often also worthwhile. A short course of oral corticosteroids can be helpful when pain is severe. Physical therapy is of uncertain benefit, as is intermittent neck traction. If these measures fail and there is persistent radicular pain for more than 2 months or a significant progressive neurologic deficit, surgical treatment may be necessary.

▶ Cervical Spondylosis

This is an important cause of pain in the neck and arms, sometimes accompanied by a segmental motor or sensory deficit in the arms or by spastic paraparesis. It is discussed in Chapter 9, Motor Disorders.

HERPES ZOSTER (SHINGLES)

This viral disorder becomes increasingly common with advancing age, causing an inflammatory reaction in one or more of the dorsal root or cranial nerve ganglia, in the affected root or nerve itself, and in the CSF. There seems to be spontaneous reactivation of varicella virus that remained latent in sensory ganglia after previous infection. Herpes zoster is common in patients with lymphoma, especially after regional radiotherapy.

The initial complaint is of a burning or shooting pain in the involved dermatome, followed within 2 to 5 days by the development of a vesicular erythematous rash. The pain may diminish in intensity as the rash develops. The rash becomes crusted and scaly after a few days and then fades, leaving small anesthetic scars. Secondary infection is common. The pain and dysesthesias may last for several weeks or, in some instances, persist for many months (**postherpetic neuralgia**) before subsiding.

Postherpetic neuralgia is most likely to occur in the elderly, when the rash is severe, with a longer duration of the rash before medical consultation, and with involvement of the first division of the trigeminal (V) nerve. The increased incidence and severity of postherpetic neuralgia with age may reflect an age-related reduction in virus-specific cell-mediated immunity. It is not clear whether immune compromise secondary to HIV infection or connective tissue disease predisposes to postherpetic neuralgia.

Pain is exacerbated by touching the involved area. Superficial sensation is often impaired in the affected dermatome, and focal weakness and atrophy can also occur. Signs are usually limited to one dermatome, but more are occasionally involved. Mild pleocytosis and an increased protein concentration sometimes occur in the CSF. The most commonly involved sites are the **thoracic dermatomes**, but involvement of the first division of the trigeminal (V) nerve, also common, is especially distressing and may lead to corneal scarring and anesthesia, as well as to a variety of other ocular complications.

Facial (VII) nerve palsy occurring in association with a herpetic eruption that involves the ear, palate, pharynx, or neck is called **Ramsay Hunt syndrome. Other rare complications** of herpes zoster include other motor neuropathies, meningitis, encephalitis, myelopathy, and cerebral angiopathy.

Unless otherwise contraindicated, the administration of **live-attenuated zoster vaccine** to patients over the age of 50 years is an important approach to preventing the occurrence of herpes zoster and reducing the risk of post-herpetic neuralgia. There is no specific treatment once herpes zoster has developed. Analgesics provide symptomatic relief—acetaminophen or nonsteroidal anti-inflammatory drugs for mild pain, and opioid analgesics when pain is more severe. Antiviral therapy (with oral acyclovir, valacyclovir, or famciclovir for 1 week) speeds recovery of the cutaneous lesions and helps the acute pain; they are generally used when patients are seen within 72 hours of symptom onset or new skin lesions are continuing to develop. It is unsettled whether their use reduces the incidence of postherpetic neuralgia. Corticosteroids are of uncertain value and do not affect the incidence of postherpetic neuralgia. Although postherpetic neuralgia can be very distressing, duloxetine (60 mg once daily) or pregabalin (150 mg increasing after 1 week to 300 mg daily in divided doses; maximum, 600 mg daily) may be helpful for relief of pain. It sometimes responds also to treatment with carbamazepine, up to 1,200 mg/d; phenytoin 300 mg/d; gabapentin, up to 3,600 mg/d; or amitriptyline 10 to 100 mg at bedtime.

Attempts at relieving postherpetic neuralgia by peripheral nerve section are generally unrewarding, but treatment with topically applied local anesthetics is sometimes helpful, as is topically applied capsaicin cream, perhaps because of depletion of pain-mediating peptides from peripheral sensory neurons. Intrathecal methylprednisolone may be helpful for intractable pain.

Movement Disorders

11

(Continued on Next Page)

Movement disorders (sometimes called **extrapyramidal disorders**) impair the regulation of voluntary motor activity without directly affecting strength, sensation, or cerebellar function. They include **hyperkinetic** disorders associated with abnormal, involuntary movements and **hypokinetic** disorders characterized by poverty of movement. Movement disorders result from dysfunction of deep subcortical gray matter structures termed the **basal ganglia.** Although there is no universally accepted anatomic definition of the basal ganglia, for clinical purposes they may be considered to comprise the caudate nucleus, putamen, globus pallidus, subthalamic nucleus, and substantia nigra. The putamen and the globus pallidus are collectively termed the **lentiform nucleus**; the combination of lentiform nucleus and caudate nucleus is designated the **corpus striatum**.

The basic circuitry of the basal ganglia consists of three interacting neuronal loops (**Figure 11-1**). The first is a **corticocortical loop** that passes from the cerebral cortex, through the caudate and putamen, the internal segment of the globus pallidus, and the thalamus, and then back to the cerebral cortex. The second is a **nigrostriatal loop** connecting the substantia nigra with the caudate and putamen. The third, a **striatopallidal loop**, projects from the caudate and putamen to the external segment of the globus pallidus, then to the subthalamic nucleus, and finally to the internal segment of the globus pallidus. In some movement disorders (eg, Parkinson disease), a discrete site of pathology within these pathways can be

identified; in other cases (eg, essential tremor), the precise anatomic abnormality is unknown.

TYPES OF ABNORMAL MOVEMENTS

Categorizing an abnormal movement is generally the first step toward arriving at the neurologic diagnosis. Abnormal movements can be classified as tremor, chorea, athetosis or dystonia, ballismus, myoclonus, or tics. They can arise in a variety of contexts, such as in degenerative disorders or with structural lesions. In many disorders, abnormal movements are the sole clinical features.

TREMOR

A *tremor* is a rhythmic oscillatory movement best characterized by its relationship to voluntary motor activity, that is, according to whether it occurs at rest, during maintenance of a particular posture, or during movement. The major causes of tremor are listed in **Table 11-1**. Tremor is enhanced by emotional stress and disappears during sleep. Tremor that occurs when the limb is at rest is generally referred to as **static tremor** or **rest tremor**. If present during sustained posture, it is called a **postural tremor**; although this tremor may continue during movement, movement does not increase its severity. When present during movement but not at rest, it is generally called an **intention** or **kinetic tremor**. Both postural and intention tremors are also called **action tremors**.

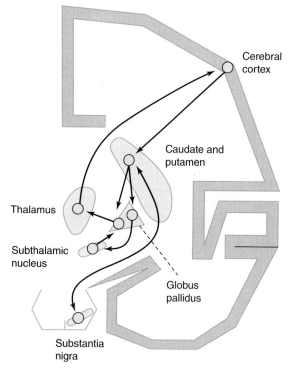

▲ **Figure 11-1.** Basic neuronal circuitry of the basal ganglia.

Table 11-1. Causes of Tremor.

Postural tremor
Physiologic tremor
Enhanced physiologic tremor
Anxiety or fear
Excessive physical activity or sleep deprivation
Sedative drug or alcohol withdrawal
Drug toxicity (eg, lithium, bronchodilators, sodium valproate, tricyclic antidepressants)
Heavy metal poisoning (eg, mercury, lead, arsenic)
Carbon monoxide poisoning
Thyrotoxicosis
Familial (autosomal dominant) or idiopathic (benign essential) tremor
Dystonic tremor
Cerebellar disorders
Wilson disease
Intention tremor
Brainstem or cerebellar disease
Drug toxicity (eg, alcohol, anticonvulsants, sedatives)
Wilson disease
Dystonic tremor
Rest tremor
Parkinsonism
Wilson disease
Heavy metal poisoning (eg, mercury)
Dystonic tremor

POSTURAL TREMOR

▶ Physiologic Tremor

An **8- to 12-Hz** tremor of the outstretched hands is a normal finding. Its physiologic basis is uncertain.

▶ Enhanced Physiologic Tremor

Physiologic tremor may be enhanced by fear or anxiety. A more conspicuous postural tremor may also be found after excessive physical activity or sleep deprivation. It can complicate treatment with certain drugs (notably lithium, tricyclic antidepressants, sodium valproate, and bronchodilators), is often conspicuous in patients with alcoholism or in alcohol or drug withdrawal states, and is common in thyrotoxicosis. It can also result from poisoning with a number of substances, including mercury, lead, arsenic, and carbon monoxide. There is no specific treatment.

▶ Other Causes

The most common type of abnormal postural tremor is **benign essential tremor**, which may be familial. Postural tremor may be conspicuous in patients with Wilson disease or cerebellar disorders. A postural tremor of the hands that is indistinguishable from essential tremor may occur in patients with dystonia. The designation **dystonic tremor** refers to a postural or intention tremor that occurs in a part of the body already affected by dystonia. It is a part of the dystonia and is most prominent when an attempt is made to oppose the dystonic posturing.

ASTERIXIS

Asterixis may be associated with postural tremor, but is itself more properly considered a form of **myoclonus** (discussed later) than tremor. It is seen most commonly in patients with **metabolic encephalopathy** and resolves with clearing of the encephalopathy.

To detect asterixis, the patient holds the arms outstretched with fingers and wrists extended. Episodic cessation of muscular activity causes sudden flexion at the wrists followed by a return to extension, so that the hands flap in a regular or, more often, an irregular rhythm. A similar phenomenon may be demonstrable at the ankles.

INTENTION (KINETIC) TREMOR

Intention or kinetic tremor occurs during activity. If the patient is asked to touch his or her nose with a finger, for example, the arm exhibits tremor during movement, often more marked as the target is reached. This form of tremor is sometimes mistaken for limb ataxia, but the latter has no rhythmic oscillatory component.

Intention tremor results from a lesion affecting the **superior cerebellar peduncle**. Because it is often very coarse, it can lead to severe functional disability. No satisfactory medical treatment exists, but stereotactic surgery of the contralateral ventrolateral nucleus of the thalamus or high-frequency thalamic stimulation through an implanted device is sometimes helpful when patients are severely incapacitated.

Intention tremor can occur—with other signs of cerebellar involvement—as a manifestation of toxicity of certain sedative or anticonvulsant drugs (eg, phenytoin) or alcohol; it is also seen in patients with Wilson disease.

REST TREMOR

▶ Parkinsonism

Rest tremor usually has a frequency of **4 to 6 Hz** and is characteristic of parkinsonism, whether the disorder is idiopathic or secondary (ie, postencephalitic, toxic, or drug induced in origin). The rate of the tremor, its relationship to activity, and the presence of rigidity or hypokinesia usually distinguish the tremor of parkinsonism from other forms of tremor. Tremor in the hands may appear as a "**pill-rolling**" maneuver—rhythmic, opposing circular movements of the thumb and index finger. There may be alternating flexion and extension of the fingers or hand or alternating pronation and supination of the forearm; in the feet, rhythmic alternating flexion and extension are common. Parkinsonism is discussed in more detail later.

▶ Other Causes

Less common causes of rest tremor include Wilson disease and poisoning with heavy metals such as mercury.

CHOREA

The word **chorea** denotes rapid irregular muscle jerks that occur involuntarily and unpredictably in different parts of the body. In florid cases, the often forceful involuntary movements of the limbs and head and the accompanying facial grimacing and tongue movements are unmistakable. Voluntary movements may be distorted by superimposed involuntary ones. In mild cases, however, patients may exhibit no more than a persistent restlessness and clumsiness. Power is full, but there may be difficulty in maintaining muscular contraction such that, for example, handgrip is relaxed intermittently (**milkmaid grasp**). The gait becomes irregular and unsteady, with the patient suddenly dipping or lurching to one side or the other (**dancing gait**). Speech often becomes irregular in

volume and tempo and may be explosive in character. In some patients, athetotic movements or dystonic posturing (see later) may also be prominent. Chorea disappears during sleep.

The pathologic basis of chorea is unclear, but some cases are associated with cell loss in the caudate nucleus and putamen. Dopaminergic drugs can provoke chorea. Causes of chorea are shown in **Table 11-2** and are discussed later. When chorea is due to a treatable medical disorder, such as polycythemia vera or thyrotoxicosis, treatment of the primary disorder abolishes it.

Table 11-2. Causes of Chorea.

Hereditary
Huntington disease
Huntington disease-like (HDL) disorders
Dentatorubral-pallidoluysian atrophy
Benign hereditary chorea
Wilson disease
Paroxysmal choreoathetosis
Familial chorea with associated acanthocytosis
Static encephalopathy (cerebral palsy) acquired antenatally or perinatally (eg, from anoxia, hemorrhage, trauma, kernicterus)
Sydenham chorea
Chorea gravidarum
Drug toxicity
Levodopa and other dopaminergic drugs
Antipsychotic drugs
Lithium
Phenytoin
Oral contraceptives
Others (eg, anticholinergics, baclofen, carbamazepine, digoxin, felbamate, lamotrigine, valproate, certain recreational drugs)
Miscellaneous medical disorders
Thyrotoxicosis, hypoparathyroidism, Addison disease
Hypocalcemia, hypomagnesemia, hyponatremia, hypernatremia
Hyperglycemia, hypoglycemia
Polycythemia vera
Hepatic cirrhosis
Systemic lupus erythematosus, primary antiphospholipid syndrome
Encephalitis or meningoencephalitis (various viruses including human immunodeficiency virus, *Mycoplasma pneumoniae*, *Mycobacterium tuberculosis*, *Borrelia burgdorferi*, *Treponema pallidum*, *Toxoplasma gondii*, other organisms)
Paraneoplastic syndrome
Cerebrovascular disorders
Vasculitis
Ischemic or hemorrhagic stroke
Subdural hematoma
Structural lesions of the subthalamic nucleus

HEMIBALLISMUS

Hemiballismus is unilateral chorea that is especially violent because the proximal muscles of the limbs are involved. It is due most often to vascular disease in the contralateral **subthalamic nucleus** and commonly resolves spontaneously in the weeks after its onset. It is sometimes due to other types of structural disease; in the past, it was an occasional complication of thalamotomy. Pharmacologic treatment is similar to that for chorea (discussed later).

DYSTONIA & ATHETOSIS

The term **athetosis** generally denotes abnormal movements that are slow, sinuous, and writhing in character. When the movements are so sustained that they are better regarded as abnormal postures, the term **dystonia** is used, and many now use the terms interchangeably. In dystonia, excessive or inappropriate contraction of muscles (often agonists and antagonists) leads to sustained abnormal postures of the affected region of the body. The abnormal movements and postures may be generalized (involving the trunk and at least two other sites) or restricted in distribution, such as to the neck (torticollis), hand and forearm (writer's cramp), or mouth (oromandibular dystonia). With restricted dystonias, two or more contiguous body regions (eg, upper and lower face) may be affected (**segmental dystonia**), or the disturbance may be limited to localized muscle groups so that only a single body region is involved (**focal dystonia**). By international consensus, dystonia is now classified along a **clinical axis** that includes age at onset, body distribution, temporal pattern, and associated features such as other movement disorders or neurologic features and along an **etiologic axis** that includes nervous system pathology and inheritance. Dystonia may be isolated (ie, occurring without other neurologic symptoms and signs apart from tremor) or secondary (**Table 11-3**), in which case other clinical features are present.

FACTORS INFLUENCING DYSTONIA

The abnormal movements are not present during sleep. They are generally enhanced by emotional stress and by voluntary activity. In some cases, abnormal movements or postures occur only during voluntary activity and sometimes only during specific activities such as writing, speaking, or chewing.

ETIOLOGY

Table 11-3 lists some of the conditions in which these movement disorders are encountered. Perinatal anoxia, birth trauma, and kernicterus from hyperbilirubinemia are the most common causes. In these circumstances, abnormal movements usually develop before 5 years of age. Careful questioning usually discloses a history of abnormal early development and often of seizures. Examination may

Table 11-3. Causes of Dystonia and Athetosis.

Inherited dystonias
Autosomal dominantly inherited disorders
Isolated generalized torsion dystonia and formes frustes
Huntington disease
Myoclonic dystonia
Dystonia-parkinsonism
Dopa-responsive dystonia
Dentatorubral-pallidoluysian atrophy
Neuroferritinopathy (neurodegeneration with brain iron-accumulation 3: NBIA3)
Spinocerebellar degenerations
Autosomal or X-linked recessively inherited disorders
Neurodegeneration with brain iron accumulation 1
Lubag
Chorea-acanthocytosis
Lysosomal storage disorders (eg, Pelizaeus-Merzbacher disease, Krabbe disease, metachromatic leukodystrophy)
Mitochondrionopathies
Leber hereditary optic atrophy
Acquired dystonias
Static perinatal encephalopathy (cerebral palsy)
Parkinson disease
Progressive supranuclear palsy
Wilson disease
Drugs
Levodopa and dopamine agonists
Antipsychotic drugs
Anticonvulsants
Calcium-channel blockers
Serotonin reuptake inhibitors
Others (see text)
Toxins (eg, methanol, manganese, carbon monoxide, carbon disulphide)
Infections: viral, postviral, bacterial, other
Vascular: ischemic anoxia; hemorrhage
Neoplastic disease
Psychogenic

reveal signs of cognitive dysfunction or a pyramidal deficit in addition to the movement disorder.

Dystonic movements and postures are the cardinal features of **isolated torsion dystonia** (discussed later). Torsion dystonia may also occur as a manifestation of Wilson disease or Huntington disease or as a sequela of encephalitis.

Acute dystonic posturing may result from treatment with dopamine receptor antagonist drugs (discussed later).

Lateralized dystonia may occasionally relate to focal intracranial disease, but the clinical context in which it occurs usually identifies the underlying cause.

MYOCLONUS

Myoclonic jerks are sudden, rapid, twitchlike muscle contractions. They can be classified according to their distribution, relationship to precipitating stimuli, site of origin (**Table 11-4**), or etiology. **Generalized myoclonus** has a widespread distribution, whereas **focal** or **segmental myoclonus** is restricted to a particular part of the body. Myoclonus can be spontaneous, or it can be brought on by sensory stimulation, arousal, or the initiation of movement (**action myoclonus**). Myoclonus may occur as a normal phenomenon (**physiologic myoclonus**) in healthy persons, as an isolated abnormality (**essential myoclonus**), or as a manifestation of epilepsy (**epileptic myoclonus**). It can also occur as a feature of a variety of degenerative, infectious, and metabolic disorders (**symptomatic myoclonus**) affecting the cerebral cortex, brainstem, or spinal cord. Myoclonus is sometimes manifest not by a sudden twitchlike muscle contraction but by a sudden loss of muscle activity (**negative myoclonus**). This is best seen as **asterixis**, discussed earlier. Careful clinical evaluation—noting the age of onset, character and distribution of myoclonus, precipitating stimuli and relieving factors, family history, and presence of any associated symptoms and signs—may suggest the cause and limit unnecessary investigations.

GENERALIZED MYOCLONUS

Causes are summarized in **Table 11-5**. Physiologic myoclonus includes the myoclonus that occurs upon falling asleep or awakening (**nocturnal myoclonus**) as well as **hiccup**. Essential myoclonus is a benign condition that occurs in the absence of other neurologic abnormalities and is sometimes inherited. Epileptic myoclonus may be impossible to differentiate clinically from nonepileptic forms. They may

Table 11-4. Anatomic Origin of Myoclonus.

Cortical
Cerebral anoxia (Lance–Adam syndrome)
Metabolic and toxic disorders (eg, uremia, dialysis syndrome, lithium, levodopa)
Neurodegenerative, infective, traumatic, vascular, and neoplastic diseases involving the cerebral cortex (eg, Alzheimer disease, Jakob–Creutzfeldt disease, Parkinson disease, and Parkinson-plus syndromes)
Epilepsies and epilepsia partialis continua
Cortical reflex myoclonus

Subcortical and brainstem
Exaggerated startle (eg, hereditary, static encephalopathies, brainstem encephalitis, multiple sclerosis, paraneoplastic disorders)
Essential, myoclonus-dystonia, and ballistic overflow myoclonus (hereditary or sporadic)
Reticular reflex myoclonus (caudal brainstem lesions; eg, uremia, posthypoxic)
Palatal myoclonus (dentate-olivary lesions)

Spinal
Propriospinal myoclonus (eg, trauma, tumor, idiopathic)
Segmental myoclonus (eg, trauma, infective, inflammatory, tumor, compressive, vascular lesions, idiopathic)

Peripheral
Hemifacial spasm (microvascular compression, tumor, inflammatory)
Peripheral nerve or plexus injury (physical injury, tumor)

Psychogenic

Table 11-5. Causes of Myoclonus.

Physiologic myoclonus
Nocturnal myoclonus
Hiccup

Essential myoclonus (hereditary or sporadic)

Epileptic myoclonus

Symptomatic myoclonus
Degenerative disorders
Storage diseases (eg, Lafora body disease, lipidoses, ceroid-lipofuscinosis)
Pantothenate kinase-associated neurodegeneration
Wilson disease
Huntington disease
Myoclonus dystonia
Alzheimer disease
Parkinson disease and Parkinson-plus disorders
Spinocerebellar degenerations
Infectious disorders
Creutzfeldt–Jakob disease
HIV-associated dementia
Subacute sclerosing panencephalitis
Viral encephalitis
Whipple disease
Metabolic disorders
Drug intoxications (eg, penicillin, antidepressants, bismuth, levodopa, anticonvulsants)
Drug withdrawal (ethanol, sedatives)
Hypoglycemia
Hyperosmolar nonketotic hyperglycemia
Hyponatremia
Hepatic encephalopathy
Uremia, dialysis syndrome
Hypoxia (Lance–Adams syndrome)
Focal brain or nerve damage
Head injury
Stroke
Tumors
Peripheral nerve or plexus injury (physical injury, tumor)

be distinguished electrophysiologically, however, by the duration of the electromyographic burst associated with the jerking, by demonstrating an electroencephalographic (EEG) correlate related temporally to the jerks, or by determining whether muscles involved in the same jerk are activated synchronously.

FOCAL OR SEGMENTAL MYOCLONUS

Focal or segmental myoclonus can arise from lesions affecting the cerebral cortex, brainstem, spinal cord, or peripheral nerve. It can result from many of the same disturbances that produce symptomatic generalized myoclonus (see Table 11-5). Metabolic disorders such as hyperosmolar nonketotic hyperglycemia can cause **epilepsia partialis continua**, in which a repetitive focal epileptic discharge occurs from the contralateral sensorimotor cortex and leads to segmental myoclonus. Brainstem involvement of the dentatorubroolivary pathway by stroke, multiple sclerosis, tumors, or other disorders can produce **palatal myoclonus,** which may be associated with an audible click or synchronous movements of ocular, facial, or other bulbar muscles. Rhythmic vertical oscillation of the soft palate occurs that is best regarded as a tremor. An irritative lesion of a peripheral or cranial nerve may lead to myoclonus, as exemplified by hemifacial spasm (discussed in Chapter 9, Motor Disorders). Segmental myoclonus is usually unaffected by external stimuli and persists during sleep.

PROPRIOSPINAL MYOCLONUS

Propriospinal myoclonus arises in the spinal cord and then spreads up and down the cord, leading to a brief bodily contraction. Electromyographic surface recordings may be necessary to show the spread of muscle activity in an orderly sequence and may help to localize the site of origin of the myoclonus. The disorder may be idiopathic or secondary to diverse pathology that in some cases is revealed by imaging. Propriospinal myoclonus may also have a psychogenic basis.

TREATMENT

Although myoclonus can be difficult to treat, cortical myoclonus in particular sometimes responds to anticonvulsant drugs such as valproic acid 250 to 500 mg orally three times daily or levetiracetam titrated up to 500 to 1,500 mg orally twice daily. It may also respond to piracetam (not available in the United States). Benzodiazepines such as clonazepam 0.5 mg orally three times daily, gradually increased to as much as 12 mg/d, may help all types of myoclonus. A combination of medications is often necessary. **Postanoxic action myoclonus** is remarkably responsive to 5-hydroxytryptophan, the precursor of the neurotransmitter 5-hydroxytryptamine (serotonin). The 5-hydroxytryptophan is increased gradually to a maximum of 1 to 1.5 mg/d orally and may be combined with carbidopa (maximum,

400 mg/d orally) to inhibit metabolism in peripheral tissues. Localized myoclonus, regardless of origin, may respond to botulinum toxin injections. A variety of other medications have been used to treat different types of myoclonus, including carbamazepine, primidone, topiramate, zonisamide, diazepam, and—for essential myoclonus—anticholinergic agents, with anecdotal reports of benefit.

TICS

Tics are sudden, recurrent, quick, coordinated abnormal movements that can usually be imitated without difficulty. The same movement occurs repeatedly and can be suppressed voluntarily for short periods, although doing so may cause anxiety. Tics tend to worsen with stress, diminish during voluntary activity or mental concentration, and disappear during sleep.

CLASSIFICATION

Tics can be classified into four groups depending on whether they are simple or multiple and transient or chronic as follows:

1. **Transient simple tics** are common in children, usually terminate spontaneously within 1 year (often within a few weeks), and generally require no treatment.
2. **Chronic simple tics** can develop at any age but often begin in childhood, and treatment is unnecessary in most cases. The benign nature of the disorder must be explained to the patient.
3. **Persistent simple or multiple tics** of childhood or adolescence generally begin before 15 years of age. There may be single or multiple motor tics, and often vocal tics, but complete remission occurs by the end of adolescence.
4. The syndrome of **chronic multiple motor and vocal tics** is generally referred to as **Gilles de la Tourette syndrome**, after the French physician who described its clinical features. It is discussed in detail later. Tics also may occur with levodopa or amphetamine use and after chronic neuroleptic use (tardive tic), after head trauma or viral encephalitis, and in autistic children. They can occur in association with degenerative disorders of the basal ganglia, such as Huntington disease, and are well described in neuroacanthocytosis, when they may have a self-mutilating character.

BRADYKINESIA & HYPOKINESIA

Bradykinesia (slowed movement) and **hypokinesia** or **akinesia** (poverty or lack of movement) are major features of parkinsonism and may be quite disabling. Manifestations include a fixity of facial expression (the so-called **masked facies**, with reduced blinking, widened palpebral fissures, and an apparently impassive appearance) and a paucity of spontaneous movement of the limbs (eg, a reduced arm swing on walking). Some patients have "**freezing**," that is, a temporary inability to move. Such symptoms are difficult for patients to describe and are often attributed erroneously to weakness.

These phenomena are tested clinically by, for example, asking the patient to make repetitive alternating movements of each extremity in turn. This can involve tapping of the index or third finger on the pad of the thumb, pronation and supination of the raised arm (as if screwing a light bulb into the ceiling), opening and closing of the fist, stomping with the foot on the ground, and tapping the foot on the floor while the heel is maintained on the ground. A progressive reduction in amplitude or speed of the movements, irregularity in rhythm, or arrests in movement indicate abnormality. Activity should be continued until at least 15 repetitions have occurred, and sometimes for longer. Abnormalities must be distinguished from the slowness of movement without fatiguing and decrement that may occur in patients with pyramidal or cerebellar dysfunction (often with an irregular rhythm in the latter context). The inexpressive face of depressed patients may simulate the masked facies of parkinsonism and should be distinguished by the lack of other extrapyramidal findings and the abnormal affect.

CLINICAL EVALUATION OF PATIENTS

HISTORY

AGE AT ONSET

The age at onset of a movement disorder may suggest the underlying cause. For example, onset in infancy or early childhood suggests birth trauma, kernicterus, cerebral anoxia, or an inherited disorder; abnormal facial movements developing in childhood are more likely to represent tics than other involuntary movements; and tremor presenting in early adult life is more likely to be of the benign essential variety than due to Parkinson disease.

The age at onset can also influence the prognosis. In **isolated torsion dystonia**, for example, progression to severe disability is much more common when symptoms develop in childhood rather than later life. Conversely, **tardive dyskinesia** is more likely to be permanent and irreversible when it develops in the elderly than during adolescence.

MODE OF ONSET

Abrupt onset of dystonic posturing in a child or young adult suggests a drug-induced reaction; a more gradual onset in an adolescent suggests a chronic disorder such as isolated torsion dystonia or Wilson disease. Similarly, the abrupt onset of severe chorea or ballismus suggests a vascular cause, and abrupt onset of severe parkinsonism

suggests a neurotoxic cause; more gradual, insidious onset suggests a degenerative process.

COURSE

The manner of progression from onset may also be helpful diagnostically. For example, Sydenham chorea usually resolves within about 6 months after onset and therefore should not be confused with other varieties of chorea that occur in childhood.

MEDICAL HISTORY

▶ Drug History

An accurate account of all drugs taken by the patient over the years is important, because many movement disorders are iatrogenic. Neuroleptic drugs may lead to abnormal movements developing either while patients are taking them or after their use has been discontinued, and the dyskinesia may be irreversible, as discussed later.

Reversible dyskinesia may develop in patients taking certain other drugs, including oral contraceptives, levodopa, and phenytoin. Several drugs, especially lithium, tricyclic antidepressants, valproic acid, and bronchodilators, can cause tremor. Serotonin reuptake inhibitors have been associated with a number of movement disorders including parkinsonism, akathisia, chorea, dystonia, and bruxism.

▶ General Medical History

1. Chorea may be symptomatic of rheumatic fever, thyroid disease, systemic lupus erythematosus, polycythemia, hypoparathyroidism, or cirrhosis of the liver.

2. Movement disorders, including tremor, chorea, hemiballismus, dystonia, and myoclonus, may occur in patients with acquired immunodeficiency syndrome (AIDS). Opportunistic infections such as cerebral toxoplasmosis or cryptococcosis are often responsible, and infection with human immunodeficiency virus type 1 (HIV-1) may also have a direct pathogenic role.

3. A history of birth trauma or perinatal distress may suggest the cause of a movement disorder that develops during childhood.

4. Encephalitis lethargica, epidemic in the 1920s, was often followed by a wide variety of movement disorders, including parkinsonism. Various other viral encephalitides (Japanese encephalitis, West Nile, St Louis, herpes simplex, dengue, mumps, measles) may be accompanied or followed by movement disorders.

▶ Family History

Some movement disorders have an inherited basis and a complete family history must be obtained, supplemented if possible by personal scrutiny of close relatives. Any possibility of consanguinity should be noted.

EXAMINATION

Clinical examination indicates the nature of the abnormal movements, the extent of neurologic involvement, and the presence of coexisting disease; these in turn may suggest the diagnosis.

Psychiatric illness or cognitive impairment raises the possibility that the movement disorder is related to that or its treatment with psychoactive medication—or that the patient has a disorder with both abnormal movements and behavioral disturbances, such as Huntington disease or Wilson disease.

Focal motor or sensory deficits raise the possibility of a structural space-occupying lesion, as does papilledema. Kayser–Fleischer rings suggest Wilson disease. Signs of vascular, hepatic, or metabolic disease may suggest other causes for a movement disorder, such as acquired hepatocerebral degeneration or vasculitis.

INVESTIGATIVE STUDIES

BLOOD & URINE TESTS

1. Serum and urine **copper** and serum **ceruloplasmin** levels are important in diagnosing Wilson disease.
2. **Complete blood count and sedimentation rate** are helpful in excluding polycythemia, vasculitis, or systemic lupus erythematosus, any of which can occasionally lead to a movement disorder. A wet film of the blood may reveal circulating acanthocytes.
3. **Blood chemistries** may reveal hepatic dysfunction related to Wilson disease or acquired hepatocerebral degeneration; hyperthyroidism or hypocalcemia as a cause of chorea; or a variety of metabolic disorders associated with myoclonus.
4. **Serologic tests** are helpful for diagnosing movement disorders caused by systemic lupus erythematosus or lupus anticoagulant syndrome. Neurosyphilis and HIV-1 infection should always be excluded by appropriate serologic tests in patients with neurologic disease of uncertain etiology.

ELECTROPHYSIOLOGIC TESTS

An EEG may help in evaluating myoclonus and in distinguishing paroxysmal dyskinesias from seizures; otherwise, it is of limited usefulness. Electromyography and somatosensory evoked potentials may help to determine the level of neural involvement in myoclonus.

IMAGING

In some patients, intracranial calcification may be found by skull X-rays or computed tomography (CT) scans; the significance of this finding, however, is not always clear. CT scans or magnetic resonance imaging (MRI) may also reveal a tumor or other lesion associated with focal dyskinesia or dystonia or with symptomatic myoclonus, caudate atrophy due to Huntington disease, or basal ganglia abnormalities associated with Wilson disease. Positron emission tomography (PET) using ^{18}F-dopa can monitor the loss of nigrostriatal projections in Parkinson disease and may be helpful diagnostically in patients with incomplete parkinsonian syndromes, but is not widely available. Dopamine transporter imaging (DaT scan) using single-photon emission computed tomography (SPECT) can also be used for this purpose.

GENETIC STUDIES

Recombinant DNA technology has been used to generate probes for genes that determine certain inheritable movement disorders, such as Huntington disease and Wilson disease. Their use may be limited, however, by the genetic heterogeneity of some diseases, imprecise gene localization by certain probes, ethical concerns about adverse psychologic reactions to the presymptomatic diagnosis of fatal disorders, and the potential for misuse of such information by prospective employers, insurance companies, and government agencies.

PSYCHOLOGIC EVALUATION

Cognitive and affective disturbances can be documented and characterized by neuropsychologic evaluation. This may be helpful in diagnosing certain disorders such as Huntington disease or diffuse Lewy body dementia. Some movement disorders, such as Gilles de la Tourette syndrome, are associated with behavioral abnormalities such as attention deficit disorder and obsessive-compulsive disorder. The findings also may be important in guiding decisions regarding invasive interventions such as deep brain stimulation, which is contraindicated in patients with atypical parkinsonian syndromes or in classic Parkinson disease when significant dementia or major depression is also present.

SELECTED MOVEMENT DISORDERS

The more common and well-defined diseases or syndromes characterized by abnormal movements are discussed here together with the principles of their treatment.

FAMILIAL OR ESSENTIAL TREMOR

PATHOGENESIS

A postural and kinetic tremor may be prominent in otherwise normal subjects. Although the pathophysiologic basis of this disorder is uncertain, it often has a familial basis with an autosomal dominant mode of inheritance. Several genes or gene loci have been implicated, but the disorder is genetically heterogeneous and in many instances genetic associations are lacking. There is evidence of involvement of olivocerebellar and cerebello-thalamo-cortical pathways. Decreased levels of $GABA_A$ and $GABA_B$ receptors have been found postmortem in the dentate nucleus. Patients with essential tremor have a higher risk of developing Parkinson disease than the general population.

CLINICAL FINDINGS

Symptoms may develop in the teenage or early adult years but often do not appear until later. The tremor typically involves one or both hands, the head, the voice, or some combination of these, but the legs tend to be spared. Examination usually reveals no other gross abnormalities, but some patients may have mild ataxia, slight cogwheel rigidity, or personality disturbances. Although the tremor may increase with time, it often leads to little disability other than cosmetic and social embarrassment. In occasional cases, tremor interferes with the ability to perform fine or delicate tasks with the hands; handwriting is sometimes severely impaired. Speech is affected when the laryngeal muscles are involved. A small quantity of alcohol sometimes provides remarkable but transient relief; the mechanism is not known. The diagnosis is made on clinical grounds by the type of tremor and absence of other causes of tremor or neurologic abnormalities. A DaT scan is normal, whereas it is abnormal in Parkinson disease.

TREATMENT

If treatment is warranted to reduce tremor amplitude because of disability or social limitations, **propranolol**, 40 to 160 mg orally twice daily, can be prescribed but will need to be taken indefinitely. Other beta-blockers, such as atenolol and sotalol, have also been used. If tremor is particularly disabling under certain predictable circumstances, a single oral dose of 40 to 120 mg of propranolol can be taken in anticipation of the precipitating circumstances.

Primidone is also effective, but patients are often particularly sensitive to it; it is therefore introduced more gradually than when used for epilepsy. Patients are started on 50 mg/d, and the daily dose is increased by 50 mg every 2 weeks until benefit occurs or side effects limit further increments. A dose of 100 or 150 mg three times a day is often effective. There is no evidence that high doses (exceeding 750 mg daily) provide any added benefit.

Occasional patients respond to alprazolam, up to 3 mg/d in divided doses. Some patients reportedly benefit from gabapentin (1,200 mg/d), topiramate (400 mg/d), zonisamide (up to 200 mg daily), or intramuscular injections of botulinum toxin. When tremor is disabling and unresponsive to pharmacologic measures, surgical measures may be necessary. High-frequency **thalamic stimulation** by an implanted electrode is effective and has a low morbidity. Benefit is maintained over the years in most patients with severe disability. Thalamotomy may be helpful but has a significantly higher morbidity than thalamic stimulation. Transcranial focused ultrasound thalamotomy may also reduce the amplitude of tremor and improve the quality of life, and remains an option for those who prefer to avoid a surgical procedure.

PARKINSONISM

Parkinsonism occurs in all ethnic groups; in the United States and Western Europe it has a prevalence of 1 to 2 per 1,000 population, with an approximately equal sex distribution. The disorder becomes increasingly common with advancing age. It is characterized by tremor, hypokinesia, rigidity, and abnormal gait and posture.

ETIOLOGY

▶ Idiopathic

The most common variety of parkinsonism occurs without obvious cause; this idiopathic form is called **Parkinson disease** or **paralysis agitans** when there are no atypical features, it is not secondary to some known cause, and there is a sustained response to treatment with dopaminergic medication. During a preclinical phase extending back for several years before the development of the motor deficit, hyposmia, constipation, anxiety, depression, and rapid-eye-movement (REM) sleep behavior disorder may be present.

▶ Encephalitis

In the first half of the 20th century, parkinsonism often developed in patients with a history of von Economo encephalitis lethargica, but such cases of **postencephalitic parkinsonism** are becoming rare, although parkinsonism still occasionally follows other encephalitic illnesses.

▶ Drug- or Toxin-Induced Parkinsonism

1. **Therapeutic drugs**—Many drugs, such as phenothiazines, butyrophenones, metoclopramide, reserpine, and tetrabenazine, can cause a reversible parkinsonian syndrome (see later). This is usually reversible by withdrawing the offending medication, although symptoms and signs may take many months to resolve.

2. **Toxic substances**—Environmental toxins such as manganese dust or carbon disulfide can lead to parkinsonism; manganese used in the home manufacture of methcathinone appears to have been responsible for parkinsonism in intravenous users of this illegal stimulant. The disorder may also appear as a sequela of severe carbon monoxide poisoning and rarely after exposure to pesticides or fumes during welding.

3. **MPTP (1-methyl-4-phenyl-1,2,5,6-tetrahydropyridine)**—A drug-induced form of parkinsonism occurred in individuals who synthesized and self-administered a meperidine analogue, MPTP. This compound is metabolized to a toxin that selectively destroys dopaminergic neurons in the substantia nigra and adrenergic neurons in the locus ceruleus and induces a severe form of parkinsonism in humans and nonhuman primates. The ability of this drug to reproduce neurochemical, pathologic, and clinical features of Parkinson disease suggests that an environmental toxin could be responsible for the idiopathic disorder. MPTP-induced parkinsonism has been used as a model to assist in the development of new drugs for treatment of this disease.

▶ Vascular Parkinsonism

Multiple subcortical white-matter infarcts may lead to symptoms and signs suggestive of parkinsonism, usually accompanied by brisk tendon reflexes and extensor plantar responses. Tremor is often relatively inconspicuous and, in some patients, abnormalities of gait are especially evident ("lower-body parkinsonism"). The MRI findings help to suggest or support the diagnosis, and management is focused on preventing stroke. The response to antiparkinsonian medication is usually disappointing.

▶ Post-traumatic Parkinsonism

Boxers and those in certain other contact sports, such as football, may develop a syndrome of dementia (dementia pugilistica), behavioral and psychiatric disturbances, parkinsonism, and pyramidal and cerebellar deficits from recurrent head trauma leading to a chronic traumatic encephalopathy. There is no satisfactory treatment.

▶ Familial & Genetic Parkinsonism

Rarely, parkinsonism occurs on a familial basis. Approximately 3% of cases arise from a single genetic cause, and it is often not possible to distinguish these from the idiopathic disorder. Early onset and a familial incidence favor a genetic cause. Susceptibility loci are being identified. Autosomal dominant parkinsonism may result from mutations of one of several genes, including α-synuclein (*SNCA*), leucine-rich repeat kinase 2 (*LRRK2*), vacuolar protein sorting-associated protein 35 (*VPS35*), and, possibly, ubiquitin carboxyl-terminal esterase L1 (*UCHL1*) and DNA J heat shock protein family (Hsp40) member **C13** (*DNAJC13*). Mutations in *PARKIN*, *DJ1*, and *PINK1* cause early onset, autosomal recessive, and sporadic juvenile-onset parkinsonism. Several other genes or chromosomal regions have been implicated in familial forms of the disease or as susceptibility factors, including the gene for beta glucosidase (*GBA*), the enzyme deficient in the lysosomal storage disorder Gaucher disease.

▶ Parkinsonism Associated With Other Neurologic Diseases

Parkinsonism that occurs in association with symptoms and signs of other neurologic disorders is considered briefly in the later section on differential diagnosis.

PATHOLOGY

Idiopathic parkinsonism (Parkinson disease) is a **proteinopathy** characterized by the misfolding and aggregation of **α-synuclein**. It is thus also referred to as a synucleinopathy. Histopathologic examination at advanced stages shows loss of pigmentation and cells in the **substantia nigra** and other brainstem centers, cell loss in the globus pallidus and putamen, and filamentous eosinophilic intraneural inclusion granules (**Lewy bodies**) containing α-synuclein in the basal ganglia, brainstem, spinal cord, and sympathetic ganglia. The distribution of Lewy bodies is more widespread than originally appreciated, with early involvement of the lower brainstem (eg, dorsal motor nucleus of the vagus [X] nerve), olfactory bulb, and enteric nervous system, and subsequent spread to the locus ceruleus, substantia nigra, transentorhinal cortex, hippocampus, and neocortex. Lewy bodies are not seen in postencephalitic parkinsonism; instead there may be nonspecific neurofibrillary degeneration in a number of diencephalic structures, as well as changes in the substantia nigra.

PATHOGENESIS

As in other neurodegenerative proteinopathies (discussed in Chapter 5, Dementia & Amnestic Disorders), the disease is thought to be triggered by protein misfolding and aggregation. In Parkinson disease, the protein involved is α-synuclein. Abnormal protein may subsequently spread from cell to cell and thereby propagate the disease to contiguous parts of the nervous system. The disease has also been linked to the microbiome, ie, the bacterial content of the gut, and this association is being investigated further. Abnormalities of mitochondrial function are well described in Parkinson disease and may play a role in pathogenesis. Other possible factors include the inappropriate production of reactive oxygen species and the occurrence of an inflammatory response in the absence of infection.

The motor manifestations of Parkinson disease appear to result from altered patterns of inhibition and excitation within the basal ganglia and its connections via direct and indirect pathways (**Figure 11-2**). Dopamine and acetylcholine act as neurotransmitters in this region. In idiopathic parkinsonism, the normal balance between these two antagonistic neurotransmitters is disturbed because of dopamine depletion in the dopaminergic nigrostriatal system (**Figure 11-3**). Other neurotransmitters, such as norepinephrine, are also depleted in the brains of patients with parkinsonism, but the clinical relevance of this deficiency is less clear.

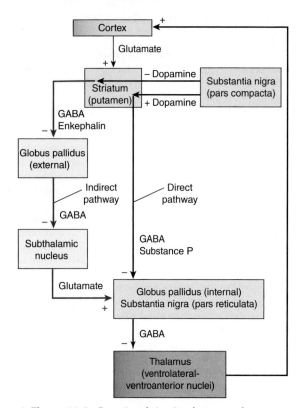

▲ **Figure 11-2.** Functional circuitry between the cerebral cortex, basal ganglia, and thalamus. The major neurotransmitters and their excitatory (+) or inhibitory (–) effects are indicated. In Parkinson disease, there is degeneration of the pars compacta of the substantia nigra, leading to overactivity in the indirect pathway (red) and increased glutamatergic output from the subthalamic nucleus (red). (Used with permission from Aminoff MJ. Pharmacologic management of parkinsonism and other movement disorders. In: Katzung BG, Masters SB, Trevor AJ, eds. *Basic and Clinical Pharmacology.* 11th ed. New York, NY: McGraw-Hill; 2009.)

CLINICAL FINDINGS

▶ Tremor

The **4- to 6-Hz** tremor of parkinsonism is characteristically most conspicuous **at rest**; it increases at times of emotional stress and often improves during voluntary activity. It commonly begins with rhythmic, opposing circular movements of the thumb and index finger ("pill-rolling"); as rhythmic flexion–extension of the fingers, hand, or foot; or as rhythmic pronation–supination of the forearm. It frequently involves the lower jaw and chin as well. Although it may ultimately be present in all limbs, it is not uncommon for the tremor to be confined to one limb, or both

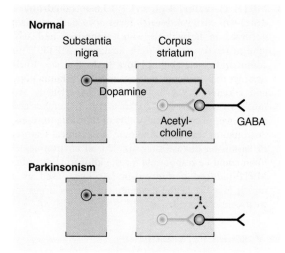

▲ **Figure 11-3.** Schematic representation of the sequence of neurons involved in parkinsonism. **Top:** Dopaminergic neurons (red) originating in the substantia nigra normally inhibit the GABAergic output from the striatum (caudate and putamen), whereas cholinergic neurons (green) exert an excitatory effect. **Bottom:** In parkinsonism, there is a selective loss of dopaminergic neurons (dashed, red). This leads to increased inhibitory output from the striatum. (Used with permission from Aminoff MJ. Pharmacologic management of parkinsonism and other movement disorders. In: Katzung BG, Trevor AJ, eds. *Basic and Clinical Pharmacology.* 13th ed. New York, NY: McGraw-Hill; 2015.)

limbs on one side, for months or years before it becomes more generalized. In some patients, tremor never becomes prominent.

▶ Rigidity

Rigidity or increased tone (ie, increased resistance to passive movement) is characteristic of parkinsonism. The disturbance in tone is responsible for the **flexed posture** of many patients. The resistance is typically uniform throughout the range of movement at a particular joint and affects agonist and antagonist muscles alike—in contrast to spasticity, where it is often greatest at the beginning of the passive movement (clasp-knife phenomenon) and more marked in some muscles than others. In some instances, the rigidity in parkinsonism is described as **cogwheel rigidity** because of ratchet-like interruptions of passive movement that may be due, in part, to the presence of tremor.

▶ Hypokinesia

The most disabling feature of parkinsonism is hypokinesia (sometimes called **bradykinesia** or **akinesia**)—a slowness of voluntary movement and a reduction in automatic movement, such as swinging the arms while walking. The patient's face is relatively immobile (**hypomimia** or **mask-like facies**), with widened palpebral fissures, infrequent blinking, a certain fixity of facial expression, and a smile that develops and fades slowly. The voice is soft (**hypophonia**) and poorly modulated. Fine or rapidly alternating movements are impaired, but power is not diminished if time is allowed for it to develop. The handwriting is small (**micrographia**), tremulous, and hard to read.

Abnormal Gait & Posture

The patient finds it difficult to get up from bed or an easy chair and adopts a flexed posture on standing (**Figure 11-4**). It is often difficult to start walking, so the patient may lean farther and farther forward while walking in place before being able to advance. The gait itself is characterized by small, shuffling steps and absence of the arm swing that normally accompanies locomotion; there is generally some unsteadiness on turning, and there may be difficulty in stopping. Retained arm swing, wide-based gait, or marked imbalance at an early stage suggests a nonparkinsonian disorder. In advanced cases, the patient

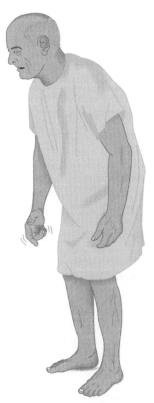

▲ **Figure 11-4.** Typical flexed posture of a patient with parkinsonism.

tends to walk with increasing speed to prevent a fall (**festinating gait**) because of the altered center of gravity that results from the abnormal posture.

Other Motor Abnormalities

There is often mild **blepharoclonus** (fluttering of the closed eyelids) and occasionally **blepharospasm** (involuntary closure of the eyelids). The patient may drool, perhaps because of impairment of swallowing. There is typically no alteration in the tendon reflexes (although a mild hyperreflexia may occur on the affected side in asymmetric parkinsonism), and the plantar responses are flexor. Repetitive tapping (approximately twice per second) over the bridge of the nose produces a sustained blink response (**Myerson sign**); the response is not sustained in normal subjects.

Nonmotor Manifestations

Anosmia is an early symptom (but may arise from many other causes, and is therefore not a specific indicator of Parkinson disease). **Cognitive decline**, executive dysfunction, and **personality changes** are common, as are **depression** and **anxiety** (Table 11-6). **Apathy** may be conspicuous. A sense of **fatigue** may be prominent, and some patients complain of pain or sensory disturbances. **Dysautonomic symptoms** include urinary urgency and urge incontinence, and constipation; postural hypotension relates most commonly to dopaminergic therapy or inactivity but may also reflect baroreflex failure or denervation of cardiac muscle. Pathologic involvement of the medulla may relate to these

Table 11-6. Nonmotor Symptoms in Parkinson Disease.

Affective disorders
Depression
Anxiety
Apathy
Fatigue
Cognitive disorders
Mild cognitive impairment
Dementia
Sleep disorders
Excessive daytime sleepiness
Insomnia
Sleep fragmentation
Vivid dreams
REM sleep behavior disorder
Anosmia
Autonomic disturbances
Constipation
Bladder dysfunction
Postural hypotension
Seborrheic dermatitis
Sensory disturbances or pain

dysautonomic changes. **Sleep disorders**, including REM behavior disorder, are common, and there may be excessive daytime somnolence. Frequent awakenings occur during nocturnal sleep; difficulty in turning over in bed, nocturia, involuntary movements (especially tremor or dystonia), and pain can make it difficult to settle down again. Seborrheic dermatitis may occur.

DIFFERENTIAL DIAGNOSIS

The diagnosis may be difficult to make in mild cases. Some degree of slowing is normal in the elderly, and certain otherwise normal people have a deliberate slowness about them.

▶ Depression

Depression may be accompanied by a somewhat expressionless face, poorly modulated voice, and reduction in voluntary activity; it can thus simulate parkinsonism. Moreover, the two diseases often coexist. A trial of antidepressant drug treatment may be helpful in some instances.

▶ Essential (Benign Familial) Tremor

This was considered separately (see earlier). An early age at onset, a family history of tremor, the relationship of the tremor to activity, a beneficial effect of alcohol on the tremor, and a lack of other neurologic signs distinguish this disorder from parkinsonism. Furthermore, essential tremor commonly affects the head (causing a nod or head shake); parkinsonism typically affects the lower jaw and chin. Dopamine transporter imaging (DaT scan) using single-photon emission computed tomography (SPECT) can be used as needed to distinguish between essential tremor (normal findings) and Parkinson disease.

▶ Parkinson-Plus Syndromes

This group of disorders is characterized by parkinsonism plus clinical evidence of more widespread disease from degeneration in other neuronal systems. Depending on the disorder, they are either synucleinopathies or tauopathies. They typically respond poorly to dopaminergic medication and have a poorer prognosis than Parkinson disease. These disorders include diffuse **Lewy body disease**, **multisystem atrophy**, **progressive supranuclear palsy**, and **corticobasal degeneration**, which are all discussed later in this chapter.

▶ Dystonia

A **dystonic tremor** may also be mistaken for parkinsonism, particularly when the dystonia is mild or unrecognized.

▶ Wilson Disease

Wilson disease (discussed later) can lead to a parkinsonian syndrome, but other varieties of abnormal movements are usually present as well. Moreover, the early age at onset and the presence of Kayser–Fleischer rings should distinguish Wilson disease from Parkinson disease, as should abnormalities in serum and urinary copper and serum ceruloplasmin.

▶ Huntington Disease

Huntington disease may occasionally be mistaken for parkinsonism when it presents with rigidity and akinesia, but a family history of Huntington disease or an accompanying dementia, if present, should suggest the correct diagnosis, which can be confirmed by genetic studies.

▶ Creutzfeldt–Jakob Disease

This prion disease may be accompanied by parkinsonian features, but dementia is usually present, myoclonic jerks are common, and ataxia is sometimes prominent; there may be pyramidal or cerebellar signs and visual disturbances, and the EEG findings of periodic discharges are usually characteristic.

▶ Normal Pressure Hydrocephalus

This condition leads to a gait disturbance (often mistakenly attributed to parkinsonism), urinary incontinence, and dementia. CT scanning reveals dilation of the ventricular system of the brain without cortical atrophy. The disorder may follow head injury, intracranial hemorrhage, or meningoencephalitis, but the cause is often obscure. Surgical shunting procedures to bypass any obstruction to the flow of cerebrospinal fluid (CSF) are often beneficial. Normal pressure hydrocephalus is discussed in more detail in Chapter 5, Dementia & Amnestic Disorders.

TREATMENT

Early parkinsonism requires no drug treatment, but it is important to discuss with the patient the nature of the disorder and the availability of medical treatment if symptoms become more severe, and to encourage activity. Treatment of the motor symptoms, when indicated, is directed toward restoring the dopaminergic–cholinergic balance in the striatum by blocking the effect of acetylcholine with anticholinergic drugs or by enhancing dopaminergic transmission (**Figure 11-5**).

▶ Anticholinergic Drugs

Muscarinic anticholinergic drugs are more helpful in alleviating **tremor** and **rigidity** than in ameliorating hypokinesia, but are generally less effective than dopaminergic drugs (see later). A number of preparations are available, and individual patients tend to favor different drugs. Among the most commonly prescribed drugs are trihexyphenidyl and benztropine (**Table 11-7**). Treatment is started with a small dose of one of the anticholinergics; the

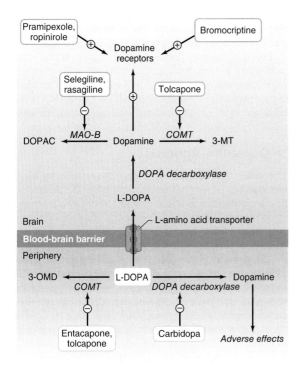

▲ Figure 11-5. Pharmacologic basis of antiparkinsonian dopaminergic therapy. (Used with permission from Aminoff MJ. Pharmacologic management of parkinsonism and other movement disorders. In: Katzung BG, Trevor AJ, eds. *Basic and Clinical Pharmacology*. 13th ed. New York, NY: McGraw-Hill; 2015.)

Table 11-7. Drugs Used in the Treatment of Parkinson Disease.

Drug	Total Daily Dose (mg)[1]
Anticholinergics	
Benztropine (Cogentin)	1-6
Trihexyphenidyl (Artane)	6-20
Amantadine (Symmetrel)	100-300
Levodopa (Sinemet; Stalevo; Parcopa; Rytary)	300-1,000[2]
Dopamine agonists	
Ergolides	
Bromocriptine (Parlodel)[3]	15-30
Nonergolides	
Pramipexole (Mirapex)	1.5-4.5
Ropinirole (Requip)	8-24
Rotigotine (Neupro)	2-8
Apomorphine (Apokyn)[4]	2-6
MAO-B inhibitors	
Selegiline (Eldepryl)	10
Rasagiline (Azilect)	0.5-1
COMT inhibitors	
Entacapone (Comtan)	600-1,000
Tolcapone (Tasmar)	300-600

[1]Doses are range for total daily maintenance; all drugs are administered in divided doses unless an extended-release formulation or a 24-hour skin patch (rotigotine) is used. Introduction is at a lower dose, which is gradually increased. Drug interactions are common; the addition of one drug may mandate reduction of another. Psychoactive side effects are common with all of these agents.
[2]Refers to the levodopa component of the commercially available carbidopa/levodopa combination (eg, 25/250 represents 250 mg of levodopa).
[3]Rarely used.
[4]Administered by subcutaneous injection.

dosage is then gradually increased until benefit occurs or side effects limit further increments. If treatment is not helpful, the drug is withdrawn and another anticholinergic preparation is tried. Anticholinergic drugs are best avoided in the elderly because of their side effects, which include dry mouth, constipation, urinary retention, defective pupillary accommodation, and confusion.

▶ Amantadine

Amantadine can be given for mild parkinsonism either alone or in combination with an anticholinergic agent. Its precise mode of therapeutic action is unclear, but its pharmacologic effects include blockade of NMDA-preferring glutamate and muscarinic cholinergic receptors and stimulation of dopamine release. Amantadine improves all the motor features of parkinsonism, its side effects (restlessness, confusion, skin rashes, edema, disturbances of cardiac rhythm) are relatively uncommon, its effects are exerted rapidly, and it is given in a standard dose of 100 mg orally twice daily. Unfortunately, however, many patients fail to respond to this drug, or its benefit is short-lived. Amantadine may also be useful in reducing the sense of extreme fatigue experienced by some patients and for iatrogenic dyskinesias in patients with advanced disease (100 mg two or three times daily).

▶ Levodopa

Levodopa, which is converted in the body to dopamine (see Figure 11-5), ameliorates all the major clinical features of parkinsonism and, unlike the anticholinergic drugs, is often particularly helpful against **hypokinesia**. **Carbidopa** is a drug that reduces the extracerebral metabolism of levodopa to dopamine by inhibiting dopa decarboxylase (see Figure 11-5), but it does not cross the blood–brain barrier. Accordingly, when levodopa is given with carbidopa, the breakdown of levodopa is limited outside the brain. Carbidopa is generally combined with levodopa in a fixed proportion (1:10 or 1:4) as carbidopa/levodopa. There remains disagreement about the best time to introduce it. Concerns that levodopa may lose its effectiveness with time (as opposed to with advance of the disease) are misplaced, but response fluctuations commonly occur after it has been used for several years and may be particularly disabling. These may relate to the disease itself or to the duration of levodopa treatment. Many physicians therefore defer the introduction of levodopa for as long as possible or use dopamine agonists (discussed later) in conjunction with it to keep the levodopa dose low.

Treatment is started with a small dose, such as carbidopa/levodopa 10/100 mg or 25/100 mg orally three times daily, and the dose is gradually increased, depending on the response. Many patients ultimately require carbidopa/levodopa 25/250 (mg) three or four times daily. Carbidopa should total at least 75 mg/d. The medication is best taken about 30 to 45 minutes before meals or 2 hours after meals to maximize absorption and uptake into the brain. A tablet of carbidopa/levodopa (25/100, 10/100, 25/250) that disintegrates in the mouth and is then swallowed with the saliva (Parcopa) is also available and is best taken about 1 hour before meals.

The most common side effects of levodopa are nausea, vomiting, hypotension, abnormal movements (dyskinesias), restlessness, and confusion. Cardiac arrhythmias and sleep disturbances occur occasionally. The incidence of nausea, vomiting, hypotension, and cardiac irregularities is reduced when levodopa is taken with carbidopa. The late dyskinesias and behavioral side effects of levodopa occur as dose-related phenomena, but reduction in dose may diminish any therapeutic benefit. Treatment with olanzapine, quetiapine, or risperidone may relieve confusion and psychotic mental disturbances without blocking the effects of levodopa or exacerbating parkinsonism. Pimavanserin is a novel atypical antipsychotic agent specifically approved for the treatment of the psychosis of Parkinson disease. Clozapine, a dibenzodiazepine derivative that does not block the therapeutic effects of dopaminergic medication, may also relieve confusion and psychotic mental disturbances and, in some instances, the dyskinesias, but requires regular monitoring of the leukocyte count.

Another late complication of levodopa therapy or consequence of advancing disease is response fluctuation such as the **wearing-off effect**, in which deterioration occurs shortly before the next dose is to be taken, or the **on–off phenomenon**, in which abrupt but transient fluctuations in the severity of parkinsonism occur at frequent intervals during the day, apparently without any relationship to the last dose of levodopa. Such fluctuations may be disabling and may relate to discontinuous (pulsatile) levels of cerebral dopamine. They can be controlled only partly by varying the dosing intervals; restricting dietary protein intake; use of a controlled-release preparation of carbidopa/levodopa or of a novel extended-release formulation of carbidopa/levodopa (Rytary); addition of entacapone,

selective monoamine oxidase type B inhibitors, or dopamine agonists to the medication regimen; or administration of carbidopa/levodopa via portable intraduodenal pump. They often respond well to deep brain stimulation.

Levodopa therapy (either alone or in conjunction with carbidopa) is contraindicated in patients with narrow-angle glaucoma or psychotic illness and should be avoided in patients receiving monoamine oxidase type A (MAO-A) inhibitors. It should also be used with care in patients with active peptic ulcers or suspected malignant melanomas.

► Dopamine Agonists

The older agonists are ergot derivatives such as **bromocriptine**, which stimulates dopamine D_2 receptors. Bromocriptine is less effective than levodopa in relieving the symptoms of parkinsonism but is also less likely to cause dyskinesias. It is now used infrequently, as more effective dopamine agonists are available.

The newer dopamine agonists are not ergot derivatives. They seem to be as effective as the older agonists but are without their potential ergot-related adverse effects and may be used in early or advanced Parkinson disease. **Pramipexole** is started at 0.125 mg three times daily; the daily dose is doubled after 1 week and again after another week; it is then increased by 0.75 mg each week according to response and tolerance. A common maintenance dose is between 0.5 and 1.5 mg three times daily. **Ropinirole** is started at 0.25 mg three times daily, and the total daily dose increased at weekly intervals by 0.75 mg until the fourth week and by 1.5 mg thereafter. Most patients need between 2 and 8 mg three times daily for benefit. Rotigotine is given as a transdermal patch applied to a clean and healthy area of skin and replaced every 24 hours; skin reactions may occur at the application site. Adverse effects of these medications include fatigue, somnolence, nausea, peripheral edema, dyskinesias, confusion, hallucinations, and orthostatic hypotension. An irresistible urge to sleep at inappropriate times sometimes occurs and may lead to injury. Disturbances of impulse control may lead to such behaviors as compulsive gambling or abnormal sexual activity. Extended-release preparations of both pramipexole and ropinirole are available.

Apomorphine hydrochloride, a nonselective dopamine receptor agonist administered by subcutaneous injection, may help rescue patients with advanced parkinsonism and severe "off" episodes of akinesia despite optimized oral therapy. Side effects include severe nausea and vomiting, somnolence, hallucinations, chest pain, and hyperhidrosis; dyskinesias may be enhanced. It should not be prescribed by physicians who are unfamiliar with its potential complications and interactions.

► Catechol-O-Methyltransferase Inhibitors

Catechol-O-methyltransferase (COMT) is one of two principal enzymes involved in the metabolic breakdown of dopamine (see Figure 11-5); the other is monoamine oxidase, discussed later. COMT inhibitors may be used to reduce the dose requirements of and any response fluctuations to levodopa. Their use improves levodopa transport into the blood and across the blood–brain barrier and thus leads to more sustained plasma levels of levodopa. Side effects include diarrhea, confusion, dyskinesias, and abnormalities of liver function tests. Two of these inhibitors are in widespread use. **Tolcapone** is taken in a daily dose of 100 or 200 mg three times daily. Acute hepatic necrosis has occurred in rare instances in patients receiving this medication; accordingly, **entacapone** (200 mg) taken with carbidopa/levodopa up to five times daily is generally preferred.

A commercial preparation named **Stalevo** is now available that combines levodopa with both carbidopa and entacapone. It provides the convenience of simplifying the drug regime and requiring the consumption of fewer tablets, and is available in three combinations: Stalevo 50 (50 mg levodopa plus 12.5 mg carbidopa and 200 mg entacapone), Stalevo 100 (100 mg, 25 mg, and 200 mg, respectively), and Stalevo 150 (150 mg, 37.5 mg, and 200 mg, respectively). More sustained plasma levels of levodopa may lead to more continuous delivery of levodopa to the brain, with a theoretical reduction in the risk of response fluctuations and dyskinetic complications. However, initiating levodopa therapy with Stalevo rather than carbidopa/levodopa fails to delay the time of onset or reduce the frequency of dyskinesia; indeed, dyskinesias may occur sooner and with increased frequency.

▶ Monoamine Oxidase Inhibitors

Selegiline, an irreversible monoamine oxidase type B (MAO-B) inhibitor, inhibits the metabolic breakdown of dopamine (see Figure 11-5). It thus enhances the antiparkinsonian effect of levodopa and may reduce mild on–off fluctuations in responsiveness. Some clinical studies suggest that selegiline may also delay the progression of Parkinson disease, although the evidence is incomplete in this regard; when used for neuroprotection, selegiline is best kept for patients with mild disease. The dose is 5 mg orally twice daily, usually given early in the day to avoid insomnia.

Rasagiline is a more potent and selective, well-tolerated, irreversible MAO-B inhibitor that is taken in a dose of 0.5 or 1 mg once daily. It is effective in the initial treatment of early parkinsonism and in addition as adjunctive therapy in patients with more advanced disease and response fluctuations to levodopa. It may also slow disease progression, although the evidence for this is ambiguous.

Safinamide, another monoamine oxidase B inhibitor, was approved by the FDA while this book was in production. It reduces response fluctuations to levodopa, diminishing off-periods in patients with wearing-off effect or on-off phenomenon. It is not effective as monotherapy for Parkinson disease. Patients are started on 50 mg orally once daily, increased after 2 weeks to 100 mg once daily.

Patients treated with monoamine oxidase B inhibitors should not take meperidine, tramadol, methadone, propoxyphene, cyclobenzaprine, St. John's wort, the antitussive dextromethorphan, or other monoamine oxidase inhibitors. There is a theoretical risk of precipitating acute toxic interreactions of the serotonin syndrome type in patients receiving tricyclic antidepressants or serotonin reuptake inhibitors. The adverse effects of levodopa, especially dyskinesias, mental changes, nausea, and sleep disorders, may be increased.

▶ Ablative Surgery

Surgical treatment of parkinsonism by **thalamotomy** or **pallidotomy** was often undertaken when patients became unresponsive to pharmacologic measures or developed intolerable adverse reactions to antiparkinsonian medication. The rate of significant complications was less than 5% after unilateral pallidotomy or thalamotomy, but approximately 20% or more after bilateral procedures. Ablative surgery has now largely been replaced by high-frequency stimulation of target structures, with a significant reduction in morbidity.

▶ Deep Brain Stimulation

High-frequency stimulation of the **globus pallidus internus** or **subthalamic nucleus** may help all the cardinal motor features of parkinsonism to a similar degree as ablative surgery, and it reduces the time spent in the off-state in patients with response fluctuations. Gait disturbances and akinesia may be helped by stimulation of the **pedunculopontine nucleus**. Deep brain stimulation has the advantage of being reversible, of having a much lower morbidity than ablative surgical procedures (especially when bilateral procedures are contemplated), and of causing minimal damage to the brain. It is thus preferred over ablative procedures. Candidates should have classic Parkinson disease (rather than atypical parkinsonism), be cognitively intact and cooperative, have previously responded well to pharmacologic treatment, have developed response fluctuations with a significant amount of off-time, and have realistic expectations of the procedure.

▶ Cellular Therapies

Autologous or fetal adrenal medullary tissue or fetal substantia nigra has been transplanted to the putamen or caudate nucleus in the belief that the transplanted tissue would continue to synthesize and release dopamine. In two controlled trials involving intracerebral transplantation of human embryonic mesencephalic tissue containing dopaminergic neurons, dyskinetic complications occurred and were sometimes incapacitating. Moreover, Lewy body pathology sometimes spreads to the transplanted tissue.

Research is currently focused on potential cellular therapies involving neural stem cells, but much work needs to be done before clinical trials can commence in Parkinson disease.

▶ Protective Therapy

Attempts have been made to slow the progression of Parkinson disease by influencing the mechanisms involved in cell death. In addition to treatment with monoamine oxidase inhibitors such as selegiline or rasagiline (which also have antiapoptotic properties), candidate therapies include those that enhance mitochondrial function or cell energetics, limit glutamate toxicity, inhibit inflammatory responses, or have antiapoptotic effects. However, the results of clinical trials have been disappointing. **Isradipine**, a calcium channel antagonist, has neuroprotective properties in animal models of Parkinson disease; a clinical trial of its efficacy in patients is currently under way.

▶ General Measures, Physical Therapy, & Aids for Daily Living

Cognitive abnormalities and psychiatric symptoms may be helped by rivastigmine (3-12 mg daily), donepezil (5-10 mg daily), or memantine (5-10 mg daily); psychosis or hallucinations by adjustment of dopaminergic regimen or addition of atypical antipsychotics (eg, quetiapine); excessive daytime sleepiness by modafinil (100-400 mg daily); REM sleep behavior disorder by clonazepam (0.5-2 mg at night); and a hyperactive bladder by oxybutynin (5-15 mg daily) or tolterodine (2-4 mg daily). Constipation may respond to stool softeners or osmotic laxatives and fatigue to amantadine. Physical therapy and speech therapy (Lee Silverman technique) are beneficial to many patients, and the quality of life can often be improved with simple aids to daily living. Such aids may include extra rails or banisters placed strategically about the home for additional support, table cutlery with large handles, nonslip rubber table mats, devices to amplify the voice, and chairs that gently eject the occupant at the push of a button.

LEWY BODY DISEASE

CLINICAL FINDINGS

Up to 15% of all patients with dementia have diffuse Lewy body disease (also discussed in Chapter 5, Dementia & Amnestic Disorders), which typically has its age of onset between 50 and 85 years. Cognitive changes leading to dementia are conspicuous and usually precede or occur shortly after the appearance of parkinsonian deficits. Cognitive function may fluctuate markedly over the 24-hour period. Visual hallucinations are common but may not be distressing. Many patients have unexplained periods of markedly increased confusion or delirium. Parkinsonian deficits become increasingly severe with

time, but tremor is often relatively inconspicuous compared with bradykinesia and rigidity. Postural hypotension and syncope are common. The disorder is characterized pathologically by the occurrence of Lewy bodies diffusely in cortical and subcortical structures. In some instances, mutations in the α-synuclein or β-synuclein genes have been described; mutations in other genes may also be implicated.

DIFFERENTIAL DIAGNOSIS

Parkinson disease differs in that cognitive function is preserved until a later stage, and motor involvement is more likely to be asymmetric in onset, with more conspicuous tremor. The marked variability over short periods of time and the accompanying motor deficit differentiate Lewy body disease from Alzheimer disease. Imaging in Lewy body disease reveals generalized cortical atrophy.

TREATMENT

Management of Lewy body disease is difficult because levodopa induces hallucinations and exacerbates the cognitive and behavioral disturbances while providing only limited benefit to the motor disturbance. Anticholinergic drugs are best avoided because they also may exacerbate cognitive dysfunction. The dementia and behavioral abnormalities often respond favorably to cholinesterase inhibitors. Antipsychotic medication is usually poorly tolerated; if necessary, however, low doses of atypical antipsychotics, such as quetiapine (up to 50 mg daily), can be prescribed. Education and support of caregivers are important.

MULTISYSTEM ATROPHY

CLINICAL FINDINGS

Multiple system atrophy (MSA) is a progressive neurodegenerative disorder (a **synucleinopathy**) with multisystem motor abnormalities and often a dysautonomia. It is more common in men and occurs usually in the sixth decade. One subtype of MSA, referred to as **MSA-P**, is associated with neuronal loss in the putamen, globus pallidus, and caudate nucleus and presents with bradykinesia and rigidity. Anterocollis is often especially conspicuous. Another type (**MSA-C**) is associated with cerebellar degeneration (see Chapter 8, Disorders of Equilibrium). When autonomic insufficiency is a conspicuous accompaniment, the eponymous designation of **Shy-Drager syndrome** is sometimes used. This latter syndrome is characterized by parkinsonian features, autonomic insufficiency (leading to postural hypotension, anhidrosis, disturbance of sphincter control, and impotence), and signs of more widespread neurologic involvement (pyramidal or lower motor neuron signs and often a cerebellar deficit). MRI reveals a hypointense putamen with a hyperintense rim.

DIFFERENTIAL DIAGNOSIS

The autonomic and multisystem—often symmetric—motor findings with marked anterocollis distinguish the disorder from classic Parkinson disease.

TREATMENT

There is no treatment for the motor deficit (although a modest response to antiparkinsonian agents occurs occasionally), but postural hypotension may respond to a liberal salt diet, fludrocortisone 0.1 to 0.5 mg/d, midodrine (an α-adrenergic receptor agonist) 10 mg three times daily, wearing waist-high elastic hosiery, and sleeping with the head up at night. Droxidopa, a precursor of norepinephrine taken orally, is also helpful for the treatment of neurogenic postural hypotension.

PROGNOSIS

The disease follows a progressive course leading to death over about 8 to 10 years.

PROGRESSIVE SUPRANUCLEAR PALSY

PATHOGENESIS

Progressive supranuclear palsy is an idiopathic, usually sporadic, degenerative disorder, a **tauopathy** (see Chapter 5, Dementia & Amnestic Disorders) that primarily affects subcortical gray matter regions of the brain. There is much overlap clinically and pathologically with corticobasal degeneration (discussed later). The principal neuropathologic finding is neuronal degeneration with the presence of **neurofibrillary tangles** in the midbrain, pons, basal ganglia, and dentate nuclei of the cerebellum. Associated neurochemical abnormalities include decreased concentrations of dopamine and its metabolite homovanillic acid in the caudate nucleus and putamen. There may be a genetic predisposition to the disorder.

CLINICAL FINDINGS

Men are affected twice as often as women, and the disorder has its onset between ages 45 and 75 years. The classic clinical features are gait disturbance with early falls, supranuclear ophthalmoplegia, pseudobulbar palsy, axial dystonia with or without extrapyramidal rigidity of the limbs, and dementia.

Supranuclear ophthalmoplegia is characterized by prominent failure of voluntary **vertical gaze**, with later paralysis of horizontal gaze; oculocephalic and oculovestibular reflexes are preserved. Vertical saccades may initially be slowed. Postural instability, marked akinesia, and unexplained falls also occur early and may precede vertical gaze palsies. In addition, the neck often assumes an extended posture (**axial dystonia in extension**), with resistance to passive flexion. Rigidity of the limbs and bradykinesia may mimic Parkinson disease, but tremor is less common or conspicuous. A coexisting **pseudobulbar palsy** produces facial weakness, dysarthria, dysphagia, and often exaggerated jaw jerk and gag reflexes; there may also be exaggerated and inappropriate emotional responses (**pseudobulbar affect**). Hyperreflexia, extensor plantar responses, and cerebellar signs are sometimes seen. The **dementia** of progressive supranuclear palsy is characterized by forgetfulness, slowed thought processes, alterations of mood and personality, and impaired calculation and abstraction. **Sleep disturbances**, especially insomnia, are common.

Some patients with pathologically verified disease have pure akinesia or a clinical phenotype resembling Parkinson disease; in others, disease resembles corticobasal degeneration, with dystonia, apraxia, and cortical sensory loss.

MRI may show **midbrain atrophy** (hummingbird sign).

DIFFERENTIAL DIAGNOSIS

Parkinson disease differs from the classic form of progressive supranuclear palsy in that voluntary downward and horizontal gaze are not usually lost, axial posture tends to be characterized by flexion rather than extension, tremor is common, the course is less fulminant, and antiparkinsonian medications are more often effective.

TREATMENT

Dopaminergic preparations may benefit rigidity and bradykinesia, especially in the first 1 or 2 years. Anticholinergics such as amitriptyline 50 to 75 mg orally at bedtime or benztropine 6 to 10 mg/d orally can improve speech, gait, and pathologic laughing or crying. Pseudobulbar affect is best treated with a commercial preparation containing dextromethorphan and quinidine sulfate (20 mg/10 mg capsules; commercially available as Nuedexta). Methysergide 8 to 12 mg/d orally may ameliorate dysphagia. There is no treatment for the dementia. Treatment is supportive. Physical and occupational therapy may be helpful.

PROGNOSIS

The disorder typically follows a progressive course, with death from aspiration or inanition within 2 to 12 (usually 6-10) years.

CORTICOBASAL DEGENERATION

CLINICAL FINDINGS

Corticobasal degeneration is a rare, nonfamilial, degenerative disorder, a **tauopathy** that occurs in middle-aged or elderly persons of either sex. It is characterized pathologically by the presence of abnormal intracellular filamentous deposits containing tau protein. It sometimes simulates Parkinson disease when bradykinesia and rigidity are conspicuous features. Postural-action tremor may also occur, but the usual cause of profound disability is **limb apraxia** and **clumsiness** rather than extrapyramidal deficits. Other clinical features include speech disturbances (aphasic, apraxic, or dysarthric), acalculia, cortical sensory deficits (eg, neglect syndromes), stimulus-sensitive myoclonus, alien limb phenomenon (the tendency for a limb to move semipurposefully, involuntarily, and without the knowledge of its owner), dysphagia, postural disturbances, dystonic features, and ultimately cognitive decline and behavioral changes. Frontal release signs, brisk tendon reflexes, and extensor plantar responses may also be encountered. There is increased saccadic latency, but saccades are of normal velocity.

Some pathologically verified cases present with a frontal behavioral-spatial disorder, a nonfluent/agrammatic variant of primary progressive aphasia, or the phenotype of progressive supranuclear palsy.

DIFFERENTIAL DIAGNOSIS

The disorder is distinguished from Parkinson disease by the marked apraxia that often leads to a useless limb, difficulty in opening or closing the eyes, or speech disturbances. The presence of pyramidal and cortical deficits in addition to any extrapyramidal dysfunction also helps in this regard, but definitive diagnosis can be made only at autopsy. MRI may show cortical, callosal, and midbrain atrophy and enlargement of the third ventricle. SPECT reveals hypoperfusion in regions of the frontal and parietal lobes.

TREATMENT

No specific therapy exists, and treatment is generally supportive. Antiparkinsonian medication is sometimes helpful for treating bradykinesia and rigidity, but often the response is disappointing. There is no treatment for the limb apraxia. Botulinum toxin may help focal dystonic features. Physical therapy is sometimes worthwhile.

PROGNOSIS

The disorder follows a progressive course, leading to increasing disability and dependence. Death typically follows within 10 years, often sooner, from aspiration pneumonia.

HUNTINGTON DISEASE

EPIDEMIOLOGY

Huntington disease is a hereditary disorder of the nervous system characterized by the gradual onset and subsequent progression of chorea and dementia. It occurs throughout the world and in all ethnic groups. Its prevalence rate is approximately 5 per 100,000 population. Symptoms usually do not appear until adulthood (typically between 30 and 50 years of age), by which time these patients have often started families of their own; thus, the disease continues from one generation to the next.

GENETICS

Huntington disease is an autosomal dominant disorder due to a mutation in the **huntingtin** gene (*HTT*). The disease shows complete penetrance, so that offspring of an affected individual have a 50% chance of developing it. Additional features of the inheritance of Huntington disease include **anticipation**, meaning that there is a trend toward earlier onset in successive generations, and **paternal descent**, which refers to the tendency for anticipation to be most pronounced in individuals who inherit the disease from their father. Both phenomena relate to the unstable nature of the mutation responsible for Huntington disease: expansion of a CAG trinucleotide repeat that codes for a polyglutamine tract. The repeat can expand during gametogenesis, especially in the male germline. This leads to an abnormal protein with longer and longer polyglutamine tracts. Normal subjects have between 9 and 37 CAG repeats, whereas nearly all patients with Huntington disease have more than 40. The age of disease onset depends on the length of the CAG repeat, but genetic polymorphisms are also associated with age of onset.

When a positive family history cannot be obtained, this may be because of the early death of a parent; moreover, relatives often conceal the familial nature of the disorder. In addition, a certain degree of eccentric behavior, clumsiness, or restlessness may be regarded as normal by lay people and medical personnel unfamiliar with the disorder. Therefore, the family history should not be regarded as negative until all close relatives of the patient have been examined personally. Nevertheless, apparently sporadic cases are occasionally encountered.

PATHOLOGY

Postmortem examination reveals cell loss, particularly in the cerebral cortex and corpus striatum (**Figure 11-6**). In the latter region, medium-sized spiny neurons that contain γ-aminobutyric acid (GABA) and enkephalin and project to the external segment of the globus pallidus are affected earliest, but other classes of neurons are eventually involved as well. Biochemical studies have shown that concentrations of the inhibitory neurotransmitter GABA, its biosynthetic enzyme glutamic acid decarboxylase (GAD), and acetylcholine and its biosynthetic enzyme choline acetyltransferase are all reduced in the basal ganglia of patients with the disease. The concentration of dopamine is normal or slightly increased. Changes in the concentrations of certain neuropeptides in the basal ganglia have also been found.

Normal

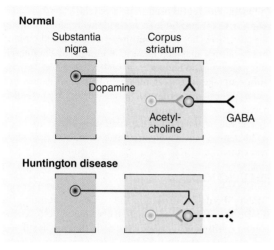

▲ **Figure 11-6.** Schematic representation of the sequence of neurons involved in Huntington disease. **A:** Dopaminergic neurons (red) originating in the substantia nigra normally inhibit the GABAergic output from the striatum (caudate and putamen), whereas cholinergic neurons (green) exert an excitatory effect. **B:** In Huntington disease, GABAergic neurons (black) are preferentially lost, resulting in reduced inhibitory output from the striatum. (Used with permission from Aminoff MJ. Pharmacologic management of parkinsonism and other movement disorders. In: Katzung BG, Trevor AJ, eds. *Basic and Clinical Pharmacology*. 13th ed. New York, NY: McGraw-Hill; 2015.)

PET has shown reduced glucose utilization, even in an anatomically normal caudate nucleus.

CLINICAL FINDINGS

Symptoms usually begin in the fourth or fifth decade, and the disease is progressive, with an average life span after onset of approximately 15 years.

▶ Initial Symptoms

Either abnormal movements or intellectual changes may be the initial symptom, but ultimately both are present. Neurodegeneration commences many years earlier and may be accompanied by subtle cognitive, psychiatric, or motor changes that are only apparent in retrospect.

1. **Dementia**—The earliest mental changes often consist of irritability, moodiness, and antisocial behavior, but a more obvious dementia subsequently develops. This is characterized at an early stage by selective and progressive impairment of attention and executive function, consistent with frontostriatal pathology.

2. **Chorea**—Movement disturbance may be characterized initially by no more than an apparent fidgetiness

or restlessness, but grossly abnormal choreiform or choreoathetoid movements are eventually seen. When severe, they may interfere with speech, swallowing, and gait. Other motor disturbances include the inability to sustain voluntary movements such as tongue protrusion. Saccadic eye movements are characteristically slowed.

3. **Atypical forms**—Especially in cases developing during childhood—but occasionally in adult-onset cases as well—the clinical picture is dominated by progressive rigidity and akinesia, with little or no chorea. This is known as the **Westphal variant**, and the correct diagnosis is suggested by the accompanying dementia and positive family history. Epilepsy and cerebellar ataxia are frequent features of the juvenile form but not of adult cases.

▶ Genetic Testing

Genetic testing provides a definitive means of establishing the diagnosis and permits presymptomatic detection of the disease. It should be preceded and followed by genetic counseling.

▶ Imaging

CT scanning or MRI often demonstrates atrophy of the cerebral cortex and caudate nucleus in established cases. Reduction in striatal metabolic rate may be demonstrated by PET.

DIFFERENTIAL DIAGNOSIS

Conditions that should be considered in the differential diagnosis of Huntington disease are listed in Table 11-2. **Tardive dyskinesia** (discussed later), which is most common, can usually be identified from the history. Laboratory studies can exclude most medical disorders associated with chorea. Other hereditary disorders with chorea are considered later.

Huntington disease-like (HDL) disorders resemble Huntington disease but are not associated with abnormal CAG trinucleotide repeat number of the huntingtin gene. Autosomal dominant (HDL1 and HDL2) and recessive forms (HDL3) have been described. HDL1 is associated with a 192-nucleotide insertion, resulting in an expanded octapeptide repeat, in the prion protein gene (*PRNP*). HDL2 is caused by an expanded CAG/CTG repeat in the junctophilin-3 gene (*JPH3*).

Benign hereditary chorea is inherited in an autosomal dominant manner or occurs de novo. It is characterized by choreiform movements that develop in early childhood, do not progress during adult life, and are not associated with dementia. An autosomal recessive form may also exist. In patients with mutations in the gene (*NKX2-1*) coding for thyroid transcription factor-1, hypothyroidism and pulmonary abnormalities may also be present (brain–thyroid–lung syndrome).

Familial chorea sometimes occurs in association with circulating acanthocytes (spiny red blood cells), but examination of a wet blood film will clearly distinguish this disorder, discussed later. Other clinical features of **chorea-acanthocytosis** include orolingual ticlike dyskinesias, vocalizations, mild intellectual decline, seizures, peripheral neuropathy, and muscle atrophy. Parkinsonian features are sometimes present. Unlike certain other disorders associated with circulating acanthocytes, there is no disturbance of β-lipoprotein concentration in the peripheral blood.

Paroxysmal choreoathetosis may occur on a familial basis, but the intermittent nature of the symptoms and their relationship to movement or emotional stress usually distinguish this disorder from Huntington disease.

Wilson disease can be distinguished from Huntington disease by the mode of inheritance, the presence of Kayser–Fleischer rings, and abnormal serum copper and ceruloplasmin levels.

Dentatorubral-pallidoluysian atrophy, another dominantly inherited CAG repeat disorder that is clinically similar to Huntington disease, is distinguished by genetic testing. It is uncommon except in those of Japanese ancestry.

Neuroferritinopathy (NBIA2) is considered later. Although characterized by progressive chorea and dystonia with onset in adults having a positive family history, cognitive function is relatively preserved, MRI is characteristically abnormal, and the mutant gene (*FTL1*) is distinct from the Huntingtin gene.

The age at onset of symptoms usually distinguishes Huntington disease from certain rare inherited childhood disorders characterized by choreoathetosis.

When the early symptoms constitute progressive intellectual failure, it may not be possible to distinguish Huntington disease from other varieties of dementia unless the family history is characteristic or the movement disorder becomes noticeable.

TREATMENT & PROGNOSIS

There is no cure for Huntington disease, which, as a rule, terminates fatally 10 to 20 years after clinical onset. There is no treatment for the dementia, but the movement disorder may respond to drugs that interfere with dopaminergic inhibition of striatal output neurons. These include drugs that deplete dopamine from nerve terminals, such as reserpine 0.5 to 5 mg/d orally or tetrabenazine 12.5 to 50 mg orally three times daily, and dopamine D_2-receptor–blocking drugs such as haloperidol 0.5 to 4 mg orally four times daily or atypical antipsychotic agents such as quetiapine. Deutetrabenazine, a selective inhibitor of the vesicular monoamine 2 transporter (VMAT2) that modulates dopamine release, was approved by the FDA for chorea while this book was in press. A dose of 6 mg/d is increased gradually depending on response and tolerance up to 24 mg twice daily. Side effects include sedation, diarrhea, fatigue, and an increased risk of depression and suicidality.

Quetiapine is also used to treat psychosis or disruptive behavior, as is olanzapine or risperidone. In some patients, clozapine can be tried but necessitates weekly blood counts. Drugs that potentiate GABAergic or cholinergic neurotransmission are generally ineffective. Selective serotonin reuptake inhibitors may help to reduce depression, aggressiveness, and agitation. Social services are helpful in management.

The role of deep brain stimulation is uncertain, but it has been used successfully in a small number of patients to treat chorea.

PREVENTION

Patients should be advised of the risk of transmitting the disease to offspring, and living offspring should receive genetic counseling. The use of genetic markers for detection of presymptomatic Huntington disease may present ethical concerns about adverse psychologic reactions or potential misuse of such information by others to the individual's detriment.

DENTATORUBRAL-PALLIDOLUYSIAN ATROPHY

This disorder, which is inherited in an autosomal dominant manner, is rare except in Japan. It is characterized by dementia, choreoathetosis, ataxia, and myoclonic epilepsy. The mutant gene, atrophin 1 (*ATN1*), is distinct from that in Huntington disease, despite the similarity of clinical phenotype. Mutant *ATN1* contains an expanded CAG repeat, the size of which correlates with age at onset and disease severity. Treatment is symptomatic, as for Huntington disease.

SYDENHAM CHOREA & PANDAS

Sydenham chorea occurs principally in children and adolescents as a complication of a previous group A hemolytic streptococcal infection. It is the most common cause of chorea developing acutely in children. The underlying pathologic feature is probably an arteritis. In approximately 30% of cases, it appears 2 or 3 months after an episode of rheumatic fever or polyarthritis, but in other patients no such history can be obtained. There is usually no recent history of sore throat and no fever. The disorder may have an acute or insidious onset, usually subsiding within the following 4 to 6 months. It may recur during pregnancy (**chorea gravidarum**), however, or in patients taking oral contraceptive preparations.

Sydenham chorea is characterized by abnormal choreiform movements that are sometimes unilateral and, when mild, may be mistaken for restlessness or fidgetiness. There may be accompanying behavioral changes, with the child becoming irritable or disobedient. Obsessive-compulsive symptoms and emotional lability also occur. In

30% of cases there is evidence of cardiac involvement, but the sedimentation rate and antistreptolysin O titer are usually normal. The diagnosis is supported by the presence of other manifestations of rheumatic fever and by the absence of any other cause for the chorea such as systemic lupus erythematosus. Cerebral MRI or CT findings are usually normal. PET and SPECT studies show reversible basal ganglia hypermetabolism.

The traditional treatment is bed rest, sedation, and prophylactic antibiotic therapy even if there are no other signs of acute rheumatism. A course of intramuscular penicillin is generally recommended, and continuous prophylactic oral penicillin daily or intramuscular benzathine penicillin G monthly until approximately age 20 years is also frequently advised to prevent streptococcal infections. If necessary, chorea can be treated with haloperidol, risperidone, or other dopamine receptor–blocking drugs, or with valproic acid or carbamazepine, depending on its severity. In severe cases unresponsive to other measures, a course of corticosteroids may be effective. The prognosis is essentially that of the cardiac complications.

PANDAS (pediatric autoimmune neuropsychiatric disorders associated with streptococcal infections) is the acronym used to refer to the association of obsessive-compulsive or tic disorders of variable severity with streptococcal infections in children. In addition, dystonia, chorea, and dystonic choreoathetosis may be sequelae of streptococcal infection. The etiology is unclear but may be similar to that of Sydenham chorea, relating to poststreptococcal autoimmunity.

ISOLATED GENERALIZED TORSION DYSTONIA

Dystonia is classified by phenomenology and etiology. Idiopathic (or primary) generalized torsion dystonia is characterized by dystonic movements and postures and an absence of other neurologic signs. The birth and developmental histories are normal. Before the diagnosis can be made, other possible causes of dystonia must be excluded on clinical grounds and by laboratory investigations.

PATHOGENESIS

Isolated generalized torsion dystonia is typically inherited as an autosomal dominant disorder with variable penetrance of 30% to 40%. Molecular genetic techniques permit identification of carriers of the responsible deletion in torsin 1A, an ATP-binding protein, but there is some evidence of genetic heterogeneity. Other dystonic disorders (discussed later) occur as autosomal or X-linked recessive disorders. Changes in the concentrations of norepinephrine, serotonin, and dopamine occur in a variety of brain regions, but their role in the pathogenesis of dystonia is uncertain. Onset may be in childhood or later life, and the disorder remains as a lifelong affliction. The diagnosis is made on clinical grounds.

CLINICAL FINDINGS

▶ History

When onset is in childhood, a family history is usually obtainable. Symptoms generally commence in the legs. Progression is likely, and the disorder typically leads to severe disability from generalized dystonia.

With onset in adult life, a positive family history is less likely. The initial symptoms are usually in the arms or axial structures. Generalized dystonia may ultimately develop in approximately 20% of patients with adult-onset dystonia, but severe disability does not usually occur.

▶ Examination

The disorder is characterized by abnormal movements and postures that are typically exacerbated by voluntary activity. For example, the neck may be twisted to one side (**torticollis**), the arm held in a hyperpronated position with the wrist flexed and fingers extended, the leg held extended with the foot plantar-flexed and inverted, or the trunk held in a flexed or extended position. There is often facial grimacing, and other characteristic facial abnormalities may also be encountered, including **blepharospasm** (spontaneous, involuntary forced closure of the eyelids for a variable time; difficulty in eye opening; repetitive blinking) and **oromandibular dystonia**. This consists of spasms of the muscles about the mouth, causing, for example, involuntary opening or closing of the mouth; pouting, pursing, or retraction of the lips; retraction of the platysma muscle; and roving or protruding movements of the tongue. The combination of blepharospasm and oromandibular dystonia is sometimes referred to as **Meige syndrome**.

DIFFERENTIAL DIAGNOSIS

Other causes of dystonia (see Table 11-3) must be distinguished before a diagnosis of isolated torsion dystonia is made. A normal developmental history before the onset of abnormal movements, an absence of other neurologic signs, and normal results of laboratory investigations, are important. Drug-induced dystonia can generally be excluded by the history. Imaging may reveal acquired brain lesions. Genetic testing in conjunction with genetic counseling is helpful by obviating the need for other diagnostic studies and facilitating further management in patients with isolated torsion dystonia that begins before 30 years of age or in older subjects with a positive family history.

TREATMENT

The abnormal movements may be helped, at least in part, by drugs. A dramatic response to levodopa suggests a variant of classic torsion dystonia, discussed separately later. Anticholinergic drugs given in the highest doses that can be tolerated (typically, trihexyphenidyl 40-50 mg/d orally in divided doses) may be very effective. Diazepam is occasionally helpful. Phenothiazines, haloperidol, or tetrabenazine may be worthwhile; however, at effective doses, these drugs usually lead to mild parkinsonism. Baclofen and carbamazepine are sometimes helpful, at least anecdotally. Stereotactic thalamotomy may help patients with predominantly unilateral dystonia involving the limbs, but—especially when performed bilaterally for generalized dystonia—may lead to major side effects such as hemiparesis, dysphagia, and dysarthria. Deep brain stimulation of the globus pallidus internus has benefitted a number of patients and should be considered in medically refractory cases. Potential adverse events include infection at the stimulator site, broken leads, hemorrhage, affective changes, and dysarthria.

COURSE & PROGNOSIS

Approximately one-third of patients eventually become confined to chair or bed, and another one-third are affected only mildly. In general, severe disability is more likely to occur when the disorder commences in childhood.

DOPA-RESPONSIVE DYSTONIA

This disorder (Segawa syndrome) is inherited in an autosomal dominant manner with incomplete penetrance (*GCH1* gene) or, rarely, as an autosomal recessive trait (*TH* gene). Symptom onset is typically in childhood but may occur later. Girls are affected more commonly than boys. Disabling dystonia may be accompanied by bradykinesia and rigidity that sometimes leads to a mistaken diagnosis of juvenile Parkinson disease; diurnal worsening of symptoms is common. Extensor plantar response or other evidence of upper motor neuron involvement may occur. Some patients have focal dystonias or minor functional deficits, whereas others become chair-bound if untreated. Remarkable recovery occurs with low doses of levodopa, to which patients are particularly sensitive. Because of the wide variation in age and manner of presentation, all children with an unexplained extrapyramidal motor disorder and all patients with symptoms that might relate to dopa-responsive dystonia probably merit a trial of levodopa therapy.

DYSTONIA-PARKINSONISM

An X-linked recessive form of dystonia-parkinsonism (sometimes called *lubag*) has been identified in men from the Philippines and relates to mutations of *TAF1* gene at Xq13.1 Female heterozygotes are reported to have mild dystonia or chorea. The response to pharmacotherapy is often disappointing. Another variety with autosomal dominant inheritance has been described in patients of differing ethnic origin, with rapid evolution of symptoms and signs over hours, days, or weeks, but slow progression thereafter; a rostrocaudal (face, arm, leg) gradient of

involvement may be noted. The disorder relates to mutation in the gene encoding the alpha-3 subunit of N,K-ATPase (*ATP1A3*) on chromosome 19q13. It may first manifest during childhood or adulthood, often after a period of stress. Levodopa therapy is ineffective.

MYOCLONIC DYSTONIA

This is an autosomal dominant disorder with incomplete penetrance and variable expression, related to mutations in the *DRD2* or *SGCE* gene. Patients exhibit rapid jerks in addition to more sustained abnormal postures. The legs are often spared. The jerks may respond to alcohol. The EEG is normal. The disorder appears to be distinct from classic isolated torsion dystonia. It usually begins before 20 years of age and has a benign, slowly progressive course over many years. Genetic studies suggest that myoclonic dystonia and essential myoclonus are allelic disorders.

LOCALIZED TORSION DYSTONIA

Some of the dystonic features of generalized torsion dystonia may occur as localized phenomena. They are probably best regarded as dystonias that occur as formes frustes of the more generalized disorder in patients with a positive family history or that represent a localized manifestation of its adult-onset form when there is no family history. In addition, localized adult-onset dystonia may exhibit autosomal dominant inheritance. Localized dystonias can be divided into focal (ie, involving a single body region), segmental (ie, affecting two or more contiguous regions), or multifocal dystonias (ie, involving at least two noncontiguous regions).

Both **blepharospasm** and **oromandibular dystonia** (both described earlier) can occur as isolated focal dystonias. Familial blepharospasm inherited as an autosomal dominant trait has been described, but the gene remains unmapped. Blepharospasm often responds well to treatment with botulinum toxin.

Spasmodic dysphonia is a focal dystonia of the laryngeal muscles. The adductor type is most common, and the excessive adduction of the vocal cords during speech causes the voice to sound tight and strained, with occasional speech arrests. In abductor spasmodic dysphonia, the vocal cords are abducted inappropriately during speech, resulting in a breathy, whispery voice. Treatment by injection of botulinum toxin into the laryngeal muscles is effective in treating the spasmodic dysphonia, especially the adductor type.

Spasmodic torticollis (cervical dystonia) usually begins in the fourth or fifth decade and is characterized by a tendency for the neck to turn to one side. This often occurs episodically in early stages, but eventually the neck is held continuously to one side. In other patients, the head may be tilted to the side (laterocollis), flexed forward (anterocollis), or extended backward (retrocollis); often, a combination of abnormal movements and postures occurs. Sensory tricks (eg, light touch of the face) may help to reduce the intensity of symptoms. Neck and shoulder pain are common, and a head tremor may be present. Although the disorder is usually lifelong, spontaneous remission does occur occasionally, especially in the first 18 months after onset. Medical treatment is generally unsatisfactory. A trial of the drugs used for more generalized torsion dystonias is worthwhile. The most effective treatment, however, is with local injection of botulinum toxin into the overactive muscles; benefit lasts for up to several months, after which the injection is repeated as needed. Selective section of the spinal accessory (XI) nerve and the upper cervical nerve roots may help patients in whom the neck is markedly deviated to the side, but recurrence of the abnormal posture is frequent. Deep brain stimulation (DBS) of the globus pallidus internus is helpful in many patients with cervical dystonia whose response to botulinum toxin is unsatisfactory.

Writer's cramp is characterized by dystonic posturing of the hand and forearm when the hand is used for writing and sometimes for other tasks (eg, playing the piano or using a screwdriver or table cutlery). Anticholinergic medications, baclofen, or benzodiazepines may help occasionally. Injections of botulinum toxin into the involved muscles are often helpful, but hand or arm weakness may be a troublesome consequence. Patients may have to learn to use the other hand for writing or other fine motor tasks, although in some cases this hand also becomes affected. The use of a pen with a large handle is sometimes worthwhile; in other instances, patients may use a keyboard.

COMBINED DYSTONIA

A large group of disorders are characterized by dystonia combined with other neurologic features, such as dementia, ataxia, dyskinesias, or parkinsonism. This includes Wilson disease, which is discussed separately.

In **idiopathic basal ganglia calcification (Fahr disease)**, calcification of the basal ganglia is associated with some combination of dystonia, parkinsonism, chorea, ataxia, and behavioral disturbances. Autosomal dominant inheritance occurs in some families (primary familial brain calcification), but there is genetic heterogeneity. Intracranial calcification may also occur idiopathically but as an incidental finding, without clinical accompaniments.

Neurodegeneration with brain iron accumulation (NBIA) refers to a group of inherited disorders with iron accumulation in the basal ganglia. Clinical manifestations include extrapyramidal and pyramidal deficits, neuropsychiatric changes, and ocular abnormalities. Age of onset, mode of inheritance, and rate of progression varies. Genetic testing identifies particular disorders. **Pantothenate kinase-associated neurodegeneration** (or **NBIA1**) is characterized by gait abnormalities, dystonia, spasticity, hyperreflexia, extensor plantar responses, behavioral changes, dysarthria, dysphagia, and ocular abnormalities (eg, retinal

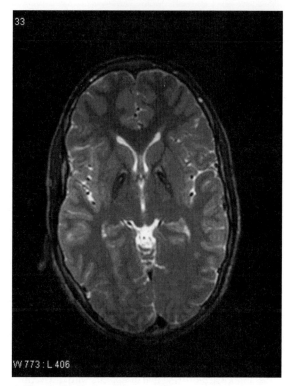

33

W 773 : L 406

▲ **Figure 11-7.** Pantothenate kinase-associated neurodegeneration (formerly Hallervorden–Spatz disease) showing the "eye of the tiger" sign. T2-weighted image shows bilateral symmetric hyperintense signal changes in the anterior medial globus pallidus representing gliosis, demyelination, neuronal loss, and axonal swelling. The surrounding hypointensity in the globus pallidus is secondary to iron deposition. (Used with permission from A. DiBernardo.)

degeneration, gaze palsies, optic atrophy). It typically presents in childhood. Deposition of iron and other pigments in the globus pallidus leads to a characteristic MRI appearance on T2-weighted MRI called the "eye of the tiger" sign (**Figure 11-7**). The disorder has autosomal recessive inheritance and results from mutations in the gene for pantothenate kinase 2 (*PANK2*). **Neuroferritinopathy (NBIA3)** is a rare, adult-onset, dominantly inherited, progressive disorder related to mutations in the ferritin light chain gene (*FTL*). It is characterized initially by chorea, dystonia (predominantly in the legs), parkinsonism, or some combination of these, with deficits subsequently becoming generalized. Cognitive features may be subtle initially, but disinhibition and emotional lability are common even at an early stage. An action-specific facial dystonia (involving symmetric frontalis and platysma contraction, giving a startled appearance) is characteristic. MRI shows excess iron in the basal ganglia, and later cavitation in the caudate and putamen.

Chorea-acanthocytosis is characterized by some combination of dystonia, chorea, orofacial dyskinesias, parkinsonism, tics, hyporeflexia, amyotrophy, and cognitive abnormalities. Dysexecutive syndromes, obsessive-compulsive disorder, depression, and psychosis may all occur. The peripheral blood contains circulating acanthocytes (spiny red cells) but a normal lipid profile. The disorder has autosomal recessive inheritance and is caused by mutation in the *VPS13A* gene.

Certain **mitochondrionopathies** may also be associated with dystonia, such as Leber hereditary optic atrophy.

PSYCHOGENIC DYSTONIA

Dystonia may occur as a somatoform or conversion disorder. Anxiety, depression, a personality disorder, or some combination of these and other psychiatric disturbances may be present. However, anxiety and depression are common consequences of dystonia that has an organic basis. Features that help to support a diagnosis of psychogenic dystonia include variable and inconsistent findings, findings that are incongruent with those of organic dystonia, a known psychologic precipitating factor, excessive pain, a prior history of somatoform disorder, other psychogenic signs (eg, nonanatomic sensory loss), multiple somatizations, abnormal posturing that disappears with distraction, lack of sensory tricks (to relieve the dystonia) and overflow dystonia, onset in the lower limbs in adults, and an impairment of function that is out of proportion to the dystonia and is selective in a manner that is difficult to explain (eg, limits the ability to work but not the ability to dress and attend to other activities of daily living). Symptoms may be relieved by psychotherapy, suggestion, or treatment with a placebo. Video surveillance may reveal a discrepancy between reported disability and the patient's actual clinical state. Treatment is of the underlying psychiatric disorder.

PAROXYSMAL DYSKINESIAS

In this group of disorders, dystonia and dyskinesias occur episodically, often on a familial basis (**Table 11-8**). The familial disorders are classified by whether they are induced by movement, as discussed later. Paroxysmal dyskinesias may also occur with basal ganglia pathology, multiple sclerosis, cerebral palsy, thyroid dysfunction, or idiopathic hypoparathyroidism; an MRI, EEG, and laboratory studies may then be necessary to clarify the nature of the underlying disorder. Treatment is of the underlying disorder. **Hypnogenic paroxysmal dyskinesia** is a form of frontal lobe epilepsy characterized by intermittent dystonia and choreoathetoid movements during sleep; it responds well to antiseizure medication.

PAROXYSMAL NONKINESIGENIC DYSKINESIA

Dystonia, chorea, and athetosis lasting from a few minutes to several hours characterize this disorder, which is inherited as an autosomal dominant trait with incomplete penetrance. Affected patients are likely to harbor mutations in

Table 11-8. Paroxysmal Dyskinesias.

	Paroxysmal Nonkinesigenic Dyskinesia	Paroxysmal Kinesigenic Choreoathetosis	Paroxysmal Exercise-Induced Dyskinesia
Gene	*MR1*	*PRRT2*	*SLC2A1*
Inheritance	AD	AD or sporadic	Sporadic or ?AD
Precipitants	Caffeine; alcohol; fatigue; stress; hunger; menstruation	Sudden movement or startle	Exercise (eg, walking for 30 minutes) or physical exertion
Usual age at onset	Before 30 years	Before 20 years	Before 30 years
Duration of episodes	Minutes, hours	Seconds, minutes	Minutes, hours (commonly 5-30 minutes)
Frequency	1-3/day; may be long episode-free intervals	Variable; may be many/day	1/day–1/month
Manifestations	Choreoathetosis; dystonia. May be unilateral and then generalize	Choreoathetosis; dystonia. Usually unilateral	Dystonia in exercised limbs. May be unilateral
Treatment	Sleep; clonazepam (anticonvulsants sometimes helpful)	Anticonvulsants (carbamazepine; phenytoin)	Usually unhelpful
Secondary causes (uncommon)	Multiple sclerosis; trauma; endocrinopathy; vascular disease	Multiple sclerosis; trauma; endocrinopathy	Trauma; insulinoma

AD, autosomal dominant.

the myofibrillogenesis regulator 1 (*MR1*) gene. Attacks may occur several times daily and are precipitated by caffeine, alcohol, fatigue, hunger, and emotional stress but not by movement. Onset may be in childhood or early adulthood. Examination between episodes is normal. Treatment is with clonazepam.

PAROXYSMAL KINESIGENIC CHOREOATHETOSIS

This disorder occurs on a sporadic basis or as an autosomal dominant trait. The gene (*PRRT2*) has been mapped to chromosome 16. There may be a history of convulsions in infancy. Attacks begin in the first or second decade, last for seconds to minutes, and are precipitated by sudden movement. They often respond to anticonvulsant medication, especially carbamazepine.

PAROXYSMAL EXERCISE-INDUCED DYSKINESIAS

In this rare disorder, which may be sporadic or familial, dystonia is brought on by exercise (as opposed to the initiation of movement) and affects the exercised limb. Onset is usually before 30 years of age; attacks last for several minutes to hours and are poorly responsive to medication. The disorder has been related to mutations in the solute carrier family 2 (facilitated glucose transporter), member 1 gene (*SLC2A1*). Pharmacologic treatment is usually unhelpful.

WILSON DISEASE

PATHOGENESIS

Wilson disease is an autosomal recessive disorder of copper metabolism that produces neurologic and hepatic dysfunction. The affected gene (*ATP7B*) codes for the beta polypeptide of copper-transporting ATPase. Although the precise nature of the biochemical abnormality in Wilson disease is unknown, its pathogenesis appears to involve decreased binding of copper to the transport protein **ceruloplasmin**. As a result, large amounts of unbound copper enter the circulation and are subsequently deposited in tissues, including the brain, liver, kidney, and cornea. Studies of mitochondrial function and aconitase activity suggest that free radical formation and oxidative damage, perhaps through mitochondrial copper accumulation, are important in pathogenesis.

CLINICAL FINDINGS

▶ Mode of Presentation

Wilson disease usually presents in childhood or young adult life. The average age at onset is approximately 11 years for patients presenting with hepatic dysfunction and 19 years for those with initial neurologic manifestations, but the disease may begin as late as the sixth decade. Hepatic and

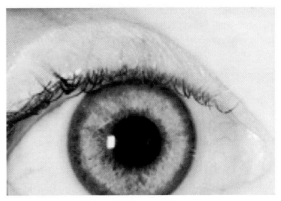

▲ **Figure 11-8.** Kayser–Fleischer ring in Wilson disease. This corneal ring is brown and located at the outer edge of the gray-blue iris. Its darkness increases as the outer border (limbus) of the cornea is approached. (Used with permission from Marc Solioz. From Usatine R, Smith MA, Mayeaux EJ Jr, Chumley H, Tysinger J, eds. *The Color Atlas of Family Medicine.* New York, NY: McGraw-Hill; 2008.)

neurologic presentations are about equally common, and most patients, if untreated, eventually develop both types of involvement. Rare presentations include joint disease, fever, hemolytic anemia, and behavioral disturbances.

▶ Non-Neurologic Findings

Ocular and hepatic abnormalities are the most prominent non-neurologic manifestations of Wilson disease. The most common ocular finding is **Kayser–Fleischer rings** (**Figure 11-8**): bilateral brown corneal rings that result from copper deposition in Descemet membrane. The rings are present in virtually all patients with neurologic involvement but may be detectable only by slit lamp examination. Hepatic involvement leads to chronic cirrhosis, which may be complicated by splenomegaly, esophageal varices with hematemesis, or fulminant hepatic failure. Splenomegaly may cause hemolytic anemia and thrombocytopenia.

▶ Neurologic Findings

Neurologic findings reflect the disproportionate involvement of the caudate nucleus, putamen, cerebral cortex, and cerebellum. Neurologic signs include resting or postural tremor, choreiform movements of the limbs, facial grimacing, rigidity, hypokinesia, dysarthria, dysphagia, abnormal (flexed) postures, and ataxia. Seizures may occur. Psychologic disorders include dementia, characterized by mental slowness, poor concentration, and memory impairment; disorders of affect, behavior, or personality; and (rarely) psychosis with hallucinations. There is a tendency for a dystonic or parkinsonian picture with hyperreflexia and extensor plantar responses to predominate when the disease begins before 20 years of age and for older patients to exhibit wild tremor, chorea, or ballismus. Symptoms may progress rapidly, especially in younger patients, but are more often gradual in development with periods of remission and exacerbation.

DIFFERENTIAL DIAGNOSIS

When Wilson disease presents as a neurologic disorder, other conditions that must be considered in the differential diagnosis include other causes of movement disorders, multiple sclerosis, and juvenile-onset Huntington disease.

INVESTIGATIVE STUDIES

Investigation may reveal abnormal liver function blood tests, aminoaciduria as a result of renal tubular damage, and a Coombs-negative hemolytic anemia. The levels of **serum copper** and **ceruloplasmin** (an a_2-globulin to which 90% of the circulating copper is bound) are low, and 24-hour **urinary copper excretion** is generally increased. Liver biopsy reveals a huge excess of copper; it also usually reveals cirrhosis. No single laboratory feature is reliable in isolation. Brain CT scanning or MRI (**Figure 11-9**) may show cerebrocortical atrophy and abnormalities in the basal ganglia. The MRI abnormalities include the "face of the giant panda" sign in the midbrain and sometimes a "face of the miniature panda" in the pontine tegmentum.

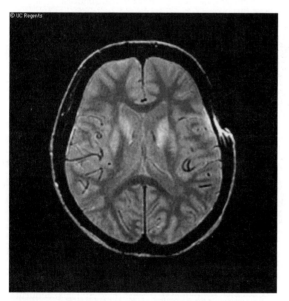

▲ **Figure 11-9.** MRI of a 31-year-old woman with Wilson disease. T2 hyperintensity involving the basal ganglia and thalamus bilaterally is shown. Other images showed T2 hyperintensity of the dorsal midbrain and central pons, T1 shortening involving the basal ganglia bilaterally, and diffuse cerebral atrophy. (Used with permission from A. Gean.)

TREATMENT

Treatment involves establishing a negative copper balance, arresting the accumulation of copper in the tissues, and removing excess copper from affected organs. The optimal means of removing copper from the brain and other organs is disputed. Most physicians use **penicillamine**, a copper-chelating agent that promotes extraction of copper from tissue deposition sites, even though instances of penicillamine-induced worsening have been described. Treatment should be started as early as possible and customarily employs approximately 1.5 g/d of orally administered penicillamine, taken in divided doses about 1 to 2 hours before meals to maximize absorption. The response to treatment may take several months and can be monitored by serial slit lamp examinations and blood chemistries. Side effects of penicillamine include nausea, nephrotic syndrome, myasthenia gravis, arthropathy, pemphigus, diverse blood dyscrasias, and a lupuslike syndrome.

Trientine hydrochloride, another chelating agent, can be given in a daily dose of 1 to 1.5 g (divided into two or three doses) and is less likely than penicillamine to cause drug reactions or neurologic deterioration. Treatment with **tetrathiomolybdate** may be even more effective in preserving neurologic function, but it is still undergoing clinical trials of its safety and efficacy.

Restriction of dietary copper (to less than 2 mg daily) is important but is insufficient as sole treatment. Administration of **zinc acetate** (150 mg/d orally in divided doses) or **zinc sulfate** or **gluconate** decreases copper absorption. The main advantage of zinc is low toxicity compared with that of other anticopper agents, although it may cause gastric irritation when introduced.

Treatment must be continued for the lifetime of the patient. Most patients treated early can expect a complete or nearly complete recovery. Liver transplantation may be required in cases with fulminant hepatic failure.

Siblings of affected patients should be screened for presymptomatic Wilson disease with neurologic and slit lamp examinations and determination of serum ceruloplasmin levels. If no abnormalities are found, serum copper and urinary copper excretion should be assayed and liver biopsy performed if necessary. Mutation analysis allows for screening family members when the index case has a known mutation. If these investigations reveal preclinical Wilson disease, therapy should be instituted as described previously for symptomatic disease.

DRUG-INDUCED MOVEMENT DISORDERS

PARKINSONISM

Parkinsonism frequently complicates treatment with dopamine-depleting agents such as reserpine or dopamine-receptor antagonists such as phenothiazines or

Table 11-9. Antipsychotic Drug-Induced Extrapyramidal Side Effects.

Drug		Relative EPS Risk[1]
First-generation (typical) antipsychotics		
Fluphenazine	Prolixin	High
Haloperidol	Haldol	High
Perphenazine	Trilafon	High
Thiothixene	Navane	High
Trifluoperazine	Stelazine	High
Chlorpromazine	Thorazine	Intermediate
Thioridazine	Mellaril	Intermediate
Second- & third-generation (atypical) antipsychotics		
Risperidone	Risperdal	Intermediate
Aripiprazole	Abilify	Low
Clozapine	Clozaril	Low
Olanzapine	Zyprexa	Low
Quetiapine	Seroquel	Low
Ziprasidone	Geodon	Low

[1]EPS, extrapyramidal symptoms (dystonia, parkinsonism, akathisia, tardive dyskinesia).

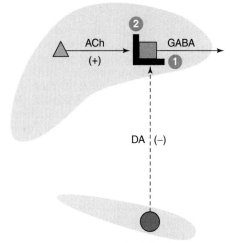

Caudate and putamen

Substantia nigra

▲ **Figure 11-10.** Mechanisms and treatment of drug-induced parkinsonism. Symptoms result from pharmacologic blockade of dopamine receptors by antipsychotic drugs (1), which mimics the degeneration of nigrostriatal dopamine (DA) neurons seen in idiopathic parkinsonism (dashed line). Symptoms may be relieved by the administration of muscarinic anticholinergic drugs (2) or by substituting an antipsychotic drug with anticholinergic properties. These measures restore the normal balance between dopaminergic and cholinergic (ACh) transmission in the striatum.

butyrophenones. With antipsychotic drugs, the risk of this complication is greatest when the agents used are potent D_2-receptor antagonists with little anticholinergic effect, such as piperazine phenothiazines, butyrophenones, and thioxanthenes (**Table 11-9**). In addition, women and elderly patients appear to be at somewhat increased risk. Tremor is relatively uncommon. Hypokinesia tends to be symmetric and the most conspicuous neurologic feature. These points, and the history of drug ingestion, often suggest the iatrogenic nature of the disorder. Signs usually develop within 3 months after starting the offending drug and disappear over weeks or months after discontinuance.

Depending on the severity of symptoms and the necessity for continuing antipsychotic drug therapy, several strategies are available for treating drug-induced parkinsonism. These include slow tapering and eventual withdrawal of the antipsychotic drug, substituting an antipsychotic agent less likely to cause extrapyramidal reactions (see Table 11-9), or adding an anticholinergic drug such as trihexyphenidyl or benztropine (**Figure 11-10**). Levodopa is of no help if the neuroleptic drugs are continued; it may be helpful if these drugs are discontinued but may then aggravate the psychotic disorder for which they were originally prescribed.

ACUTE DYSTONIA OR DYSKINESIA

Acute dystonia or dyskinesia (such as blepharospasm, torticollis, or facial grimacing) is an occasional complication of dopamine receptor antagonist treatment, generally occurring within 1 week after introduction of such medication and often within 48 hours. Men and younger patients show increased susceptibility to this complication. The pathophysiologic basis of the disturbance is unclear, but intravenous treatment with an anticholinergic drug (eg, benztropine 2 mg or diphenhydramine 50 mg) usually alleviates it.

AKATHISIA

Akathisia is a state of motor restlessness characterized by an inability to sit or stand still, which is relieved by moving about. It is a very common movement disorder induced by chronic treatment with antipsychotic drugs and occurs more often in women than in men. It may be seen as a tardive phenomenon after the discontinuation of neuroleptics. Akathisia is treated in the same manner as drug-induced parkinsonism.

TARDIVE DYSKINESIA

Tardive dyskinesia may develop after long-term treatment with antipsychotic dopamine receptor antagonist drugs or with metoclopramide. It occurs more commonly with the older, first-generation drugs than with more recently developed "atypical" antipsychotic agents (see Table 11-9). It is common in chronically institutionalized psychiatric patients, and the risk of developing tardive dyskinesia appears to increase with advancing age. It often first manifests after a reduction in dose or withdrawal of the offending drug and—at this stage—may resolve after a few weeks or months if the drug is discontinued, especially in young patients.

▶ Pathogenesis

The underlying pathophysiology is unknown. Drug-induced supersensitivity of striatal dopamine receptors has been proposed but is unlikely to be responsible for several reasons. Supersensitivity always accompanies chronic antipsychotic drug treatment, whereas tardive dyskinesia does not. Supersensitivity may occur early in the course of treatment, whereas tardive dyskinesia does not develop for at least 3 months. In addition, supersensitivity is invariably reversible when drugs are discontinued; tardive dyskinesia is not.

The clinical features of tardive dyskinesia, particularly its persistent nature, are more suggestive of an underlying degenerative abnormality. Such an abnormality may involve GABA neurons, because GABA and its synthesizing enzyme, glutamic acid decarboxylase, are depleted in the basal ganglia after chronic treatment of animals with antipsychotic drugs, and GABA levels in cerebrospinal fluid (CSF) are decreased in patients with tardive dyskinesia.

▶ Pathology

No consistent pathologic features have been found in the brains of patients with tardive dyskinesia, although inferior olive atrophy, degeneration of the substantia nigra, and swelling of large neurons in the caudate nucleus have been described in some cases.

▶ Clinical Findings

The clinical disorder is characterized by abnormal choreoathetoid movements that are often especially conspicuous about the face and mouth in adults and tend to be more obvious in the limbs in children. The onset of dyskinesia is generally not until months, or years, after the start of treatment with the responsible agent. Tardive dyskinesia may be impossible to distinguish from such disorders as Huntington disease or isolated torsion dystonia unless a history of drug exposure is obtained.

▶ Prevention

Tardive dyskinesia is easier to prevent than to cure. Metoclopramide should not be prescribed for more than 3 months. Antipsychotic drugs should be prescribed only on clear indication, and their long-term use should be monitored, with periodic drug holidays to determine whether the need for treatment continues. Drug holidays may also help to unmask incipient dyskinesias—which, curiously, tend to worsen when the drug is withdrawn. Antipsychotic medication should be gradually withdrawn when possible when dyskinesia appears during a drug holiday, as this may allow remission to occur. Anticholinergic drugs should not be prescribed to protect patients from developing tardive dyskinesia as they may actually worsen the disorder.

▶ Treatment

Treating the established disorder is generally unsatisfactory, although the disorder may resolve spontaneously after withdrawal of the causal medication, especially in children or young adults. Antidopaminergic agents such as haloperidol or phenothiazines suppress the abnormal movements, but their use for this purpose is not recommended because they may aggravate the underlying disorder. Treatment with reserpine 0.25 mg, gradually increased to 2 to 4 mg/d orally, or tetrabenazine 12.5 mg, gradually increased to as much as 200 mg/d orally, taken in divided doses, may be helpful, as may treatment with deutetrabenazine, which was approved by the FDA while this book was in press.

A number of other pharmacologic approaches have been suggested and may help in individual cases; these include treatment with carbamazepine, baclofen, valproate, lithium, clonazepam, and alprazolam. Calcium-channel blockers have also been advocated. However, evidence of benefit with these various drugs is inconclusive. Anticholinergic drugs should be avoided except in patients with tardive dystonia (see later), as they may exacerbate the dyskinesia.

Occasional patients with severe dyskinesia have been treated with deep brain stimulation of the globus pallidus or subthalamic nucleus. In patients requiring continued treatment for psychosis, clozapine, risperidone, olanzapine, or quetiapine should be used in place of the typical antipsychotics.

OTHER TARDIVE SYNDROMES

A variety of other late and often persistent movement disorders may appear during the course of antipsychotic drug treatment.

Tardive dystonia is usually segmental in distribution, affecting two or more contiguous body parts, such as the face and neck or arm and trunk. It is less often focal; when this is the case, the head and neck are particularly apt to be affected, producing blepharospasm, torticollis, or oromandibular dystonia. Generalized dystonia is least common and tends to occur in younger patients. Treatment is as for tardive dyskinesia, except that anticholinergic drugs may also be helpful; focal dystonias may also respond to local injection of botulinum A toxin.

Tardive akathisia (characterized by a feeling of restlessness and a need to move about, with an inability to sit or stand still) can also occur; it is treated in the same manner as drug-induced parkinsonism.

Tardive tic, a drug-induced disorder resembling Gilles de la Tourette syndrome (see later), is characterized by multifocal motor and vocal tics. It can be treated in the same manner as Gilles de la Tourette syndrome if symptoms do not remit spontaneously.

Tardive tremor and **tardive myoclonus** may also occur but are much less common than the other tardive syndromes.

Rabbit syndrome is a neuroleptic-induced disorder characterized by rhythmic vertical movements about the mouth, resembling the chewing movements of a rabbit; the tongue is spared. Anticholinergic drugs may be helpful in its treatment.

NEUROLEPTIC MALIGNANT SYNDROME

This rare complication of treatment with antipsychotic drugs (neuroleptics) is manifested by **rigidity**, **fever**, **altered mental status**, and **autonomic dysfunction**. Haloperidol is implicated most often, but the syndrome can complicate treatment with any antipsychotic drug; whether concomitant treatment with lithium or anticholinergic drugs increases the risk is uncertain. Symptoms typically develop over 1 to 3 days and can occur at any time during the course of treatment.

The differential diagnosis includes infection, which must be excluded in any febrile patient. Neuroleptic malignant syndrome resembles malignant hyperthermia (see Chapter 9, Motor Disorders), but the latter disorder develops over minutes to hours rather than days and is associated with the administration of inhalational anesthetics or neuromuscular blocking agents rather than antipsychotics.

Treatment of neuroleptic malignant syndrome includes withdrawal of antipsychotic drugs, lithium, and anticholinergics; reduction of body temperature with antipyretics and artificial cooling; and rehydration. When significant hyperthermia is present, patients are best managed in an intensive care unit. Dantrolene may be beneficial, as may dopamine agonists, levodopa preparations, or amantadine, especially for hyperthermic patients and those not responding adequately to supportive measures and withdrawal of the causal medication. The mortality rate is as high as 20%.

The response to resumption of antipsychotic therapy after an episode of neuroleptic malignant syndrome is unpredictable, but recurrence may certainly occur and mandates careful monitoring of patients in these circumstances.

OTHER DRUG-INDUCED MOVEMENT DISORDERS

Levodopa produces a wide variety of abnormal movements as a dose-related phenomenon in patients with parkinsonism. They can be reversed by withdrawing the medication or reducing the dose. **Chorea** may also develop in patients receiving a variety of other medications, including dopamine agonists, anticholinergic drugs, buspirone, phenytoin, carbamazepine, amphetamines, methylphenidate, lithium, and oral contraceptives; it resolves with discontinuance of the responsible drug. **Dystonia** has resulted from administration of dopamine agonists, lithium, serotonin reuptake inhibitors, carbamazepine, and metoclopramide; and **postural tremor** from administration of theophylline, caffeine, lithium, thyroid hormone, tricyclic antidepressants, valproic acid, and isoproterenol.

GILLES DE LA TOURETTE SYNDROME

Gilles de la Tourette syndrome, characterized by chronic—typically lifelong—multiple motor and verbal tics, is of unknown cause and does not relate to social class, ethnic group, perinatal abnormalities, birth trauma, or birth order. Symptoms begin before 21 years of age, most often by the age of 11, and the course is one of remission and relapse. Most cases are sporadic, although there is occasionally a family history, and partial expression of the trait may occur in siblings or offspring of patients. Inheritance has been attributed to an autosomal dominant gene with variable penetrance, but inheritance is complex, and risk alleles have been difficult to identify. The prevalence in the United States has been estimated to be 0.05%, and the disorder is more common in males than females.

PATHOGENESIS

The pathogenesis is obscure, but the corticostriato-thalamocortical pathways seem to be involved. Dopaminergic excess in the brains of patients with Gilles de la Tourette syndrome has been postulated, mainly because of the beneficial effects that dopamine-blocking drugs can have on the tics. The administration of dopamine receptor agonists often fails to produce the exacerbation of symptoms that might be anticipated from this hypothesis, however.

Analysis of linkage in a two-generation pedigree has led to the identification of a rare mutation in the *HDC* gene encoding histidine decarboxylase, the rate-limiting enzyme in histamine biosynthesis. Such findings suggest a role for histaminergic neurotransmission in the pathogenesis and modulation of Gilles de la Tourette syndrome and tics. No structural basis for the clinical disorder has been recognized.

CLINICAL FINDINGS

The first signs consist of motor tics in 80% of cases and vocal (phonic) tics in 20%; there may be either a single or multiple tics. When the initial sign is a motor tic, it commonly involves the face, as in sniffing, blinking, or forced eye closure. It is generally not possible to make the diagnosis at this stage.

All patients ultimately develop a number of different motor tics and involuntary vocal tics, the latter commonly consisting of grunts, barks, hisses, throat-clearing or coughing, and the like. Vocal tics sometimes take the form of verbal utterances including **coprolalia** (vulgar or obscene speech), which occurs eventually in approximately half of all patients. There may also be **echolalia** (parroting the speech of others), **echopraxia** (imitation of others' movements), and **palilalia** (repetition of words or phrases).

The motor tics may consist of simple movements such as blinking, facial grimacing, or sniffing, but more complicated movements or movement sequences may also develop, such as a bizarre series of hopping, jumping, and kicking; body gyrations; and complex obscene gestures. The tics vary over time in severity, character, and the muscle groups involved. In 40% to 50% of cases, some of the tics involve self-mutilation with such activities as severe nail-biting or hair-pulling, picking at the nose, or biting the lips or tongue. **Sensory tics**, consisting of pressure, tickling, and warm or cold sensations, also occur. The tics, which can often be suppressed temporarily by intense volitional effort, are typically followed by a sense of relief.

Behavioral disorders, including **obsessive-compulsive disorder**, **attention deficit disorder**, **learning difficulties**, and **impulse control disorders**, are common in patients with Gilles de la Tourette syndrome, but their precise relationship to the tic disorder is uncertain.

Examination usually reveals no other abnormalities, and the history is therefore of paramount importance. Videotaping of the patient in the home environment may be helpful. There is a higher than expected incidence of left-handedness or ambidexterity. In approximately 50% of cases, the EEG shows minor nonspecific abnormalities of no diagnostic relevance.

DIFFERENTIAL DIAGNOSIS

The differential diagnosis includes the various movement disorders that can present in childhood. Other disorders characterized by tics (see earlier discussion) are distinguished by resolution of the tics by early adulthood, by the restricted number of tics, or by the context in which the tics occur. A psychogenic disorder may be diagnosed erroneously because of the variability of the tics, their exacerbation by stress, and their suppression with voluntary effort. Laboratory tests are typically normal, but examination of a wet blood film for acanthocytes, thyroid function tests, and serum copper and ceruloplasmin determination should be considered to exclude other causes. Imaging studies usually are unnecessary unless there are abnormalities other than tics on neurologic examination.

Wilson disease can simulate Gilles de la Tourette syndrome; it must be excluded because it responds well to medical treatment. In addition to a movement disorder, Wilson disease produces hepatic involvement, Kayser–Fleischer corneal rings, and abnormalities of serum copper and ceruloplasmin, which are absent in Gilles de la Tourette syndrome.

Sydenham chorea can be difficult to recognize if there is no recent history of rheumatic fever or polyarthritis and no clinical evidence of cardiac involvement, but this disorder is a self-limiting one, usually clearing in 3 to 6 months.

Bobble-head syndrome, which can be difficult to distinguish from Gilles de la Tourette syndrome, is characterized by rapid, rhythmic bobbing of the head in children with progressive hydrocephalus.

COMPLICATIONS

Gilles de la Tourette syndrome is often unrecognized for years, the tics being attributed to psychiatric illness or attention-seeking behavior, or mistaken for some other form of abnormal movement. They may also be mistaken for a general medical disorder, as when sniffing and throat clearing are attributed to allergies. Indeed, in many cases the correct diagnosis is finally made by the family rather than the physician. In consequence, patients are often subjected to unnecessary and expensive treatment before the true nature of the disorder is recognized. Psychiatric disturbances, sometimes culminating in suicide, may occur because of the cosmetic and social embarrassment produced by the tics. Drug therapy can lead to a number of side effects, as discussed next.

TREATMENT

Treatment is symptomatic and, if effective, must be continued indefinitely. Education of the patient, family members, and teachers is important. Extra break periods at school and additional time for test taking are often helpful. Cognitive behavioral therapy or other forms of behavioral intervention may be helpful. When tics are mild and nondisruptive, pharmacologic measures may not be needed.

Clonidine, an alpha$_2$-adrenergic receptor agonist, has been reported to ameliorate motor or vocal tics in roughly 50% of children so treated. It may act by reducing activity in noradrenergic neurons arising in the locus ceruleus. It is started in a dose of 2 to 3 µg/kg/d, increasing after 2 weeks to 4 µg/kg/d and then, if necessary, to 5 µg/kg/d taken to a daily maximum of 0.3 or 0.4 mg in divided doses. It may cause an initial transient fall in blood pressure. The most frequent side effect is sedation. Other adverse reactions include reduced or excessive salivation and diarrhea. **Guanfacine** can also be used, starting with 0.5 mg at bedtime and increasing to a maximum of 2 mg twice daily. These alpha-adrenergic agonists have less troublesome side effects than the typical antipsychotics, which are the only therapies for this disorder approved by the US Food and Drug Administration. There are reports that topiramate or tetrabenazine may also be helpful.

Atypical **antipsychotics**, including risperidone and aripiprazole, are sometimes beneficial, and may be preferred over the typical agents. When a typical antipsychotic is required, haloperidol is generally regarded as the drug of choice. It is started at a low daily dose (0.25 mg), which is gradually increased by 0.25 mg every 4 or 5 days until there is maximum benefit with a minimum of side effects or until side effects limit further increments. A total daily dose of 2 to 8 mg is usually optimal, but higher doses are sometimes necessary. Side effects include extrapyramidal movement disorders, sedation, dryness of the mouth, blurred vision, and gastrointestinal disturbances. Pimozide, another dopaminergic-receptor antagonist, may be helpful in patients who are either unresponsive to or cannot tolerate haloperidol. Treatment is started with 1 mg/d and the dose is increased by 1 mg every 5 days; most patients require 7 to 16 mg/d. Phenothiazines such as fluphenazine are also sometimes helpful. Dopamine-depleting drugs such as **tetrabenazine** can also be used as the initial symptomatic treatment for patients with troublesome tics.

Injection of **botulinum toxin A** at the site of the most problematic focal tics may be worthwhile.

Treatment of any associated attention deficit disorder may include the use of a clonidine patch, guanfacine, methylphenidate, dextroamphetamine, desipramine, or atomoxetine, whereas obsessive-compulsive disorder may require selective serotonin reuptake inhibitors or clomipramine.

Patients occasionally respond favorably to clonazepam or carbamazepine, but diazepam, barbiturates, phenytoin, and cholinergic agonists (eg, deanol) are usually not helpful.

Neurosurgical treatment, for example, by prefrontal leucotomy, anterior cingulotomy, or thalamotomy, has not been helpful, but bilateral deep brain stimulation of various target sites has reportedly been worthwhile in otherwise intractable cases.

ACQUIRED HEPATOCEREBRAL DEGENERATION

Acquired hepatocerebral degeneration produces a neurologic disorder associated with extrapyramidal, cerebellar, and pyramidal signs as well as dementia. Extrapyramidal signs include rigidity, rest tremor, chorea, athetosis, and dystonia. This condition is discussed in Chapter 5, Dementia & Amnestic Disorders.

RESTLESS LEGS SYNDROME

Restless legs syndrome is characterized by an unpleasant creeping, crawling, itching, or tingling discomfort that is perceived as arising deep within the legs and occasionally in the arms as well. Symptoms tend to occur when patients

are relaxed, especially while lying down or sitting, and lead to a need to move about. They are often particularly troublesome at night and may delay the onset of sleep. A sleep disorder associated with periodic movements during sleep may also occur and can be documented by polysomnographic recording. The cause is unknown, although the disorder may have a genetic predisposition; several genetic loci have been associated with the syndrome. The disorder seems especially common among pregnant women and is not uncommon among uremic or diabetic patients with neuropathy. Most patients, however, have no obvious predisposing cause.

Symptoms sometimes resolve after correction of coexisting iron-deficiency anemia or reduction of caffeine intake, and they may respond to treatment with drugs such as gabapentin, pregabalin, dopamine agonists (pramipexole, ropinirole, or rotigotine), levodopa, or opiates. Benzodiazepines (especially clonazepam 0.5 to 2 mg daily) are also sometimes helpful, especially in those requiring treatment only intermittently. However, the decision to initiate treatment should be based, at least in part, on the frequency of symptoms.

Gabapentin is taken once or twice daily, typically in the evening and before sleep. It is started at 300 mg daily, and the dose is then built up depending on response and tolerance (to approximately 1,800 mg daily). Pregabalin, 150 to 300 mg daily taken in divided doses, is often also effective.

Dopaminergic therapy is the treatment of choice for severe cases but carries the risk of **augmentation**. The term *augmentation* refers to the earlier onset or greater intensity of symptoms, a reduced latency to symptom onset when at rest, and a briefer response to medication. Augmentation seems to occur especially in relation to levodopa therapy (levodopa/carbidopa 100/25 or 200/50 taken approximately 1 hour before bedtime), prompting many to use a dopamine agonist in place of levodopa when dopaminergic therapy is required. When augmentation occurs in patients receiving levodopa, the daily dose should be divided; alternatively, a dopamine agonist should be substituted (pramipexole 0.125-0.75 mg or ropinirole 0.25-4.0 mg once daily). When augmentation occurs with an agonist, the daily dose should be divided or the patient switched to another agonist or to other medications. Dopamine agonists are best avoided in patients with a history of impulse control disorder or addiction.

If opiates are required, those with long half-lives or low addictive potential are preferred. Oxycodone is often effective; the dose varies with the patient. Opiate treatment is best reserved for patients with otherwise intractable symptoms or for those requiring treatment only intermittently.

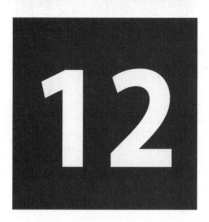

Seizures & Syncope

EPISODIC LOSS OF CONSCIOUSNESS

Consciousness is lost when the function of both cerebral hemispheres or the brainstem reticular activating system is compromised. Episodic dysfunction of these anatomic regions produces transient, and often recurrent, loss of consciousness. There are two major causes of episodic loss of consciousness: seizures and syncope.

SEIZURES

Seizures are disorders characterized by temporary neurologic signs or symptoms resulting from **abnormal, paroxysmal, and hypersynchronous electrical neuronal activity** in the brain.

SYNCOPE

Syncope is loss of consciousness due to **reduced blood flow to both cerebral hemispheres or the brainstem**. It can result from pancerebral hypoperfusion caused by vasovagal reflexes, orthostatic hypotension, or decreased cardiac output, or from selective hypoperfusion of the brainstem resulting from vertebrobasilar ischemia.

APPROACH TO DIAGNOSIS

Seizures and syncope have different causes, diagnostic approaches, and treatment.

First determine whether the setting in which the event occurred, or associated symptoms or signs, suggests a direct result of a disease requiring prompt attention, such as **hypoglycemia**, **meningitis**, **head trauma**, **cardiac arrhythmia**, or **acute pulmonary embolism**. Assess the number of spells and their similarity or dissimilarity. If all spells are identical, then a single pathophysiologic process can be assumed. Major differential features should be ascertained as discussed below.

EVENTS AT ONSET OF SPELL

Prodromal Symptoms (Aura)

Inquire about prodromal and initial symptoms. A witness may be critical. The often brief, stereotyped premonitory symptoms (aura) at the onset of some seizures may localize the central nervous system (CNS) abnormality responsible for seizures. Note that more than one type of aura may occur in an individual patient. A sensation of fear, olfactory or gustatory hallucinations, or visceral or déjà vu sensations are commonly associated with seizures originating in the temporal lobe. Progressive light-headedness, dimming of vision, and faintness suggest decreased cerebral blood flow (eg, simple faints, cardiac arrhythmias, orthostatic hypotension).

Posture When Loss of Consciousness Occurs

Orthostatic hypotension and simple faints occur in the upright or sitting position. Episodes that also or only occur in the recumbent position suggest seizure or cardiac arrhythmia as a likely cause, although syncope induced by strong emotional stimuli (eg, phlebotomy) can also occur in recumbency.

Relationship to Physical Exertion

Syncope induced by exertion is usually due to cardiac arrhythmias or outflow obstruction (eg, aortic stenosis, obstructive hypertrophic cardiomyopathy, or atrial myxoma).

Focal Symptoms

Focal motor or sensory phenomena (eg, involuntary jerking of one hand, hemifacial paresthesias, or forced head turning) suggest a seizure originating in the contralateral frontoparietal cortex. A sensation of fear, olfactory or gustatory hallucinations, or visceral or déjà vu sensations are commonly associated with seizures originating in the temporal lobe.

EVENTS DURING THE SPELL

Tonic Stiffening & Clonic Movement

Generalized tonic–clonic (grand mal, or major motor) seizures are characterized by loss of consciousness, accompanied initially by tonic stiffening and subsequently by clonic (jerking) movements of the extremities (see Figure 12-2).

Flaccidity

Cerebral hypoperfusion usually produces flaccid unresponsiveness.

Brief Stiffening or Jerking

Loss of consciousness from hypoperfusion rarely lasts more than 10 to 20 seconds and is not followed by postictal confusion unless severe and protracted brain ischemia has occurred. Cerebral hypoperfusion can also result in stiffening or jerking movements, especially if hypoperfusion is prolonged, for example, because the patient is prevented from falling or otherwise assuming a recumbent posture. This phenomenon, sometimes referred to as **convulsive syncope**, is self-limited and does not require anticonvulsant treatment.

EVENTS AFTER THE SPELL

Prompt Recovery of Consciousness

Recovery from a simple faint is characterized by a prompt return to consciousness, with full lucidity, within 20 to 30 seconds.

Postictal Confusion

A period of confusion, disorientation, or agitation (**postictal state**) follows a generalized tonic–clonic seizure. The period of confusion usually lasts minutes. Although such behavior is often strikingly evident to witnesses, it may not be recalled by the patient.

Prolonged Confusion

Prolonged alteration of consciousness (**prolonged postictal state**) may follow status epilepticus. It may also occur after a single seizure in patients with diffuse structural cerebral disease (eg, dementia, other cognitive impairment, head trauma, or encephalitis), metabolic encephalopathy, or continuing nonconvulsive seizures.

Tongue Biting

Biting of the lateral aspect of the tongue is highly specific for generalized tonic–clonic seizure and may be noted by the patient after such a spell.

Urinary Incontinence

Incontinence of urine can occur during either seizure or syncope. Fecal incontinence is an uncommon result of a seizure.

SEIZURES

A seizure is a transient disturbance of cerebral function caused by an abnormal neuronal discharge. **Epilepsy**, a group of disorders characterized by **recurrent seizures**, is a common cause of episodic loss of consciousness defined as two unprovoked seizures or as a single seizure when clinical factors or investigations suggest an above average risk of recurrence. The prevalence of epilepsy in the general population is about 2-3%, but the lifetime probability of experiencing a seizure is approximately 10%.

An actively convulsing patient or a reported seizure in a known epileptic usually poses no diagnostic difficulty. However, because most seizures occur outside the hospital and are unobserved by medical personnel, the diagnosis most often must be established retrospectively. The two historic features most suggestive of a seizure are the **aura** associated with seizures of focal onset and the **postictal confusional state** that follows generalized tonic–clonic seizures.

ETIOLOGY

Seizures can result from either primary CNS dysfunction, an underlying metabolic derangement, or systemic disease. This distinction is critical, because therapy must be directed at the underlying disorder as well as at seizure control. A list of common neurologic and systemic disorders that produce seizures is presented in **Table 12-1**. The age of the patient may help in establishing the cause of seizures (**Figure 12-1**).

The **genetic** contribution to epilepsy and its response to treatment is complex. A single epileptic syndrome (eg, juvenile myoclonic epilepsy) can result from mutations in several different genes; conversely, mutations in a single gene (eg, *SCN1A* sodium channel subunit) can cause several epilepsy phenotypes. Genes implicated in susceptibility to epilepsy include those coding for sodium, calcium, potassium, and chloride channels; nicotinic cholinergic, GABA, and G protein-coupled receptors; and enzymes.

Table 12-1. Common Causes of New-Onset Seizures.

Primary neurologic disorders
Benign febrile convulsions of childhood
Idiopathic/cryptogenic seizures
Cerebral dysgenesis
Symptomatic epilepsy
Head trauma
Stroke or vascular malformations
Mass lesions
CNS infections
Encephalitis
Meningitis
Cysticercosis
HIV encephalopathy
Systemic disorders
Hypoglycemia
Hyponatremia
Hyperosmolar states
Hypocalcemia
Uremia
Hepatic encephalopathy
Porphyria
Drug toxicity
Drug withdrawal
Global cerebral ischemia
Hypertensive encephalopathy
Eclampsia
Hyperthermia

PRIMARY NEUROLOGIC DISORDERS

Benign Febrile Convulsions

Benign febrile convulsions occur in 2% to 5% of children aged 6 months to 5 years, usually during the first day of a

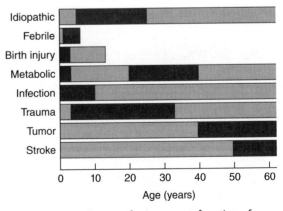

▲ **Figure 12-1.** Causes of seizures as a function of age at onset. Bars show the range of ages at which seizures from a given cause typically begin; darker shading indicates peak incidence.

febrile illness (temperature > 100.4°F or 38°C), and in the absence of CNS infection (meningitis or encephalitis). There may be a family history of benign febrile convulsions or other types of seizures. Mutations in several genes have been linked to febrile convulsions, including the G protein-coupled receptor *MASS1*; the inositol monophosphatase *IMPA2*; *SCN1A*, *SCN1B*, and *SCN2A* sodium channel subunits; *KCNQ2*, *KCNQ3*, and *KCNA1* potassium channel subunits; and *GABRG2* and *GABRD* GABA receptor subunits.

Benign febrile convulsions usually last for less than 10 to 15 minutes and lack focal features. Approximately two-thirds of patients experience a single seizure, and fewer than one-tenth have more than three. Seizures occurring during the first hour of fever in children younger than 18 months or in children with a family history of febrile seizures are associated with an increased risk for recurrence; 90% of recurrences occur within 2 years of the initial episode. Any MRI abnormality increases the risk of subsequent febrile status. The differential diagnosis includes meningitis and encephalitis (see Chapter 4, Confusional States); if present, these entities should be treated as described elsewhere in this volume.

Because benign febrile convulsions are usually self-limited, treatment is often unnecessary; prolonged convulsions (≥15 minutes) can be aborted with diazepam 0.3 mg/kg orally, intramuscularly, or intravenously or 0.6 mg/kg rectally, or by buccal midazolam (0.5 mg/kg; maximum, 10 mg). Such treatment may decrease the risk of recurrence. When recurrence does occur and parents are particularly anxious, intermittent oral diazepam at the onset of febrile illness may prevent further recurrences. The probability of developing a chronic seizure disorder is 2% to 6% and is highest in patients with persistent neurologic abnormalities; prolonged, focal, or multiple seizures; or a family history of nonfebrile seizures. Long-term administration of phenobarbital or valproic acid to reduce the risk of subsequent afebrile seizures is generally not indicated, as the risk of nonfebrile seizures is unaltered and anticonvulsant drug use is associated with significant morbidity.

▶ Idiopathic (Cryptogenic) Seizures

These account for two-thirds of new-onset seizures in the general population. The age range of onset is broad, from the second to the seventh decade (see Figure 12-1). The risk of recurrence in the next 5 years is approximately 35% after a first unprovoked seizure. A second seizure increases the risk of recurrence to approximately 75%. Most recurrences occur in the first year. Genes implicated in idiopathic generalized epilepsy include the mitochondrial NAD-dependent malic enzyme *ME2* and the *CACNA1A* and *CACNB4* calcium channel subunits.

▶ Head Trauma

Head trauma is a common cause of epilepsy, particularly when it occurs perinatally or is associated with a **depressed** **skull fracture** or **intracerebral or subdural hematoma**. Seizures that occur within the first week after nonpenetrating head injuries are not predictive of a chronic seizure disorder, however. Although patients with serious head injuries are often treated prophylactically with anticonvulsant drugs, a resultant reduction in the incidence of posttraumatic seizures in patients so treated has not been consistently observed.

▶ Stroke

Stroke affecting the cerebral cortex produces seizures in 5% to 15% of patients and can occur after **thrombotic** or **embolic** infarction or intracerebral **hemorrhage** (see Chapter 13, Stroke). As in head trauma, early seizures are not necessarily indicative of chronic epilepsy, and long-term anticonvulsant therapy may not be required. Even without rupturing, **vascular malformations** may be associated with seizures, presumably as a result of their irritative effects on adjacent brain tissue.

▶ Mass Lesions

Mass lesions, such as brain **tumors** (Table 6-4) or **abscesses** (Table 3-7), can present with seizures. Glioblastomas, astrocytomas, and meningiomas are the most common tumors associated with seizures, reflecting their high prevalence among tumors that affect the cerebral hemispheres.

▶ Meningitis or Encephalitis

Bacterial (eg, *Haemophilus influenzae* or tuberculous), **viral** (eg, herpes simplex), **fungal**, or **parasitic** (eg, cysticercosis) infections (see Chapter 4, Confusional States) can also cause seizures. Seizures in patients with AIDS are most often related to HIV-associated dementia, but also occur with toxoplasmosis or cryptococcal meningitis.

▶ Developmental Anomalies

Cortical dysgenesis and **neuronal migration disorders** can predispose to epilepsy.

SYSTEMIC DISORDERS

Metabolic and other systemic disorders, including drug-overdose and drug-withdrawal syndromes, may be associated with seizures that abate with correction of the underlying abnormality. In these cases, the patient is not considered to have epilepsy. Many of these disorders are discussed in detail in Chapter 4, Confusional States.

1. **Hypoglycemia** can produce seizures, especially with serum glucose levels of 20 to 30 mg/dL, but neurologic manifestations of hypoglycemia are also related to the rate at which serum glucose levels fall.

2. **Hyponatremia** may be associated with seizures at serum sodium levels less than 120 mEq/L (mean 110mEq/L) or at higher levels after a rapid decline.

3. **Hyperosmolar states**, including both hyperosmolar nonketotic hyperglycemia and hypernatremia, may lead to seizures when serum osmolality rises above approximately 330 mOsm/L.

4. **Hypocalcemia** with serum calcium levels in the range of 4.3 to 9.2 mg/dL can produce seizures with or without tetany.

5. **Uremia** can cause seizures, especially when it develops rapidly, but this tendency correlates poorly with absolute serum urea nitrogen levels.

6. **Hepatic encephalopathy** is sometimes accompanied by generalized or multifocal seizures.

7. **Porphyria** is a disorder of heme biosynthesis that produces both neuropathy (see Chapter 9, Motor Disorders) and seizures. The latter may be difficult to treat because most anticonvulsants can exacerbate the metabolic abnormalities. Case reports attest to the safety and efficacy of gabapentin, lorazepam, and levetiracetam in porphyria.

8. **Drug overdose** can exacerbate epilepsy or cause seizures in nonepileptic patients. Generalized tonic-clonic seizures are most common, but focal or multifocal partial seizures can also occur. The drugs most frequently associated with seizures are antidepressants, antipsychotics, cocaine, insulin, isoniazid, lidocaine, and methylxanthines (**Table 12-2**).

9. **Drug withdrawal**, especially withdrawal from ethanol or sedative drugs, may be accompanied by one or more generalized tonic-clonic seizures that usually resolve spontaneously. Alcohol withdrawal seizures occur within 48 hours after cessation or reduction of ethanol intake in 90% of cases and are characterized by brief flurries of one to six attacks that resolve within 12 hours. Acute abstinence from sedative drugs can also produce seizures in patients habituated to more than 600 to 800 mg/d of secobarbital or equivalent doses of other short-acting sedatives. Seizures from sedative drug withdrawal typically occur 2 to 4 days after abstinence but may be delayed for up to 1 week. Focal seizures are rarely due to alcohol or sedative drug withdrawal alone; such occurrences suggest an additional focal cerebral lesion that requires evaluation.

10. **Global cerebral ischemia** (see Chapter 13, Stroke) from cardiac arrest, cardiac arrhythmias, or hypotension may produce, at onset, a few tonic or tonic-clonic movements that resemble seizures, but they probably reflect abnormal brainstem activity instead. Global ischemia may also be associated with spontaneous myoclonus (see Chapter 11, Movement Disorders) or, after consciousness returns, with myoclonus precipitated by movement (action myoclonus). Partial or generalized tonic-clonic seizures also occur; these may be manifested only by subtle movements of the face or eyes and must be recognized and treated. Nonetheless, isolated seizures after global cerebral ischemia do not necessarily indicate a poor outcome.

11. **Hypertensive encephalopathy** (see Chapter 4, Confusional States) may be accompanied by generalized tonic-clonic or partial seizures.

12. **Eclampsia** refers to the occurrence of seizures or coma in a pregnant woman with hypertension, proteinuria, and edema (**preeclampsia**). As in hypertensive encephalopathy in nonpregnant patients, cerebral edema, ischemia, and hemorrhage may contribute to neurologic complications. Magnesium sulfate has been widely used to treat eclamptic seizures and for this purpose may be superior to anticonvulsants such as phenytoin.

13. **Hyperthermia** can result from infection, exposure (heat stroke), hypothalamic lesions, or drugs such as phencyclidine, as well as anticholinergics or neuroleptics (**neuroleptic malignant syndrome**; see Chapter 11, Movement Disorders) and inhalational anesthetics or neuromuscular blocking agents (**malignant hyperthermia**; see Chapter 9, Motor Disorders). Clinical features of severe hyperthermia (42°C, or 107°F) include seizures, confusional states or coma, shock, and renal failure. Treatment is with antipyretics and artificial cooling to reduce body temperature immediately to 39°C (102°F) and anticonvulsants and more specific therapy (eg, antibiotics for infection,

Table 12-2. Major Categories of Drugs Reported to Cause Seizures.

Antibiotics (quinolones, penicillins, isoniazid)
Anticholinesterases (organophosphates, physostigmine)
Antidepressants (tricyclic, monocyclic, heterocyclic; selective serotonin reuptake inhibitors)
Antihistamines
Antipsychotics (phenothiazines, butyrophenones, atypicals)
Chemotherapeutics (etoposide, ifosfamide, cisplatin)
Cyclosporine, FK 506 (tacrolimus)
Hypoglycemic agents (including insulin)
Hypo-osmolar parenteral solutions
Lithium
Local anesthetics (bupivacaine, lidocaine, procaine, etidocaine)
Methylxanthines (theophylline, aminophylline)
Narcotic analgesics (fentanyl, meperidine, pentazocine, propoxyphene)
Phencyclidine
Sympathomimetics (amphetamines, cocaine, ecstasy[1], ephedrine, phenylpropanolamine, terbutaline)

[1]Methylenedioxymethamphetamine (MDMA).

dantrolene for malignant hyperthermia) where indicated. Patients who survive may be left with ataxia as a result of the special vulnerability of cerebellar neurons to hyperthermia.

NONEPILEPTIC SEIZURES

Attacks that resemble seizures (nonepileptic seizures or psychogenic seizures) may be manifestations of a psychiatric disturbance such as conversion disorder, somatization disorder, factitious disorder with physical symptoms, or malingering.

Nonepileptic seizures usually can be distinguished both clinically and by the electroencephalographic (EEG) findings. In patients with nonepileptic seizures resembling tonic–clonic attacks, there may be warning and preparation before the attack; there is usually no tonic phase, and the clonic phase consists of wild thrashing movements during which the patient rarely comes to harm or is incontinent. Ictal eye closure is common. In some instances, there are abnormal movements of all extremities without loss of consciousness; in others, there is shouting, uttering of obscenities, or goal-directed behavior during apparent loss of consciousness. There is no postictal confusion after the attack, nor are there abnormal clinical signs. The EEG, if recorded during an episode, does not show organized seizure activity, and postictal slowing does not occur. The differential diagnosis should include frontal lobe seizures, which may be marked by unusual midline movements (eg, pelvic thrusting or bicycling) and by very brief postictal states. Ictal EEG abnormalities may escape detection as well.

It is important to appreciate that many patients with nonepileptic seizures also have genuine epileptic attacks that require anticonvulsant medications, but these should be prescribed at an empirically appropriate dose. Psychiatric referral may be helpful.

CLASSIFICATION & CLINICAL FINDINGS

CLASSIFICATION

Seizures are classified as follows:

▶ Generalized Seizures

1. **Tonic–clonic** (grand mal)
2. **Absence** (petit mal)
3. **Other types** (tonic, clonic, myoclonic, atonic)

▶ Partial (Focal) Seizures

1. **Simple partial** (with preservation of consciousness; focal onset aware seizure)
2. **Complex partial** (focal impaired awareness seizure, temporal lobe, psychomotor, or focal seizures with dyscognitive features)

3. **Partial seizures with secondary generalization** (focal to bilateral tonic clonic)

GENERALIZED SEIZURES

▶ Generalized Tonic–Clonic Seizures

Generalized tonic–clonic seizures are attacks in which consciousness is lost, usually without aura or other warning. When a warning does occur, it usually consists of nonspecific symptoms.

1. **Tonic phase**—The initial manifestations are unconsciousness and tonic contraction of limb muscles for 10 to 30 seconds, producing first flexion and then extension, particularly of the back and neck (**Figure 12-2**). Tonic contraction of the muscles of respiration may produce an expiration-induced vocalization (cry or moan) and cyanosis, and contraction of masticatory muscles may cause tongue trauma. The patient falls to the ground and may be injured.

2. **Clonic phase**—The tonic phase is followed by a clonic (alternating muscle contraction and relaxation) phase of symmetric limb jerking that persists for an additional 30 to 60 seconds or longer. Ventilatory efforts return immediately after cessation of the tonic phase, and cyanosis clears. The mouth may froth with saliva. With time, the jerking becomes less frequent, until finally all movements cease and the muscles are flaccid. Sphincteric relaxation or detrusor muscle contraction may produce urinary incontinence.

3. **Recovery**—As the patient regains consciousness, there is postictal confusion and often headache. Full orientation commonly takes 10 to 30 minutes or even longer in patients with status epilepticus (see next section) or preexisting structural or metabolic brain disorders. Physical examination during the postictal state is usually otherwise normal in idiopathic epilepsy or seizures of metabolic origin, except that plantar responses may be transiently extensor (Babinski sign). The pupils always react to light, even when the patient is unconscious.

4. **Status epilepticus**—Status epilepticus is defined arbitrarily as a seizure continuing for 5 to 30 minutes or more without ceasing spontaneously or as seizures recurring so frequently that full consciousness is not restored between successive episodes. Status epilepticus is a medical emergency because it can lead to permanent brain damage from hyperpyrexia, circulatory collapse, or excitotoxic neuronal damage if untreated.

▶ Absence (Petit Mal) Seizures

These are genetically transmitted seizures that always begin in childhood and rarely persist into adolescence. Genes linked to childhood absence epilepsy include the voltage-gated calcium channel and $GABA_A$ receptor

Tonic phase

Clonic phase

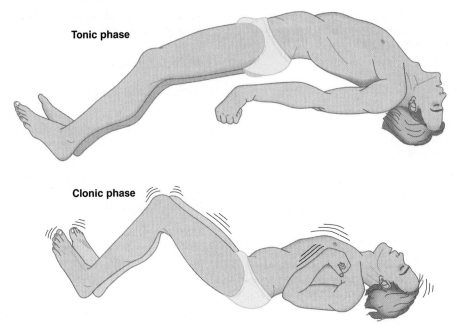

▲ **Figure 12-2.** Generalized tonic–clonic seizure, illustrating the appearance of the patient in the tonic (stiffening) and clonic (shaking) phases.

subunits, malic enzyme 2, and inhibin alpha precursor. The spells are characterized by brief loss of consciousness (for 5-10 seconds) without loss of postural tone. Subtle motor manifestations, such as eye blinking or a slight head turning, are common. More complex automatic movements (automatisms) are uncommon. Full orientation is present immediately after seizure cessation.

There may be as many as several hundred spells daily, leading to impaired school performance or social interactions, so that children may be mistakenly thought to be mentally retarded. The spells are characteristically inducible by hyperventilation or by intermittent photic stimulation. The EEG pattern during a seizure is that of **3-Hz spike-wave activity** (**Figure 12-3**). In most patients with

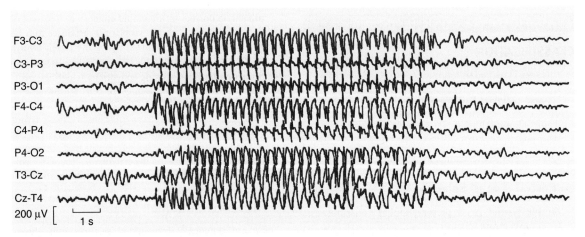

F3-C3

C3-P3

P3-O1

F4-C4

C4-P4

P4-O2

T3-Cz

Cz-T4

200 μV

1 s

▲ **Figure 12-3.** EEG of a patient with typical absence (petit mal) seizures, showing a burst of generalized 3-Hz spike-wave activity (center of record) that is bilaterally symmetric and bisynchronous. Odd-numbered leads indicate electrode placements over the left side of the head; even numbers, over the right side.

normal intelligence and normal background activity on EEG, absence spells occur only during childhood; uncommonly, the attacks continue into adult life, either alone or in association with other types of seizures.

Other Types of Generalized Seizures

These include tonic seizures (not followed by a clonic phase), clonic seizures (not preceded by a tonic phase), and myoclonic seizures.

1. **Tonic seizures** are characterized by continuous muscle contraction that can lead to fixation of the limbs and axial musculature in flexion or extension; they are a cause of drop attacks. The accompanying arrest of ventilatory movements leads to cyanosis. Consciousness is lost, and there is no clonic phase to these seizures.

2. **Clonic seizures** are characterized by repetitive clonic jerking accompanied by loss of consciousness. There is no initial tonic component.

3. **Myoclonic seizures** are characterized by sudden, brief, shock-like contractions that may be localized to a few muscles or one or more extremities or may have a more generalized distribution causing falls. Juvenile myoclonic epilepsy is the most common cause, with onset usually in adolescence. Not all myoclonic jerks have an epileptic basis, however, as discussed in Chapter 11, Movement Disorders. There is a family history of seizures in one-third of patients with myoclonic seizures. The disorder is genetically heterogeneous, with linkage in different families to the calcium channel beta4 subunit, CASR calcium channel sensor receptor, GABA$_A$ receptor alpha one and delta subunits, and myoclonin1. Myoclonic seizures may also be associated with a variety of rare hereditary neurodegenerative disorders, including Unverricht-Lundborg disease (cystatin B mutations), Lafora body disease (laforin mutations), neuronal ceroid lipofuscinosis, and mitochondrial encephalomyopathy (myoclonus epilepsy with ragged red fibers on skeletal muscle biopsy).

4. **Atonic seizures** result from loss of postural tone, sometimes after a myoclonic jerk, leading to a fall or drop attack. They are most common in developmental disorders such as the Lennox–Gastaut syndrome.

PARTIAL SEIZURES

Focal Onset Aware Seizures (Simple Partial Seizures)

Focal seizures begin with motor, sensory, or autonomic phenomena, depending on the cortical region affected. For example, clonic movements of a single muscle group in the face, a limb, or the pharynx may occur and may be self-limited; they may be recurrent or continuous or may spread to involve contiguous regions of the motor cortex (**Jacksonian march**).

Autonomic symptoms may consist of pallor, flushing, sweating, piloerection, pupillary dilatation, vomiting, borborygmi, or hypersalivation. Psychic symptoms include distortions of memory (eg, déjà vu, the sensation that a new experience is familiar), forced thinking or labored thought processes, cognitive deficits, affective disturbances (eg, fear, depression, an inappropriate sense of pleasure), hallucinations, or illusions. During focal onset aware seizure, consciousness is preserved unless and until the seizure discharge spreads to other areas of the brain, producing tonic–clonic seizures (**focal to bilateral tonic–clonic seizures; secondary generalization**). The **aura** is the portion of the seizure that precedes loss of consciousness and of which the patient retains some memory. The aura is sometimes the sole manifestation of the epileptic discharge.

In the postictal state, a focal neurologic deficit such as hemiparesis (**Todd paralysis**) may persist for 30 minutes to 36 hours and indicates an underlying focal brain lesion.

Focal Impaired Awareness Seizures (Complex Partial Seizures)

Seizures formerly called complex partial, temporal lobe, limbic, or psychomotor seizures are now descriptively referred to as focal impaired awareness seizures. These are partial seizures in which consciousness, responsiveness, or memory is impaired. Risk factors include prolonged febrile seizures of childhood, head trauma, or brain infections. Many causes are unknown. The seizure discharge usually arises from the temporal lobe or medial frontal lobe but can originate elsewhere. The symptoms take many forms but are usually stereotyped for the individual patient. Seizures may begin with an **aura**. Epigastric sensations are most common, but affective (fear), psychic (déjà vu), and sensory (olfactory hallucinations) symptoms also occur. Consciousness is then impaired. Seizures generally persist for 1 to 3 minutes; those originating in the frontal lobe are briefer. The motor manifestations are characterized by coordinated involuntary motor activity, termed **automatisms**, which take the form of orobuccolingual movements in approximately 75% of patients and other facial or neck or hand movements in approximately 50%. Sitting up or standing, fumbling with objects, and bilateral limb movements are less common. With frontal lobe origin, bicycling movement or pelvic thrusting can occur. Involvement of both sides of the brain, previously called secondary generalization, is now termed focal to bilateral tonic-clinic seizure. A postictal confusional state of approximately 15 minutes follows, but the patient may not be completely normal for hours.

DIAGNOSIS

The diagnosis of seizures is based on clinical recognition of one of the seizure types described previously. The EEG can be a helpful confirmatory test in distinguishing seizures

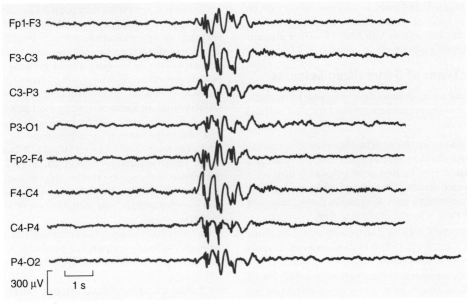

Fp1-F3

F3-C3

C3-P3

P3-O1

Fp2-F4

F4-C4

C4-P4

P4-O2

300 μV ⌊ 1 s

▲ **Figure 12-4.** EEG of a patient with idiopathic (primary generalized) epilepsy. A burst of generalized epileptiform activity (**center**) is seen on a relatively normal background. These findings, obtained at a time when the patient was not experiencing seizures, support the clinical diagnosis of epilepsy. Odd-numbered leads indicate electrode placements over the left side of the head; even numbers, over the right side.

from other causes of loss of consciousness (**Figure 12-4**). However, a normal or nonspecifically abnormal interictal EEG never excludes the diagnosis of epilepsy. Specific EEG features that suggest epilepsy include abnormal spikes, polyspike discharges, and spike-wave complexes.

A standard diagnostic evaluation of patients with recent onset of seizures is presented in **Table 12-3**. Metabolic and toxic disorders that can cause seizures (see Table 12-1) should be excluded because they do not require anticonvulsants.

Seizures with a clearly focal onset or those that begin after the age of 25 years require prompt evaluation to exclude the presence of a structural brain lesion. Magnetic resonance imaging (MRI) is essential for this purpose (computed tomography [CT] scan is not adequate). If no cause is found, the decision to begin chronic anticonvulsant therapy should be based on the probability of recurrence. After a single generalized tonic–clonic seizure, recurrence of one or more seizures can be expected within 3 to 4 years in 30% of untreated adult patients (**Figure 12-5**).

TREATMENT

PRINCIPLES OF TREATMENT

Therapy should be directed toward the cause of the seizures, if known (see Table 12-1). Seizures associated with meta- bolic and systemic disorders usually respond poorly to

anticonvulsants but cease with correction of the underlying abnormality. Acute withdrawal from alcohol and other seda- tive drugs produces self-limited seizures that, in general, require no anticonvulsant drug therapy. Acute head trauma

Table 12-3. Evaluation of a New Seizure Disorder in a Stable Patient.

History (including medications and drug exposure)
General physical examination
Complete neurologic examination
Blood studies
Fasting glucose
Serum electrolytes
Serum calcium
Renal function studies
Hepatic function studies
Complete blood count
Serum FTA-ABS
EEG (abnormal in 20-60% of first EEGs; 60-90% with repeated EEGs)
Brain MRI (especially with abnormal neurologic examination, progressive disorder, or onset of seizures after age 25 years)

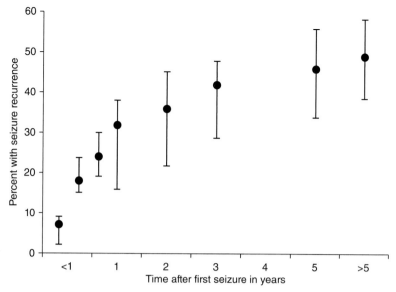

Figure 12-5. Percentages of patients with a first seizure experiencing a recurrent seizure over time. (Used with permission from Krumholz A, Wiebe S, Gronseth GS, et al. Evidence-based guideline management of an unprovoked first seizure in adults. *Neurology.* 2015;84(16):1705-1713.)

and other structural brain lesions that result in seizures must be diagnosed and treated appropriately, and the associated seizures controlled by anticonvulsant drug therapy. Idiopathic epilepsy is treated with anticonvulsant medications.

There are four key principles of management:

1. **Establish the diagnosis of epilepsy before starting drug therapy**—Therapeutic trials of anticonvulsant drugs intended to establish or reject a diagnosis of epilepsy may yield incorrect diagnoses.

2. **Choose the right drug for the seizure type**—Absence seizures, for example, do not respond to most drugs used for focal onset or generalized seizures.

3. **Modulate treatment according to seizure control, rather than the serum drug levels**—Control of seizures is achieved at different drug levels in different patients.

4. **Evaluate one drug at a time**—In most cases, seizures can be controlled with a single drug. Therefore, beginning therapy with multiple drugs may expose patients to increased drug toxicity without added therapeutic benefit.

ANTICONVULSANT DRUGS

Most anticonvulsant drugs act by potentiating inhibitory (GABAergic) synaptic transmission, inhibiting excitatory (glutamatergic) synaptic transmission, or attenuating postsynaptic propagation of action potentials through sodium channel blockade. Drugs acting at GABAergic synapses

and their molecular targets are illustrated in **Figure 12-6**; those acting at glutamatergic synapses and their molecular targets are illustrated in **Figure 12-7**.

Commonly used anticonvulsant drugs and their dosages and methods of administration are listed in **Table 12-4**.

TREATMENT STRATEGIES

Most patients with epilepsy fall into one of the following treatment categories.

▶ New Seizures

Most epileptologists do not recommend chronic anticonvulsant drug treatment after a single seizure unless an underlying cause is found that is not correctable and is likely to produce recurrent seizures (eg, primary or metastatic brain tumor). However, recurrent seizures (two or more, greater than two hours apart) do require anticonvulsant treatment; if such therapy is to be administered, the oral loading schedules presented in Table 12-4 can be used. Note that starting a drug at its daily maintenance dose produces stable serum drug levels only after approximately five half-lives have elapsed. Therefore, loading doses should only be given to achieve therapeutic drug levels promptly in patients with frequent seizures.

1. **Focal seizures with impaired consciousness or focal to bilateral tonic–clonic seizures**—As appropriate drugs of first choice for treating these seizure types, **levetiracetam, lamotrigine,** or **sodium valproate** are preferred;

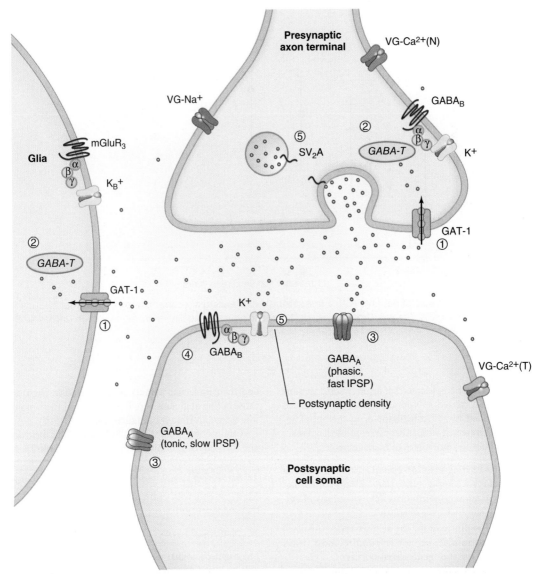

▲ **Figure 12-6.** Known and potential sites of action of anticonvulsant drugs at inhibitory GABAergic synapses: (1) GABA transporters (tiagabine); (2) GABA transaminase (vigabatrin); (3) GABA$_A$ receptors (benzodiazepines, barbiturates); and (4) GABA$_B$ receptors. Abbreviations: GABA-T, GABA transaminase; GAT, GABA transporter; VG, voltage-gated ion channel; (N) and (T), calcium channel subtypes. Small circles in the intercellular space represent GABA molecules. (Used with permission from Katzung BG, Masters SB, Trevor AJ. eds. *Basic and Clinical Pharmacology.* 11th ed. New York, NY: McGraw-Hill; 2009.)

phenytoin, carbamazepine, oxcarbazepine, topiramate, or **zonisamide** are also appropriate. Aside from ethosuximide (and perhaps rufinamide), all currently available seizure medications have demonstrated efficacy in treating partial seizures. As none of the newest medications (including lacosamide, perampanel, and eslicarbazepine) have demonstrated superior efficacy or

side-effect profiles, they should not be used for initial therapy. Gabapentin is usually not used for initial seizure treatment because its short half-life is a significant limitation. Tiagabine, vigabatrin, barbiturates, and benzodiazepines are not used for initial treatment because of their side-effect profiles. In limited comparative trials, lamotrigine is superior to carbamazepine.

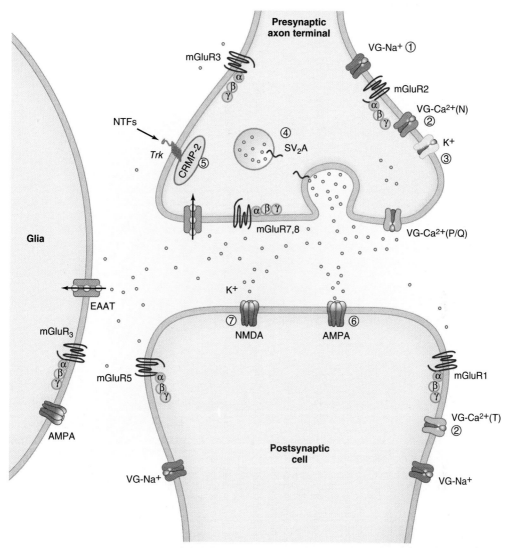

▲ **Figure 12-7.** Known and potential sites of action of anticonvulsant drugs at excitatory glutamatergic synapses: (1) voltage-gated sodium channels (phenytoin, carbamazepine, lamotrigine); (2) voltage-gated calcium channels (ethosuximide, lamotrigine, gabapentin, pregabalin); (3) voltage-gated potassium channels (retigabine); (4) synaptic vesicle glycoprotein 2A (levetiracetam, brivaracetam); (5) collapsin-related mediator protein-2; (6) AMPA-preferring glutamate receptors (phenobarbital, topiramate, lamotrigine, perampanel); (7) NMDA-preferring glutamate receptors (felbamate). Abbreviations: EAAT, excitatory amino acid transporter; mGluR, metabotropic glutamate receptor; (N), (P/Q), and (T), calcium channel subtypes; NTFs, neurotrophic factors. Small circles in the intercellular space represent glutamate molecules. (Used with permission from Katzung BG, Masters SB, Trevor AJ. eds. *Basic and Clinical Pharmacology.* 11th ed. New York, NY: McGraw-Hill; 2009.)

2. **Generalized seizures—Valproic acid** is effective for all types of primary generalized seizures, but is not recommended as the initial treatment in women of childbearing age because of its potential teratogenicity. However, in comparative trials, valproate is better tolerated than topiramate and more effective than lamotrigine. Levetiracetam, topiramate, lamotrigine, and zonisamide can also be used successfully in generalized epilepsies.

3. **Absence seizures—**Absence attacks of the petit mal variety are treated with **sodium valproate** or **ethosuximide**. The former has the advantage of also providing

Table 12-4. Summary of Anticonvulsant Drug Therapy.

Drug	Usual Preparation	Loading or Initial Dose[1]	Maintenance Dose[1]	Serum Half-Life (Normal Renal and Hepatic Function)	Therapeutic Serum Levels	Indications
Phenytoin (Dilantin)	100 mg; 30, 50 mg also available	Oral loading: 1,000 mg in two to four divided doses over 12-24 h / Intravenous loading: 1,000-1,500 mg (15-18 mg/kg) not exceeding 50 mg/min / Fosphenytoin is prodrug form for intramuscular or intravenous use	300-400 mg/d in a single dose or divided doses	Oral: 18-24 h / Intravenous: 12 h / Kinetics are dose dependent and may vary widely	10-20 µg/mL	F, G, S
Carbamazepine (Tegretol)	200, 300 mg; XR: 100, 200, 400 mg	100 mg twice daily; increase by 200 mg/d to maintenance dose	400-1,600 mg/d in three or four doses, or in two doses in XR form	12-18 h (monotherapy)	4-12 µg/mL	F, S
Oxcarbazepine (Trileptal)	150, 300, 600 mg	300 mg twice daily	600-2,400 mg/d in two doses	8-10 h	12-30 µg/mL*	F, S
Phenobarbital (Luminal)	15, 30, 60, 100 mg	180 mg twice daily for 3 days or same as maintenance dose	90-180 mg/d in a single dose	3-5 days	20-40 µg/mL	F, G, S
Valproic acid (Depakote, Depakene)	250 mg	Same as maintenance dose	750-3,000 mg/d in two or three doses	6-18 h	50-150 µg/mL	G, M, A, F, S
Ethosuximide (Zarontin)	250 mg	15 mg/kg/d, then increase by 25 mg/d at weekly intervals to maintenance dose	15-40 mg/kg/d in two or three doses	24-36 h (children); 60 h (adults)	40-100 µg/mL	A
Clonazepam (Klonopin)	0.5, 1, 2 mg	Children: 0.01-0.03 mg/kg/d in two or three divided doses / Adults: 0.5 mg/d	Children: 0.01-0.02 mg/kg/d in two or three doses / Adults: 1.5-2.0 mg/d in two or three doses	20-40 h	0.02-0.10 µg/mL	F, G
Gabapentin (Neurontin)	100, 300, 400 mg	300 mg three times daily	900-4,800 mg/d in three doses	5-7 h	Not established	F, S
Lamotrigine (Lamictal)	50, 100, 200 mg	25 mg twice daily then slowly increase[2]	200-500 mg/d in two doses[2]	12-60 h[2]	5-15 µg/mL*	G, F, S, A, LGS
Levetiracetam (Keppra)	250, 500, 750 mg	250-500 mg twice daily	1,000-3,000 mg/d in two doses	8-10 h	10-40 µg/mL*	G, F, M
Vigabatrin (Sabril)	500 mg	500 mg twice daily; increase by 500 mg every week to maintenance dose	2-4 g/d in two doses	5-8 h	Not established	F
Topiramate (Topamax)	25, 100, 200 mg	25 mg/d; increase by 25-50 mg every 2 weeks to maintenance dose	100-400 mg/d in two doses	16-30 h	4-12 mg/mL*	G, F, S, A

Drug	Strengths/Forms	Initial/Titration	Maintenance dose	Half-life	Therapeutic level	Seizure type
Tiagabine (Gabitril)	4, 12, 16, 20 mg	4 mg/d; increase by 4-8 mg every week to maintenance dose	12-56 mg/d in three doses	5-13 h	Not established	F, S
Zonisamide (Zonegran)	100 mg	100 mg/d	300-600 mg/d in one or two doses	52-69 h	10-40 mg/mL*	G, F, S, M
Pregabalin (Lyrica)	25, 50, 75, 100, 150, 200, 225, 300 mg	100-150 mg/d in two divided doses	150-600 mg/d	6 h	Not established	F
Eslicarbazepine (Aptiom)	200, 400, 600, 800 mg	400 mg/d; increase by 400 mg/d every week to maintenance dose	1,200 mg/d	13-20 h	Not established	F
Lacosamide (Vimpat)	50, 100, 150, 200 mg, 10 mL sol, IV	50 mg twice daily; increase by 100 mg/d every week to maintenance dose	400 mg in two divided doses	13 h	Not established	F
Perianal (Fycompa)	2, 4, 6, 8, 10, 12 mg	2 mg at night (4 mg when added to enzyme-inducing AED), increase by 2 mg/d every week to maintenance dose	8-12 mg at bedtime	105 h	Not established	F
Rufinamide (Banzel)	200, 400 mg	200-1,600 mg in two divided doses, increase by 400-800 mg qod to max 3,200 mg	3,200 mg in two divided doses	6-10 h	Not established	LGS
Brivaracetam (Briviact)	10, 25, 50, 75, 100 mg	50 mg twice daily	adjusted to 50-200 mg/d	9 h	Not established	F

A, absence; F, focal (partial); G, generalized tonic–clonic; LGS, (Adult) Lennox–Gastaut Syndrome; M, myoclonic; S, secondarily generalized tonic–clonic; *, provisional.

[1]Given orally unless indicated otherwise.

[2]Varies depending on interaction with co-administered anticonvulsant drugs; loading dose is 25 mg every other day for 2 weeks when taking valproic acid.

protection against tonic–clonic seizures but has caused fatalities from hepatic damage in children younger than 10 (usually <2) years of age. Levetiracetam, topiramate, zonisamide, and lamotrigine may also be used for absence seizures. As with valproate, they provide protection against tonic–clonic seizures as well.

4. **Myoclonic seizures**—These are treated with **sodium valproate, levetiracetam, zonisamide,** or **clonazepam.**

Recurrent Seizures on Drug Therapy

1. **Determining serum levels of drugs**—Blood levels of anticonvulsant drugs the patient has been taking should be measured in samples taken just before a scheduled dose. For a single breakthrough seizure, no acute change in medication is mandated, even if there has been no interruption of drug therapy and anticonvulsant drug levels are in the therapeutic range, but a slight increase in prescribed dose may be considered. If the history or serum drug levels suggest that treatment has been interrupted, the prescribed drug should be started again as for new seizures.

2. **Changing to a different drug**—A different anticonvulsant should be introduced only if seizures continue to occur after maximum therapeutic benefit has been achieved with the initial drug. This means that blood levels of the drug are in the therapeutic range and that drug toxicity precludes further dosage increments. An anticonvulsant that has failed to alter seizure frequency should be discontinued gradually once therapeutic levels of the new drug have been achieved. Transition to monotherapy with a different drug is recommended twice before trials of two-drug combination therapy. As second monotherapy or combination therapeutic agents, lamotrigine or sodium valproate (alone or in combination) are preferred; levetiracetam, zonisamide, or topiramate are also appropriate. After failure of two appropriate anticonvulsants at therapeutic plasma concentrations, patients are deemed medically refractory. Drug recommendations in special circumstances are addressed below (**Table 12-5**).

Table 12-5. Drugs in Special Circumstances.

Elderly*	Lamotrigine	Levetiracetam	Gabapentin
Renal disease	Lamotrigine	Levetiracetam	
Liver failure	Levetiracetam		
Immunosuppression	Levetiracetam		
Brain tumor, RT, chemo	Levetiracetam		
Depression	Levetiracetam	Valproate (men)	

*All drugs at lower doses than standard.

3. **Treating refractory seizures**—In some patients, disabling seizures persist despite trials of major anticonvulsants, alone and in combination, at the highest doses the patient can tolerate. When no treatable cause can be found, seizures are not due to a progressive neurodegenerative disease, and medical treatment has been unsuccessful for at least 2 years, evaluation for possible **surgical therapy** should be considered.

Presurgical evaluation begins with a detailed history and neurologic examination to explore the cause of seizures and their site of origin within the brain and to document the adequacy of prior attempts at medical treatment. MRI and electrophysiologic studies are performed to identify the epileptogenic zone within the brain. Several electrophysiologic techniques can be used: **EEG**, in which cerebral electrical activity is recorded noninvasively from the scalp; **intracranial or invasive EEG**, in which activity is recorded from electrodes inserted into the brain (depth electrodes) or placed over the brain surface (subdural electrodes); and **electrocorticography**, which involves intraoperative recording from the surface of the brain. When an epileptogenic zone can be identified in this manner and its removal is not expected to produce undue neurologic impairment, surgical excision may be indicated.

Patients with focal impaired awareness seizure (complex partial seizures) arising from a single temporal lobe are the most frequent surgical candidates; unilateral anterior temporal lobectomy or stereotaxic laser interstitial thermal therapy (with fewer neurocognitive effects) abolishes seizures and auras in approximately 50% of these patients and significantly reduces their frequency in another 25%. Hemispherectomy and corpus callosum section are also sometimes used to treat intractable epilepsy.

Left **vagal (X) nerve stimulation** has been shown to reduce seizure frequency by as much as 50% in adults and children with refractory epilepsy. Response rates increase over 12-18 months. The mechanism of action is unknown, but afferent responses from the vagus are received in the nucleus tractus solitarius in the medulla and project widely.

Transcranial magnetic stimulation and deep brain stimulation are evolving experimental treatments.

As **diet therapy**, the ketogenic diet (4:1 fat/carbohydrate) has been used for a century in the pediatric epileptic population. Resultant ketone bodies may affect GABA synthesis or glutamate release. The diet is difficult to maintain but the Atkins diet may produce a similar reduction in seizure frequency (50% seizure reduction in one-third of patients).

Multiple Seizures or Status Epilepticus

1. **Early management**—Status epilepticus is a medical emergency because of its potential for causing irreversible brain injury and death.

a. Immediate attention should be given to ensure that the airway is patent and the patient is positioned to prevent aspiration of stomach contents.

b. The laboratory studies listed in **Table 12-6** should be ordered without delay.

c. Dextrose (50 mL of 50% solution) should be given intravenously.

d. Meningitis and encephalitis should be considered, especially if fever and meningeal signs are present, and a lumbar puncture performed if indicated. Note that **postictal pleocytosis** is detectable in cerebrospinal fluid (CSF) in approximately 2% of patients with single generalized tonic–clonic seizures (and approximately 15% of those with status epilepticus) in the absence of infection. The white blood cell count may be as high as 80/μL, with either polymorphonuclear or mononuclear predominance. Serum protein content may be slightly elevated, but glucose concentration is normal, and Gram stain is negative. The postictal pleocytosis resolves in 2 to 5 days.

Table 12-6. Emergency Evaluation of Serial Seizures or Status Epilepticus.

Treatment with anticonvulsants should be instituted immediately (Table 12-7), while the following measures are taken.

Vital signs:
  Blood pressure: exclude hypertensive encephalopathy and shock
  Temperature: exclude hyperthermia
  Pulse: exclude life-threatening cardiac arrhythmia

Draw venous blood for serum glucose, calcium, electrolytes, hepatic and renal function studies, complete blood count, erythrocyte sedimentation rate, and toxicology
Insert intravenous line
Administer glucose (50 mL of 50% dextrose) intravenously
Obtain any available history

Rapid physical examination, especially for:
  Signs of trauma
  Signs of meningeal irritation or systemic infection
  Papilledema
  Focal neurologic signs
  Evidence of metastatic, hepatic, or renal disease

Arterial blood gases
Lumbar puncture, unless the cause of seizures has already been determined or signs of increased intracranial pressure or focal neurologic signs are present
ECG
Calculate serum osmolality: 2 (serum sodium concentration) + (serum glucose/20) + (serum urea nitrogen/3); normal range, 270-290 mOsm/L
Urine sample for toxicology

2. **Drug therapy to control seizures**—Every effort must be made to establish a precise etiologic diagnosis so that treatment of the underlying disorder can be started. Because generalized seizure activity per se damages the brain if it persists for more than 2 hours, drug therapy to terminate seizures should be instituted immediately. An outline for rapid pharmacologic control of multiple seizures is presented in **Table 12-7**.

3. **Management of hyperthermia**—The systemic physiologic consequences of status epilepticus are related to increased motor activity and high levels of circulating catecholamines; they include hyperthermia (temperature elevation to 42-43°C [108-109°F] in the absence of infection), lactic acidosis (pH < 7.00), and peripheral blood leukocytosis (elevation to 30,000 cells/μL). These derangements resolve after cessation of the seizures. Only hyperthermia, which is known to increase the risk of brain damage from status epilepticus, requires specific attention. Severe hyperthermia must be treated with a cooling blanket and, if necessary, the induction of motor paralysis with a neuromuscular blocking agent. Mild or moderate hyperthermia (101-102°F), not requiring specific intervention, may persist for 24 to 48 hours after seizure cessation. Lactic acidosis resolves spontaneously over 1 hour and should not be treated. Infection should, of course, be excluded.

DISCONTINUING ANTICONVULSANTS

Patients (usually children) with epilepsy who are seizure-free on medication for 2 to 5 years may wish to discontinue anticonvulsant drugs. In patients with normal intelligence and a normal neurologic examination, the risk of seizure recurrence may be as low as 25%. Risk factors for recurrence include slowing or spikes (maximum risk with both present) on EEG. When anticonvulsants are to be withdrawn, one drug is eliminated at a time by tapering the dose slowly over approximately 6 weeks. Recurrence of seizures has been reported in approximately 20% of children and 40% of adults after medication withdrawal, in which case prior medication should be reinstituted at the previously effective levels.

COMPLICATIONS OF EPILEPSY & ANTICONVULSANT THERAPY

▶ Complications of Epilepsy

When the diagnosis of epilepsy is made, the patient should be warned against working around moving machinery or at heights and reminded of the risks of swimming alone. The issue of driving must also be addressed. Many state governments have notification requirements when a diagnosis of epilepsy is made.

Sudden unexpected death in epilepsy (SUDEP) affects 1 in 1000 epileptic patients yearly; if seizures are uncontrolled, the risk of death after a generalized seizure is 1 in

Table 12-7. Drug Treatment of Status Epilepticus in Adults.

Drug	Dosage/Route	Advantages/Disadvantages/Complications
Lorazepam or midazolam or diazepam or diazepam gel	0.1 mg/kg IV at rate not greater than 2 mg/min 10 mg IM 10 mg IV over 2 minutes 0.2 mg/kg rectally	Fast acting. Effective half-life 15 minutes for diazepam and 14 h for lorazepam. Abrupt respiratory depression or hypotension in 5%, especially when given in combination with other sedatives. Seizure recurrence in 50% of patients; therefore, must add maintenance drug (fosphenytoin, phenytoin, or phenobarbital).
Proceed immediately to fosphenytoin or phenytoin		
Fosphenytoin or phenytoin	Fosphenytoin: 1000-1500 mg (20 mg/kg) IV at 150 mg (phenytoin equivalents)/min in saline or dextrose solution Phenytoin: 1000-1500 mg (20 mg/kg) slowly at rate not greater than 50 mg/min (cannot be given in dextrose solution)	Peak serum concentration 10-20 minutes after IV infusion. Little or no respiratory depression. Drug levels in the brain are therapeutic at completion of infusion. Effective as a maintenance drug. Hypotension and cardiac arrhythmias can occur.
If seizures persist, another 10 mg/kg of fosphenytoin or phenytoin can be administered; if seizures still continue, proceed immediately to phenobarbital		
Phenobarbital	1000-1500 mg (20 mg/kg) IV slowly (50 mg/min)	Peak brain levels within 30 minutes. Effective as maintenance drug. Respiratory depression and hypotension common at higher doses. (Intubation and ventilatory support should be immediately available.)
If the above is ineffective, proceed immediately to general anesthesia		
Propofol or pentobarbital or midazolam	1-2 mg/kg IV bolus and 2-10 mg/kg/h infusion 15 mg/kg IV slowly, followed by 0.5-4 mg/kg/h 0.2 mg/kg IV slowly, followed by 0.75-10 µg/kg/min	Intubation and ventilatory support required. Hypotension is a limiting factor. Pressors may be required to maintain blood pressure (dopamine up to 10 µg/kg/min).

IM, intramuscular; IV, intravenous.

150. SUDEP accounts for 8-17% of all deaths in patients with epilepsy. The cause is uncertain but appears to be seizure related and caused by either a heart rhythm abnormality or an abnormality in breathing.

Decreased bone mineral density, which may lead to **osteoporosis**, occurs with use of P450-inducing anticonvulsants (phenobarbital, phenytoin, carbamazepine, and primidone) and probably with valproate as well. The newer anticonvulsants are safer. The need for periodic assessment of bone mineral density in the setting of these agents is controversial.

Side Effects of Anticonvulsant Drugs

The side effects of anticonvulsant drug therapy are summarized in **Table 12-8.** Nearly all anticonvulsant drugs may lead to **blood dyscrasias,** and some have **hepatic toxicity.** For this reason, a complete blood count and liver function tests should be obtained before initiating administration of these drugs and at intervals during the course of treatment. *The authors recommend performing these tests twice in the first weeks to months and every 6 to 12 months thereafter.* Lamotrigine has a 1:1000 incidence of Stevens–Johnson syndrome in the first 8 weeks. Most anticonvulsant drugs (especially barbiturates) affect cognitive function to some degree, even in therapeutic doses.

Drug Interactions

A variety of drugs alter the absorption or metabolism of anticonvulsants when given concomitantly. The changes in anticonvulsant levels are summarized in **Table 12-9**. Some anticonvulsants (carbamazepine, primidone, phenytoin, phenobarbital, topiramate, felbamate, and oxcarbazepine) that induce the cytochrome P450 system may lead to reduced effectiveness of oral contraceptives. Oral contraceptive medications may decrease the plasma concentration of lamotrigine.

Epilepsy & Anticonvulsant Therapy in Pregnancy (Oral contraceptives have greater failure rate than non oral)

1. **Teratogenic effects of epilepsy**—The incidence of stillbirth, microcephaly, mental retardation, and seizure disorders is increased in children born to epileptic mothers.

2. **Teratogenic effects of anticonvulsant treatment**—Anticonvulsant therapy during pregnancy is also associated with a greater than normal frequency of congenital malformations, especially cleft palate, cleft lip, and cardiac anomalies. Such malformations are about

Table 12-8. Side Effects of Anticonvulsant Drugs.

Drug	Dose Related	Idiosyncratic	Drug	Dose Related	Idiosyncratic
Phenytoin	Diplopia Ataxia Hirsutism Coarse facial features Polyneuropathy Osteoporosis Megaloblastic anemia Sedation	Skin rash Fever Lymphoid hyperplasia Hepatic dysfunction Blood dyscrasia Stevens–Johnson syndrome Gingival hyperplasia	Lamotrigine	Dizziness Ataxia Insomnia Diplopia	Skin rash in 1-2% (frequency increased by concomitant valproic acid therapy and reduced by gradual build-up of dose) Stevens–Johnson syndrome May worsen myoclonic seizures
Carbamazepine	Diplopia Ataxia Osteoporosis Hyponatremia	Skin rash Blood dyscrasia Hepatic dysfunction Stevens–Johnson syndrome	Levetiracetam	Depression Mood changes Dizziness Fatigue Insomnia	
Oxcarbazepine	Hyponatremia	Skin rash			
Phenobarbital	Sedation Insomnia Behavioral disturbance Diplopia Ataxia Osteoporosis	Skin rash Stevens–Johnson syndrome Dupuytren's contracture	Vigabatrin	Sedation Vertigo Psychosis	Peripheral visual constriction (irreversible)
Valproic acid	Gastrointestinal distress Tremor Sedation Weight gain Hair loss Thrombocytopenia	Hepatic dysfunction Peripheral edema Pancreatitis Teratogenesis	Topiramate	Anorexia Mental slowing Paresthesia Anxiety Weight loss	Renal stones Glaucoma Teratogenesis
Ethosuximide	Gastrointestinal distress Sedation Ataxia Headache	Skin rash Blood dyscrasia	Tiagabine	Dizziness Sedation Nausea	Rash
			Zonisamide	Drowsiness Anorexia Depression	Nephrolithiasis Skin rash
Clonazepam	Sedation Diplopia Ataxia Behavioral disturbance Hypersalivation		Eslicarbazepine	Dizziness Diplopia	
			Lacosamide	Dizziness Memory alteration Mood dysfunction	AV block
Gabapentin and pregabalin	Drowsiness Fatigue Drugged sensation Weight gain	Rash, edema	Perampanel	Somnolence Dizziness	Psychosis Behavioral disturbances

Table 12-9. Some Major Anticonvulsant Drug Interactions.

Drug	Levels Increased By	Levels Decreased By
Phenytoin	Benzodiazepines Chloramphenicol Disulfiram Ethanol Isoniazid Phenylbutazone Sulfonamides Topiramate Trimethoprim Warfarin Zonisamide	Carbamazepine Phenobarbital Pyridoxine Vigabatrin
Carbamazepine	Erythromycin Felbamate[1] Isoniazid Propoxyphene Valproic acid	Phenobarbital Phenytoin Oxcarbazepine Zonisamide
Phenobarbital	Primidone Valproic acid	—
Valproic acid	—	Topiramate Tiagabine Lamotrigine Phenytoin Carbamazepine
Ethosuximide	Valproic acid	—
Clonazepam	—	—
Gabapentin	—	—
Lamotrigine	Valproic acid	Carbamazepine Phenobarbital Phenytoin
Vigabatrin	—	—
Topiramate	—	Carbamazepine Phenytoin Valproic acid
Tiagabine	—	Carbamazepine Phenytoin Phenobarbital
Zonisamide	Lamotrigine	Carbamazepine Phenytoin
Ezogabine	—	Phenytoin Carbamazepine
Eslicarbazepine	—	Phenytoin Carbamazepine Phenobarbital
Perampanel	—	Phenytoin Carbamazepine Oxcarbazepine
Lacosamide	Eslicarbazepine	—

[1]Levels of the parent compound are diminished, but levels of active metabolite increase.

twice as common in the offspring of medicated than of unmedicated epileptic mothers, but because patients with more severe epilepsy are more likely to be treated, it is difficult to know whether epilepsy or its treatment is the more important risk factor.

3. **Differences in teratogenesis among anticonvulsants—** In women unexposed to anticonvulsant drugs, congenital malformations occur in 1.1%. Among women using common anticonvulsants, malformations occur in 2.2-9% of births. The relative risk (highest to lowest) is associated with valproic acid, phenobarbital, topiramate, carbamazepine, phenytoin, levetiracetam, and lamotrigine. Topiramate exposure in the first trimester is associated with oral cleft malformations. From current data, the safest anticonvulsants in pregnancy are lamotrigine and levetiracetam.

4. **Folate deficiency—**Several anticonvulsants can lower serum folate levels. As dietary deficiency of folic acid is associated with neural tube defects, folate supplementation (1 mg/d) should be provided for all women of childbearing age who take antiepileptic drugs.

5. **Withdrawing anticonvulsants before pregnancy—** When an epileptic patient who has been seizure free for several years is contemplating pregnancy, an attempt should be made to assess whether anticonvulsant drugs can be safely withdrawn before conception. In contrast to generalized tonic–clonic seizures, partial and absence seizures present little risk to the fetus, and it may be possible to tolerate imperfect control of these seizures during pregnancy to avoid fetal drug exposure. If anticonvulsant therapy is continued during pregnancy, it is best to maintain treatment with a single drug that has been shown effective for the patient's seizures, using a dose that avoids clinical toxicity. Status epilepticus is treated as described previously for nonpregnant patients.

6. **Anticonvulsant levels in pregnancy—**Plasma levels of anticonvulsant drugs may **decrease** during pregnancy because of the patient's enhanced drug metabolism, and higher doses may be required to maintain control of seizures. It is therefore important to monitor drug levels closely in this setting. This is particularly important with lamotrigine as the dose often needs to be doubled or tripled during a pregnancy to maintain adequate blood levels.

PROGNOSIS

After a single unprovoked seizure, less than half of patients will have a recurrence over 3 to 5 years (ie, develop epilepsy). If a second seizure occurs, however, the subsequent recurrence rate approaches 75%, and anticonvulsants therefore should be started. In prospective assessment, 47% are seizure free on the first agent, 13% with a second drug added, and 4% with a third or multiple drugs. At the onset of treatment, patients should be seen every few months to monitor seizure frequency and make dose adjustments.

SYNCOPE

Syncope is episodic loss of consciousness associated with loss of postural tone. The pathophysiology, involving global hypoperfusion of the brain or brainstem, is distinct from that of seizures. The most common causes of syncope are given in **Table 12-10**.

VASOVAGAL SYNCOPE (SIMPLE FAINTS)

Vasovagal syncope occurs in all age groups. Genetic factors may be relevant. Precipitating factors include emotional stimulation, pain, the sight of blood, fatigue, medical instrumentation, blood loss, or prolonged motionless standing. Vagally mediated decreases in arterial blood pressure and heart rate combine to produce CNS hypoperfusion and subsequent syncope. Cerebral ischemia resulting in brief tonic–clonic movements can occur.

Vasovagal episodes generally begin while the patient is in a standing or seated position and only rarely in a horizontal position (eg, with phlebotomy or intrauterine device insertion). A prodrome lasting 30 to 60 seconds usually precedes syncope and can include marked facial pallor, lassitude, yawning, light-headedness, nausea, diaphoresis, salivation, blurred vision, and tachycardia.

Table 12-10. Common Causes of Syncope and Their Prevalence.

	Percentage of Patients
Neurally mediated causes	
Vasovagal	8-41
Situational Micturition Defecation Swallow Cough	1-8
Carotid sinus syncope	0.45
Orthostatic hypotension	4-10
Decreased cardiac output Obstruction to flow	1-8
Arrhythmias	4-38
Neurologic and psychiatric diseases	3-32
Unknown	13-41

Used with permission from Simon RP. Syncope. In: Goldman L, Ausiello DA, eds. *Cecil Textbook of Medicine.* 23rd ed. Philadelphia, PA: Saunders; 2008:2687-2691. Originally adapted from Kapoor W. Approach to the patient with syncope. In: Braunwald E, Goldman L, eds. *Primary Cardiology.* 2nd ed. Philadelphia, PA: Saunders; 2003.

The patient, who then loses consciousness and falls to the ground, is pale and diaphoretic and has dilated pupils. Breathing continues. The eyes remain open and there is an upward turning of the globes. Bradycardia replaces tachycardia as consciousness is lost. During unconsciousness, abnormal movements may occur, particularly if the patient remains relatively vertical; these are mainly tonic or opisthotonic, but seizure-like tonic–clonic activity is occasionally seen, which can lead to a misdiagnosis of epilepsy. Urinary incontinence may also occur.

The patient recovers consciousness very rapidly (20-30 seconds) after assuming the horizontal position, but residual nervousness, dizziness, headache, nausea, pallor, diaphoresis, and an urge to defecate may be noted. A postictal confusional state, characteristic of seizures, with disorientation and agitation either does not occur or is very brief (<30 seconds). Syncope may recur, especially if the patient stands within the next 30 minutes.

Reassurance and a recommendation to avoid precipitating factors are usually the only treatment necessary.

Recurrent vasovagal syncope (also termed **neurally mediated or neurocardiogenic syncope**) can be diagnosed by inducing syncope during head-up tilt-testing. The bradycardia and hypotension of syncope can be ameliorated by the alpha-agonist midodrine (2.5 to 10 mg three times daily) or with the alpha-beta adrenergic agonist droxidopa (100 mg three times daily initially). Tilt-training may have benefit. Artificial pacing is ineffective.

CARDIOVASCULAR SYNCOPE

A cardiovascular cause is suggested when syncope occurs in a recumbent position, during or after physical exertion, or in a patient with known heart disease. Loss of consciousness related to cardiac disease is most often due to an abrupt decrease in cardiac output with resultant cerebral hypoperfusion. Such cardiac dysfunction can result from cardiac arrest, rhythm disturbances (either brady- or tachyarrhythmias), cardiac inflow or outflow obstruction, intracardiac right-to-left shunts, leaking or dissecting aortic aneurysms, or acute pulmonary embolism (**Table 12-11**). The diagnosis is established by electrophysiologic study and/or long-term event recording. Event monitors triggered by the patient at the onset of symptoms may be helpful; implantable loop recorders, providing continuous EKG recording for up to 3 years, have a high diagnostic yield in unexplained syncope.

CARDIAC ARREST

Cardiac arrest (ventricular fibrillation or asystole) from any cause will result in loss of consciousness in 3 to 5 seconds if the patient is standing or within 15 seconds if the patient is recumbent. Seizure like activity and urinary and fecal incontinence may be seen as the duration of cerebral hypoperfusion increases.

Table 12-11. Cardiovascular Causes of Syncope.

Cardiac arrest
Cardiac dysrhythmias
Tachyarrhythmias
Supraventricular
Paroxysmal atrial tachycardia
Atrial flutter
Atrial fibrillation
Accelerated junctional tachycardia
Postural tachycardia syndrome (POTS)
Ventricular
Ventricular tachycardia
Torsade de pointes
Ventricular fibrillation
Brugada syndrome
Mitral valve prolapse (click-murmur syndrome)
Prolonged QT-interval syndromes
Bradyarrhythmias
Sinus bradycardia
Sinus arrest
Second- or third-degree heart block
Implanted pacemaker failure or malfunction
Sick sinus syndrome (tachycardia-bradycardia syndrome)
Drug toxicity (eg, digitalis, quinidine, procainamide, propranolol, phenothiazines, tricyclic antidepressants, potassium)
Cardiac inflow obstruction
Left atrial myxoma or thrombus
Tight mitral stenosis
Constrictive pericarditis or cardiac tamponade
Restrictive cardiomyopathies
Tension pneumothorax
Cardiac outflow obstruction
Aortic stenosis
Pulmonary stenosis
Hypertrophic cardiomyopathy
Dissecting aortic aneurysm
Severe pulmonary vascular disease
Pulmonary hypertension
Acute pulmonary embolus

TACHYARRHYTHMIAS

▶ Supraventricular Tachyarrhythmias

Supraventricular tachyarrhythmias (**atrial or junctional tachycardia**, **atrial flutter**, or **atrial fibrillation**) may be paroxysmal or chronic. Syncope is preceded most often by sudden brief palpitations or less often by dizziness or dyspnea.

Heart rates faster than 160 to 200/min reduce cardiac output by decreasing the ventricular filling period or inducing myocardial ischemia. Prolonged tachycardia of 180 to 200 beats or more per minute will produce syncope in 50% of normal persons in the upright posture; in patients with underlying heart disease, a heart rate of

135/min may impair cardiac output enough to induce loss of consciousness. Patients with sinus node dysfunction may develop profound bradycardia or even asystole on termination of their tachyarrhythmias. The diagnosis is established when arrhythmias are demonstrated during a symptomatic episode.

The **postural tachycardia syndrome** (POTS) is a systemic disorder that occurs predominantly in women 15-45 years old. Its major symptom is an orthostatic increase in heart rate of 30 or more beats per minute, generally without significant change in blood pressure, occurring on standing from a supine position. Associated symptoms include palpitation, tremulousness, gastrointestinal symptoms, fatigue, sleep disturbances, and migraine. Symptoms are accentuated by dehydration, alcohol, and exercise. The induced heart rate increase diminishes with age.

▶ Ventricular Tachyarrhythmias

Ventricular tachyarrhythmias (**idiopathic ventricular tachycardia** or multiform, frequent, or paired **premature ventricular contractions**) are found on prolonged ECG monitoring in some patients with syncope. The syncope associated with ventricular tachycardia is characterized by a very brief prodrome (<5 seconds). The duration of syncope and of the arrhythmia are closely linked. Frequent or repetitive premature ventricular contractions alone do not often coincide with syncopal symptoms but are predictive of sudden death. Elevation of the ST segment in the right precordium of young adults, without structural heart disease (**Brugada syndrome**), predisposes to ventricular arrhythmias and sudden death. Multiple genes, particularly involving sodium channels, have been implicated.

▶ Mitral Valve Prolapse

Mitral valve prolapse (**click-murmur syndrome**) is a common disorder that can be associated with ventricular tachyarrhythmias and resultant syncope in a small number of patients. Other symptoms include nonexertional chest pain, dyspnea, and fatigue. The ECG may be normal or show nonspecific ST-T wave changes or frequent premature ventricular contractions. Diagnosis is by echocardiography.

▶ Prolonged QT Syndrome

The congenital prolonged QT-interval syndrome consists of paroxysmal ventricular arrhythmias (often torsades de pointes), syncope (usually during exercise), and sudden death. It is inherited as an autosomal recessive condition associated with deafness or as an autosomal dominant form without deafness. Cardiac events are most common during the early teenage years to the mid-twenties. Genes implicated in prolonged QT syndrome include potassium channels (*KCNE1, KCNE2, KCNH2, KCNJ2, KCNJ5,*

KCNQ1), sodium channels (*SCN4B*, *SCN5A*), calcium channels (*CACNA13*), A kinase anchor protein 9 (*AKAP9*), ankyrin 2 (*ANK2*), caveolin 3 (*CAV3*), and α-1 syntrophin (*SNTA1*). Sporadic cases also occur. Antiarrhythmic drugs and electrolyte disorders (hypomagnesemia, hypocalcemia, hypokalemia) can also produce QT prolongation. Hereditary cases may respond to β-blockers.

BRADYARRHYTHMIAS

▶ Sinoatrial Node Disease

Sinoatrial node disease (ie, **sick sinus syndrome**), a disorder of older adults, is commonly associated with syncope caused by profound sinus bradycardia, prolonged sinus pauses, or sinus arrest with a slow atrial, junctional, or idioventricular escape rhythm. The diagnosis is by electrocardiographic rhythm identification. Sick sinus syndrome may be inherited as an autosomal recessive or dominant disorder, caused by mutations in the type V voltage-gated sodium channel alpha subunit (*SCN5A*) or hyperpolarization-activated cyclic nucleotide-gated potassium channel 4 (*HCN4*) genes, respectively. Patients should be evaluated promptly by a cardiologist, as a permanent pacemaker is necessary in many cases. In **tachycardia-bradycardia syndrome**, a form of sick sinus syndrome, both types of arrhythmias occur.

▶ Complete Heart Block

Complete heart block (**third-degree atrioventricular block**) is a common cause of bradyarrhythmia producing recurrent syncope without prodrome. Permanent atrioventricular conduction abnormalities are easily noted on a routine ECG, but intermittent (paroxysmal) conduction abnormalities may not be present on a random tracing. A normal PR interval on an ECG obtained after the episode does not exclude the diagnosis of transient complete heart block.

Patients with syncope and documented or suspected complete heart block should be hospitalized promptly. Patients with acute inferior myocardial infarctions are at high risk for atrioventricular block.

CARDIAC INFLOW OBSTRUCTION

Atrial or ventricular **myxomas** and atrial **thrombi** usually present with embolic events, but they may also produce a left ventricular inflow or outflow obstruction that results in a sudden decrease in cardiac output, followed by syncope. A history of syncope occurring with change in position is classic but uncommon. Echocardiography can confirm the diagnosis. Surgical removal of the myxoma is indicated.

Constrictive pericarditis or **pericardial tamponade** presents with dyspnea, thoracic pain, and signs of cardiac failure. Here, any maneuver or drug that decreases heart rate or venous return can result in suddenly inadequate cardiac output and syncope.

CARDIAC OUTFLOW OBSTRUCTION

▶ Aortic Stenosis

Loss of consciousness from congenital or acquired severe aortic stenosis usually occurs after exercise and is often associated with dyspnea, angina, and diaphoresis. The pathophysiology may involve acute left ventricular failure resulting in coronary hypoperfusion and subsequent ventricular fibrillation, or abrupt increases in left ventricular pressure that stimulate baroreceptors, leading to peripheral vasodilation. Echocardiography can help confirm the diagnosis.

Symptomatic aortic stenosis requires valve replacement; without treatment, survival after syncope from aortic stenosis is 18 months to 3 years.

▶ Pulmonary Stenosis

Most pulmonic valve disorders are congenital. Severe pulmonary stenosis can produce syncope, associated with dyspnea and angina, especially after exertion. A hemodynamic process similar to that occurring in aortic stenosis is responsible. Diagnosis is by echocardiology.

HYPERTROPHIC CARDIOMYOPATHY

Hypertrophic cardiomyopathy comprises a group of congenital cardiomyopathies inherited as autosomal dominant disorders of variable severity. Many different genes have been implicated. Symptoms usually begin between the second and fourth decades. Dyspnea is the most common presenting complaint and can be associated with chest pain and palpitations. Syncope occurs in 30% of patients, is the presenting complaint in 10% of patients, and characteristically develops during or after exercise, but orthostatic and posttussive episodes also occur. Syncope may be due to left ventricular outflow obstruction, inflow obstruction, or transient arrhythmias. The diagnosis can be confirmed by echocardiography. Propranolol may control symptoms; an implantable cardioverter defibrillator may terminate potentially fatal ventricular arrhythmias.

DISSECTING AORTIC ANEURYSM

Although acute onset of severe chest or back pain is the most common presenting symptom, approximately 5% to 10% of patients with acute aortic dissections (usually proximal dissection) present with isolated syncope. In 15% of patients, the dissection is painless. Other neurologic abnormalities (stroke, coma, spinal cord ischemia) may or may not be present. Cardiac tamponade is present and may be etiologic in the majority of patients presenting with syncope. A transthoracic echocardiogram is diagnostic.

PULMONARY HYPERTENSION & PULMONARY EMBOLUS

Syncope, often exertional, may be the presenting symptom of pulmonary hypertension. A history of exertional dyspnea is usual, and blood gas analysis shows hypoxemia, even at rest. Syncope is the presenting symptom in approximately 20% of patients experiencing massive pulmonary embolism. The mechanism of syncope is pulmonary vascular occlusion with attenuated cardiac output resulting in reduced cerebral perfusion. Tachy- and bradyarrhythmias may be associated. Upon recovery, such patients are hypotensive, often complain of pleuritic chest pain, dyspnea, and apprehension. Hypotension, tachycardia, tachypnea, hemoptysis, and arterial hypoxemia (O_2 saturations are an inadequate screen) frequently accompany these large emboli. Venous thrombosis is a common embolic source; in some cases, embolization may be induced by defecation.

CEREBROVASCULAR SYNCOPE

Cerebrovascular disease (Chapter 13, Stroke) is an often suspected but actually uncommon cause of episodic unconsciousness.

BASILAR ARTERY INSUFFICIENCY

Basilar artery transient ischemic attacks usually occur after the sixth decade; males with ischemic heart disease and hypertension are most commonly affected. Syncopal attacks occur in about 10% and occur among other symptoms of brainstem ischemia: diplopia, vertigo, ataxia, dysphagia, dysarthria, paresthesias, and drop attacks. Syncopal episodes are typically sudden in onset and brief in duration (seconds to minutes), but when consciousness is lost, recovery is frequently prolonged (30-60 minutes or longer). Isolated unconsciousness without other symptoms of brainstem ischemia is rarely due to basilar artery insufficiency. Two-thirds of patients have recurrent attacks, and strokes eventually occur in approximately one-fifth of all cases. Basilar artery symptoms can also be due to associated subclavian steal. Treatment is discussed in Chapter 13, Stroke.

SUBCLAVIAN STEAL SYNDROME

The subclavian steal syndrome results from subclavian or innominate artery stenosis that causes retrograde blood flow in the vertebral artery, diverting flow from the brainstem and producing hypoperfusion. Sudden turning of the head in the direction of the affected side can induce symptoms of vertigo, syncope, and intermittent claudication of the upper extremity. The degree of subclavian artery stenosis that produces symptoms is variable, but even minor (~40%) stenosis may sometimes do so. A difference between blood pressures measured in the two arms is nearly always found, the average difference being a 45 mm Hg decrease in systolic pressure in the arm supplied by the stenotic vessel. Cerebrovascular risk factors should be modified; stroke is rare. Arteriography and revascularization procedures may be considered.

MIGRAINE

In ~10% of patients with migraine, syncope occurs during the headache, often on rapid rising to a standing position, suggesting that loss of consciousness is due to orthostatic hypotension; autonomic neuropathy may coexist. The headache can precede or follow the syncopal spell. Migraine without syncope occurs in the majority. Syncopal migraine has both more prolonged unconsciousness and more prolonged recovery than syncope alone. A familial association between migraine and syncope occurs. In some patients, **basilar migraine** produces symptoms similar to those of basilar artery transient ischemic attacks. Antimigraine prophylactic agents (see Chapter 6, Headache & Facial Pain) are often effective in preventing attacks.

TAKAYASU DISEASE

Takayasu disease, sometimes referred to as **pulseless arteritis,** is a panarteritis of the aorta and its major branches that is most prevalent in young Asian women. Symptoms of claudication are most common, followed by fatigue, headache, visual disturbances, and dyspnea. Syncope occurs in 10%; precipitating factors include exercise, standing, or head movement. Vascular examination shows an absent or diminished pulse, a blood pressure difference between extremities, bruits, hypertension, stroke, heart failure, and aortic regurgitation. The erythrocyte sedimentation rate and C reactive protein may be elevated. Angioplasty is the treatment of choice although medical approaches include corticosteroids or methotrexate.

CAROTID SINUS SYNCOPE

Carotid sinus syncope is uncommon. Men are affected twice as often as women, and most affected individuals are more than 60 years old. Drugs known to predispose to carotid sinus syncope include propranolol, digitalis, and methyldopa. Carotid sinus syncope is diagnosed when carotid sinus massage for 10 seconds (on either side and in supine and upright postures) results in a mixture of bradycardia/hypotension (carotid sinus hypersensitivity) and reproduces spontaneous syncope. Carotid sinus hypersensitivity without syncope is common in older men. Treatment for symptomatic patients is with pacing.

Carotid sinus syncope may be mistakenly diagnosed when symptoms result from compression of a normal carotid artery contralateral to an occluded internal carotid artery. Carotid sinus massage should not be performed in patients with recent TIA or stroke or with carotid bruit.

ORTHOSTATIC HYPOTENSION

Orthostatic hypotension patients represent approximately 15% of syncope patients. Symptomatic orthostasis occurs more often in men than in women, is most common in the sixth and seventh decades, but may appear even in teenagers. Loss of consciousness usually occurs upon rapidly rising to a standing position, standing motionless for a prolonged period (especially after exercise), or standing after prolonged recumbency (especially in the elderly).

Numerous conditions can produce orthostatic hypotension (**Table 12-12**), which generally results from either **hypovolemia** or **autonomic dysfunction**. The latter may be due to drugs, autonomic neuropathy, or CNS disorders affecting sympathetic pathways in the hypothalamus, brainstem, or spinal cord.

Orthostatic hypotension may also be a feature of neurodegenerative disorders. **Idiopathic orthostatic hypotension** is associated with isolated degeneration of postganglionic sympathetic neurons. In **multisystem atrophy (Shy-Drager syndrome)**, degeneration of preganglionic sympathetic neurons occurs in combination with parkinsonian, pyramidal, cerebellar, or lower motor neuron signs. These disorders are discussed in Chapter 11, Movement Disorders.

The diagnosis of classic orthostatic hypotension is established by demonstrating a decline in blood pressure of at least 20 mm Hg systolic or 10 mm Hg diastolic within 3 minutes of the patient standing from a lying position. Severe orthostatic intolerance associated with heart rate increases (>120/min) without significant hypotension or syncope is termed **postural orthostatic tachycardia syndrome** (POTS) and is most common in young women (see above).

A detailed general physical and neurologic examination and laboratory studies (hematocrit, stool occult blood, serum glucose and electrolytes, FTA-ABS, nerve conduction studies) should be directed toward establishing the cause of the disorder. Any medication (particularly diuretics, venodilators such as nitrates, and vasodilators such as α-agonists) that might be responsible for orthostatic hypotension should be discontinued if possible. The patient should be instructed to stand up gradually, to elevate the head of the bed on blocks, and to use waist-high elasticized support hosiery. Rapid ingestion of 500 mL of water on awakening prior to getting out of bed increases blood pressure for an hour. Other therapy is dictated by the specific cause of hypotension.

After discontinuing hypotension-inducing medications, enhancing hydration, and adding dietary salt, patients with continued symptoms can be treated with regimens that include midodrine (starting at 2.5 mg two or three times daily increasing to 10 mg tid as needed) and droxidopa as blood pressure enhancers. Pyridostigmine and fludrocortisone are next-line agents, and low-dose atomoxetine may be effective with central autonomic failure.

MISCELLANEOUS CAUSES OF SYNCOPE

COUGH SYNCOPE

Cough (tussive) syncope occurs chiefly in middle-aged men with chronic obstructive pulmonary disease but has also been reported in children. Coughing, which need not be prolonged, immediately precedes unconsciousness. Cough syncope may occur while the patient is supine. Prodromal symptoms are absent, and the duration of unconsciousness is brief—often only a few seconds. Full recovery of consciousness occurs promptly. A history of similar episodes is common, and symptoms may be reproduced by having the patient cough on request. The cause may be a decrease in cerebral blood flow from increased intracranial pressure, which results from the transmission of cough-induced, markedly increased intrathoracic pressure to the intracranial compartment via the spinal fluid or venous connections. Other data support a baroreflex-mediated fall in total peripheral resistance induced by coughing.

Table 12-12. Causes of Orthostatic Hypotension.

Hypovolemia or hemorrhage

Adrenal insufficiency

Drug-induced hypotension
Antidepressants (tricyclics, monoamine oxidase inhibitors)
α and β receptor blockers
Antihypertensives
Dopaminergic drugs (dopamine agonists, levodopa)
Calcium channel antagonists
Diuretics
Vasodilators (nitroglycerin, sildenafil)
Phenothiazines

Polyneuropathies
Amyloid neuropathy
Diabetic neuropathy
Guillain–Barré syndrome
Porphyric neuropathy

Other neurologic disorders
Idiopathic orthostatic hypotension
Multiple sclerosis
Parkinsonism (Parkinson disease, Lewy body dementia, multisystem atrophy)
Posterior fossa tumor
Spinal cord injury with paraplegia
Surgical sympathectomy
Syringomyelia/syringobulbia
Tabes dorsalis
Wernicke encephalopathy

Cardiac pump failure

Prolonged bed rest

The condition is usually benign, and there is no specific treatment except for antitussive drugs such as dextromethorphan. Syncopal spells with a pathophysiology similar to that of coughing include **laughter**-induced syncope and syncope induced by **sneezing** or **weightlifting**.

MICTURITION & DEFECATION SYNCOPE

Micturition syncope is a cerebral hypoperfusion event occurring almost exclusively in men, probably because of the standing position for urination, and is due to peripheral pooling of blood plus vagally induced bradycardia. Episodes can occur immediately before, during, or after micturition. They are more likely to occur at night after the prolonged recumbency of sleep. Urination in a sitting position usually eliminates the symptoms. Syncope during defecation occurs most often in older women and at night, but it can occur throughout the day. The etiology is speculative, but vasodilation and bradycardia following distension of the rectum has been suggested. Border-zone cerebral ischemia has been reported.

GLOSSOPHARYNGEAL NEURALGIA

Glossopharyngeal neuralgia (see Chapter 6, Headache & Facial Pain) is a rare syndrome characterized by intermittent, agonizing, paroxysmal pain localized to the tonsillar pillar or occasionally to the external auditory meatus. The pain is triggered by contact with or movement of the tonsillar pillars, especially during swallowing or talking. Syncope results from activation of a glossopharyngeal-vagal reflex arc, producing transient bradyarrhythmia leading to cerebral hypoperfusion. Carbamazepine 400 to 1000 mg/d orally will prevent pain and bradycardia in most patients. Microvascular decompression of cranial nerve IX or X has been suggested.

PSYCHOGENIC SYNCOPE

Psychogenic syncope is a diagnosis of exclusion and is often made erroneously. Recording an episode with an implantable loop recorder may be required. Suggestive clinical features are lack of any prodrome, possible secondary gain, bizarre postures and movements, lack of pallor, frequent spells, and a prolonged period of apparent unresponsiveness. Eyes are closed during episodes. Psychogenic spells rarely occur when the patient is alone and are rarely associated with incontinence or injury. Most patients are young or have a well-documented history of conversion disorder. Without such a history, diagnosis after the third decade is suspect.

The EEG during psychogenic unconsciousness is normal, without the slowing that typically occurs with cerebral hypoperfusion and follows unconsciousness from a seizure. Caloric testing (see Chapter 3, Coma), which produces nystagmus in conscious patients and tonic eye deviation in unconscious patients, can distinguish psychogenic unresponsiveness from coma caused by a metabolic or structural lesion. Establishing a diagnosis of psychogenic pseudosyncope has been associated with a decrease in frequency of episodes.

NARCOLEPSY

Severe episodes of daytime sleepiness, occurring in the setting of adequate nighttime sleep, can mimic syncope. In narcolepsy, a sporadic disorder with an onset between ages 10 and 20, induced sleep episodes are brief and follow a fixed pattern in a given patient. REM sleep is disordered, and REM elements occur during wakefulness. These elements include sleep paralysis and hypnogogic hallucinations-described as dreaming while awake (both occurring at the transition between sleep and waking), as well as motor paralysis of cataplexy (evolving over many seconds, lasting 1-2 minutes, affecting the face and neck before trunk and limbs, and induced by emotion, usually laughing). A decrease in hypocretin neurons of the lateral hypothalamus and a decrease in CSF hypocretin are found in most narcolepsy and all cataplectic patients. A narcolepsy diagnosis is made by history and nocturnal polysomnography to exclude nocturnal sleep disorders, document two or more sleep onset REM periods, and show brief sleep latencies (less than eight minutes). Narcolepsy treatment begins with brief naps in the morning and afternoon. Modafinil (100-400 mg each morning or 200 mg bid) is the first-line pharmacologic therapy. Cataplexy can be attenuated by tricyclic antidepressants (clomipramine 10-150 mg/d). Sleep paralysis and hypnogogic hallucinations are usually addressed by education.

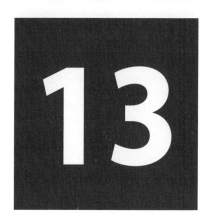
(Continued on Next Page)

Stroke is the fifth leading cause of death in the United States (after heart disease, cancer, chronic lung disease, and injuries and accidents) and the most common disabling neurologic disorder. Approximately 800,000 new strokes occur and approximately 130,000 people die from stroke in the United States each year.

The incidence of stroke increases with age; approximately two-thirds of all strokes occur in those older than 65 years. Modifiable risk factors for stroke include systolic or diastolic hypertension, atrial fibrillation, diabetes, dyslipidemia, physical inactivity, and obstructive sleep apnea (**Table 13-1**). Genetic, usually polygenic, factors also contribute to stroke risk. The incidence of stroke has decreased in recent decades, largely because of improved treatment of hypertension, dyslipidemia, and diabetes and reduction in smoking.

APPROACH TO DIAGNOSIS

Stroke is a syndrome with four key features:

1. **Sudden onset**—The sudden onset of symptoms is documented by the history.
2. **Focal involvement of the central nervous system**—The site of involvement is suggested by symptoms and signs, pinpointed more precisely by neurologic examination, and confirmed by imaging studies (computed tomography [CT] or magnetic resonance imaging [MRI]).
3. **Lack of rapid resolution**—The duration of neurologic deficits is documented by the history. The classic definition of stroke requires that deficits persist for at least 24 hours (to distinguish stroke from transient ischemic attack, discussed later). However, any such time point is arbitrary, and transient ischemic attacks usually resolve within 1 hour.
4. **Vascular cause**—A vascular cause may be inferred from the acute onset of symptoms and often from the patient's age, the presence of risk factors for stroke, and the occurrence of symptoms and signs referable to the territory of a particular cerebral blood vessel. Investigative studies can often identify a more specific etiology, such as arterial thrombosis, cardiogenic embolus, or clotting disorder.

ACUTE ONSET

Strokes begin abruptly. Neurologic deficits may be maximal at onset or may progress over seconds to hours (or occasionally days).

Table 13-1. Risk Factors for Stroke.

Nonmodifiable risk factors
Increased age
Male sex
Low birth weight
Family history of stroke
Modifiable risk factors
Vascular
Hypertension (BP >140 mm Hg systolic or >90 mm Hg diastolic)
Cigarette smoking
Asymptomatic carotid stenosis (>60% diameter)
Peripheral artery disease
Cardiac
Atrial fibrillation (with or without valvular disease)
Congestive heart failure
Coronary artery disease
Endocrine
Diabetes mellitus
Postmenopausal hormone therapy (estrogen ± progesterone)
Oral contraceptive use
Metabolic
Dyslipidemia
High total cholesterol (top 20%)
Low HDL cholesterol (<40 mg/dL)
Obesity (especially abdominal)
Hematologic
Sickle cell disease
Lifestyle
Physical inactivity
Obstructive sleep apnea

BP, blood pressure; HDL, high-density lipoprotein.
Data from Goldstein LB, et al. Guidelines for the primary prevention of stroke. A guideline for healthcare professionals from the American Heart Association/American Stroke Association. *Stroke.* 2011;42:517-584.

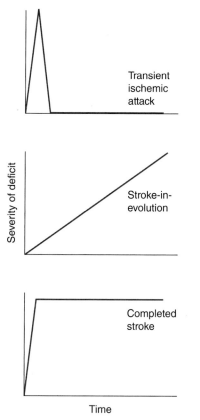

Figure 13-1. Time course of cerebral ischemic events. A transient ischemic attack (TIA) produces neurologic deficits that resolve completely within a short period, usually within 1 hour. Stroke-in-evolution, or progressing stroke, causes deficits that continue to worsen while the patient is observed. Completed stroke is defined by the presence of persistent deficits; it does not necessarily imply that the entire territory of the involved vessel is affected or that no improvement has occurred since the onset.

A stroke that is actively progressing as a direct consequence of the underlying vascular disorder (but not because of associated cerebral edema) or has done so in recent minutes is termed **stroke in evolution** or **progressing stroke** (Figure 13-1).

Focal cerebral deficits that develop slowly (over weeks to months) suggest a cause other than stroke, such as tumor or inflammatory or degenerative disease.

FOCAL INVOLVEMENT

Stroke produces focal symptoms and signs that correlate with the area of the brain supplied by the affected blood vessel.

In **ischemic stroke**, occlusion of a blood vessel interrupts the flow of blood to a specific region of the brain, interfering with neurologic functions dependent on that region and producing a more or less stereotyped pattern of deficits.

Hemorrhage produces a less predictable pattern of focal involvement because complications such as increased intracranial pressure, cerebral edema, compression of brain tissue and blood vessels, or dispersion of blood through the subarachnoid space or cerebral ventricles can impair brain function at sites remote from the hemorrhage.

Global cerebral ischemia (usually from cardiac arrest) and **subarachnoid hemorrhage** (discussed in Chapter 6, Headache & Facial Pain) affect the brain in more diffuse fashion and produce global cerebral dysfunction; the term *stroke* is not usually applied in these cases.

In most cases of stroke, the history and neurologic examination provide enough information to localize the lesion to **one side of the brain** (eg, to the side opposite a hemiparesis or hemisensory deficit or to the left side if aphasia is present) and to the **anterior or posterior cerebral circulation**.

ANTERIOR (CAROTID) CIRCULATION

The anterior cerebral circulation supplies most of the **cerebral cortex** and **subcortical white matter**, **basal ganglia**, and **internal capsule**. It consists of the internal carotid artery and its branches: the **anterior choroidal**, **anterior cerebral**, and **middle cerebral arteries**. The middle cerebral artery in turn gives rise to deep, penetrating **lenticulostriate** branches (**Figure 13-2**). The specific territory of each of these vessels is listed in **Table 13-2**.

Anterior circulation strokes are commonly associated with symptoms and signs of hemispheric dysfunction (**Table 13-3**), such as **aphasia**, **apraxia**, or **agnosia** (described in Chapter 1, Neurologic History & Examination). They also often produce hemiparesis, hemisensory disturbances, and visual field defects, but these can occur with posterior circulation strokes as well.

POSTERIOR (VERTEBROBASILAR) CIRCULATION

The posterior cerebral circulation supplies the **brainstem**, **cerebellum**, **thalamus**, and portions of the **occipital** and **temporal lobes**. It consists of the paired **vertebral arteries**, the **basilar artery**, and their branches: the **posterior inferior cerebellar**, **anterior inferior cerebellar**, **superior cerebellar**, and **posterior cerebral arteries** (see Figure 13-2). The posterior cerebral artery also gives off **thalamoperforate** and **thalamogeniculate** branches. Areas supplied by these arteries are listed in Table 13-2.

Posterior circulation strokes produce symptoms and signs of brainstem or cerebellar dysfunction or both (see Table 13-3), including **coma**, **drop attacks** (sudden

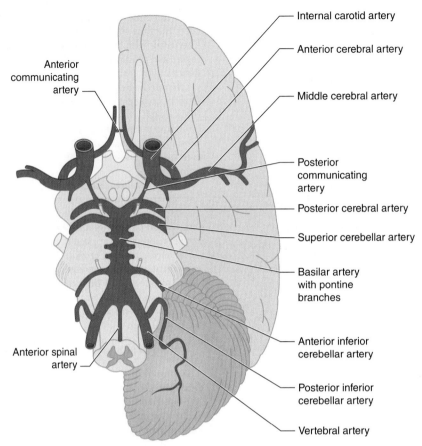

▲ Figure 13-2. Major cerebral arteries. The anterior and posterior cerebral circulations arise anterior and posterior to the posterior communicating arteries, respectively. The circle of Willis is formed by the anterior communicating, anterior cerebral, internal carotid, posterior communicating, and posterior cerebral arteries. (Used with permission from Waxman S. *Clinical Neuroanatomy.* 26th ed. New York, NY: McGraw-Hill; 2010.)

collapse without loss of consciousness), **vertigo, nausea** and **vomiting, cranial nerve palsies, ataxia,** and **crossed sensorimotor deficits** that affect the face on one side of the body and the limbs on the other. Hemiparesis, hemisensory disturbances, and visual field deficits also occur, but are not specific to posterior circulation strokes.

DURATION OF DEFICITS

Stroke produces neurologic deficits that persist. When symptoms and signs resolve completely after brief periods (usually within 1 hour) without evidence of cerebral infarction, the term **transient ischemic attack (TIA)** is used (see Figure 13-1). About 15% of strokes are preceded by TIAs. Recurrent TIAs with identical clinical features (stereotypic TIAs) are usually caused by thrombosis or embolism arising from the same site within the cerebral circulation. TIAs that differ in character from event to event suggest

recurrent emboli from distant (eg, cardiac) or multiple sites. Although TIAs do not themselves produce lasting neurologic dysfunction, they are important to recognize because 3-10% of patients with TIAs will have a stroke within 2 days and 9-17% will have a stroke within 90 days—and because this risk may be reduced with treatment.

VASCULAR ORIGIN

Although hypoglycemia, other metabolic disturbances, trauma, and seizures can produce focal central neurologic deficits that begin abruptly and last for at least 24 hours, the term *stroke* is used only when such events are caused by vascular disease.

The underlying pathologic process in stroke can be either **ischemia** or **hemorrhage**, usually arising from an arterial lesion. Ischemia and hemorrhage account for approximately 90% and 10% of strokes, respectively. It may

Table 13-2. Territories of the Principal Cerebral Arteries.

Artery	Territory
Anterior circulation	
Internal carotid artery branches	
Anterior choroidal	Hippocampus, globus pallidus, lower internal capsule
Anterior cerebral	Medial frontal and parietal cortex and subjacent white matter, anterior corpus callosum
Middle cerebral	Lateral frontal, parietal, occipital, and temporal cortex and subjacent white matter
Lenticulostriate branches	Caudate nucleus, putamen, upper internal capsule
Posterior circulation	
Vertebral artery branches	
Posterior inferior cerebellar	Medulla, lower cerebellum
Basilar artery branches	
Anterior inferior cerebellar	Lower and middle pons, anterior cerebellum
Superior cerebellar	Upper pons, lower midbrain, upper cerebellum
Posterior cerebral	Medial occipital and temporal cortex and subjacent white matter, posterior corpus callosum, upper midbrain
Thalamoperforate branches	Thalamus
Thalamogeniculate branches	Thalamus

Table 13-3. Symptoms and Signs of Anterior and Posterior Circulation Ischemia.

Symptom or Sign	Incidence (%)[1]	
	Anterior	Posterior
Headache	25	3
Altered consciousness	5	16
Aphasia[2]	20	0
Visual field defect	14	22
Diplopia[2]	0	7
Vertigo[2]	0	48
Dysarthria	3	11
Drop attacks[2]	0	16
Hemi- or monoparesis	38	12
Hemisensory deficit	33	9

[1]Most patients have multiple symptoms and signs.
[2]Most useful distinguishing features.
Modified from Hutchinson EC, Acheson EJ. *Strokes: Natural History, Pathology and Surgical Treatment.* Philadelphia, PA: Saunders; 1975.

not be possible to distinguish the two by history and neurologic examination, but CT scan or MRI permits definitive diagnosis. Among ischemic strokes, about 35% are attributed to **large artery occlusion**, 25% to **small artery occlusion**, 20% to **cardiac embolism**, 15% to unknown causes (**cryptogenic**), and 5% to other processes.

ISCHEMIA

Interruption of blood flow to the brain deprives neurons, glia, and vascular cells of glucose and oxygen. Unless blood flow is promptly restored, this leads to death of brain tissue (**infarction**) within the **ischemic core**, where flow is typically less than 20% of normal. The pattern of cell death depends on the severity of ischemia. With mild ischemia, as in cardiac arrest with rapid reperfusion, **selective vulnerability** of certain neuronal populations may be

observed. More severe ischemia produces **selective neuronal necrosis**, in which most or all neurons die but glia and vascular cells are preserved. Complete, permanent ischemia, such as occurs in stroke without reperfusion, causes **pannecrosis**, affecting all cell types and resulting in chronic cavitary lesions.

Where ischemia is incomplete (20-40% of normal blood flow)—as in the ischemic **border zone** or **penumbra**—cell damage is potentially reversible and cell survival may be prolonged. However, unless blood flow is restored, by recanalization of the occluded vessel or collateral circulation from other vessels, reversibly damaged cells begin to die as well, and the infarct expands. Death of penumbral tissue is associated with a worse clinical outcome.

Brain edema is another determinant of stroke outcome. Ischemia leads to vasogenic edema as fluid leaks from the intravascular compartment into brain parenchyma. Edema is usually maximal approximately 2 to 3 days after stroke and may be sufficiently severe that it produces a mass effect that causes herniation (displacement of brain tissue between intracranial compartments) and death.

Two pathogenetic mechanisms can produce ischemic stroke—thrombosis and embolism. However, the distinction is often difficult or impossible to make on clinical grounds.

▶ Thrombosis

Thrombosis produces stroke by occluding large cerebral arteries (especially the internal carotid, middle cerebral, or basilar), small penetrating arteries (as in lacunar stroke), cerebral veins, or venous sinuses. Symptoms typically evolve over minutes to hours. Thrombotic strokes are often preceded by TIAs, which tend to produce similar symptoms because they affect the same territory.

Embolism

Embolism produces stroke when cerebral arteries are occluded by the distal passage of clot from the heart, aortic arch, or large cerebral arteries. Emboli in the anterior cerebral circulation most often occlude the middle cerebral artery or its branches, because most hemispheric blood flow is through this vessel. Emboli in the posterior cerebral circulation usually lodge at the apex of the basilar artery or in the posterior cerebral arteries. Embolic strokes often produce neurologic deficits that are maximal at onset. When TIAs precede embolic strokes, especially those arising from a cardiac source, symptoms typically vary between attacks because different vascular territories are affected.

HEMORRHAGE

Hemorrhage may interfere with cerebral function through a variety of mechanisms, including destruction or compression of brain tissue, compression of vascular structures, and edema. Intracranial hemorrhage is classified by its location as intracerebral, subarachnoid, subdural, or epidural, all of which—except subdural hemorrhage—are usually caused by arterial bleeding.

Intracerebral Hemorrhage

Intracerebral hemorrhage causes symptoms by destroying or compressing brain tissue. Unlike ischemic stroke, intracerebral hemorrhage tends to cause more severe headache and depression of consciousness, as well as neurologic deficits that do not necessarily correspond to the distribution of any single blood vessel.

Subarachnoid Hemorrhage

Subarachnoid hemorrhage leads to cerebral dysfunction due to increased intracranial pressure, resulting hypoperfusion, direct destruction of tissue, and toxic constituents of subarachnoid blood. Subarachnoid hemorrhage may be complicated by vasospasm (leading to ischemia), rebleeding, extension of blood into brain tissue (producing an intracerebral hematoma), or hydrocephalus. Subarachnoid hemorrhage usually presents with headache rather than focal neurologic deficits, and is therefore discussed in Chapter 6, Headache & Facial Pain.

Subdural or Epidural Hemorrhage

Subdural or epidural hemorrhage produces a mass lesion that can compress the underlying brain. These hemorrhages are typically traumatic in origin and usually present with headache or altered consciousness. Because of their importance as causes of coma, subdural and epidural hemorrhages are discussed in Chapter 3, Coma.

FOCAL CEREBRAL ISCHEMIA

PATHOPHYSIOLOGY

The pathophysiology of focal cerebral ischemia is complex, as it evolves over time, affects the brain nonuniformly, and targets multiple cell types. Nevertheless, several potentially important underlying mechanisms have been identified, some of which are likely to operate early and others later in the course of stroke. Moreover, some mechanisms contribute to ischemic injury, whereas others promote tissue survival or repair.

INJURY MECHANISMS

Energy Failure

Neurons rely on oxidative metabolism to generate adenosine triphosphate (ATP) for their high energy demands. Reduction of blood flow interferes with the delivery of two key substrates for this process—oxygen and glucose—causing ATP levels to fall. Cells can compensate to a limited extent by generating ATP via glycolysis but, without prompt reperfusion, they cease to function and eventually die. Like other ischemic injury mechanisms, energy failure is most pronounced in the ischemic core and less so in the surrounding penumbra.

Ion Gradients

A major use of cellular energy is the maintenance of transmembrane ion gradients. With energy failure, these are dissipated. Na^+/K^+-ATPase, which accounts for the majority of neuronal energy expenditure and is responsible for maintaining high intracellular K^+ concentrations, fails to do so. K^+ leaks from cells and depolarizes adjacent cells, activating voltage-gated ion channels and neurotransmitter release. Extracellular K^+ and neurotransmitter glutamate trigger cortical spreading depression, leading to further neuron and astrocyte depolarization. This consumes additional energy and may extend the infarct.

Calcium Dysregulation

Intracellular Ca^{2+} is normally maintained at low levels, but ischemic elevation of extracellular K^+ causes membrane depolarization and triggers influx of extracellular Ca^{2+} into neurons. Catabolic enzymes are activated, mitochondrial function is compromised, and cell death pathways are mobilized.

Excitotoxicity

Excitotoxicity refers to the neurotoxic effects of excitatory neurotransmitters, especially glutamate. Ischemia promotes excitotoxicity by stimulating neuronal glutamate release, reversing astrocytic glutamate uptake, and activating glutamate receptor-coupled ion channels. Influx of Ca^{2+} through these channels contributes to Ca^{2+} dysregulation and activates neuronal nitric oxide synthase, generating potentially neurotoxic nitric oxide.

Oxidative & Nitrosative Injury

Some toxic effects of ischemia are mediated by highly reactive oxidative and nitrosative compounds, including superoxide and nitric oxide, which act primarily during the reperfusion phase that follows ischemia. Their effects include inhibiting mitochondrial enzymes and function, damaging DNA, activating ion channels, causing covalent modification of proteins, and triggering cell death pathways.

Cell Death Cascades

Ischemic cell death occurs most rapidly in the infarct core and more slowly in the penumbra and during reperfusion. Rapid cell death involves necrosis, in which cells and organelles swell, membranes rupture, and cellular contents spill into the extracellular space, whereas more delayed (programmed) cell death (eg, apoptosis) predominates in the penumbra and during reperfusion.

Inflammation

Cerebral ischemia triggers an inflammatory response that involves both resident and blood-borne cells of the innate immune system. The former include astrocytes and microglia, and the latter neutrophils, lymphocytes, and monocytes. Adaptive immune responses emerge later in the course. Molecular mediators of ischemia-induced inflammation include adhesion molecules, cytokines, chemokines, and proteases. Although the early inflammatory response to ischemia exacerbates injury, subsequent inflammatory events may be neuroprotective or contribute to repair.

SURVIVAL & REPAIR MECHANISMS

Collateral Circulation

The first line of defense against ischemia is collateral circulation, which, if adequate, can bypass an arterial occlusion. The cerebral circulation contains numerous collateral pathways, accounting for the observation that patients with total occlusion of a major vessel are sometimes asymptomatic. However, this is not always the case, especially when occlusion is abrupt. Collateral routes for cerebral blood flow during arterial occlusion include the following:

1. **Bilateral vertebral artery occlusion**—anterior spinal artery
2. **Common carotid artery occlusion**—contralateral common carotid artery via ipsilateral external carotid artery or vertebral artery via ipsilateral occipital artery
3. **Internal carotid artery occlusion**—ipsilateral external carotid artery via ophthalmic artery or circle of Willis
4. **Middle cerebral artery occlusion**—ipsilateral anterior or posterior cerebral artery via leptomeningeal anastomoses

Inhibitory Neurotransmitters

Enhanced tonic inhibition mediated through extrasynaptic $GABA_A$ receptors may mitigate excitotoxic injury early in the course of stroke. However, persistent inhibition may impair recovery.

Transcriptional Hypoxia Response

Hypoxia activates transcription of proteins that promote cell survival and tissue recovery, including glycolytic enzymes, erythropoietin, and vascular endothelial growth factor. Other cytoprotective proteins induced after ischemia include antiapoptotic proteins, growth factors, and heat-shock proteins.

Neurogenesis

Cerebral ischemia stimulates neurogenesis and some new neurons migrate to ischemic brain regions. Here they may promote survival and repair by releasing growth factors, suppressing inflammation, or other effects.

Angiogenesis

Ischemia also stimulates capillary sprouting to enhance local blood supply. The impact of this process (angiogenesis) in the acute phase of stroke is uncertain, but it may help to protect against subsequent ischemic episodes.

Ischemic Tolerance

Ischemia may provide paradoxical protection against subsequent ischemia through ischemic tolerance, in which mild ischemia preconditions brain tissue and confers relative ischemia resistance. Ischemic tolerance involves extensive changes in gene expression and numerous molecular mediators.

Repair Mechanisms

Most patients recover to some extent after stroke, reflecting a capacity for postischemic repair and the brain's innate plasticity. Plastic changes occur in the peri-infarct region and at remote sites, such as the contralateral cerebral hemisphere, and include changes in gene expression, increased neuronal excitability, axonal sprouting, synaptogenesis, somatotopic reorganization, and formation of new neuronal circuits.

PATHOLOGY

LARGE ARTERY OCCLUSION

On gross inspection, a recent infarct from large artery occlusion is a swollen, softened area of brain that usually involves both gray and white matter (**Figure 13-3**).

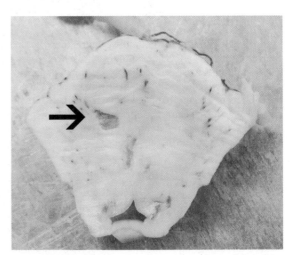

▲ **Figure 13-4.** Lacunar infarct in the pons (arrow). (Used with permission from Kemp WL, Burns DK, Brown TG. *Pathology: The Big Picture*. New York, NY: McGraw-Hill; 2008. Fig. 11-15.)

Microscopy shows acute ischemic changes in neurons (shrinkage, microvacuolization, dark staining), destruction of glial cells, necrosis of small blood vessels, disruption of nerve axons and myelin, and accumulation of interstitial fluid. Perivascular hemorrhages may be observed. Depending on the interval between infarction and death, cerebral edema may also be present. Edema is maximal during the first 4-5 days after stroke and can cause herniation of the cingulate gyrus across the midline or of the temporal lobe below the tentorium (see Chapter 3, Coma). In the chronic phase, the infarct site appears as a cavitary lesion.

SMALL ARTERY OCCLUSION

Infarcts from small artery occlusion rarely cause death, so only chronic lesions are usually found at autopsy. These include **lacunes**, or small cavities up to ~15 mm in diameter, usually located in subcortical white (eg, internal capsule) or deep gray (eg, basal ganglia or thalamus) matter (**Figure 13-4**); **white matter (including periventricular) lesions** showing punctate or confluent myelin rarefaction, gliosis, and axonal loss; and **microbleeds**. Small vessel occlusion may be associated with atherosclerosis, **lipohyalinosis** (collagenous thickening and inflammation of the vessel wall), or **fibrinoid necrosis** (vessel-wall destruction with perivascular inflammation).

CLINICAL-ANATOMIC CORRELATION

Infarction in the distribution of different cerebral arteries produces distinctive clinical syndromes, which can facilitate anatomic and etiologic diagnosis and help guide treatment.

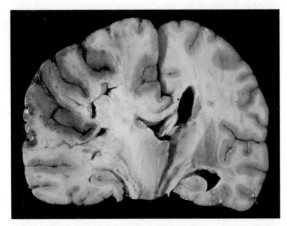

A

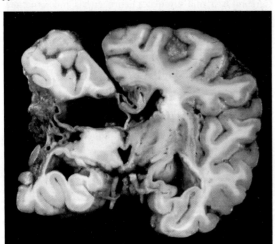

B

▲ **Figure 13-3.** Large vessel (left middle cerebral artery) ischemic stroke in the acute and chronic phases. Acutely (**A**), there is discoloration of the ischemic tissue, edema, mass effect, and, in this case, herniation of the cingulate gyrus across the midline. Over time (**B**), necrotic brain tissue gives way to a cavitary lesion. (Used with permission from Reisner HM. *Pathology: A Modern Case Study*. New York, NY: McGraw-Hill; 2015. Fig. 21-19.)

ANTERIOR CEREBRAL ARTERY

▶ Anatomy

The anterior cerebral artery supplies the parasagittal cerebral cortex (**Figures 13-5** and **13-6**), which includes portions of motor and sensory cortex related to the contralateral leg, the so-called bladder inhibitory or micturition center, and the anterior corpus callosum.

▶ Clinical Syndrome

Anterior cerebral artery strokes produce contralateral paralysis and sensory loss exclusively or primarily affecting the leg. There may also be abulia (apathy), disconnection syndromes such as the alien hand (involuntary performance of complex motor activity), transcortical expressive aphasia (see Chapter 1, Neurologic History & Examination), and urinary incontinence.

MIDDLE CEREBRAL ARTERY

▶ Anatomy

The middle cerebral artery supplies most of the remainder of the cerebral hemisphere and deep subcortical structures (see Figures 13-5 and 13-6). Cortical branches include the **superior division**, which supplies motor and sensory representation of the face, hand, and arm, and the **expressive language (Broca) area** of the dominant hemisphere (**Figure 13-7**). The **inferior division** supplies the visual radiations, visual cortex related to macular vision, and the **receptive language (Wernicke) area** of the dominant hemisphere. **Lenticulostriate** branches of the most proximal portion (stem) of the middle cerebral artery supply the basal ganglia and motor fibers to the face, hand, arm, and leg as they descend in the genu and posterior limb of the internal capsule.

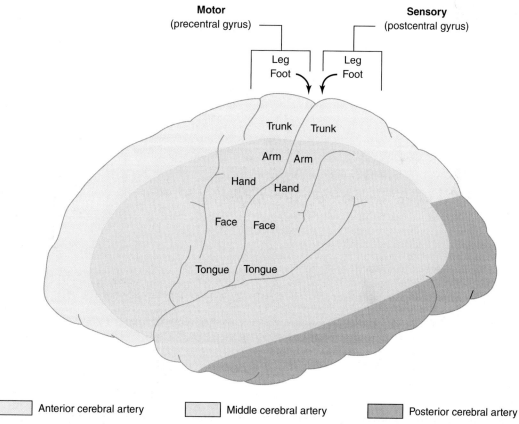

Figure 13-5. Arterial supply of the primary motor and sensory cortex (lateral view). The middle cerebral artery supplies areas related to face and upper limb function, whereas the anterior cerebral artery supplies areas related to lower limb function. This explains why middle cerebral artery strokes affect the face and arm most severely, whereas anterior cerebral artery strokes affect the leg. (Used with permission from Waxman S. *Clinical Neuroanatomy*. 26th ed. New York, NY: McGraw-Hill; 2010.)

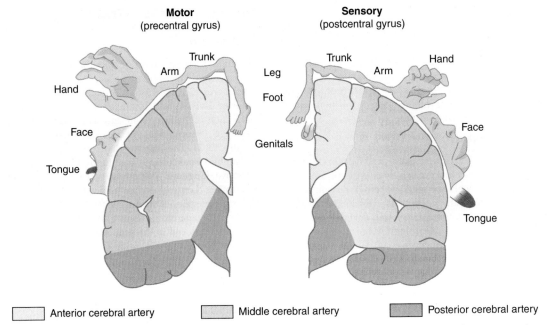

Figure 13-6. Arterial supply of the primary motor and sensory cortex (coronal view). (Used with permission from Waxman S. *Clinical Neuroanatomy*. 26th ed. New York, NY: McGraw-Hill; 2010.)

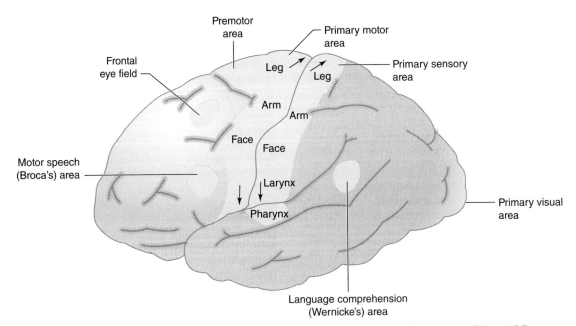

Figure 13-7. Anatomic basis of middle cerebral artery syndromes. Stroke in the distribution of the middle cerebral artery causes hemiparesis affecting primarily face and arm (due to involvement of the primary motor area), hemisensory deficit affecting primarily face and arm (due to involvement of the primary sensory area), gaze preference toward the affected hemisphere (due to involvement of the frontal eye field), aphasia if the dominant hemisphere is affected (due to involvement of Broca area, Wernicke area, or both), and hemianopia (due to involvement of the optic radiations leading to the primary visual area. (Used with permission from Waxman S. *Clinical Neuroanatomy*. 26th ed. New York, NY: McGraw-Hill; 2010.)

Clinical Syndrome

Depending on the site of involvement, several clinical syndromes can occur.

1. **Superior division stroke** results in contralateral hemiparesis that affects the face, hand, and arm but spares the leg, and contralateral hemisensory deficit in the same distribution, but no homonymous hemianopia. If the dominant hemisphere is involved, there is Broca (expressive) aphasia, which is characterized by impaired language expression with intact comprehension.

2. **Inferior division stroke** results in contralateral homonymous hemianopia that may be denser inferiorly, impaired cortical sensory functions (eg, graphesthesia and stereognosis) on the contralateral side of the body, and disorders of spatial thought (eg, anosognosia [unawareness of deficit], neglect of the contralateral limbs and contralateral side of external space, dressing apraxia, and constructional apraxia). If the dominant hemisphere is involved, Wernicke (receptive) aphasia occurs and is manifested by impaired comprehension and fluent but often nonsensical speech. With involvement of the nondominant hemisphere, an acute confusional state may occur.

3. **Occlusion at the bifurcation or trifurcation of the middle cerebral artery** combines the features of superior and inferior division stroke, including contralateral hemiparesis and hemisensory deficit involving the face and arm more than leg, homonymous hemianopia, and—if the dominant hemisphere is affected—global (combined expressive and receptive) aphasia.

4. **Occlusion of the stem of the middle cerebral artery** occurs proximal to the origin of the lenticulostriate branches, resulting in a clinical syndrome similar to that seen after occlusion at the trifurcation. In addition, however, involvement of the internal capsule causes paralysis of the contralateral leg, so hemiplegia and sensory loss affect the face, hand, arm, and leg.

INTERNAL CAROTID ARTERY

Anatomy

The internal carotid artery arises at the bifurcation of the common carotid artery in the neck. In addition to the anterior and middle cerebral arteries, it also gives rise to the ophthalmic artery, which supplies the retina.

Clinical Syndrome

Internal carotid artery occlusion may be asymptomatic, or cause strokes of highly variable severity, depending on the adequacy of collateral circulation. Symptomatic occlusion results in a syndrome similar to that of middle cerebral artery stroke (contralateral hemiplegia, hemisensory deficit, and homonymous hemianopia, together with aphasia if the dominant hemisphere is involved). Monocular blindness is also common.

POSTERIOR CEREBRAL ARTERY

Anatomy

The paired posterior cerebral arteries arise from the tip of the basilar artery (**Figure 13-8**) and supply the occipital cerebral cortex, medial temporal lobes, posterior corpus callosum, thalamus, and rostral midbrain. Emboli in the basilar artery tend to lodge at its apex and occlude one or both posterior cerebral arteries; subsequent fragmentation can produce asymmetric or patchy posterior cerebral artery infarction.

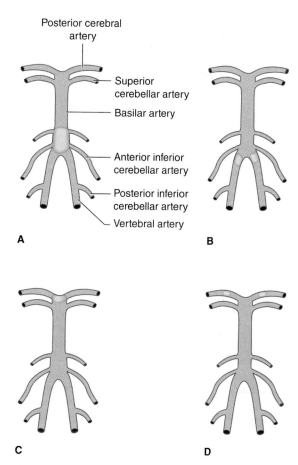

▲ **Figure 13-8.** Sites of thrombotic and embolic occlusions in the vertebrobasilar circulation. (**A**) Thrombotic occlusion of the basilar artery. (**B**) Thrombotic occlusion of both vertebral arteries. (**C**) Embolic occlusion at the apex of the basilar artery. (**D**) Embolic occlusion of both posterior cerebral arteries.

Clinical Syndrome

Posterior cerebral artery occlusion produces homonymous hemianopia affecting the contralateral visual field, except that macular vision may be spared. In contrast to visual field defects from infarction in the middle cerebral artery territory, those caused by posterior cerebral artery occlusion may be denser superiorly. With occlusion near the origin of the posterior cerebral artery at the level of the midbrain, ocular abnormalities may occur, including vertical gaze palsy, oculomotor (III) nerve palsy, internuclear ophthalmoplegia, and vertical skew deviation of the eyes. Involvement of the occipital lobe of the dominant hemisphere may cause anomic aphasia (difficulty in naming objects), alexia without agraphia (inability to read without impairment of writing), or visual agnosia. The last is failure to identify objects presented in the left side of the visual field, caused by a lesion of the corpus callosum that disconnects the right visual cortex from language areas of the left hemisphere. Bilateral posterior cerebral artery infarction may result in cortical blindness, memory impairment (from temporal lobe involvement), or inability to recognize familiar faces (prosopagnosia), as well as a variety of exotic visual and behavioral syndromes.

BASILAR ARTERY

Anatomy

The basilar artery arises from the junction of the paired vertebral arteries (see Figure 13-8) and courses over the ventral surface of the brainstem to terminate at the level of the midbrain, where it bifurcates to form the posterior cerebral arteries. Branches of the basilar artery supply the occipital and medial temporal lobes, medial thalamus, posterior limb of the internal capsule, brainstem, and cerebellum.

Clinical Syndromes

1. **Thrombosis**—Thrombotic occlusion of the basilar artery or both vertebral arteries (see Figure 13-8) is often incompatible with survival. It causes bilateral symptoms and signs of brainstem and cerebellar dysfunction from involvement of multiple branch arteries (**Figure 13-9**). Temporary occlusion of one or both vertebral arteries, leading to transient brainstem dysfunction, can also result from rotating the head in patients with cervical spondylosis.

   Basilar thrombosis usually affects the proximal basilar artery (see Figure 13-8), which supplies the pons. Involvement of the dorsal pons (tegmentum) produces unilateral or bilateral abducens (VI) nerve palsy; horizontal eye movements are impaired, but vertical nystagmus and ocular bobbing may be present. The pupils are constricted due to involvement of descending sympathetic pupillodilator fibers, but may be reactive.

Hemiplegia or quadriplegia is usually present, and coma is common. A CT or MRI brain scan will differentiate between basilar occlusion and pontine hemorrhage.

In some patients, the ventral pons (basis pontis) is infarcted and the tegmentum is spared. Such patients remain conscious but quadriplegic (**locked-in syndrome**). Locked-in patients may be able to open or move their eyes vertically on command. A normal conventional electroencephalogram (EEG) further distinguishes the locked-in state from coma (see Chapter 3, Coma).

Stenosis or occlusion of the subclavian artery proximal to the origin of the vertebral artery can lead to the **subclavian steal syndrome**, in which blood is diverted from the vertebral artery into the distal subclavian artery with physical activity of the ipsilateral arm. The resulting brainstem ischemia can mimic basilar thrombosis, but is not predictive of stroke.

2. **Embolism**—Emboli in the basilar artery usually lodge at its apex (see Figure 13-8). Interruption of blood flow to the ascending reticular formation in the midbrain and thalamus produces immediate loss or impairment of consciousness. Unilateral or bilateral oculomotor (III) nerve palsies are characteristic. Hemiplegia or quadriplegia with decerebrate or decorticate posturing results from involvement of the cerebral peduncles in the midbrain. Thus, the **top of the basilar syndrome** may be confused with midbrain damage caused by transtentorial uncal herniation. Less commonly, an embolus may lodge more proximally, producing a syndrome indistinguishable from basilar thrombosis.

   Smaller emboli may occlude the rostral basilar artery transiently before fragmenting and passing into one or both posterior cerebral arteries (see Figure 13-8). In such cases, portions of the midbrain, thalamus, and temporal and occipital lobes can be infarcted. Patients may display visual (homonymous hemianopia, cortical blindness), visuomotor (impaired convergence, paralysis of upward or downward gaze, diplopia), and behavioral (especially confusion) abnormalities without prominent motor dysfunction. Sluggish pupillary responses are a helpful sign of midbrain involvement.

LONG CIRCUMFERENTIAL VERTEBROBASILAR BRANCHES

Anatomy

The long circumferential branches of the vertebral and basilar arteries are the posterior inferior cerebellar, anterior inferior cerebellar, and superior cerebellar arteries (see Figure 13-2). They supply the dorsolateral brainstem, including dorsolateral cranial nerve nuclei (V, VII, and

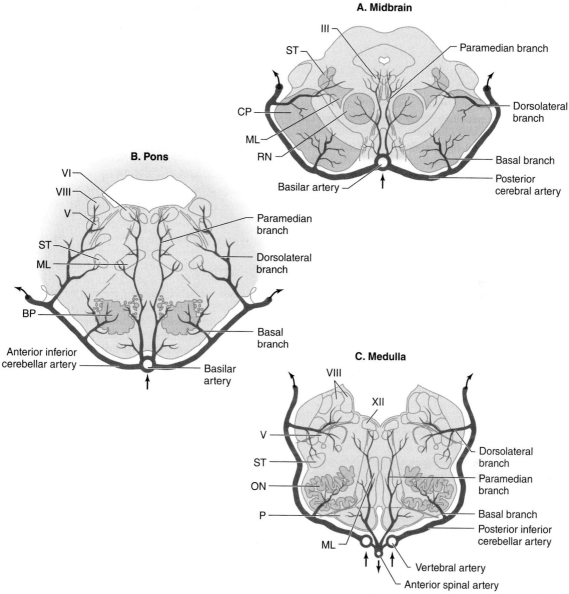

▲ **Figure 13-9.** Arterial supply of the brainstem. **(A)** Midbrain: The basilar artery gives off paramedian branches that supply the oculomotor (III) nerve nucleus and red nucleus (RN). A larger branch, the posterior cerebral artery, courses laterally around the midbrain on each side, giving off a basal branch that supplies the cerebral peduncle (CP) and a dorsolateral branch supplying the spinothalamic tract (ST) and medial lemniscus (ML). The posterior cerebral artery continues (**upper arrows**) to supply the thalamus, occipital lobe, and medial temporal lobe. **(B)** Pons: Paramedian branches of the basilar artery supply the abducens (VI) nucleus and medial lemniscus (ML). Each anterior inferior cerebellar artery gives off a basal branch to descending motor pathways in the basis pontis (BP) and a dorsolateral branch to the trigeminal (V) nucleus, vestibular (VIII) nucleus, and spinothalamic tract (ST), before passing to the cerebellum (**upper arrows**). **(C)** Medulla: Paramedian branches of the vertebral arteries supply descending motor pathways in the pyramid (P), the medial lemniscus (ML), and the hypoglossal (XII) nucleus. Another paired branch, the posterior inferior cerebellar artery, gives off a basal branch to the olivary nuclei (ON) and a dorsolateral branch that supplies the trigeminal (V) nucleus, vestibular (VIII) nucleus, and spinothalamic tract (ST), on its way to the cerebellum (**upper arrows**). (Used with permission from Waxman S. *Clinical Neuroanatomy*. 26th ed. New York, NY: McGraw-Hill; 2010.)

VIII) and pathways entering and leaving the cerebellum in the cerebellar peduncles.

Clinical Syndromes

Occlusion of a circumferential branch produces infarction in the dorsolateral medulla or pons.

1. **Posterior inferior cerebellar artery occlusion** results in the **lateral medullary (Wallenberg) syndrome** (see Chapter 8, Disorders of Equilibrium). The presentation varies, but can include ipsilateral cerebellar ataxia, Horner syndrome, and facial sensory deficit; contralateral impaired pain and temperature sensation; and nystagmus, vertigo, nausea, vomiting, dysphagia, dysarthria, and hiccup. The motor system is characteristically spared because of its ventral location in the brainstem.

2. **Anterior inferior cerebellar artery occlusion** leads to infarction of the lateral portion of the caudal pons and produces many of the same features. Horner syndrome, dysphagia, dysarthria, and hiccup do not occur, but ipsilateral facial weakness, gaze palsy, deafness, and tinnitus are common.

3. **Superior cerebellar artery occlusion** causes lateral rostral pontine infarction and resembles anterior inferior cerebellar artery lesions, but impaired optokinetic nystagmus (nystagmus evoked by tracking a moving object) or skew deviation (vertical dysconjugacy) of the eyes may occur, hearing is unaffected, and contralateral sensory loss may involve touch, vibration, and position as well as pain and temperature sense.

LONG PENETRATING PARAMEDIAN VERTEBROBASILAR BRANCHES

Anatomy

Long penetrating paramedian arteries supply the medial brainstem, including the medial portion of the cerebral peduncle, sensory pathways, red nucleus, reticular formation, and midline cranial nerve nuclei (III, IV, VI, XII).

Clinical Syndrome

Occlusion of a long penetrating artery causes paramedian infarction of the brainstem and results in contralateral hemiparesis if the cerebral peduncle is affected. Associated cranial nerve involvement depends on the level of the brainstem at which occlusion occurs. Occlusion in the **midbrain** results in ipsilateral oculomotor (III) nerve palsy, which may be associated with contralateral tremor or ataxia from involvement of pathways connecting the red nucleus and cerebellum. Ipsilateral abducens (VI) and facial (VII) nerve palsies are seen with lesions in the **pons**, and hypoglossal (XII) nerve involvement may occur with lesions in the **medulla**.

SHORT BASAL VERTEBROBASILAR BRANCHES

Anatomy

Short branches arising from the long circumferential arteries (discussed previously) penetrate the ventral brainstem to supply the brainstem motor pathways.

Clinical Syndrome

The most striking finding is contralateral hemiparesis caused by corticospinal tract involvement in the cerebral peduncle or basis pontis. Cranial nerves (eg, III, VI, VII) that emerge from the ventral surface of the brainstem may be affected as well, giving rise to ipsilateral cranial nerve palsies.

LACUNAR INFARCTION

Anatomy

Small vessel occlusion affecting penetrating arteries deep in the brain may cause infarcts in the putamen or, less commonly, the thalamus, caudate nucleus, pons, posterior limb of the internal capsule, or other sites (**Figure 13-10**). These are referred to as **lacunar infarcts** or **lacunes**.

Clinical Syndromes

Many lacunar infarcts are not recognized clinically and are detected only as incidental findings on imaging studies or at autopsy. In other cases, however, they produce distinctive clinical syndromes. Lacunar strokes develop over hours to days. Headache is absent or minor, and the level of consciousness is unchanged. Hypertension and diabetes are thought to predispose to lacunar stroke, but these and other cardiovascular risk factors may be absent. The prognosis for recovery from a lacunar stroke is good, but recurrent stroke is common. Although a variety of deficits can be produced, there are four classic and distinctive lacunar syndromes.

1. **Pure motor hemiparesis** consists of hemiparesis affecting the face, arm, and leg to a roughly equal extent, without associated disturbance of sensation, vision, or language. Lacunes that produce this syndrome are usually located in the contralateral internal capsule or pons. Pure motor hemiparesis also may be caused by internal carotid or middle cerebral artery occlusion, subdural hematoma, or intracerebral mass lesions.

2. **Pure sensory stroke** is characterized by hemisensory loss, which may be associated with paresthesia, and results from lacunar infarction in the contralateral thalamus. It may be mimicked by occlusion of the posterior cerebral artery or by a small hemorrhage in the thalamus or midbrain.

3. **Ataxic hemiparesis**, sometimes called **ipsilateral ataxia and crural (leg) paresis**, comprises pure motor

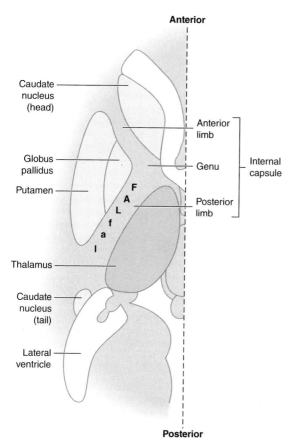

Caudate
nucleus
(head)

Anterior
limb

Genu — Internal
capsule

Globus
pallidus

Putamen

F
A
L
f
a
l

Posterior
limb

Thalamus

Caudate
nucleus
(tail)

Lateral
ventricle

Anterior

Posterior

▲ **Figure 13-10.** Arterial supply of deep cerebral structures involved in lacunar infarction. The basal ganglia (caudate nucleus, putamen, and globus pallidus; light blue) and internal capsule are supplied by the anterior circulation (lenticulostriate branches of the middle and the anterior choroidal artery). The thalamus (dark blue) is supplied by the posterior circulation (thalamoperforate and thalamogeniculate branches of the posterior cerebral artery). Descending motor fibers to the face (F), arm (A), and leg (L) and ascending sensory fibers from face (f), arm (a), and leg (l) are shown in the posterior limb of the internal capsule. (Used with permission from Waxman S. *Clinical Neuroanatomy.* 26th ed. New York, NY: McGraw-Hill; 2010.)

hemiparesis combined with ataxia of the hemiparetic side and usually affects the leg predominantly. Symptoms result from a lesion in the contralateral pons, internal capsule, or subcortical white matter.

4. **Dysarthria-clumsy hand syndrome** consists of dysarthria, facial weakness, dysphagia, and mild weakness and clumsiness of the hand on the side of facial involvement. Lacunes causing this syndrome are located in the contralateral pons or internal capsule. Infarcts or small intracerebral hemorrhages at a variety of locations can

produce a similar syndrome, however. In contrast to the lacunar syndromes described earlier, premonitory TIAs are unusual.

ETIOLOGY

Focal cerebral ischemia can result from underlying disorders that primarily affect the blood, blood vessels, or heart (**Table 13-4**).

VASCULAR DISORDERS

▶ Atherosclerosis

Atherosclerosis of the large extracranial arteries in the neck and at the base of the brain and of smaller intracranial arteries is the most common cause of focal cerebral

Table 13-4. Conditions Associated With Focal Cerebral Ischemia.

Vascular disorders
Atherosclerosis
Hypertension
Diabetes mellitus
Vasculitis
Giant cell arteritis
Systemic lupus erythematosus
Polyarteritis nodosa
Primary angiitis of the central nervous system
Syphilitic arteritis
AIDS
Other vasculopathies
Fibromuscular dysplasia
Carotid or vertebral artery dissection
Multiple progressive intracranial occlusions (moyamoya)
Drug abuse
Migraine
Reversible cerebral vasoconstriction syndrome
Venous or sinus thrombosis
Rare Mendelian disorders
Cardiac disorders
Atrial fibrillation
Myocardial infarction
Mechanical prosthetic heart valves
Dilated cardiomyopathy
Rheumatic mitral stenosis
Infective endocarditis
Nonbacterial thrombotic endocarditis
Atrial myxoma
Paradoxical embolus
Hematologic disorders
Hemoglobinopathies
Hypercoagulable states
Myeloproliferative disorders
Secondary polycythemia

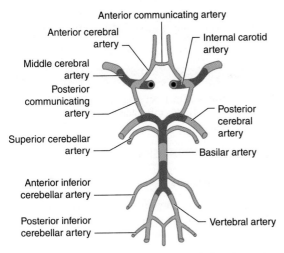

▲ Figure 13-11. Sites of predilection (dark red areas) for atherosclerosis in the intracranial arterial circulation, reflecting preferential involvement of arterial branch points and curvatures.

ischemia. Within the cerebral circulation, the sites of predilection (**Figure 13-11**) are the origin of the common carotid artery, the internal carotid artery just above the common carotid bifurcation and within the cavernous sinus, the origin of the middle cerebral artery, the vertebral artery at its origin and just above where it enters the skull, and the basilar artery.

The pathogenesis of atherosclerosis is incompletely understood, but endothelial cell dysfunction is thought to be an early step (**Figure 13-12**). This tends to occur at sites of low or disturbed blood flow, such as curvatures and branch points of large and medium-sized arteries. Endothelial dysfunction allows adhesion and subendothelial migration of circulating monocytes and intramural accumulation of lipids. Inflammation ensues, and engulfment of lipids by monocyte-derived macrophages produces lipid-laden foam cells, which contribute to an early atheromatous lesion, the **fatty streak**.

At this stage, growth and chemotactic factors released by endothelial cells and macrophages stimulate proliferation of intimal smooth muscle cells and migration of additional smooth muscle cells to the intima from the tunica media. These cells secrete extracellular matrix constituents, leading to the formation of a **fibrous cap** over the **atherosclerotic plaque,** in which a necrotic core develops (**Figure 13-13**). In some cases, fractures in the cap lead to **plaque rupture,** a serious complication associated with the release of procoagulant factors and subsequent thrombosis. Possible outcomes include thrombotic occlusion of the vessel lumen or embolization.

Major risk factors for atherosclerosis leading to stroke include systolic or diastolic hypertension, elevated serum

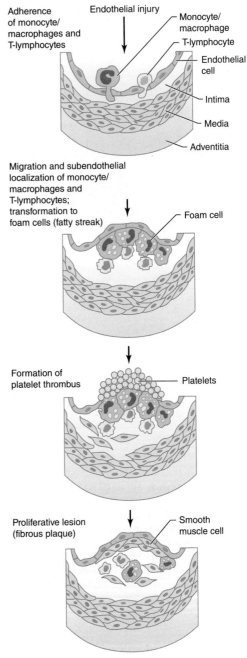

▲ Figure 13-12. Arterial lesion in atherosclerosis. Endothelial injury permits entry of low-density lipoprotein cholesterol and circulating mononuclear cells into the vessel wall, where they form a fatty streak. The subsequent attachment of platelets and proliferation of smooth muscle cells within this lesion leads to production of a fibrous plaque, which may encroach on the arterial lumen or rupture to occlude the vessel and provide a source of emboli.

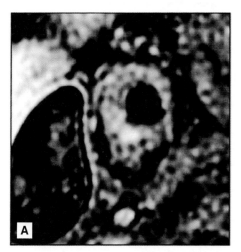

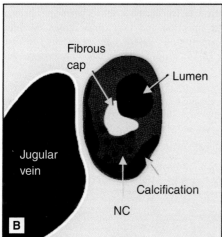

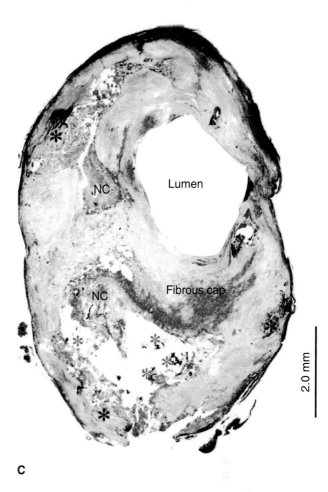

Figure 13-13. In vivo imaging and histopathology of common carotid artery atheroma. Contrast-enhanced black blood MRI of an atherosclerotic common carotid artery (**A**) shows a narrowed lumen, thick fibrous cap, hemorrhagic necrotic core (NC), and focal calcification, as outlined in the schematic (**B**). The corresponding Movat pentachrome-stained endarterectomy section (**C**) shows the same features (*, calcification). (Used with permission from Wasserman BA, Wityk RJ, Trout HH 3rd, Virmani R. Low-grade carotid stenosis: looking beyond the lumen with MRI. *Stroke.* 2005;36:2504-2513.)

LDL cholesterol, and diabetes mellitus. Treatment of atherosclerotic cerebrovascular disease is discussed under *Prevention & Treatment* later in this chapter.

▶ Hypertension

Hypertension, commonly (but not universally) defined as systemic blood pressure >140 mm Hg systolic or >90 mm Hg diastolic, is a major risk factor for stroke. Screening and treatment for hypertension have had key roles in reducing stroke incidence in recent decades. Blood pressure should be measured with the patient seated and relaxed for 5 minutes before three readings are taken at 1-minute intervals, and calculated as the average of the last two readings. Values obtained in the clinic may be confounded by sampling error or patient anxiety, however, leading to spuriously low (**masked hypertension**) or high (**white coat hypertension**) readings. Consequently, 24-hour ambulatory or automated unattended blood pressure measurement is sometimes used to improve diagnostic accuracy.

Chronic hypertension causes degenerative changes in the walls of small arteries and arterioles; such changes include **lipohyalinosis** (collagenous thickening and inflammation) and **fibrinoid necrosis** (degeneration with perivascular inflammation). In the cerebral circulation, these effects are most pronounced in penetrating small arteries and arterioles of the subcortical white matter, basal ganglia, thalamus, pons, and cerebellum. Hypertensive vascular disease predisposes to both ischemic stroke (see *Lacunar Infarction* earlier in this chapter) and intracerebral hemorrhage (see *Hypertensive Hemorrhage* later in this chapter).

Diabetes

Type 1 and type 2 diabetes mellitus is associated with an increased risk of both ischemic stroke and intracerebral hemorrhage. Diabetes affects large and medium-sized arteries, which exacerbates atherosclerosis, as well as small arteries and arterioles, such as those involved in lacunar infarction (discussed earlier in this chapter). It has been difficult to demonstrate a beneficial effect of glycemic control on stroke incidence in diabetics, but treatment of diabetes is indicated to prevent other adverse effects. Antihypertensive drugs and statins can reduce stroke risk in diabetic as in non-diabetic patients.

Vasculitis

Vasculitis is an uncommon cause of stroke but is important to recognize because it is treatable. Stroke can result from either primary central nervous system vasculitis or systemic vasculitis, and may be the earliest manifestation of the disease.

1. **Primary central nervous system vasculitis** is an idiopathic inflammatory disease that affects small arteries and veins in the brain and spinal cord and can cause transient or progressive multifocal ischemia. Clinical features include headache, hemiparesis and other focal neurologic abnormalities, and cognitive disturbances. The cerebrospinal fluid (CSF) may show elevated protein and lymphocytic pleocytosis, but the erythrocyte sedimentation rate is typically normal. Diagnosis is by angiography, which shows focal and segmental narrowing of small arteries and veins, or brain biopsy. Differential diagnosis includes reversible cerebral vasoconstriction syndrome (discussed later in this chapter). Treatment is discussed in Chapter 4, Confusional States.

2. **Giant cell (temporal) arteritis** produces inflammatory changes that affect branches of the external carotid, cervical internal carotid, posterior ciliary, extracranial vertebral, and intracranial arteries. Inflammatory changes in the arterial wall stimulate platelet adhesion and aggregation, leading to thrombosis or distal embolism. Physical examination may show tender, nodular, or pulseless temporal arteries. Laboratory findings include an increased erythrocyte sedimentation rate and evidence of vascular stenosis or occlusion on angiography or color duplex ultrasonography. Definitive

diagnosis is by temporal artery biopsy. Giant cell arteritis should be considered in patients with transient monocular blindness or transient cerebral ischemic attacks—especially the elderly—because corticosteroid therapy can prevent its complications, notably permanent blindness. Treatment is discussed in Chapter 6, Headache & Facial Pain.

3. **Systemic lupus erythematosus** is associated with a vasculopathy that involves small cerebral vessels and leads to multiple microinfarcts, but true vasculitis is absent. Libman-Sacks endocarditis accompanying systemic lupus may also be a source of cardiogenic emboli.

4. **Polyarteritis nodosa** is a segmental vasculitis of small- and medium-sized arteries that affects multiple organs. Transient symptoms of cerebral ischemia, including typical spells of transient monocular blindness, can occur.

5. **Syphilitic arteritis** occurs within 5 years after primary syphilitic infection and may cause stroke. Medium-sized penetrating vessels are typically involved (**Figure 13-14**), producing punctate infarcts in the deep

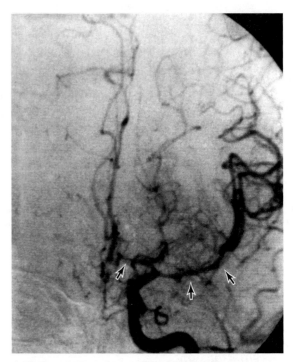

▲ **Figure 13-14.** Left carotid angiogram (AP projection) in syphilitic arteritis showing marked narrowing of the proximal middle cerebral artery (**two right arrows**) and anterior cerebral artery (**left arrow**). (Used with permission from the BMJ Group. From Lowenstein DH, Mills C, Simon RP. Acute syphilitic transverse myelitis: unusual presentation of meningovascular syphilis. *Genitourin Med.* 1987;63:333-338.)

cerebral white matter that can be seen on CT scan or MRI. Treatment (discussed in Chapter 4) is important to prevent tertiary neurosyphilis (general paresis or tabes dorsalis).

6. **AIDS** is associated with an increased incidence of TIAs and ischemic stroke. In some cases, cerebrovascular complications of AIDS are related to endocarditis or opportunistic infections, such as toxoplasmosis or cryptococcal meningitis.

▶ Other Vasculopathies

1. **Fibromuscular dysplasia** produces segmental medial fibroplasia of large (especially renal, carotid, and vertebral) arteries and is associated with arterial dissection (see below) and aneurysms. Familial cases suggest autosomal dominant inheritance with incomplete penetrance. Stroke is most common in children and young and middle-aged adults, especially females. A characteristic "string-of-beads" appearance on angiography is diagnostically helpful. Symptomatic carotid artery disease is usually treated with antiplatelet drugs and intraluminal dilation of the affected vessel.

2. **Carotid or vertebral artery dissection** may occur spontaneously or in response to minor trauma, and is most common in middle age. It results from medial degeneration followed by hemorrhage into the vessel wall, and causes stroke by occluding the vessel or predisposing to thromboembolism. Carotid dissection may be accompanied by prodromal transient hemispheric ischemia or monocular blindness, jaw or neck pain, visual abnormalities that mimic those seen in migraine, or Horner syndrome. Vertebral dissection may produce headache, neck pain, and signs of brainstem dysfunction. Treatment is with antiplatelet drugs, sometimes combined with endovascular repair.

3. **Multiple progressive intracranial arterial occlusions (moyamoya)** produce bilateral narrowing or occlusion of the distal internal carotid arteries and adjacent anterior and middle cerebral artery trunks. Reactive arteriogenesis leads to a fine network of collateral channels at the base of the brain, which can be seen by angiography (**Figure 13-15**). Moyamoya may be idiopathic (moyamoya disease) or due to atherosclerosis, sickle cell disease, or other arteriopathies. It is most common in children and middle-aged adults, and more common in females than males, but occurs in all ethnic groups, and may be sporadic or inherited. Children tend to present with ischemic strokes and adults with intracerebral, subdural, or subarachnoid hemorrhage. Treatment includes antiplatelet drugs and surgical revascularization procedures.

4. Drug abuse, **especially involving** cocaine, amphetamines, other stimulants (eg, phenylpropanolamine,

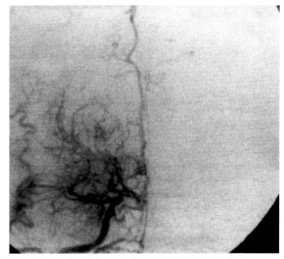

A

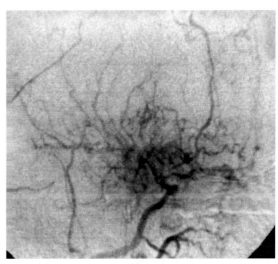

B

▲ **Figure 13-15.** Carotid angiogram in moyamoya. The middle cerebral artery and its branches are replaced by a diffuse capillary pattern that has been likened to a "puff of smoke". (**A**) AP view. (**B**) Lateral view.

ephedrine, or ecstasy), or heroin, is a risk factor for stroke. Intravenous drug users may develop infective endocarditis leading to embolic stroke, but stroke also occurs in drug users without endocarditis, including those who take drugs only orally, intranasally, or by inhalation. In these cases, stroke typically has its onset within hours of drug use. Cocaine hydrochloride and amphetamines are most often associated with intracerebral hemorrhage, whereas stroke from alkaloidal (crack) cocaine use is usually ischemic; proposed mechanisms include drug-induced endothelial dysfunction leading to a prothrombotic state, vasospasm, rupture of preexisting aneurysms or vascular malformations, and vasculitis. Stroke has also been reported after use of synthetic cannabinoids.

5. Migraine with (but not without) aura is a rare cause of ischemic stroke, most common in women, patients less than 65 years old, smokers, and oral contraceptive users. Both thrombotic and cardioembolic mechanisms have been proposed. Migraineurs exhibit a higher incidence of subclinical white matter lesions in the posterior circulation, patent foramen ovale, and cervical artery dissection, but their relationship to clinical stroke is uncertain. Sporadic or familial (autosomal dominant) hemiplegic migraine is associated with focal cerebral edema during attacks and with cerebellar atrophy, but not with stroke.

6. **Reversible cerebral vasoconstriction syndrome** is characterized by recurrent **thunderclap headache** (excruciating pain that reaches peak severity within 1 minute of onset), multifocal construction of cerebral arteries and, in most cases, spontaneous resolution within 3 months. Women are affected more often than men, and recent use of vasoconstrictor drugs, especially serotonergic antidepressants, is common. Focal neurologic symptoms and signs, including hemiparesis, aphasia, visual disturbances and seizures are present in about one-half of cases. CT or MRI may show multiple lesions, including hemispheric borderzone infarctions, subarachnoid hemorrhage, intracerebral hemorrhage and vasogenic edema. Angiography is abnormal bilaterally, with concentric smooth tapering and segmental dilatation the most frequent findings. Cerebrospinal fluid is usually normal. Treatment is with nimodipine (eg, 60 mg orally every 4-8 hours for 4-12 weeks); corticosteroids appear to be unhelpful and possibly harmful. Differential diagnosis includes primary central nervous system vasculitis (discussed earlier in this chapter) and aneurysmal subarachnoid hemorrhage (see Chapter 6, Headache & Facial Pain), but neither produces recurrent thunderclap headache. Borderzone infarction or vasogenic edema on CT or MRI also argues against these diagnoses.

7. Venous or sinus thrombosis (**Figure 13-16**) is an uncommon cause of stroke. It affects young women most often and may be associated with a predisposing condition, such as otitis or sinusitis, pregnancy and the puerperium, dehydration, cancer, or coagulopathy. Clinical features include headache, papilledema, impaired consciousness, seizures, and focal neurologic deficits. CSF pressure is typically increased, and in cases of septic thrombosis, pleocytosis may occur. A CT scan may show edema, infarct, hemorrhage, or filling defect in the superior sagittal sinus (delta sign). MRI with MR angiography is the most definitive diagnostic test.

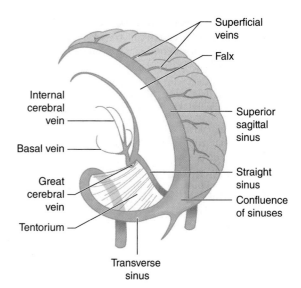

▲ **Figure 13-16.** Major cerebral veins and venous sinuses subject to thrombotic occlusion. (Used with permission from Waxman S. *Clinical Neuroanatomy.* 26th ed. New York, NY: McGraw-Hill; 2010.)

Treatment is with anticoagulants and, for septic thrombosis, antibiotics.

8. **Rare Mendelian disorders** may also be associated with stroke. Cerebral autosomal dominant arteriopathy with subcortical infarcts and leukoencephalopathy (**CADASIL**), due to mutations in the *NOTCH3* gene, produces small-vessel strokes, migraine, encephalopathy, and seizures. Both small- and large-vessel strokes can be seen with mutations in α-galactosidase A (**Fabry disease**, X-linked recessive); ATP-binding cassette, subfamily C, member 6 (**pseudoxanthoma elasticum**, autosomal recessive); neurofibromin (**neurofibromatosis 1**, autosomal dominant); and cystathionine β-synthase (**homocystinuria**, autosomal recessive). Arterial dissection leading to stroke may complicate autosomal dominant mutations in the type 3 collagen α-1 chain (**Ehlers–Danlos syndrome, type IV**) or fibrillin-1 (**Marfan syndrome**).

CARDIAC DISORDERS

▶ Atrial Fibrillation

Atrial fibrillation is common: its prevalence increases with age and reaches ~5% by 65 years. Formerly associated with rheumatic heart disease, it is now usually due to ischemic or hypertensive heart disease. Atrial fibrillation increases stroke risk 2- to 7-fold and, when valvular heart disease is also present, about 17-fold. Additional risk factors include age >75 years, hypertension or diabetes, and heart failure. Atrial fibrillation predisposes to embolic stroke from thrombi that form in the left atrial appendage due to stasis of blood. Treatment is with oral anticoagulants (see *Prevention & Treatment* later in this chapter). Tachycardia-bradycardia (sick sinus) syndrome is also associated with cardioembolic stroke, whereas most other arrhythmias are more likely to cause pancerebral hypoperfusion and syncope (see Chapter 12, Seizures & Syncope).

Myocardial Infarction

Myocardial infarction is followed by stroke, usually cardioembolic, within 1 month in ~2.5% of patients. Factors associated with increased risk include left ventricular dysfunction with low cardiac output, left ventricular thrombus or aneurysm, and atrial fibrillation. Treatment with aspirin, other antiplatelet drugs, warfarin, or combinations of these may reduce the risk of stroke after myocardial infarction, but is also associated with a risk for bleeding.

Prosthetic Heart Valves

Patients with prosthetic heart valves are at increased risk for embolic stroke, which varies with the composition and location of the valve. **Mechanical valves** present the highest risk and require chronic administration of warfarin, with or without aspirin. **Transcatheter valves** are associated with fewer thromboembolic complications, and antiplatelet treatment with low-dose aspirin and clopidogrel for 6 months after valve replacement is thought to be adequate. **Bioprosthetic (bovine or porcine) valves** are the least thrombogenic and are usually managed with a 3-month course of warfarin or low-dose aspirin. Mitral valve prostheses are generally associated with a higher risk of thromboembolic complications than are aortic valve prostheses.

Dilated Cardiomyopathy

Dilated cardiomyopathy can be caused by genetic disorders (eg, muscular dystrophies), drugs (eg, alcohol or cytotoxic agents), viral infection, or autoimmunity. Stroke results from embolization of intraventricular thrombi, but additional factors (eg, atrial fibrillation or valvular heart disease) may help account for this association. Neither antiplatelet therapy nor anticoagulation has been shown to be of clear benefit for patients with dilated cardiomyopathy in normal sinus rhythm.

Rheumatic Mitral Stenosis

Stroke incidence is increased in patients with rheumatic heart disease—particularly those with mitral stenosis and atrial fibrillation. Definitive diagnosis is by transthoracic or transesophageal echocardiography. Treatment includes anticoagulation and, for severe symptomatic stenosis, percutaneous mitral balloon valvuloplasty or surgical valve repair or replacement.

Infective Endocarditis

Infective (bacterial or fungal) endocarditis is associated with a 25-50% incidence of systemic embolization. Up to two-thirds of embolic events affect the brain, typically within the middle cerebral artery distribution. Factors that predispose to infectious endocarditis include intravenous drug use, hemodialysis, intravenous catheterization, valvular heart disease, and prosthetic heart valves. *Staphylococcus aureus* and *Streptococcus viridans* are the most common organisms in patients with native valves and in community-acquired endocarditis, whereas *Staphylococcus aureus* predominates in intravenous drug users, hospital-acquired infections, and recent recipients of prosthetic heart valves. Fungal endocarditis is rare, is usually caused by *Candida* or *Aspergillus*, and has a worse prognosis.

The risk of embolization in infectious endocarditis is highest with mitral valve infection and with fastidious gram-negative organisms (*Haemophilus, Aggregatibacter, Cardiobacterium, Eikenella,* or *Kingella*). Infectious endocarditis can cause cardioembolic stroke or intracerebral or subarachnoid hemorrhage from rupture of a **mycotic aneurysm**, which are most common before or soon after the onset of antibiotic treatment.

Signs of infective endocarditis include heart murmur, petechiae, subungual splinter hemorrhages, retinal Roth spots (red spots with white centers), Osler nodes (painful red or purple digital nodules), Janeway lesions (red macules on the palms or soles), and clubbing of the fingers or toes. Diagnosis is by culturing the responsible organism from the blood and imaging vegetations with echocardiography. Treatment is with antibiotics and, for recurrent emboli or large left-sided valvular vegetations, valve repair or replacement surgery. Anticoagulation, thrombolytics, and initiation of antiplatelet agents should be avoided because of the risk of intracranial hemorrhage, although long-term antiplatelet therapy may be continued in some cases if bleeding complications are absent.

Nonbacterial Thrombotic Endocarditis

Nonbacterial thrombotic (marantic) endocarditis is most frequent in patients with cancer and causes the majority of ischemic strokes in this population. The tumors most often associated with this type of stroke are adenocarcinomas of the lung, gastrointestinal tract, or prostate. Vegetations are present on the mitral or aortic valves, but associated murmurs are rare. Vegetations may be detected by transesophageal echocardiography, but failure to demonstrate vegetations does not exclude the diagnosis. Aspirin, other antiplatelet agents, and anticoagulation all appear to reduce the risk of recurrent thromboembolic events after stroke in patients with cancer.

Atrial Myxoma

Atrial myxoma, a rare benign tumor of the heart, can cause embolic stroke, especially when located in the left atrium. It usually presents in young patients and is more common in females. Multiple, bihemispheric strokes may be seen. Atrial myxoma can also obstruct left ventricular outflow, causing syncope. Diagnosis is by echocardiography. Treatment consists of surgical resection of the tumor and, in some cases, anticoagulation or antiplatelet drugs.

Paradoxical Embolus

Congenital anomalies associated with pathologic communication between the right and left sides of the heart, such as patent foramen ovale and atrial or ventricular septal defect, may permit "paradoxical" passage of emboli from the systemic venous circulation to the brain. However, patent foramen ovale is common, and its presence does not necessarily imply a causal link to stroke (see *Cryptogenic Stroke* later in this chapter).

HEMATOLOGIC DISORDERS

Hemoglobinopathies

1. **Sickle cell (hemoglobin S) disease** results from a GLU-6VAL mutation in the hemoglobin β chain gene and most commonly affects patients of West African descent. The mutation causes sickle-shaped deformation of erythrocytes when the partial pressure of oxygen in blood is reduced, resulting in vascular stasis and endothelial injury. Clinical features include hemolytic anemia and vascular occlusions, which may be extremely painful (sickle cell crisis). Homozygotes are more severely affected than heterozygotes.

   Cerebrovascular complications of sickle cell disease occur in both children and adults and include silent cerebral infarction, ischemic stroke (usually involving the intracranial internal carotid or proximal middle or anterior cerebral artery), aneurysmal subarachnoid hemorrhage, and cerebral venous or sinus thrombosis. Increased cerebral blood flow velocity on transcranial Doppler studies (which should be performed annually from age 2-16 years) can identify patients at increased risk, who may benefit from chronic transfusion therapy to maintain hemoglobin S levels <30%.

   Stroke in patients with sickle cell disease should not be assumed to be due to the hemoglobinopathy, and alternative causes (eg, cardiogenic embolus) should be sought. Acute treatment includes administration of supplemental oxygen, intravenous fluids to correct dehydration, and exchange transfusion to achieve a hemoglobin level of 10 g/L and hemoglobin S level <30%. Patients who satisfy criteria for anticoagulation or thrombolysis (see *Prevention & Treatment* later in this chapter) should be treated accordingly. Secondary prevention in patients with prior stroke involves blood transfusion every 3-4 weeks to reduce hemoglobin S levels to <30%. Hydroxyurea may be employed as an alternative or adjunct to transfusion.

2. **β-Thalassemia** can result from a variety of autosomal recessive mutations that interfere with synthesis of the hemoglobin β chain. It is most common in Mediterranean and certain South Asian populations. The disease is clinically heterogeneous, with earlier onset and more severe (β-thalassemia major) and later onset and less severe (β-thalassemia intermedia) phenotypes. Both are associated with a hypercoagulable state and splenectomy-induced thrombocytosis, which may predispose to stroke. Clinically overt ischemic stroke is more common in β-thalassemia major and silent cerebral infarction in β-thalassemia minor. Antiplatelet agents and blood transfusion may have a role in treatment.

Hypercoagulable States

Causes of hypercoagulable states that may be associated with stroke include **paraproteinemia** (especially macroglobulinemia), **estrogen therapy**, **oral contraceptives**, **postpartum and postoperative states**, **cancer**, and **antiphospholipid antibody syndrome**. Treatment is of the underlying disorder, discontinuing the suspect medication if applicable, or (for antiphospholipid antibody syndrome) administration of aspirin.

Myeloproliferative Disorders

Myeloproliferative disorders—especially **polycythemia vera** and **essential thrombocythemia**—are associated with increased risk for ischemic stroke, transient ischemic attacks, and cerebral venous or sinus thrombosis. Risk correlates poorly with increased platelet or white blood cell counts, perhaps because these disorders also affect platelet function and coagulation pathways; extremely high platelet counts paradoxically protect against thrombosis because of associated defects in von Willebrand factor. Instead, the best predictors of stroke are age >65 years, previous arterial thrombotic events, and hematocrit >45%. Treatment is with phlebotomy, aspirin, and in some cases cytoreduction.

Secondary Polycythemia

Polycythemia may occur not only in myeloproliferative disorders, but also as a complication of chronic obstructive lung disease or erythropoietin-producing tumors. Polycythemia with hematocrit >45% is associated with reduced cerebral blood flow and increased risk of stroke. Treatments include phlebotomy, antiplatelet drugs, cytoreduction with hydroxyurea, and Janus kinase 2 inhibitors.

CRYPTOGENIC STROKE

In many patients with stroke, no cause can be identified. This condition has been termed cryptogenic stroke. Compared to patients with stroke of known cause, those with cryptogenic stroke tend to be younger, have less severe impairment, and experience fewer recurrences. Cryptogenic stroke is diagnosed when imaging excludes lacunar stroke based on lesion size or location, arteries supplying the affected region show <50% luminal stenosis, high-risk cardioembolic sources (eg, atrial fibrillation, recent myocardial infarction, mechanical prosthetic heart valve, mitral stenosis, endocarditis, atrial myxoma) are absent, and no other specific cause of stroke can be identified.

Cryptogenic stroke is associated with a high incidence of **patent foramen ovale**, a congenital defect in the interatrial septum that can provide a route for paradoxical embolism from the venous circulation to the brain. Other possible etiologies of cryptogenic stroke include artery-to-artery embolism from atherosclerotic (but nonstenotic) cervical or intracranial vessels, undetected intermittent atrial fibrillation, mitral valve prolapse, and aortic stenosis or calcification.

Patients with cryptogenic stroke should be evaluated and treated for stroke risk factors (see Table 13-1) and given aspirin (eg, 325 mg orally daily). Certain patients with cryptogenic stroke and patent foramen ovale, such as those age ≤60 years with a moderate or large interatrial shunt or atrial septal aneurysm, may derive added benefit from foramenal closure. If a venous source of embolism is present in a patient with TIA or stroke and patent foramen ovale, treatment options include anticoagulation, inferior vena cava filter, and transcatheter closure of the cardiac defect.

CLINICAL FINDINGS

HISTORY

▶ Predisposing Factors

Risk factors (see Table 13-1) such as TIAs, hypertension, diabetes, dyslipidemia, ischemic or valvular heart disease, cardiac arrhythmia, cigarette smoking, and oral contraceptive use should be inquired about. Hematologic and other systemic disorders (see Table 13-4) can also increase the risk of stroke. Antihypertensive drugs can precipitate cerebrovascular symptoms if the blood pressure is lowered excessively in patients with nearly total cerebrovascular occlusion and poor collateral circulation.

▶ Onset & Course

The history should establish the time of onset of symptoms, whether similar symptoms have occurred before, and whether the clinical picture is that of TIA, stroke in evolution, or completed stroke (see Figure 13-1). The history may also suggest a thrombotic or embolic etiology:

1. **Features suggesting thrombotic stroke** include stepwise progression of neurologic deficits, antecedent TIAs with identical symptoms, and lacunar infarction.
2. **Features suggesting embolic stroke** include maximal deficit within 5 minutes of onset, impaired consciousness at onset, sudden regression of deficit, multifocal infarction, Wernicke or global aphasia without associated hemiparesis, top-of-the-basilar syndrome, hemorrhagic transformation of infarct, or associated valvular disease, cardiomegaly, arrhythmia, or endocarditis. However, none of these features is definitive.

▶ Associated Symptoms

1. **Headache** is present at onset in about 25% of patients with ischemic stroke and is especially common in intracranial arterial dissection and venous or sinus thrombosis.
2. **Seizures** can accompany the onset of stroke or follow stroke by weeks to years, but do not definitively distinguish embolic from thrombotic stroke.

PHYSICAL EXAMINATION

▶ General Physical Examination

The general physical examination should focus on searching for an underlying systemic (especially treatable) cause of cerebrovascular disease as follows:

1. The **blood pressure** should be measured to detect hypertension—a major risk factor for stroke.
2. **Comparison of blood pressure and pulse on the two sides** can reveal differences related to atherosclerotic disease of the aortic arch or coarctation of the aorta.
3. **Ophthalmoscopic examination** of the retina can provide evidence of embolization in the anterior circulation, in the form of visible embolic material in retinal blood vessels.
4. **Neck examination** may reveal the absence of carotid pulses or the presence of carotid bruits. However, reduced carotid artery pulsation in the neck is a poor indicator of internal carotid artery disease, significant carotid stenosis can occur without an audible bruit, and a loud bruit can occur without stenosis.
5. **Cardiac examination** can detect arrhythmias, or murmurs related to valvular disease, which may predispose to cardioembolic stroke.
6. **Temporal artery palpation** is useful in the diagnosis of giant cell arteritis, in which these vessels may be tender, nodular, or pulseless.
7. **Skin examination** may show signs of a coagulation disorder, such as ecchymoses or petechiae.

Neurologic Examination

Patients with cerebrovascular disorders may or may not have abnormal neurologic findings. A normal examination is expected, for example, after a TIA has resolved. Where deficits are found, the goal is to define the anatomic site of the lesion, which may suggest the cause or optimal management of stroke. For example, evidence of anterior circulation involvement may lead to angiographic evaluation for possible surgical correction of an internal carotid lesion, whereas signs that suggest vertebrobasilar or lacunar infarction will dictate a different course of action.

1. **Cognitive deficits** such as aphasia, unilateral neglect, or constructional apraxia suggest a cortical lesion in the anterior circulation and exclude vertebrobasilar or lacunar stroke. Coma implies brainstem or bihemispheric involvement.

2. **Visual field abnormalities** also exclude lacunar infarction, but hemianopia can occur with occlusion of either the middle or posterior cerebral artery, which supply the optic radiation and visual cortex, respectively. Isolated hemianopia suggests posterior cerebral artery stroke, because middle cerebral artery stroke should produce additional (motor and somatosensory) deficits.

3. **Ocular palsy, nystagmus, or internuclear ophthalmoplegia** assigns the underlying lesion to the brainstem and thus the posterior cerebral circulation.

4. **Hemiparesis** can be due to lesions in cerebral cortical regions supplied by the anterior circulation, descending motor pathways in the brainstem supplied by the vertebrobasilar system, or lacunes at subcortical or brainstem sites. Hemiparesis affecting the face, hand, and arm more than the leg is characteristic of middle cerebral artery lesions. Hemiparesis affecting the face, arm, and leg to a similar extent is consistent with large vessel stroke in the internal carotid, middle cerebral stem, or vertebrobasilar distribution, or with lacunar infarction. Crossed hemiparesis, which involves the face on one side and the rest of the body on the other, assigns the lesion to the brainstem between the facial (VII) nerve nucleus in the pons and the decussation of the pyramids in the medulla.

5. **Cortical sensory deficits** such as astereognosis or agraphesthesia, with preserved primary sensory modalities, imply a cortical deficit within the middle cerebral artery territory. Hemisensory deficits without associated motor involvement are usually lacunar. Crossed sensory deficits result from lesions in the medulla, as seen in the lateral medullary syndrome (Wallenberg syndrome, Chapter 8, Disorders of Equilibrium).

6. **Hemiataxia** usually points to a lesion in the ipsilateral brainstem or cerebellum but can also be produced by lacunar stroke in the internal capsule.

INVESTIGATIVE STUDIES

BLOOD TESTS

Blood Glucose

Hypoglycemia and hyperglycemia can both present with focal neurologic signs and masquerade as stroke. Hypoglycemia requires immediate administration of glucose to avoid permanent brain injury. Hyperglycemia (hyperosmolar nonketotic hyperglycemia or diabetic ketoacidosis) also requires prompt specific treatment.

Complete Blood Count

This can identify possible causes of stroke (eg, polycythemia, anemia from hemoglobinopathy) or suggest concomitant infection, which may complicate its course. A platelet count less than 100,000/μL contraindicates thrombolytic therapy for stroke (see later).

Coagulation Studies

Coagulation defects due to anticoagulant drugs or liver dysfunction may affect eligibility for thrombolytic therapy and other aspects of management. The prothrombin time (PT) and internationalized normal ratio (INR) are useful for detecting the effects of warfarin and liver disease, but other tests (eg, thrombin time or ecarin clotting time) may be required to detect anticoagulation by direct thrombin (dabigatran) or factor Xa (rivaroxaban, apixaban, edoxaban) inhibitors.

Inflammatory Markers

An increased erythrocyte sedimentation rate (ESR) is seen in giant cell arteritis and other systemic vasculitides.

Serologic Assay for Syphilis

A positive serum treponemal assay (FTA-ABS or MHA-TP) establishes, and a negative assay excludes, past or present syphilis infection. Positive CSF serology (VDRL) indicates untreated or inadequately treated neurosyphilis and suggests syphilitic arteritis as the cause of stroke.

Circulating Troponin Level

Myocardial infarction, which requires specific management, should be excluded by measuring troponin as a marker of myocardial ischemia, as well as by electrocardiogram.

ELECTROCARDIOGRAM (ECG)

An ECG should be obtained routinely to detect unrecognized myocardial infarction or cardiac arrhythmias, such as atrial fibrillation, which predispose to stroke.

LUMBAR PUNCTURE

Lumbar puncture (see Chapter 2, Investigative Studies) should be performed only in selected cases, to exclude subarachnoid hemorrhage (manifested by xanthochromia and red blood cells) or to document meningovascular syphilis (reactive CSF VDRL) as the cause of stroke.

BRAIN IMAGING

A **noncontrast CT scan** or **MRI** (**Figure 13-17**) should be obtained routinely (and always prior to thrombolytic therapy) to distinguish between infarction and hemorrhage as the cause of stroke, to exclude other lesions (eg, tumor or abscess) that can mimic stroke, and to localize the lesion. Noncontrast CT is usually preferred for initial diagnosis because it is widely and rapidly available. However, its sensitivity within the first 6 hours is limited, and MRI may be superior for demonstrating early infarcts and brainstem or cerebellar infarcts and for detecting thrombotic occlusion of venous sinuses.

Diffusion-weighted MRI (**DWI**) and **perfusion-weighted MRI** (**PWI**) are additional imaging techniques that may be useful for early detection and prognostication in stroke. DWI is superior to CT for detecting stroke in the first 12 hours after onset and may help predict final infarct volume in anterior circulation stroke. However, diffusion defects are sometimes seen with TIAs, and small strokes or brainstem strokes may escape detection. The difference between DWI and PWI abnormalities (**diffusion-perfusion mismatch**) may represent tissue at risk of infarction but potentially salvageable by thrombolysis, roughly corresponding to the ischemic penumbra.

VESSEL IMAGING

Imaging techniques can identify underlying causes of cerebrovascular disease (eg, carotid stenosis, vasculitis, fibromuscular dysplasia, arterial dissection, aneurysm, arteriovenous malformation), including operable extracranial carotid lesions.

Doppler ultrasonography can detect operable stenosis of the extracranial carotid artery and is noninvasive. However, it may not distinguish stenosis from occlusion and does not visualize the surrounding vascular anatomy, so is used primarily for screening.

Digital subtraction X-ray angiography is more sensitive and specific, but carries a small (<1%) risk of serious complications, including stroke.

CT angiography (CTA) and **MR angiography (MRA)** are noninvasive substitutes for digital subtraction angiography and can detect both extracranial and intracranial cerebrovascular disease with high sensitivity and specificity. CTA involves radiation exposure and may be obscured by artifact from calcium in atherosclerotic plaques.

ECHOCARDIOGRAPHY

Echocardiography is useful for demonstrating cardiac lesions that may be responsible for embolic stroke (eg, mural thrombus, valvular disease, atrial myxoma, or patent foramen ovale).

DIFFERENTIAL DIAGNOSIS

In patients presenting with focal central nervous system dysfunction of sudden onset, structural and metabolic processes that can mimic ischemic stroke must be excluded. Such a process should be suspected when the neurologic deficit does not conform to the distribution of any single cerebral artery, or when consciousness is impaired in the absence of severe focal deficits.

Disorders sometimes mistaken for ischemic stroke include intracerebral hemorrhage, subdural or epidural hematoma, subarachnoid hemorrhage, brain tumor, and brain abscess. These can be excluded by CT scan or MRI. Metabolic disturbances such as hypoglycemia and hyperosmolar nonketotic hyperglycemia may present in stroke-like fashion, but the blood glucose level is diagnostic.

PREVENTION & TREATMENT

Antithrombotic drugs used in the prevention or treatment of cerebrovascular disease are listed in **Table 13-5**. Treatment related to specific underlying vascular, cardiac, and hematologic causes of stroke (eg, anti-inflammatory, antibiotic, or antiarrhythmic drugs) was addressed earlier in this chapter in the section on *Etiology*.

PRIMARY PREVENTION

▶ **Lifestyle**

Moderate to vigorous aerobic **activity** for 30 to 40 min per day, 3 to 4 times per week, is recommended. A **diet** low in sodium and saturated fats and rich in fruits, vegetables, low-fat dairy products, and nuts may also reduce stroke risk, as may **weight** reduction in overweight or obese patients, cessation of **smoking**, and moderation of heavy **alcohol** use.

Obstructive sleep apnea is associated with atrial fibrillation and increased stroke risk. Treatment with devices that provide continuous positive airway pressure during sleep may reduce this risk, but such an effect has not been proven.

▶ **Statins**

Treatment with a statin (eg, atorvastatin 20 mg orally daily) is recommended for patients, with or without dyslipidemia, who are at high (>10%) 10-year risk for cardiovascular events, including stroke. Risk is assessed based on sex,

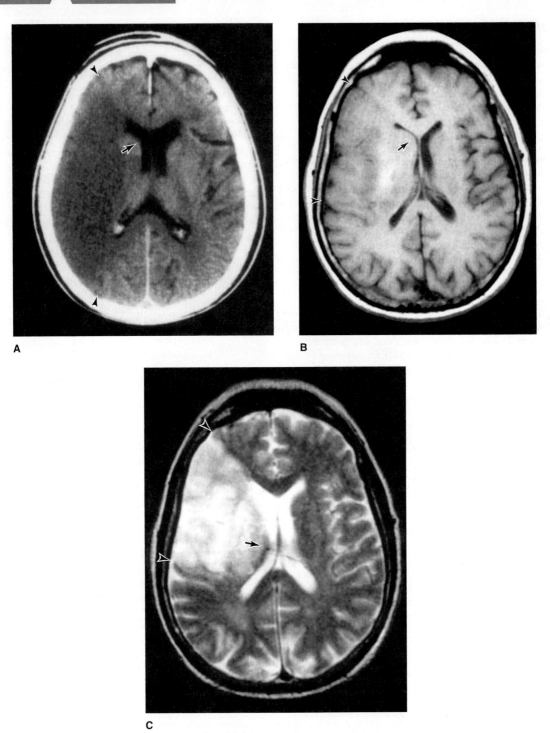

A

B

C

▲ **Figure 13-17.** Imaging studies in ischemic stroke in the right middle cerebral artery territory. (**A**) CT scan show-ing low density and effacement of cortical sulci (**between arrowheads**) and compression of the anterior horn of the lateral ventricle (**arrow**). (**B**) T1-weighted MRI scan showing loss of sulcal markings (**between arrowheads**) and compression of the anterior horn of the lateral ventricle (**arrow**). (**C**) T2-weighted MRI scan showing increased signal intensity (**between arrowheads**) and ventricular compression (**arrow**).

Table 13-5. Drugs for Thromboembolic Cerebrovascular Disease.

Drug	Route	Dosage
Anticoagulants		
Antithrombin activators		
Heparin	IV	To aPTT = 1.5-2.0 × control
Vitamin K antagonists		
Warfarin	PO	To INR = 2.5 ± 0.5
Direct thrombin inhibitors		
Dabigatran[1]	PO	150 mg bid
Direct factor Xa inhibitors		
Apixaban	PO	5 mg bid
Edoxaban	PO	60 mg qd
Rivaroxaban	PO	20 mg qd
Antiplatelet agents		
Aspirin	PO	81-325 mg/d
Aspirin/dipyridamole[2]	PO	25/200 mg bid
Clopidogrel	PO	75 mg qd
Thrombolytics		
Recombinant tissue plasminogen activator (r-tPA)	IV / IA	0.9 mg/kg once / Not established

IA, intraarterial; IV, intravenous; PO, oral.

[1]The combination of dabigatran and either simvastatin or lovastatin is associated with increased risk of major (including intracerebral) hemorrhage. A different anticoagulant or a different statin should be substituted.
[2]Extended-release formulation.

age, race, total and HDL-cholesterol, systolic blood pressure, antihypertensive therapy, diabetes, and smoking history (see http://tools.acc.org/ASCVD-Risk-Estimator/). This approach reflects the finding that statins have vasoprotective (eg, anti-inflammatory) actions in addition to their lipid-lowering effects.

Blood Pressure Control

Blood pressure should be reduced by lifestyle modification, antihypertensive drugs, or both for patients with hypertension (>140 mm Hg systolic or >90 mm Hg diastolic pressure).

Glycemic Control

Diabetes increases the risk of stroke and should be treated, although the relationship between intensity of glycemic control and stroke incidence is unclear. In addition to whatever effect glycemic control may have, stroke risk in diabetics can be reduced by statins and antihypertensive treatment.

Antiplatelet Drugs

Low-dose **aspirin** (81-100 mg/d) may reduce the risk of stroke in patients with increased (>10%) 10-year risk for such events (see http://tools.acc.org/ASCVD-Risk-Estimator/).

Anticoagulation

Anticoagulation is indicated for patients with certain cardiac disorders that predispose to stroke, assuming an acceptably low likelihood of hemorrhagic complications. Algorithms like the **CHA$_2$DS$_2$-VASc** score are sometimes used to assess stroke risk in atrial fibrillation: it assigns 2 points each for age ≥75 years and history of transient ischemic attack or stroke, and 1 point each for congestive heart failure, treated or untreated hypertension, diabetes, peripheral arterial disease or aortic plaque or history of myocardial infarction, age 65-74 years, and female sex. However, this scale does not account for all stroke risk factors, and treatment decisions should always be tailored to the individual patient. Patients with **valvular atrial fibrillation** and CHA$_2$DS$_2$-VASc score ≥2 are commonly designated to receive long-term warfarin treatment targeted to an international normalized ratio (INR) of 2.5 ± 0.5. Options for those with CHA$_2$DS$_2$-VASc score = 1 include warfarin, aspirin, and no treatment; no treatment may be indicated for a CHA$_2$DS$_2$-VASc score = 0. In patients with **nonvalvular atrial fibrillation** and CHA$_2$DS$_2$-VASc score ≥2, dabigatran, rivaroxaban, apixaban, or edoxaban can be substituted for warfarin. **Mitral stenosis** with either a history of embolism or associated left atrial thrombus is also an indication for warfarin, and certain patients should be treated with both warfarin and aspirin following **mechanical aortic or mitral valve replacement**. The role of anticoagulation in reducing stroke risk related to other cardiac disorders—such as bioprosthetic valve replacement, heart failure, severe mitral stenosis, or ST-elevation myocardial infarction with mural thrombus or apical dyskinesis—is less clear.

Asymptomatic Carotid Artery Stenosis

Asymptomatic 70% to 99% stenosis of the extracranial internal carotid artery or carotid bulb (but not total carotid occlusion) is also associated with an increased risk of stroke, and patients with asymptomatic stenosis should be treated with low-dose **aspirin** and **statins**. In some cases with >70% stenosis, carotid **endarterectomy** or carotid artery **stenting** (discussed later) may be employed, assuming that a surgical complication rate of 3% or less can be anticipated.

TRANSIENT ISCHEMIC ATTACK & ACUTE ISCHEMIC STROKE

Transient ischemic attack, or **TIA**, is an episode of focal cerebral ischemia that resolves fully and rapidly, usually within 1 hour, without evidence of cerebral infarction. The goal of treatment is to prevent subsequent stroke, which occurs in 3-10% of patients within 2 days and 9-17% within 90 days. In contrast to TIA, **acute ischemic stroke** implies a persistent focal neurologic deficit, which may be improving, stable, or worsening (stroke in evolution or progressing stroke) when the patient is seen. Evaluation and treatment are similar in both cases; the major difference is that thrombolytic therapy is not usually considered for TIA, in which the vascular occlusion that caused symptoms is thought to have resolved with the resolution of symptoms.

Several algorithms have been developed to predict the acute risk of stroke (and, therefore, the urgency of evaluation and treatment) in patients with TIA. The **ABCD2** scale, designed largely for triage in the emergency room, takes into account age, blood pressure, clinical presentation (focal weakness or speech impairment), duration of the event, and concurrent diabetes to determine the need for urgent hospital admission and diagnostic evaluation. Variants like the **ABCD3-I** scale include additional considerations, such as the occurrence of multiple TIAs and imaging findings, and are tailored for use by specialists after TIA has been diagnosed. Nevertheless, decisions regarding evaluation and treatment of patients with TIA should always be individualized.

▶ Investigative Studies

Patients with suspected TIA or acute ischemic stroke should be evaluated promptly with **blood tests** (complete blood count, prothrombin and partial thromboplastin time, erythrocyte sedimentation rate, treponemal test for syphilis, glucose) and **ECG** to identify underlying causes or mimics of cerebrovascular disease and guide subsequent therapy.

Noncontrast CT scan or **MRI** should be performed immediately to exclude intracerebral hemorrhage and other disorders that can mimic ischemic stroke.

Patients with symptoms or imaging findings consistent with anterior circulation ischemia should undergo **CT angiography** or **MR angiography** to detect clinically consistent stenosis or occlusion of the internal carotid or proximal middle cerebral artery, which may be amenable to intraarterial clot retrieval, or operable lesions in the extracranial carotid artery (discussed later in this chapter).

Echocardiography should be performed if there is a predisposing cardiac disorder or if symptoms suggest cardiogenic embolus (eg, recurrent TIAs with symptoms related to different vascular territories).

▶ Medical Treatment

1. **Blood pressure** should usually not be lowered acutely, except for patients with acute ischemic stroke in whom it is high enough (>185 mm Hg systolic or >110 mm Hg diastolic pressure) to make an otherwise suitable candidate ineligible for thrombolytic therapy (see later). When acute antihypertensive therapy is required, recommended drugs include intravenous labetalol or nicardipine.

2. **Hyperthermia**, which may adversely affect outcome, should be corrected, and any infectious cause identified.

3. **Hypoxia** (oxygen saturation ≤94%) should be treated with supplemental oxygen.

4. **Hypoglycemia** (blood glucose <60 mg/dL) should be corrected.

5. **Anticoagulation** with **heparin**, given by continuous intravenous infusion to achieve an activated partial thromboplastin time (aPTT) 1.5 to 2.5 times control, followed by **warfarin**, given orally daily to achieve an INR of 2.5 ± 0.5, or **another oral anticoagulant** (see Table 13-5), is indicated if a cardiac embolic source (eg, atrial fibrillation, mitral stenosis, or mechanical valve replacement) appears to be responsible for TIA or acute ischemic stroke.

6. **Antiplatelet therapy** with aspirin (325 mg orally once, followed by 81-325 mg orally daily) is recommended for presumed noncardiogenic TIA or acute ischemic stroke, unless the patient is to undergo thrombolysis.

7. **Statins** should be continued for patients receiving long-term statin treatment.

▶ Interventional Treatment

Interventional treatment is an option for selected patients with acute ischemic stroke, but is not used for TIA.

1. **Intravenous thrombolysis**—Intravenous administration of recombinant tissue-type plasminogen activator (r-tPA or alteplase) within 4.5 hours of the onset of symptoms can reduce disability and mortality from acute ischemic stroke. The drug is administered at 0.9 mg/kg, up to a maximum total dose of 90 mg; 10% of the dose is given as an intravenous bolus and the remainder as a continuous intravenous infusion over 60 minutes. Treatment should be started within 60 minutes of the patient's arrival at the hospital, which provides time for diagnosis and evaluation of possible contraindications. Intravenous r-tPA should be given whether or not subsequent intraarterial thrombectomy is being considered. When the appropriate expertise is not available locally, remote diagnosis of stroke and supervision of intravenous thrombolysis via telemedicine can provide care of similar quality.

Contraindications to thrombolysis are designed to avoid unnecessarily treating patients who are improving spontaneously or unlikely to benefit, or exacerbating bleeding complications (including intracerebral hemorrhage). Contraindications designed to avert unnecessary or ineffectual treatment include the presence of only minor neurologic deficits and onset of symptoms more than 6 hours prior to initiating treatment. Contraindications related to bleeding complications include recent head trauma, intracranial or spinal surgery, gastrointestinal malignancy or recent hemorrhage, current severe uncontrolled hypertension, and bleeding diathesis.

Within the first 24 hours after administration of r-tPA, anticoagulants and antiplatelet agents should not be given, blood pressure should be carefully monitored, and arterial puncture and placement of central venous lines, bladder catheters, and nasogastric tubes should be avoided.

2. **Intraarterial thrombolysis**—Intraarterial administration of r-tPA may be beneficial in patients with acute ischemic stroke who are not candidates for intravenous thrombolysis, such as those treated 4.5 to 6 hours after the onset of symptoms or with a recent history of major surgery, and patients in whom intravenous therapy is unsuccessful.

3. **Clot retrieval**—Mechanical thrombectomy with a stent retriever, typically in combination with intravenous r-tPA, can improve functional outcome for patients with stenosis or occlusion of proximal (internal carotid or proximal middle cerebral) intracranial arteries in the anterior cerebral circulation. Those who are not candidates for or who fail intravenous thrombolysis may also benefit from this procedure, which should be started within 6 hours after the onset of symptoms.

Surgical Treatment

1. **Carotid endarterectomy** (surgical removal of thrombus from a stenotic common or internal carotid artery in the neck) is indicated for patients with anterior circulation TIAs and high-grade (70-99%) extracranial internal carotid artery stenosis—and for selected patients with moderate (50-70%) stenosis—on the side appropriate to the symptoms. The net benefit of endarterectomy assumes a combined perioperative morbidity and mortality of less than 6%.

2. **Carotid artery stenting** is as effective as endarterectomy for treating extracranial carotid stenosis, assuming a similar perioperative morbidity and mortality rate. Stenting is associated with an increased risk of periprocedural stroke and death, but a decreased risk of periprocedural myocardial infarction. Considering the generally greater adverse effect of stroke than of myocardial infarction on quality of life, carotid endarterectomy probably remains superior overall, although stenting may be preferable for some (eg, younger) patients.

3. **Decompressive craniectomy with dural expansion** (loose closure of dura and skin over the bony defect), often with ventriculostomy drainage to treat hydrocephalus, can be lifesaving when cerebellar infarction causes brainstem compression and depressed consciousness. Decompressive craniectomy is also sometimes used to prevent transtentorial herniation and death in patients younger than 60 years who deteriorate within 48 hours after large hemispheric strokes.

SECONDARY PREVENTION

Secondary prevention (ie, prevention of a subsequent cerebrovascular event in patients with prior TIA or ischemic stroke) involves measures similar to those employed in primary prevention, with the following exceptions.

Statins

Treatment with a statin (eg, atorvastatin 80 mg orally daily) is recommended for all patients with prior TIA or ischemic stroke.

Blood Pressure Control

Angiotensin converting enzyme inhibitors and diuretics appear to be more effective than other antihypertensive regimens in reducing the risk of recurrent stroke.

Antiplatelet Drugs

All patients with prior non-cardioembolic TIA or ischemic stroke should receive aspirin (81-325 mg/d); aspirin/dipyridamole (25/200 mg twice daily) or clopidogrel (75 mg/d) alone are alternative options. For patients whose TIA or stroke occurred while taking aspirin, it is unclear if increasing the dose or substituting another antiplatelet drug confers additional benefit. There is no evidence that anticoagulation or the combination of antiplatelet therapy and anticoagulation is effective in this setting.

Anticoagulation

Patients with prior TIA or ischemic stroke and **valvular atrial fibrillation** or **mechanical aortic or mitral valve replacement** should be given long-term warfarin treatment targeted to an INR of 2.5 ± 0.5. Low-dose aspirin is added for patients with mechanical valves who are at low risk for bleeding complications. **Nonvalvular atrial fibrillation** should be treated with warfarin (INR 2.5 ± 0.5), apixaban, dabigatran, rivaroxaban, or edoxaban. Short-term (~3 months) anticoagulation with warfarin is indicated for prior TIA or ischemic stroke with **acute** myocardial infarction or cardiomyopathy when either is complicated by mural thrombus. Warfarin for 3 to 6 months followed by long-term low-dose aspirin is recommended for recipients of bioprosthetic valves. Either antiplatelet drugs or anticoagulation with warfarin can be used in rheumatic valvular disease without atrial fibrillation.

▶ Surgical Treatment

Surgical treatment for secondary prevention of TIA or stroke (carotid endarterectomy or stenting) is as described earlier for treatment of TIA or acute ischemic stroke.

COMPLICATIONS

Clinical complications are common after stroke and can strongly affect outcome. They may occur either early in the course or during chronic recovery.

1. **Aphasia** and **dysarthria** may respond to language and speech training and the use of communication devices.

2. **Bladder and bowel incontinence** should be investigated and addressed and indwelling urinary catheters should be removed within 24 hours after admission if possible.

3. **Cognitive impairment** following stroke may benefit from environmental enrichment, physical exercise, and limiting the use of psychoactive medications.

4. **Deep vein thrombosis** should be prophylaxed with subcutaneous low molecular weight or unfractionated heparin, with or without intermittent pneumatic compression of the legs, if ambulation is impaired.

5. **Depression** is common after stroke, with physical disability, stroke severity, prior depression, or impaired cognition carrying an increased risk. Poststroke depression may respond to antidepressants, stimulants (eg, methylphenidate), exercise, or brief psychosocial therapy.

6. **Dysphagia** is observed in about one-half of patients after stroke, and may lead to aspiration, malnutrition, and dehydration. Screening for dysphagia should be conducted early in the course and, if present, swallowing should be assessed by videofluoroscopy or fiberoptic endoscopy. When swallowing is impaired after stroke, nasogastric tube feeding should be started within 1 week and may be continued for up to 3 weeks. If tube feeding is required for a longer period, percutaneous gastrostomy should be employed.

7. **Falls** can be reduced with balance training, exercise programs, and assistive devices (eg, cane or walker).

8. **Hemiplegic shoulder pain** should be alleviated by positioning and range-of-motion exercises.

9. **Infections**, especially pneumonia and urinary tract infections, complicate stroke in 25-65% of patients. Contributing factors include both stroke-induced immunodepression and factors like aspiration and urinary catheterization. However, prophylactic antibiotic therapy does not improve outcome in patients with stroke.

10. **Osteoporosis** and associated risk of bone fractures may complicate stroke, after which bone mineral density typically declines, especially on the hemiparetic side and in nonambulatory patients. Supplementation with calcium and vitamin D may be indicated.

11. **Post-stroke central pain (Dejerine–Roussy or thalamic pain syndrome)** is most common after stroke involving the spinothalamic system in the ventral posterior thalamus. It usually begins months after stroke and is experienced in the region of a sensory deficit. Pain may respond to treatment with amitriptyline, lamotrigine, or electrical or repetitive transcranial magnetic stimulation of the motor cortex.

12. **Seizures** occur within the first few days after stroke in up to 25% of patients, most often in the first 24 hours, and especially following cortical strokes. However, routine poststroke seizure prophylaxis with anticonvulsant drugs is not recommended.

13. **Sexual dysfunction** is common after stroke, with decreased libido, erection, and ejaculation in men and impaired lubrication and orgasm in women. Interventions include addressing possible psychological factors, limiting the use of medications that interfere with sexual function, and pharmacotherapy (eg, sildenafil).

14. **Skin breakdown and contractures** should be guarded against by turning and positioning, attention to skin care, use of mattresses and cushions, and orthotic devices where indicated.

15. **Spasticity** may be relieved by botulinum toxin, oral antispasticity drugs (eg, baclofen, dantrolene, or tizanidine), or intrathecal baclofen.

REHABILITATION

Most patients show some spontaneous improvement in neurologic function in the 3 to 6 months after stroke, reflecting the adaptive plasticity of the brain. However, optimal postacute stroke care involves treatment in an inpatient rehabilitation facility. Recovery of mobility and limb function can be enhanced by training and practice. Effective rehabilitative measures include fitness and strength training, over-ground gait training, pharmacologic modulation of spasticity, speech and language therapy, and perhaps noninvasive transcortical magnetic or direct current stimulation. The efficacy of constraint-induced movement therapy is uncertain. Early commencement of rehabilitative therapy and high-intensity regimens are recommended, and patient motivation is an important factor.

PROGNOSIS

Outcome after stroke is influenced by several factors, the most important being the nature and severity of the resulting neurologic deficit and the patient's age. The cause of stroke and coexisting medical disorders also affect prognosis. About one-half of stroke survivors are discharged directly home from the hospital, whereas the remainder require at least interim care in an inpatient rehabilitation or skilled nursing facility. Roughly 50% of patients have returned to work by 6-12 months after stroke. Poststroke mortality is ~10% at 30 days, ~20% at 1 year, and ~40% at 5 years.

INTRACEREBRAL HEMORRHAGE

Intracerebral hemorrhage refers to bleeding in the brain parenchyma, as distinguished from bleeding in the epidural, subdural, or subarachnoid space surrounding the brain. Symptomatic intracerebral hemorrhage usually presents as (focal) stroke, and may be indistinguishable from ischemic stroke except by imaging studies. In contrast, epidural, subdural, and subarachnoid hemorrhages tend to affect the brain more diffusely; headache and altered consciousness are the most prominent features, while focal signs are less conspicuous. However, imaging studies are required for definitive diagnosis in these disorders as well.

Two varieties of intracerebral bleeding are observed. The best characterized—**cerebral macrobleeds**—are macroscopic, almost always symptomatic, often neurologically devastating, and most often caused by head trauma or chronic hypertension. In recent years, another type of intracerebral hemorrhage—**cerebral microbleeds**—has been recognized, based largely on imaging studies. Cerebral microbleeds are 1-10 mm in diameter, individually asymptomatic, and reflect cerebral small vessel disease. The most commonly identified causes are hypertension, which is associated with microbleeds in the deep subcortical gray matter and brainstem, and cerebral amyloid angiopathy (discussed below), which tends to produce lobar microbleeds at the cortical gray matter-white matter junction. Less frequent causes of microbleeds include CADASIL, moyamoya, and infective endocarditis (discussed earlier as causes of focal cerebral ischemia), as well as fat embolism and cerebral malaria. Microbleeds are associated with cognitive dysfunction and an increased risk of large intracerebral hemorrhages; nonlobar microbleeds are also predictive of ischemic stroke. Treatment of microbleeds involves controlling hypertension; their presence does not preclude the use of antiplatelet agents, anticoagulants, thrombolytics, or statins for treatment of concurrent ischemic cerebrovascular disease, if otherwise indicated.

Except where noted, the discussion below relates to the larger (macrobleed) variety of intracerebral hemorrhage.

HYPERTENSIVE HEMORRHAGE

EPIDEMIOLOGY

Intracerebral hemorrhage causes ~10% of strokes, independent of age. Hypertension is the most common underlying cause of nontraumatic hemorrhage.

PATHOPHYSIOLOGY

▶ Chronic Hypertension

Chronic hypertension promotes changes in the walls of penetrating small cerebral arteries and arterioles in the subcortical white matter, basal ganglia, thalamus, pons, and cerebellum. These changes consist of **lipohyalinosis** (collagenous thickening and inflammation of the vessel wall) and **fibrinoid necrosis** (vessel-wall destruction with perivascular inflammation), which are associated with ischemic (lacunar) stroke and may also lead to the development of **miliary (Charcot–Bouchard) aneurysms**, which predispose to hemorrhage.

▶ Acute Hypertension

The role of acute elevation of blood pressure in intracerebral hemorrhage is uncertain. Most patients are hypertensive after intracerebral hemorrhage, but this may be due to a combination of baseline chronic hypertension and the vasopressor response to increased intracranial pressure (Cushing reflex). Some patients with intracerebral hemorrhage have no history of hypertension and lack signs of hypertensive end-organ disease, suggesting that acute hypertension might be a precipitant, as does the occurrence of intracerebral hemorrhage following sympathomimetic drug (eg, amphetamine or cocaine) use.

▶ Hematoma Effects

Hypertensive hemorrhage causes both destruction and compression of brain tissue. In addition, breakdown products of extravasated blood may cause inflammation and secondary injury. Perihematoma edema correlates with hematoma size, which predicts a poor outcome. Increased intracranial pressure results in tamponade of the ruptured vessel, but can also lead to brain herniation and death.

▶ Hydrocephalus

Hydrocephalus may result from hematomal compression of the ventricular system or its obstruction by intraventricular or subarachnoid blood. This complication is especially common after cerebellar hemorrhage.

▶ Rebleeding

This occurs in up to ~15% of cases and is associated with clinical worsening.

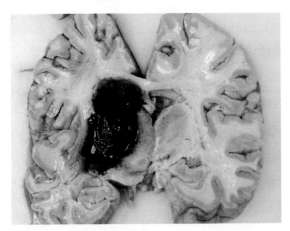

▲ **Figure 13-18.** Hypertensive intracerebral hemorrhage in the basal ganglia with mass effect effacing the adjacent ventricle. (Used with permission from Kemp WL, Burns DK, Brown TG. *Pathology: The Big Picture.* New York, NY: McGraw-Hill; 2008. Fig. 11-16.)

PATHOLOGY

Most hypertensive hemorrhages originate from long, narrow penetrating arterial branches along which lipohyalinosis, fibrinoid necrosis, and Charcot–Bouchard aneurysms are found at autopsy. These include the caudate and putaminal branches of the middle cerebral arteries, branches of the basilar artery supplying the pons, thalamic branches of the posterior cerebral arteries, branches of the superior cerebellar arteries supplying the dentate nuclei and the deep white matter of the cerebellum, and some white matter branches of the cerebral arteries, especially in the parietooccipital and temporal lobes. In the acute phase after intracerebral hemorrhage, there is edema surrounding the hematoma and often displacement of adjacent brain structures and ventricular effacement (**Figure 13-18**). About one-half of hemorrhages, especially those arising in the putamen or thalamus, extend into the ventricles. In the chronic phase following intracerebral hemorrhage, the only abnormality may be a slitlike defect corresponding to the resorbed hematoma, with pigmented margins containing hemosiderin-laden macrophages.

CLINICAL FINDINGS

Hypertensive hemorrhage occurs without warning, most commonly while the patient is awake. Headache is present in ~50% of patients and may be severe; vomiting is common. Blood pressure is elevated, so normal or low blood pressure in a patient with stroke makes the diagnosis of hypertensive hemorrhage unlikely.

After hemorrhage, increasing edema produces clinical worsening over minutes to days, and rebleeding may occur. Clinical features vary with the site of hemorrhage (**Table 13-6**).

▶ Deep Cerebral Hemorrhage

The most common sites of hypertensive hemorrhage are the **putamen** and **thalamus**, which are separated by the posterior limb of the internal capsule. This segment of the internal capsule is traversed by descending motor and ascending sensory fibers, including the optic radiations (**Figure 13-19**). Pressure from an expanding lateral (putaminal) or medial (thalamic) hematoma, therefore, produces a contralateral sensorimotor deficit.

Putaminal hemorrhage typically leads to more severe motor deficit and thalamic hemorrhage to more marked sensory disturbance. Homonymous hemianopia may occur transiently after thalamic hemorrhage and is often persistent in putaminal hemorrhage. Putaminal hemorrhage produces tonic eye deviation toward the affected side of the brain, whereas thalamic hemorrhage may cause tonic downward and medial deviation from pressure on the midbrain center for upgaze. Aphasia may occur if putaminal or thalamic hemorrhage exerts pressure on cortical language areas.

Table 13-6. Clinical Features of Hypertensive Intracerebral Hemorrhage.

Location	Coma	Pupils	Eye Movements	Sensorimotor Disturbance	Hemianopia	Seizures
Putamen	Common	Normal	Ipsilateral deviation	Contralateral hemiparesis	Common	Uncommon
Thalamus	Common	Small, sluggish	Downward and medial deviation may occur	Contralateral hemisensory deficit	May occur transiently	Uncommon
Lobar	Uncommon	Normal	Normal or ipsilateral deviation	Contralateral hemiparesis or hemisensory deficit	Common	Common
Pons	Early	Pinpoint	Absent horizontal	Quadriparesis	None	None
Cerebellum	Delayed	Small, reactive	Impaired late	Gait ataxia	None	None

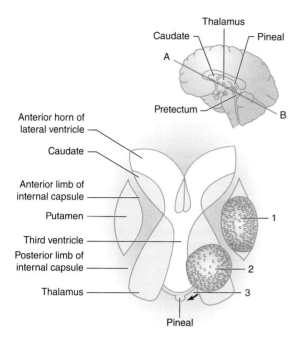

Anterior horn of
lateral ventricle

Caudate

Anterior limb of
internal capsule

Putamen

Third ventricle

Posterior limb of
internal capsule

Thalamus

Pineal

▲ **Figure 13-19.** Anatomic relationships in deep cerebral hemorrhage. **Top:** Plane of section. **Bottom:** Putaminal (1) and thalamic (2) hemorrhages can compress or transect the adjacent posterior limb of the internal capsule. Thalamic hemorrhages can also extend into the ventricles or compress the hypothalamus or midbrain upgaze center (3).

▶ Lobar Hemorrhage

Hypertensive hemorrhages also occur in subcortical white matter underlying the frontal, parietal, temporal, and occipital lobes. Symptoms and signs vary according to the location, but can include headache, vomiting, hemiparesis, hemisensory deficits, aphasia, and visual field defects. Seizures are more frequent than with hemorrhages in other locations, whereas coma is less so.

▶ Pontine Hemorrhage

Bleeding into the pons produces coma within seconds to minutes and usually death within 48 hours. Key findings are **pinpoint pupils** and absent or impaired horizontal eye movements; vertical eye movements may be preserved. There may be **ocular bobbing**—bilateral downbeating excursion of the eyes at about 5-second intervals. Patients are commonly quadriparetic with decerebrate posturing, and hyperthermia may be present. Pontine hemorrhage usually ruptures into the fourth ventricle, and often extends into the midbrain, producing midposition fixed pupils. Small pontine hemorrhages that spare the reticular activating system are associated with less severe deficits and good recovery.

▶ Cerebellar Hemorrhage

Cerebellar hemorrhage produces headache, dizziness, and vomiting of sudden onset, and **inability to stand or walk** within minutes. Patients may initially be alert or only mildly confused, but large hemorrhages lead to coma within 12 to 24 hours in most cases. When coma is present at onset, cerebellar hemorrhage may be indistinguishable from pontine hemorrhage.

Findings include impaired gaze toward or forced deviation away from the lesion, caused by pressure on the pontine lateral gaze center. **Skew deviation**, in which the eye ipsilateral to the lesion is depressed, may occur. The pupils are small and reactive. Impaired upgaze indicates **upward transtentorial herniation** of the cerebellar vermis and midbrain, and implies a poor prognosis. Ipsilateral facial weakness of lower motor neuron type occurs in ~50% of cases, but limb strength is normal. Despite prominent gait ataxia, limb ataxia is usually minimal. Plantar responses are flexor early, but become extensor with brainstem compression.

Cerebellar hemorrhage is especially important to diagnose early because it is treatable (see later). The main mistake to avoid is failing to consider the diagnosis when limb ataxia is absent and gait is not tested. Accordingly, stance and gait should be examined in any patient who presents acutely with headache, dizziness, or vomiting.

INVESTIGATIVE STUDIES

A noncontrast CT scan should be obtained to confirm the diagnosis of intracerebral hemorrhage and assess the likelihood of a cause other than chronic hypertension. Lobar hemorrhage, deep hemorrhage in an atypical location, or disproportionate subarachnoid blood or perihematomal edema should prompt a search for such alternative etiologies, using CT angiography or MR angiography to detect, for example, intracranial aneurysm or arteriovenous malformation. Conventional cerebral angiography can be used to better characterize potentially operable lesions.

Blood tests should be obtained to identify coagulopathy or thrombocytopenia as a possible cause of hemorrhage or complicating factor. Blood glucose should be measured to detect hyperglycemia or hypoglycemia, which may require treatment. Lumbar puncture yields bloody cerebrospinal fluid, but should not be performed because of the risk of brain herniation.

DIFFERENTIAL DIAGNOSIS

Putaminal, thalamic, and lobar hypertensive hemorrhages may be difficult to distinguish from infarction in the same locations. However, severe headache, nausea and vomiting, and impaired consciousness suggest hemorrhage. CT or MRI (**Figure 13-20**) provides a definitive diagnosis.

Brainstem stroke and cerebellar infarction can mimic cerebellar hemorrhage, but are readily distinguishable by

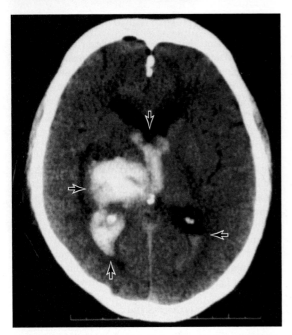

▲ **Figure 13-20.** CT scan in hypertensive intracerebral hemorrhage. Blood produces a high-density signal at the site of hemorrhage in the thalamus (**left arrow**) and extends into the third ventricle (**top arrow**) and the occipital horns of the ipsilateral (**bottom arrow**) and contralateral (**right arrow**) lateral ventricles.

CT scan or MRI. Acute peripheral vestibulopathy also produces nausea, vomiting, and gait ataxia, but not headache or impaired consciousness.

Hypertensive hemorrhage must also be distinguished from intracerebral hemorrhage due to other causes, which are discussed later in this chapter.

TREATMENT

▶ Medical

1. **Initial management** of intracerebral hemorrhage includes airway support with ventilatory assistance if required.

2. **Hypertension** should be treated by reducing systolic blood pressure to 140-179 mm Hg with intravenous nicardipine and, if needed, intravenous labetalol. This is as effective as more intensive reduction to 110-139 mm Hg in improving clinical outcome.

3. **Coagulopathy** should be reversed by clotting factor replacement with prothrombin complex concentrate or fresh frozen plasma. If coagulopathy is due to anticoagulation with warfarin, warfarin should be discontinued and vitamin K administered. Severe **thrombocytopenia** should be corrected by platelet transfusion.

4. **Hyperglycemia** and **hypoglycemia** should both be avoided and insulin or glucose administered as needed.

5. **Fever** should be suppressed with antipyretics; when an infectious cause is excluded, fever may be due to inflammation from the hematoma or its subarachnoid or intraventricular extension.

6. **Brain edema** should not be treated with corticosteroids or osmotic agents, which are ineffective in improving outcome.

7. **Seizures** may occur, especially with lobar hemorrhages, but prophylactic administration of anticonvulsants is not recommended.

▶ Surgical

1. **Cerebellar hemorrhage**—Neurologic deterioration, brainstem compression, and hydrocephalus are indications for decompressive posterior fossa surgery, which may avert a fatal outcome. Results are best in conscious patients.

2. **Lobar hemorrhage**—Surgical evacuation can also be useful for lobar hematomas, especially those larger than 30 mL in volume and located within approximately 1 cm of the brain surface. Patients with good neurologic function who begin to deteriorate are optimal candidates. Prognosis is related to the level of consciousness before surgery.

3. **Deep hemorrhage**—Surgery is not beneficial for pontine or deep cerebral hypertensive hemorrhage.

COMPLICATIONS

Complications and their treatment are similar to those described previously for ischemic stroke, except that prophylaxis of deep vein thrombosis with subcutaneous heparin is not recommended in the acute phase.

REHABILITATION

Rehabilitation is as described previously for ischemic stroke.

PROGNOSIS

Considerable return of neurologic function can occur after intracerebral hemorrhage, depending on its location and size. Mortality is 30-40% at 1 month; most deaths occur in the first few days. At discharge from the hospital, about 75% of patients have significant disability.

OTHER CAUSES

TRAUMA

Intracerebral hemorrhage is a frequent consequence of closed-head trauma. Traumatic hemorrhages may occur at (coup) or directly opposite (contrecoup) the site of impact. The most common locations are the frontal and temporal lobes. Traumatic hemorrhage is diagnosed by CT or MRI.

HEMORRHAGIC TRANSFORMATION OF CEREBRAL INFARCTS

Hemorrhage into a cerebral infarct is common and usually has no effect on outcome. Factors that predispose to hemorrhagic transformation include thrombolytic therapy, anticoagulation, cardioembolic stroke, massive infarction, cortical gray matter infarction, and thrombocytopenia. Treatment consists of discontinuing thrombolytic or anticoagulant drugs where applicable.

ANTICOAGULATION & THROMBOLYTIC THERAPY

Patients receiving anticoagulants or thrombolytic agents are at increased risk for developing intracerebral hemorrhage.

COAGULOPATHY

Intracerebral hemorrhage can complicate disorders involving either clotting factors (eg, hepatic failure, hemophilia, disseminated intravascular coagulopathy) or platelets (eg, immune thrombocytopenic purpura).

CEREBRAL AMYLOID ANGIOPATHY

Cerebral amyloid (congophilic) angiopathy is characterized by β-amyloid deposits in the walls of leptomeningeal and cortical capillaries, arterioles, and small arteries. The disorder is most common in elderly patients and typically produces lobar hemorrhage, including microbleeds, at multiple sites. Risk factors include apolipoprotein E ε4 and ε2 alleles, anticoagulation or antiplatelet therapy, head trauma, and hypertension. Rare hereditary cases (eg, amyloid βA4 precursor protein mutations) are inherited in autosomal dominant fashion.

VASCULAR MALFORMATIONS

Cerebrovascular malformations can affect arteries (saccular, or berry, **aneurysms**), veins (**cavernous malformations**), or their interconnections (**arteriovenous malformations**, or **AVMs**), and rupture can cause intracerebral hemorrhage.

AVMs are usually sporadic, but may also be features of Mendelian disorders, such as hereditary hemorrhagic telangiectasia (Osler–Weber–Rendu disease). They consist of tortuous arteries and dilated veins and arise developmentally when the intervening capillary beds fail to form, but continue to undergo remodeling throughout life **(Figure 13-21)**. They may be asymptomatic or cause hemorrhage, seizures, headache, or focal neurologic deficits. For unruptured AVMs, the risk of rupture is 1-3% per year. However, when rupture occurs it carries a 10-30% mortality rate and, for survivors, a 6% risk of re-rupture over the next year. Anticonvulsants are the treatment of choice for AVMs that present with seizures. In the case of

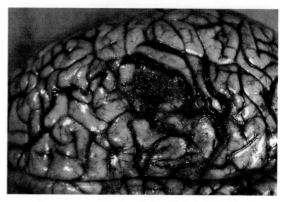

▲ **Figure 13-21.** Arteriovenous malformation (AVM) on the cortical surface with enlarged draining veins **(center)** Used with permission from Peter Anderson D.V.M., Ph.D., PEIR Digital Library Image 9386. © University of Alabama at Birmingham, Department of Pathology.

hemorrhage, however, surgical resection, endovascular embolization, or radiosurgery can prevent rebleeding.

Cavernous malformations can be sporadic or familial. In the latter case, they result from autosomal dominant mutations in one of three genes: Krev interaction trapped 1 (*KRIT1* or *CCM1*), malcavernin (*CCM2*), or programed cell death protein 10 (*PDCD10* or *CCM3*). Like AVMs, cavernous malformations can present with hemorrhage, seizures, headache, or focal neurologic deficits. The risk of bleeding is ~1% per year for previously unruptured lesions, but increases to ~5% per year once bleeding has occurred. Treatment approaches include conservative management (eg, anticonvulsants for patients presenting with seizures), microsurgical resection, and radiosurgery.

Saccular aneurysms are acquired lesions of arterial walls, located especially at branch points around the circle of Willis. When aneurysms bleed, they usually present with subarachnoid hemorrhage, but at some sites (eg, middle cerebral artery) they may bleed into brain parenchyma to produce an intracerebral hematoma. Aneurysms are discussed in detail in Chapter 6, Headache & Facial Pain.

AMPHETAMINE OR COCAINE ABUSE

Amphetamine or cocaine use can cause intracerebral hemorrhage, typically within minutes to hours after the drug is taken. Most such hemorrhages are located in subcortical white matter and may be related to acutely elevated blood pressure, rupture of a preexisting vascular anomaly, or drug-induced arteritis.

HEMORRHAGE INTO TUMORS

Bleeding into primary or metastatic brain tumors is an occasional cause of intracerebral hemorrhage. Tumors associated with hemorrhage include melanoma, lung carcinoma, glioma, breast carcinoma, renal cell carcinoma, and oligodendroglioma. Bleeding into a tumor should be considered when a patient with known cancer experiences acute neurologic deterioration; it may also be the presenting manifestation of cancer.

ACUTE HEMORRHAGIC LEUKOENCEPHALITIS

This rare monophasic demyelinating and hemorrhagic disorder typically follows respiratory infection in children. Multiple small perivascular hemorrhages are found in the brain. Clinical features include fever, headache, confusional state, and coma. CSF shows a polymorphonuclear pleocytosis, and CT or MRI may demonstrate hemorrhage. The classic clinical picture is of a fulminant course leading to death within several days, but some patients respond to corticosteroids or plasma exchange.

▼ GLOBAL CEREBRAL ISCHEMIA

ETIOLOGY

Global cerebral ischemia occurs when blood flow is inadequate to meet the metabolic requirements of the brain, as in **cardiac arrest**. Global ischemia produces more severe brain injury than does pure anoxia with preserved circulation (eg, primary respiratory arrest or carbon monoxide poisoning), presumably because it also impairs glucose delivery and removal of toxic metabolites.

PATHOLOGY

The severity of cerebral pathology is determined by the duration of global ischemia, and its distribution is governed by the preferential vulnerability of certain neuronal populations and arterial **watershed** (**borderzone**) regions. Preferentially vulnerable neurons include CA1 pyramidal neurons of the hippocampus; cerebellar Purkinje neurons; pyramidal neurons of neocortical layers 3, 5, and 6; thalamic reticular neurons; and medium-sized neurons in the caudate nucleus and putamen. Arterial watersheds are located at the borders between the anterior, middle, and posterior cerebral arteries (**Figure 13-22**). Superimposed disease of the craniocervical arteries may lead to asymmetries in the distribution of cerebral damage from global ischemia.

CLINICAL FINDINGS

BRIEF ISCHEMIA

Reversible encephalopathies are common after brief circulatory arrest. In such cases, coma persists for less than 12 hours. Transient confusion or amnesia may occur on

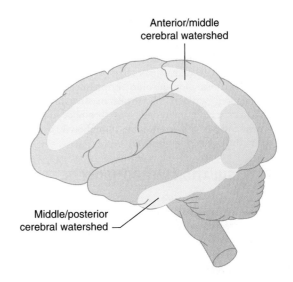

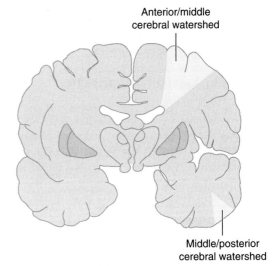

▲ **Figure 13-22.** Distribution of cerebral watershed (borderzone) infarcts (blue areas) associated with global cerebral ischemia.

awakening, but recovery is typically rapid and complete. Some patients show severe anterograde and variable retrograde amnesia and a bland, unconcerned affect with or without confabulation. This syndrome may reflect reversible bilateral damage to the thalamus or hippocampus.

PROLONGED ISCHEMIA

▶ Coma

Coma lasting for more than 12 hours after cardiac arrest may be associated with lasting focal or multifocal motor, sensory, and cognitive deficits upon awakening. It is discussed in Chapter 3, Coma.

Focal Cerebral Dysfunction

Focal neurologic signs after cardiac arrest include partial or complete cortical blindness, weakness of both arms (bibrachial paresis), and quadriparesis. **Cortical blindness** is usually transient and results from ischemia in the border zone between the middle and posterior cerebral arteries. **Bibrachial paresis (man-in-a-barrel syndrome)** results from bilateral infarction of the motor cortex in the border zone between the anterior and middle cerebral arteries.

Myoclonus & Seizures

Posthypoxic action myoclonus (Lance–Adams syndrome) after cardiac arrest produces multifocal myoclonus and is sometimes associated with signs of cerebellar disease, including dysarthria, dysmetria, ataxia, and intention tremor. It occurs in conscious patients without severe ischemic injury and typically improves over time. Treatment with clonazepam, valproic acid, or levetiracetam may be effective. **Myoclonic status**, which occurs in comatose patients, consists of generalized, bilateral, synchronous twitching that usually affects the face and trunk. It is usually, but not always, associated with a poor outcome. Partial or generalized **seizures**, including status epilepticus, are also seen after cardiac arrest, and should be treated with anticonvulsants.

Persistent Vegetative or Minimally Responsive State

Some patients who are initially comatose after cardiac arrest survive and awaken, but remain functionally decorticate and unaware of their surroundings. They typically regain spontaneous eye opening, sleep-wake cycles, roving eye movements, and brainstem and spinal cord reflexes. This **persistent vegetative** or **minimally responsive state** (see Chapter 3, Coma) is thus distinct from coma and appears to be associated with **laminar necrosis** of the neocortex. In some apparently unaware patients, however, functional MRI or EEG can demonstrate responsiveness. Most such patients have traumatic rather than ischemic brain injury, but the possibility that a patient without overt behavioral responses remains subclinically aware and responsive should always be explored. A persistent vegetative state associated with an isoelectric (flat) EEG is termed **neocortical death.** Persistent vegetative states must be distinguished from **brain death** (see Chapter 3, Coma), in which both cerebral and brainstem functions are absent.

Spinal Cord Syndromes

Spinal cord injury from hypoperfusion is usually seen only with profound cerebral involvement. Although an arterial watershed occurs at the mid-thoracic level of the cord, autopsy studies show that ischemic injury after cardiac arrest affects large neurons in the anterior horns of the lumbar spinal cord most prominently. This may be due to the large size and high metabolic activity of these neurons, and is consistent with the clinical finding of flaccid paraplegia associated with spinal cord injury after cardiac arrest.

TREATMENT

Treatment of global cerebral ischemia involves restoring cerebral circulation, eliminating arrhythmias, maintaining systemic blood pressure, correcting acid-base or electrolyte abnormalities, and detecting and treating clinical and electrographic seizures. Ventilatory assistance and supplemental oxygen may be necessary.

Induced hypothermia to 32 to 34°C for 12 to 24 hours by surface or endovascular cooling can improve 6-month survival and neurologic outcome after out-of-hospital cardiac arrest with ventricular fibrillation. However, some data suggest that maintaining temperature at 36°C may be equally effective.

Seizures, including possible electrographic seizures and status epilepticus, should be investigated by EEG and treated aggressively with anticonvulsants, but prophylactic administration of anticonvulsants is not recommended.

PROGNOSIS

Rates for survival to hospital discharge are ~10% for out-of-hospital and ~20% for in-hospital cardiac arrest. Prognosis is better for patients with ventricular fibrillation or pulseless ventricular tachycardia (~40% survival to discharge) than for asystole or pulseless electrical activity (electromechanical dissociation) (~20% survival to discharge).

The goal of neurologic prognostication after cardiac arrest is to distinguish patients with and without a chance for meaningful recovery. Meaningful recovery is excluded by **pupillary areflexia**, observed using a magnifying glass, at 72 hours after arrest or rewarming. Other signs, such as myoclonus at 24 hours, or corneal areflexia or absent or decerebrate motor responses to pain at 72 hours, are less reliable. In patients who have undergone therapeutic hypothermia, the effects of hypothermia per se, drugs administered in hypothermia protocols (eg, sedatives and paralytics), and hypothermia-induced changes in drug metabolism can delay recovery. The prognostic value of EEG, somatosensory evoked potentials, or neuroimaging findings is uncertain.

Appendix: Clinical Examination of Common Isolated Peripheral Nerve Disorders

CLINICAL EXAMINATION OF COMMON ISOLATED PERIPHERAL NERVE DISORDERS: INTRODUCTION

The accompanying illustrations are a guide for examining sensory and selected motor function of certain peripheral nerves: radial (**Figure A-1**), median (**Figure A-2**), ulnar (**Figure A-3**), fibular (peroneal) (**Figure A-4**), and femoral (**Figure A-5**). The sensory distribution of the lateral femoral cutaneous and obturator nerves is also shown (**Figures A-6 and A-7**). It is not intended to illustrate the findings of a lesion at any particular level of the nerves depicted. Sensory deficits may be less extensive than the full sensory field of a nerve because the fields of two nerves overlap, because a distal nerve lesion affects only part of the field, or because different sensory modalities are differentially involved.

Radial Nerve

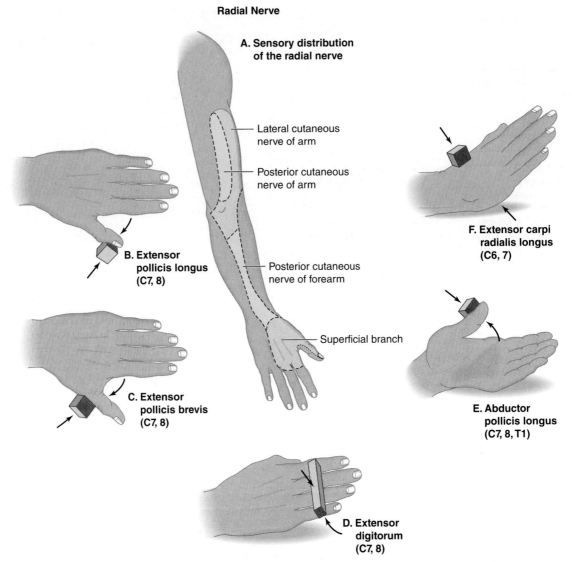

A. Sensory distribution of the radial nerve

Lateral cutaneous nerve of arm

Posterior cutaneous nerve of arm

B. Extensor pollicis longus (C7, 8)

Posterior cutaneous nerve of forearm

Superficial branch

C. Extensor pollicis brevis (C7, 8)

F. Extensor carpi radialis longus (C6, 7)

E. Abductor pollicis longus (C7, 8, T1)

D. Extensor digitorum (C7, 8)

▲ **Figure A-1.** Testing the radial nerve. **(A)** Sensory distribution: The radial nerve supplies the dorsolateral surface of the upper arm, forearm, wrist, and hand; the dorsal surface of the thumb; the dorsal surface of the index and middle fingers above the distal interphalangeal joints; and the lateral half of the dorsal surface of the ring finger above the distal interphalangeal joint. **(B)** Extensor pollicis longus: The thumb is extended at the interphalangeal joint against resistance. **(C)** Extensor pollicis brevis: The thumb is extended at the metacarpophalangeal joint against resistance. **(D)** Extensor digitorum: The fingers are extended at the metacarpophalangeal joints against resistance. **(E)** Abductor pollicis longus: The thumb is abducted (elevated in a plane at 90 degrees to the palm) at the carpometacarpal joint against resistance. **(F)** Extensor carpi radialis longus: The wrist is extended toward the radial (thumb) side against resistance.

Median Nerve

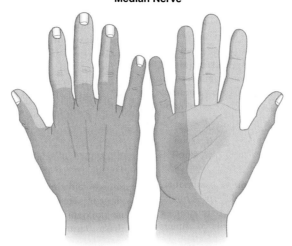

A. Sensory distribution of the median nerve

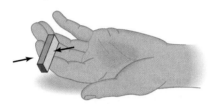

B. Flexor digitorum profundus I and II (C7, 8, T1)

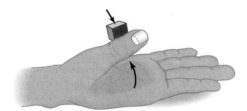

C. Abductor pollicis brevis (C8, T1)

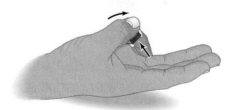

D. Opponens pollicis (C8, T1)

▲ **Figure A-2.** Testing the median nerve. **(A)** Sensory distribution: The median nerve supplies the dorsal surface of the index and middle fingers; the lateral half of the dorsal surface of the ring finger; the lateral two-thirds of the palm; the palmar surface of the thumb, index finger, and middle finger; and the lateral half of the palmar surface of the ring finger. **(B)** Flexor digitorum profundus I and II: The index and middle fingers are flexed at the distal interphalangeal joints against resistance. **(C)** Abductor pollicis brevis: The thumb is abducted (elevated at 90 degrees to the plane of the palm) at the metacarpophalangeal joints against resistance. **(D)** Opponens pollicis: The thumb is crossed over the palm to touch the little finger against resistance.

Ulnar Nerve

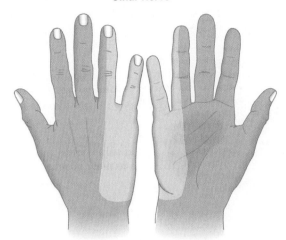

A. Sensory distribution of the ulnar nerve

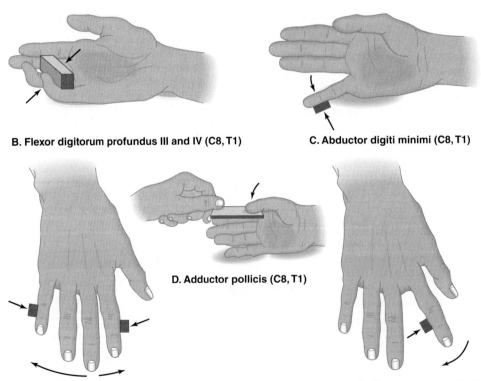

B. Flexor digitorum profundus III and IV (C8, T1)

C. Abductor digiti minimi (C8, T1)

D. Adductor pollicis (C8, T1)

E. Dorsal interossei (C8, T1)

F. First palmar interosseous (C8, T1)

▲ **Figure A-3.** Testing the ulnar nerve. **(A)** Sensory distribution: The ulnar nerve supplies the dorsal and palmar surfaces of the medial one-third of the hand, the dorsal and palmar surfaces of the little finger, and the dorsal and palmar surfaces of the medial half of the ring finger. **(B)** Flexor digitorum profundus III and IV: The index and middle fingers are flexed at the distal interphalangeal joints against resistance. **(C)** Abductor digiti minimi: The little finger is abducted against resistance. **(D)** Adductor pollicis: A piece of paper is grasped between the thumb and the palm with the thumbnail at 90 degrees to the plane of the palm while the examiner tries to pull the paper away. **(E)** Dorsal interossei: The fingers are abducted against resistance. **(F)** First palmar interosseous: The abducted index finger is adducted against resistance.

Fibular Nerve

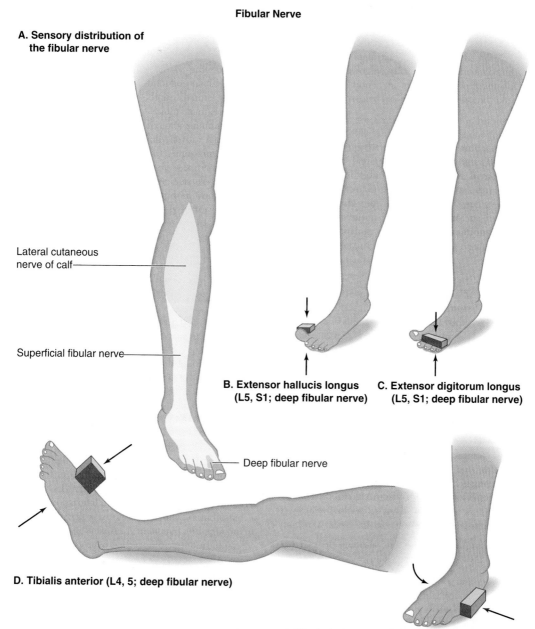

A. Sensory distribution of the fibular nerve

Lateral cutaneous nerve of calf

Superficial fibular nerve

Deep fibular nerve

B. Extensor hallucis longus (L5, S1; deep fibular nerve)

C. Extensor digitorum longus (L5, S1; deep fibular nerve)

D. Tibialis anterior (L4, 5; deep fibular nerve)

E. Fibularis (peroneus) longus and brevis (L5, S1; superficial fibular nerve)

▲ **Figure A-4.** Testing the fibular (peroneal) nerve. **(A)** Sensory distribution: The common fibular (peroneal) nerve has three main sensory branches. The lateral cutaneous nerve of the calf supplies the lateral surface of the calf, the superficial fibular (peroneal) nerve supplies the lateral surface of the lower leg and the dorsum of the foot, and the deep fibular (peroneal) nerve supplies a roughly triangular patch of skin on the dorsum of the foot between the first and second toes. **(B)** Extensor hallucis longus: The large toe is extended (dorsiflexed) against resistance. **(C)** Extensor digitorum longus: The second, third, fourth, and fifth toes are extended against resistance. **(D)** Tibialis anterior: The foot is dorsiflexed at the ankle against resistance. **(E)** Fibularis (peroneus) longus and brevis: The foot is everted (rotated laterally) at the ankle against resistance.

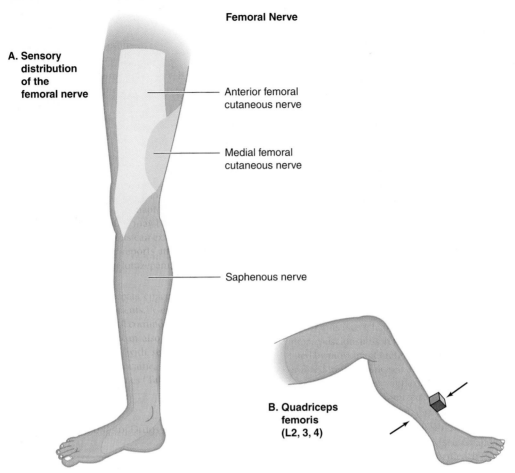

Femoral Nerve

A. Sensory distribution of the femoral nerve

Anterior femoral cutaneous nerve

Medial femoral cutaneous nerve

Saphenous nerve

B. Quadriceps femoris (L2, 3, 4)

▲ **Figure A-5.** Testing the femoral nerve. (A) Sensory distribution: The femoral nerve has three main sensory branches. The anterior femoral cutaneous nerve supplies the anterior surface of the thigh, the medial femoral cutaneous nerve supplies the anteromedial surface of the thigh, and the saphenous nerve supplies the medial surface of the lower leg, ankle, and foot. (B) Quadriceps femoris: The leg is extended at the knee against resistance.

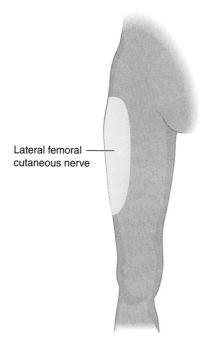

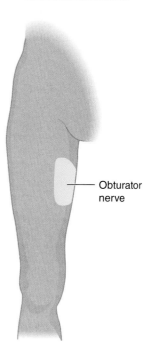

Lateral femoral cutaneous nerve

Obturator nerve

▲ **Figure A-6.** Sensory distribution of the lateral femoral cutaneous nerve.

▲ **Figure A-7.** Sensory distribution of the obturator nerve.

Index

Note: Page numbers followed by *f* and *t* indicate figures and tables, respectively.